NEONATAL DRUG FORMULARY 2002

FIFTH EDITION

DILIP R. BHATT, M.D., F.A.A.P., F.A.C.C., F.A.C.M.Q.
Clinical Associate Professor of Pediatrics, University of Southern California, Los Angeles, California; Assistant Clinical Professor of Pediatrics; Loma Linda University Medical Center, Loma Linda, California; Director of Neonatology, Pediatric Cardiology, Kaiser Permanente Fontana Medical Center, Fontana, California.

DEBORAH S. BRUGGMAN, PHARM.D.
Pediatric Pharmacist Specialist, Kaiser Permanente Los Angeles Medical Center, Los Angeles, California; Assistant Adjunct Professor of Pharmacy Practice, University of Southern California, School of Pharmacy, Los Angeles; Assistant Professor of Clinical Pharmacy, University of California, San Francisco California.

JANET C. THAYER-THOMAS, Ph.D., R.N.
Pediatric Case Manager; Nursing Care Coordinator, High Risk Infant Follow-up, Southern California Permanente Medical Group, Kaiser Permanente Los Angeles Medical Center, Los Angeles, California.

PRADIP KUMAR SHAH M.D.
Director of Neonatology, Kaiser Permanente Riverside Medical Center, Riverside California; Coordinator, High Risk Infant Follow-up, Inland Empire, Kaiser Permanente Medical Service Area (Fontana and Riverside).

DAVID BRAUN, M.D.
Regional Physician Coordinator, Perinatal Services Kaiser Permanente Southern California; Staff Neonatologist, Kaiser Permanente, Woodland Hills Medical Center, Woodland Hills, California; Clinical Instructor in Pediatrics, University of California at Los Angeles, Westwood, California.

ARMILLA A. G. HENRY, R.N., M.S.N., N.N.P.
Kaiser Permanente Riverside Medical Center, Riverside California.

Originally Developed by:

Editors: Dilip R. Bhatt, M.D.
Deborah S. Bruggman, Pharm.D.
Janet C. Thayer-Thomas, Ph.D., R.N.
Pradip Kumar Shah, M.D.
David Braun, M.D.
Armilla A. G. Henry, R.N., M.S.N., N.N.P.

Publishing: N.D.F. Los Angeles

NOTICE

Although great care has been taken in compiling and editing the information presented in this work to ensure its accuracy and thoroughness, neither the authors, Mead Johnson Nutritionals, Kaiser Foundation Hospitals or Southern California Permanente Medical Group can accept any responsibility for the continued currency of the information contained herein, for any errors or omissions, whether caused by negligence or otherwise, or for any consequences whatsoever arising from use of this information. In view of ongoing research, changes in government regulations, and the constant flow of information relating to drug reactions, the reader is urged to check the package insert of each drug for any change in indications, dosage, added warnings and precautions. This is of particular importance in regard to new or infrequently used drugs.

The popularity and apparent utility of this drug formulary is gratifying. We encourage you to send suggestions for its improvement to us.

ISBN 0-945539-02-9

Neonatal Drug Formulary 2002
Att: Dilip R. Bhatt, M.D.
P.O. Box 3240
Fontana, CA. 92334

ACKNOWLEDGEMENTS

The editors are thankful for the encouragement and aid of their colleagues in preparing this fifth edition. Extraordinary help was provided by Denise M. Caven, Executive Assistant and Project Coordinator of Thayer-Thomas and Associates, La Cañada, California and the Medical Library staffs of the Kaiser Foundation Hospitals, Southern California.

We are especially grateful to the Southern California Permanente Medical Group for their continued support of the authors. We thank Mead Johnson Nutritionals, without whom this endeavor would not have been possible. Their generous educational grants provided funding for word-processing, book publication, and production of the CD-ROM and Palm Pilot™ versions of this formulary.

For the development of the CD-ROM and Palm Pilot™ versions, we thank Orlando Chacon, Computer Specialist, Oasis Consulting, Alta Loma, California.

For Their Love and Understanding
We Dedicate This Book To Our Families

Harshida
Rajan and Meera

Dennis
Steven, Heather, and Katherine

Michael, Kevin and Kate

Shashi
Ajay and Rita

Sherri
Eric and Elisabeth

Lambert
Armilla and Breanna

CONTENTS

ABACAVIR (Ziagen)

Supplied: Tablet 300 mg
Oral solution 20 mg/mil in 240 ml

Comments: Oral solution: store at controlled room temperature of 20° C (68-77° F) Do not freeze. May be refrigerated (1)

Abacavir (Ziagen)

Dosage: Neonatal: Not approved for infants younger than 3 mo of age. For infants between 1 and 3 mo of age, a dosage of 8 mg/kg of body weight twice daily is under study.

Major Toxic Effects:
Most frequent: Nausea, vomiting, headache, fever, rash, anorexia, and fatigue.
Unusual (more severe): Approximately 5% of adults and children develop a potentially fatal hypersensitivity reaction. Symptoms include fever, fatigue, malaise, nausea, vomiting, diarrhea, and abdominal pain. Physical findings include lymphadenopathy, ulceration of mucous membranes, and maculopapular or urticarial skin rash. A hypersensitivity reaction can occur without a rash. Laboratory abnormalities include elevated liver function test results, elevated creatine phosphokinase and creatinine levels, and lymphopenia. This reaction generally occurs in the first 6 weeks of therapy. For patients suspected of having a hypersensitivity reaction, ABC should be stopped and not restarted since hypotension and death have occurred on rechallenge.

Drug Indications: No significant interactions between ABC, zidovudine (ZDV), and lamivudine (3TC).
Abacavir does not inhibit and is not metabolized by hepatic cytochrome P-450 enzymes. Thus, it should not cause changes in drug levels or clearance of agents metabolized through these pathways, such as protease inhibitors and NNRTIs.

(American Academy of Pediatrics: Report of the Committee on Infectious Diseases. Red Book 2000, p.678)

ACETAMINOPHEN (Tylenol, Tempra, Panadol)

Supplied: Suppositories 80mg, 120mg, 125mg, 325mg, 650mg
Elixir 120mg/5ml, 160mg/5ml
Liquid 160mg/5ml (alcohol free)
Infant drops 100mg/ml (alcohol free)

Administration: PO, PR

Comments: Many generic products exists, check concentration against label.

Acetaminophen (APAP, Liquiprin, Panadol, Tempra, Tylenol)

Indications and use: Analgesic-antipyretic.

Actions: Mechanism of analgesic effect is unclear. Reduction of fever is produced by direct action on the hypothalamic heat-regulating center.

Route: PO, PR
Dosage: 5-10 mg/kg/dose q4-6h as needed.

Adverse effects: Hepatic necrosis with overdosage, rash, fever, and blood dyscrasias (neutropenia, pancytopenia, leukopenia, thrombocytopenia). May be hepatotoxic with chronic use.
(Gomella: Neonatology 1999, p.550)

Acetaminophen

Dose & Route: Pediatric: 10-15 mg/kg dose
PO/PR Q4-6 hr;
Dosing by age:
0-3 mo: 40 mg/dose
4-11 mo: 80 mg/dose

Remarks: Does not possess anti-inflammatory activity. May cause hemolysis at large doses in type A G6PD deficiency.

$T_{1/2}$: 1 - 3 hrs. in neonates; metabolized in the liver. some preparations contain alcohol (7%-10%) and/or phenylalanine; all suspensions should be shaken before use.
Adjust dose in renal failure.
(Siberry: The Harriet Lane Handbook 2000, pp.615-616)

Acetaminophen

Route: PO, PR
Neonatal Dose: 40 mg 4-5 times daily.
Preterm: PO: 10 mg/kg/dose

Pediatric Dose: Give doses 4-5 times daily, not to exceed 5 doses/day.
3-5 kg: 40mg/dose
6-8 kg: 80mg
9-10 kg: 120 mg
Max: 4 g/d

Discussion: Has no anti-inflammatory effects; adjust dose for renal impairment, hepatic toxicity with serum levels >200 μg/ml
(Rudolph: Rudolph's Pediatrics 1996, p.2170)

Acetaminophen

10-15 mg/kg/dose q 6 hours as required PO.
20-25 mg/kg/dose q 6 hours as required PR.
(Truog: Management of pain in the postoperative neonate. Clin Perinatol 1989;16:74)

ACETAZOLAMIDE (Diamox)

Supplied: Tablets 125mg, 250mg
Injection, powder for 500mg/vial

Administration: IV, PO
Reconstitute each 500mg vial with at least 5ml SWFI (1).
Administer this concentration IV push over 60 seconds (2).

IM administration is painful. Reconstituted solutions retain potency for one week if refrigerated. Since this product contains no preservative, however, use within 24 hours of reconstitution (1).
Oral suspensions can be prepared with crushed tablets and suspended in flavored vehicle to help disguise bitter taste. Concentrations of 250mg/5ml more palatable than higher concentrations. Stable for approximately 1 week. (3)

Extemporaneous Compounding (Recipe)

Dosage form: Oral suspension
Made from: Tablets
Concentration: 25mg/mL
Stability: 60 days
Store: Refrigerate
Label: Shake well

Ingredient	Strength	Quantity
Acetazolamide tablets	250 mg	12
Ora-Sweet or Ora-Sweet SF		
Ora-plus		aa qs 120 mL

Instructions: Place the tablets in a mortar and reduce to a fine powder. Add approximately 20 mL of vehicle and mix to a uniform paste. Add vehicle in geometric portions to almost desired volume while mixing. Transfer to a graduate and qs to volume with vehicle. Mix well. (11)

Acetazolamide (Diamox)

Indications and use:
For use as a mild diuretic or as an anticonvulsant in refractory neonatal seizures. to decrease cerebrospinal fluid (CSF) production in posthemorrhagic hydrocephalus; also used in the treatment of renal tubular acidosis.

Actions: Carbonic anhydrase inhibitor. Appears to retard abnormal discharge from central nervous system (CNS) neurons. Beneficial effects may be related to direct inhibition of carbonic anhydrase or may be due to the acidosis produced. Also produces urinary alkalosis, useful in the treatment of renal tubular acidosis.

Route: IV, PO.

Dosage: Diuretic: 5 mg/kg/dose qd-qod
Anticonvulsant: 8-30 mg/kg/day PO divided q6-8h.
To alkalinize urine: 5 mg/kg/dose 2-3 times over 24 h
To decrease CSF production: 50-100 mg/kg/day divided q6-8h.

Elimination: Unchanged in urine. Half life is 4-10 hours.

Adverse effects: Gastrointestinal (GI) irritation, anorexia, transient hypokalemia, drowsiness, and paresthesias.

Comments: Limited clinical experience in neonates. Used as an adjunct to other medications in refractory seizures. Tolerance to diuretic effect with long-term use.

(Gomella: Neonatology 1999, p.550)

Acetazolamide

Route: Diuretic (PO, IV)

Dose: Child: 5mg/kg/dose QD-QOD

Glaucoma: Child: 20-40 mg/kg/24hr÷Q6hr IM/IV; 8-30 mg/kg/24hr÷Q6-8hr

Seizures: 8-30 mg/kg/24hr÷Q6-12hr

Max dose: 1 g/24hr.

Urine Alkalinization: 5 mg/kg/dose PO repeated BID-TID

Remarks: **Contraindicated** in hepatic failure, severe renal failure (GRF <10 ml/min), and hypersensitivity to sulfonamides.

$T_{1/2}$: 2-6hr; IM injection may be painful; bicarbonate replacement therapy may be required during ling-term use (see Citrate or Sodium Bicarbonate).

Possible side effects (more likely with long-term therapy) include GI irritation, paresthesias, excretion, hypokalemia, acidosis, reduced urate secretion, aplastic anemia, polyuria, and development of renal calculi.

(Siberry: The Harriet Lane Handbook 2000, p.616)

Acetazolamide

Diuretic:

Dose/kg: 5 mg

Route and frequency: PO, IV, qd

Comments: May cause acidosis, hypokalemia, and GI irritation

Hydrocephalus:

Dose/kg: 5 mg (titrate to max of 20 mg)

Route and frequency: q6h

(Avery: Neonatology Pathophysiology and Management of the Newborn, 1999 p.1551)

ACETYLCYSTEINE (Mucomyst, Mucosil)

Supplied: Solution 10% and 20%

Administration: Inhalation, intratracheal instillation

Unlabeled use: It has been used as an enema to treat bowel obstruction due to meconium ileus or its equivalent (1).

Acetylcysteine

Dose & Route: Meconium Ileus: 5-10 ml/kg of 10% solution PR by soft rubber catheter. This may be given up to Q6hr.

Nebulizer: 3-5 ml of 20% solution (diluted with equal volume of H_2O or sterile saline to equal 10%), or 6-10 ml of 10% solution. Administer TID-QID.

Remarks: For nebulized use, give inhaled bronchodilator 10-15 minutes prior to use and follow with postural drainage and/or suctioning after acetylcysteine administration. Prior hydration is essential for meconium ileus treatment.

May induce bronchospasm, stomatitis, drowsiness, rhinorrhea, nausea, vomiting, and hemoptysis.

(Siberry: The Harriet Lane Handbook 2000, p.617)

Acetylcysteine (Mucomyst)

Dose: Meconium Ileus Equivalent:
Infants: Contraindicated. Treatment of choice is surgical.
Children or Adults: 100-200 ml by irrigation bid.

Pulmonary Mucolytic: 6-10 ml of 10% solution by nebulization tid-qid.

Toxicity: Local irritation; may cause bronchospasm, stomatitis, rhinorrhea, nausea. Hemoptysis may occur with prolonged use.

(Benitz: The Pediatric Drug Handbook 1995, p.167)

Acetylcysteine

Dose: 5% solution of N-acetylcysteine (Mucomyst ®)...every 4h as part of their endotracheal tube toilet for a total of seven days.

Comment: N-acetylcysteine was associated with a 59±26% increase in total airway resistance by the third day of treatment ($p<0.01$). A two-fold increase in airway resistance associated with an increased frequency of bradycardia and cyanosis spells was seen in two of the infants following three days of N-acetylcysteine administration, with a rapid improvement in their condition when subsequently switched to saline.

(Bibi: Intratracheal N-acetylcysteine use in infants with chronic lung disease. Acta Paediatr 1992;81:335-339)

ACYCLOVIR (Zovirax)

Supplied: Suspension 200mg/5ml
Ointment Topical 5%
Injection, powder for 500mg/vial, 1 gm/vial
(contains 4.2mEq Na/gram)

Administration: IV, PO, TOPICAL
Ointment is for cutaneous use only, not for use in the eyes.

Use a finger barrier (glove) to apply to prevent spread of infection.

IV administration: Add 10ml SWFI to 500mg vial, or 20ml to 1 gm vial. This yields a concentration of 50mg/ml. Do not use bacteriostatic water to reconstitute as it contains parabens, which may precipitate and benzyl alcohol which is toxic to neonates. Stable for infusion in D5W or NS (2). Remove and dilute the calculated dose in an appropriate

IV solution at a volume selected for administration during each 1 hour infusion. Infusion concentrations of 7mg/ml or lower are recommended to prevent phlebitis. Use reconstituted solution within 12 hours. Once diluted for administration, use each dose within 24 hours. Refrigeration of reconstituted solutions may result in formation of a precipitate which redissolves at room temperature (1). Do not administer IM.

The recommended final concentration for administration is 7mg/ml. Administer over at least 1 hour to prevent renal tubular damage (1). Administer over 1-2 hours (6).

Compatible: Cefotaxime, dextrose, gentamicin, lorazepam, ampicillin, potassium chloride, ranitidine, sodium chloride (9).

Incompatible: Dobutamine, dopamine (9).

Acyclovir

Treatment: For recommended antiviral dosages and duration of therapy with acyclovir, valaciclovir, famciclovir, and penciclovir for different HSV infections. Neither valaciclovir nor famciclovir is approved by the US Food and Drug Administration (FDA) for use in children.

Neonatal. Parenteral acyclovir is the treatment of choice for neonatal HSV infections. Acyclovir should be administered to all neonates with HSV infection, irrespective of presenting clinical findings. The best outcome in terms of morbidity and mortality is observed among infants with disease limited to the skin, eyes, and mouth. Although most neonates treated for HSV encephalitis survive, the majority suffer substantial neurologic sequelae. Approximately 50% of neonates with disseminated disease die despite antiviral therapy. The dosage of acyclovir is 60 mg/kg per day in 3 divided doses, given intravenously for 14 days if disease is limited to the skin, eye, and mouth and for 21 days if disease is disseminated or involves the CNS. Relapse of skin, eyes, and mouth and CNS disease can occur after cessation of treatment. The optimal management of these recurrences is not established. The value of long-term suppressive or intermittent acyclovir therapy for neonates with disease of the skin, eyes, and mouth is being evaluated.

Infants with ocular involvement due to HSV infection should receive a topical ophthalmic drug (1% to 2% trifluridine, 1% iododeoxyuridine, or 3% vidarabine), as well as parenteral antiviral therapy.

Central Nervous System. Patients with HSV encephalitis should be treated for 21 days with intravenous acyclovir. Therapy is less effective in older adults than in children and patients who are comatose or semicomatose at initiation of therapy. For persons with Bell palsy, the combination of acyclovir and prednisone should be considered.

Ocular. Treatment of eye lesions should be undertaken in consultation with an ophthalmologist. several DNA inhibitor drugs, such as 1% to 2% trifluridine, 1% iododeoxyuridine, and 3% vidarabine, have proven efficacy for topical therapy of superficial keratitis. Topical corticosteroids are contraindicated in suspected HSV conjunctivitis; however, ophthalmologists may choose to use corticosteroids in conjunction with antiviral drugs to treat locally invasive infections. For children with recurrent ocular lesions, oral suppressive therapy with acyclovir (20 mg/kg every 6 hours) may be of benefit.

(American Academy of Pediatrics: Report of the Committee on Infectious Diseases. Red Book 2000, pp.313-315)

<u>Acyclovir</u> (Zovirax)

Indication: HSV encephalitis
Route: IV
Usually Recommended Dosage:
30 mg/kg per day in 3 divided doses for a minimum of 14-21 d

Indication: Neonatal HSV
Route: IV
Usually Recommended Dosage:
60 mg/kg per day in 3 divided doses for 14-21 d

Comments: Dose should be decreased in patients with impaired renal function.
Oral dosage of acyclovir in children should not exceed 80 mg/kg per day.

(American Academy of Pediatrics: Report of the Committee on Infectious Diseases. Red Book 2000, pp.675-677)

<u>Acyclovir</u>

For Herpes Simplex Virus Infections

A comparison of vidarabine with acyclovir suggests that these compounds have a similar level of activity for this disease, but vidarabine is no longer available for clinical use. Acyclovir is safe for use in newborns and is familiar to pediatricians from its other clinical uses.

The current recommendation for acyclovir treatment of neonatal HSV infections is 30 mg/kg per day in three doses, based on its demonstrated efficacy, with the usual duration of therapy being 14 to 21 days. These recent observations may result in a change to the use of 20 mg/kg per dose three times a day for 21 days.

The use of oral acyclovir is contraindicated for the treatment of acute HSV infections in newborns. Its limited oral bioavailability results in plasma and CSF concentrations of drug that are inadequate for therapeutic effects on viral replication. The high risk of progression from localized mucocutaneous infections requires the administration of intravenous acyclovir to these infants, regardless of how well they may appear at the time of diagnosis. In addition to intravenous therapy, infants with ocular involvement caused by HSV should receive one of the topical ophthalmic agents approved for this indication. Topical acyclovir is not necessary for treatment of mucocutaneous lesions caused by HSV because parenteral drug reaches these sites.

Intravenous acyclovir has been tolerated well by infants given each of the doses evaluated in the prospective studies done by the Collaborative Antiviral Study Group, including 60 mg/kg per day. Adequate hydration is necessary to minimize the risk of nephrotoxicity and dosage adjustments are necessary if renal clearance is impaired. As for all drugs the possibility of acute toxicity should be considered in any child receiving parenteral antiviral therapy and should be assessed by serially evaluating bone marrow, renal, and hepatic functions. The potential for long-term harm from these drugs remains to be defined.

(Remington: Infectious Diseases of the Fetus and Newborn Infant, 2001, pp.437-440)

<u>Acyclovir</u>

For Varicella Zoster viral infection

The antiviral drug ACV is the drug of choice for treatment of potentially severe or severe VZV infections.

Although there is little information on the use of ACV in newborns, it has been used to treat a great many infants with neonatal HSV infection. In a study in which 95 infants received ACV (30 mg/kg per day intravenously), no short- or long-term toxicity was observed.

There is little information, however, on the use of the larger dose usually employed to treat VZV infections in newborns (a dose of 1500 mg/m^2 per day is about three times that of the dose for neonatal HSV infection). for infants with severe disease, however this dosage has been employed without obvious difficulties, although there are no controlled studies. Pharmacokinetic studies have indicated that dose adjustments may be necessary in premature infants and/or those with hepatic or renal dysfunction. There are no data with regard to use of oral ACV for neonatal infections caused by VZV, and in addition, ACV is poorly absorbed when given by the gastrointestinal route. Therefore, only intravenous ACV can be recommended for treatment of severe varicella in the neonate.

(Remington: Infectious Diseases of the Fetus and Newborn Infant, 2001, p.703)

Acyclovir

Indication: For neonatal herpes simplex infection

Acyclovir is the newest anti-herpes drug found to have limited toxicity, high specificity, and greater activity against the virus than vidarabine. The drug is a deoxyguanosine analogue that is activated by a herpes-specific thymidine kinase and inhibits viral DNA polymerase and thereby viral replication. Controlled studies of herpes simplex encephalitis in adults indicate greater benefit in relation to both mortality and morbidity for acyclovir than for vidarabine. A controlled multiinstitutional study of acyclovir verus vidarabine in the treatment of neonatal herpes simplex infection demonstrated no appreciable difference in efficacy between the two. However, we prefer acyclovir because of its higher solubility and relatively low toxicity. However, renal and neurological toxicity can occur. Because acyclovir is excreted primarily by the kidneys, dose should be modified in infants with impaired renal function. Recommended dose in the term infant with normal renal function is 10 mg/kg every 8 hours, and in the premature infant less than 33 weeks of gestation, 10 mg/kg every 12 hours. Each dose is infused over 1 hour, and total duration of therapy is 3 weeks.

(Volpe: Neurology of the Newborn 2001, pp.746-747)

Acyclovir

Route: IM, IV

Dosage (mg/kg/dose) by Gestational age plus weeks of life:

≤26 Wks: 20 q12h
27-34 Wks: 20 q12h
35-42 Wks: 20 q8h
≥43 Wks: 20 q8h

(Nelson: Pocket Book of Pediatric Antimicrobial Therapy 2000-2001 p.17)

Acyclovir (Zovirax)

Classification: Antiviral agent.

Action and spectrum:

Indicated in herpes simplex and varicella-zoster viral infections. Virostatic activated in virally infected cells, inhibits viral DNA polymerase, and is a viral chain terminator. Good activity against herpes simplex (types 1 and 2) and varicella-zoster viruses. Poor activity against Epstein-Barr virus and cytomegalovirus. CSF concentrations are 50% those of plasma.

Route: Topical, IV, PO

Dosage: Topical: Apply sufficient amount to cover lesion q3h.
IV: 30-40 mg/kg/day divided q8h for 10-14 days (dilute to final concentration of 7 mg/mL and infuse over 60 minutes).

PO (varicella): 20 mg/kg/dose q6h initiated at first sign of disease. Continue for 5 days.

Adverse effects: Transient elevation of serum creatinine, thrombocytosis, jitters, rash, and hives.

Comments: Drug of choice for documented or suspected herpes encephalitis (suggest 40 mg/kg/day IV in divided doses for 14 days).

(Gomella: Neonatology 1999, p.550)

Acyclovir

Condition: Herpes simplex infection

Therapy: Acyclovir 60 mg/kg/day as 1-2 hr IV infusion div q8h x 21 days for CNS and disseminated disease, or x 14 days for other types; PLUS trifluridine ophthalmic solution topically q2h for conjunctivitis (max 9 times/day)

Comment: Larger dosages of acyclovir and more days of Rx than previously recommended may be beneficial

(Nelson: Pocket Book of Pediatric Antimicrobial Therapy 2000-2001, p.8)

Acyclovir

IMMUNOCOMPETENT:

Neonatal HSV and HSV encephalitis:

Route & Dose: All ages: 30 mg/kg/24 hr or 1500 mg/m^2/24 hr ÷ Q8 hr IV x 14-21 days. Higher doses of 45-60 mg/kg/24 hr ÷ Q8 hr IV can be used in term infants.

Mucocutaneous HSV (including genital):

Route & Dose: Initial infection:
IV: 15 mg/kg/24 hr or 750 mg/m^2/24 hr ÷ Q8 hr x 5-7 days
PO: 1200 mg/24 hr ÷ Q8 hr x 7-10 days

Recurrence:
PO: 1200 mg/24 hr ÷ Q8 hr or 1600 mg/24 hr ÷ Q12 x 5 days

Chronic suppressive therapy:
PO: 800-1000 mg/24 hr ÷ 2-5 x day for up to 1 year

Zoster:

Route & Dose: IV: 30 mg/kg/24 hr or 1500 mg/m^2/24 hr ÷ Q8 hr x 7-10 days
PO: 4000 mg/24 hr ÷ 5 x 24 hr x 5-7 days for patients ≥12 yr

Varicella:

Route & Dose: IV: 30 mg/kg/24 hr or 1500 mg/m^2/24 hr ÷ Q8 hr x 7-10 days
PO: 80 mg/kg/24 hr ÷ QID x 5 days (begin treatment at earliest signs/symptoms); **max dose**: 3200 mg/24 hr

Max dose of oral acyclovir in children = 80 mg/kg/24 hr

IMMUNOCOMPROMISED:

HSV:

Route & Dose: IV: 750-1500 mg/m^2/24 hr ÷ Q8 hr x 7-14 days
PO: 1000 mg/24 hr ÷ 3-5 times/24 hr x 7-14 days

HSV Prophylaxis:

Route & Dose: IV: 750 mg/m^2/24 hr ÷ Q8 hr during risk period
PO: 600-1000 mg/24 hr ÷ 3-5 times/24 hr during risk period

Varicella or Zoster:

Route & Dose: IV: Same as immunocompetent dosing x 7-10 days
PO: 250-600 mg/m^2/dose 4-5 times/24 hr

CMV Prophylaxis:

Route & Dose: IV: 1500 mg/m^2/24 hr ÷ Q8 hr during risk period
PO: 800-3200 mg/24 hr ÷ Q6-24 hr during risk period
Max dose of oral acyclovir in children = 80 mg/kg/24 hr

TOPICAL:

Apply 0.5 inch ribbon of 5% ointment for 4 inch square surface area 6 times a day x 7 days.

Comments: See most recent edition of the AAP Red Book for further details. Oral absorption is unpredictable (15-30%). Use ideal body weight for obese patients when calculating dosages.

Adequate hydration and slow (1 hr) IV administration are essential to prevent crystallization in renal tubules; dose alteration necessary in patients with impaired renal function.

Can cause renal impairment; has been infrequently associated with headache, vertigo, insomnia, encephalopathy, GI tract irritation, rash urticaria, arthralgia, fever, and adverse hematologic effects.

(Siberry: The Harriet Lane Handbook 2000, p.618)

ADENOSINE (Adenocard)

Supplied: 3mg/ml in 2ml and 5ml vials (preservative free)

Administration: Rapid IV Bolus only, over 1-2 seconds. To be certain the solution reaches the systemic circulation, administer either directly into a vein or, if given into an IV line, as proximal as possible AND FOLLOW WITH A RAPID SALINE FLUSH (1).

Adenosine ATP

Class: IV Purinergic agonists

Uses: Termination of reentry SVT, AV block to distinguish AFL?

Dose (Level) Adenosine: 100 μg/kg IV, up to 300 μg/kg if needed
ATP: <1yr, 2-5 mg IV; >1 yr, 2–15 mg IV

Mode of Action: Vagotonic, antiadrenergic, depress slow inward Ca^{++} current, increase K^+ conductance (hyperpolarization)

ECG/EP Changes: ↑AH

Side Effects: Sinus arrest, sinus bradycardia, flushing, nausea, headache, asthma

(Garson: The science and practice of pediatric cardiology 1998, p.2954)

Adenosine

Dosing: IV: 100-300 mcg/kg push

Warnings: Hypotension, flushing, bronchospasm

Intravenous Administration, Kinetics, Metabolites:

The drug is given as a rapid intravenous bolus. Its effects are generally seen in 7 to 20 seconds. It is a very useful therapeutic and diagnostic agent.

Dosing and Interactions:

Initial doses of 100 to 150 μg/kg are given as a rapid peripheral bolus, followed by a flush of saline. The dose may be doubled sequentially, up to a maximum of 300 μg/kg or the adult dose of 6 to 12 mg. An adequate record of the electrocardiographic tracing is essential during adenosine administration. Aminophylline interferes with the actions of adenosine. Dipyridamole and diazepam can inhibit its cellular uptake and potentiate its effects.

Side Effects: Adenosine may cause hypotension, facial flushing, and mild bronchospasm. Ventricular ectopy is not unusual and may be the mechanism of termination of some AV reciprocating tachycardias. Occasionally, atrial fibrillation results from adenosine administration during SVTs.

(Gillette: Clinical Pediatric Arrhythmias 1999,pp.231-248)

Adenosine

Uses: PSVT: diagnostically to diagnose primary atrial re-entry, some JET, causes of WCT.

Dosing: 100 μg/kg rapid bolus; increase by 50 μg/kg up to 250 μg/kg max

Acute Side Effects: Sinus arrest: AV block; PVCs; Afib (all transient)

Other Considerations:

Not useful if therapeutic theophylline; low dose in presence of dipyridamole

AFib, atrial fibrillation; AV atrioventricular; JET, junctional ectopic tachycardia; PSVT, paroxysmal supraventricular tachycardia; PVC, premature ventricular contractions; WCT, wide-complex tachycardia.

(Gillette: Clinical Pediatric Arrhythmias 1999, p.152)

Adenosine (Adenocard)

Indications and use:

Conversion to sinus rhythm of paroxysmal supraventricular tachycardia.

Actions: A purine nucleoside naturally occurring in all human cells. Slows conduction time through the atrioventricular (AV) node and interrupts reentry pathways through the AV node to restore normal sinus rhythm. Its electrophysiologic effects are mediated by depression of calcium slow-channel conduction, an increase in potassium conductance, and possibly indirect antiadrenergic effects.

Route: IV

Dosage: 0.1- 0.2 mg/kg by rapid IV push over 1-2 s.

Adverse effects: Do not use in second- or third-degree AV block. May produce a short-duration first-, second-, or third-degree heart block; hypotension; brief dyspnea; and facial flushing. Half-life is < 10 s; duration is 20-30 s. Carbamazepine increases the degree of heart block caused by adenosine. Methylxanthines (eg, caffeine and theophylline) are competitive antagonists; larger adenosine doses may be required.

(Gomella: Neonatology 1999, p.551)

Adenosine

Supraventricular tachycardia:

Route & Dose: Children: 0.1-0.2 mg/kg rapid IV push over 1-2 seconds; may increase dose by 0.05 mg/kg increments every 2 min to **max** of 0.25 mg/kg (up to 12 mg), or until termination of SVT

Max single dose: 12 mg

Comment: **Contraindicated** in 2nd and 3rd degree AV block or sick-sinus syndrome unless pacemaker placed.

Follow each dose with NS flush, $T_{1/2}$: <10 seconds.

May precipitate bronchoconstriction. Side effects include facial flushing, headache, shortness of breath, dyspnea, nausea, chest pain, lightheadedness.

(Siberry: The Harriet Lane Handbook 2000, p.619)

Adenosine

Dose/kg: 0.05 mg

Route and frequency: IVP

Titrate dose in increments of 0.05 mg/kg every 2 min to a max of 0.25 mg/kg or until termination of PSVT
(max single dose: 12 mg)

Comments: Push over 1 to 2 seconds flush with NS
Higher doses may be needed for peripheral administration vs, central administration

(Avery: Neonatology Pathophysiology and Management of the Newborn 1999, p.1551)

Adenosine

All study infants had an umbilical venous line in the right atrium and infusion of study drug was given using this line. The starting dose for adenosine was 25 μg/kg/min of adenosine base (0.1 μmol per kg/min). The placebo group received normal saline at the same calculated volume. A response to IV infusion was defined as an increase in postductal Pao_2 of ≥20 Torr compared with preinfusion value. If a response was not seen after 30 minutes of infusion, the dose was doubled to give the infant 50 μg/kg/min of adenosine base (0.2 μmol/kg/min of adenosine).

Conclusion. Data from this pilot study indicate that adenosine infusion at a dose of 50 μg/kg/min improves Pao_2 in infants with PPHN without causing hypotension or tachycardia. Larger trials are needed to determine its effects on mortality and/or need for extracorporeal membrane oxygenation in infants with PPHN.

(Konduri: Adenosine Infusion Improves Oxygenation in Term Infants With Respiratory Failure. Pediatrics 1996;97:295-300)

AGAR

Agar

The neonates in this group received 500 mg of agar (Pastagar B; Pasteur Institute, 64941) orally by spoon every 6 hours before feedings, in 10 mL of distilled water....Oral agar was given to the neonates until their bilirubin levels were decreased to 10 mg/dL....The efficacy of phototherapy in decreasing the serum bilirubin level in neonatal hyperbilirubinemia can be augmented with the use of oral agar. Oral agar can also be used as a single agent for the treatment of neonatal hyperbilirubinemia, since it is as effective as phototherapy.

(Caglayan: Superiority of Oral Agar and Phototherapy Combination in the Treatment of Neonatal Hyperbilirubinemia. Pediatrics 1993;92:86-89)

ALBUMIN (Normal Serum Albumin)

Supplied: Injection 5% in 50ml, others
Injection 25% in 10ml, 20ml, 50ml

Administration: IV

5%: (5gm/dL) contains 130 to 160 mEq of Na per liter. Administer by IV infusion and without further dilution (1).

25%: (25gm/dL) contains 130 to 160 mEq of Na per liter. May be given undiluted or diluted in NS. If sodium restriction is required, it may be administered in a carbohydrate solution such as D5W (1). Do not dilute with sterile water as a hypotonic solution which causes hemolysis may result. The hemolysis and acute renal failure that may result may be life-threatening (5).

Compatible: Blood, dextrose, parenteral nutrition, plasma, and sodium chloride (9).

Incompatible: No data available (9).

Albumin

Medications, volume expansion, and vascular access: Epinephrine in a dose of 0.01-0.03 mg/kg (0.1-0.3 mL/kg of 1:10,000 solution) should be administered if the heart rate remains <60 bpm after a minimum of 30 seconds of adequate ventilation and chest compressions. Emergency volume expansion may be accomplished with an isotonic crystalloid solution or O-negative red blood cells; albumin-containing solutions are no longer the fluid of choice for initial volume expansion. Intraosseous access can serve as an alternative route for medications/volume expansion if umbilical or other direct venous access is not readily available.

(American Academy of Pediatrics. American Heart Association: International Guidelines for Neonatal Resuscitation: An excerpt from the guidelines 2000 for cardiopulmonary resuscitation and emergency cardiovascular care: International consensus on science. Pediatrics 2000;106:1-16)

<u>Albumin, Human</u> (various)

Indications and use:
Plasma volume expander. Treatment of hypoproteinemia.

Actions: Maintains plasma colloid oncotic pressure. IV administration causes a shift of fluid from the interstitial spaces into the circulation. Serves as a carrier for may substances, such as bilirubin. Limited nutritional value.

Route: IV

Dosage: 0.5-1.0 g/kg IV (or 10-20 mL/kg of 5% IV bolus) repeated as necessary. Maximum 6 g/kg/d.

Adverse effects: Infrequent. Rapid infusion may cause vascular overload and precipitation of congestive heart failure. Hypersensitivity reactions may include chills, fever, nausea, and urticaria.

Comments: More purified than plasma protein fraction and thus less likely to cause hypotension.

(Gomella: Neonatology 1999, p.551)

<u>Albumin, Human</u> (Normal serum albumin)

Dose & Route: Hypoproteinemia:
Children: 0.5-1 g/kg/dose IV over 30-120 min.

Hypovolemia:
Children: 0.5-1 g/kg/dose IV, rapid infusion.

Max Dose: 6 g/kg/24hr or 250 g/48 hr

Remarks: Contraindicated in cases of CHF or severe anemia: rapid infusion may cause fluid overload; hypersensitivity reactions may occur; may cause rapid increase in serum sodium levels.

Caution: 25% concentration contraindicated in preterm infants due to risk of IVH. For infusion, use 5 micron filter or larger. Both 5% and 25% products are isotonic but differ in oncotic effects. Dilutions of the 25% product should be made with D5W or NS.

(Siberry: The Harriet Lane Handbook 2000, p.619)

<u>Albumin</u>

Administration: Parenteral: I.V.: Administer through a 5-micron filter or larger, do **not** give through 0.22 micron filter; too rapid infusion may result in vascular over-load

Hypoproteinemia: Infuse over 2-4 hours; for neonates, dose may be added to hyperalimentation fluid and infused over 24 hours

Hypovolemia: Rate of infusion depends on severity of hypovolemia and patient's symptoms; usually infuse dose over 30-60 minutes (faster infusion rates may be clinically necessary)

Maximum rates of I.V. infusion after initial volume replacement:
5%: 2-4 mL/minute
25%: 1 mL/minute

Monitoring Parameters:

Observe for signs of hypervolemia, pulmonary edema, and cardiac failure

Nursing Implications:

Albumin administration must be completed within 6 hours after entering container, provided that administration is begun within 4 hours of entering the container

Additional Information:

In certain conditions (eg, hypoproteinemia with generalized edema, nephrotic syndrome), doses of albumin may be followed with I.V. furosemide: 0.5-1 mg/kg/dose; albumin contains 130-160 mEq of sodium/L; osmolarity: 5% albumin = 300 mOsm/L; 25% albumin = 1500 mOsm/L

(Taketomo: Pediatric Dosage Handbook 1999-2000, pp.36-37)

<u>Albumin</u>

Albumin is available as a 25% solution in distilled water or as a 5% solution in saline. Plasma protein fraction (PPF) is a similar product except that it is subject to fewer purification steps in the fractionation process.

Dosage and Administration:

Albumin and PPF do not need to be administered through a filter. Dosage and rate of infusion depend upon the patient's clinical condition. In shock the usual dosage of 5% albumin is 500 ml in adults and 10-20 ml/kg in children.

(Lilleyman: Pediatric Hematology 1999, p.734)

ALBUTEROL (Proventil, Ventolin, Salbutamol)

Supplied: Syrup 2mg/5ml
Soln for inhalation 0.083% in 3ml, 0.5% (5mg/ml) in 20ml
Aerosol, 90mcg/actuation.

Administration: Inhalation, PO
Inhalation solution is diluted with sterile normal saline (1).

<u>Albuterol</u> (Proventil, Ventolin)

Indications and use:

Manage bronchospasm in reversible airway obstruction,

increase maximal expiratory flow in infants with respiratory distress syndrome (RDS), and improve lung mechanics in ventilator-dependent infants and those with bronchopulmonary dysplasia (BPD).

Actions: Primarily β_2-adrenergic stimulation ((bronchodilation and vasodilation) with minor β_1 stimulation (increased myocardial contractility and conduction). Duration of action is ~3-8 h.

Route: Nebulization.
Dosage: 0.5%: 0.04 mL/kg/dose (= 0.2 mg/kg/dose).
0.083%: 0.2 mL/kg/dose (= 0.2 mg/kg/dose).
Dilute in 2 mL of normal saline and give q 4-6h.

Adverse effects: Tachycardia, tremors, CNS stimulation, hypokalemia, and hypertension.
Comments: Titrate the dose to the heart rate and clinical effect.
(Gomella: Neonatology 1999, p.551)

Albuterol

Dose/kg: 0.05-0.25 mg per dose

Route & frequency: Inhalation for bronchodilation q2h to q6h

Comments: Avoid circulatory overload. Tachycardia, arrhythmias, tremor, hypokalemia, and irritable behavior have been reported.
(Avery: Neonatology Pathophysiology and Management of the Newborn 1999, p.1551)

Albuterol

Dosage: 0.1 ml/kg/dose by nebulization. Supplied as a 0.5% solution. May be used as a continuous IV infusion at 0.5 to 5 μg/kg/min.
Comments: Selective ß$_2$ agonist.
(Fanaroff: Neonatal Perinatal Medicine 1997, p.1749)

ALFENTANIL (Alfenta)

Supplied: Injection 500mcg/ml in 2ml, 5ml, 10ml, 20ml
Administration: IV
Stable in NS, D5NS, D5LR, D5W, LR
Comment: Hypotension has occurred in neonates with respiratory distress syndrome receiving alfentanil 20mcg/kg (1).

Alfentanil

Warnings: Rapid I.V. infusion may result in skeletal muscle and chest wall rigidity → impaired ventilation → respiratory distress/arrest; inject slowly over 3-5 minutes; nondepolarizing skeletal muscle relaxant may be required

Precautions: Use with caution inpatients with bradycardia

Adverse Reactions:
Cardiovascular: Bradycardia, peripheral vasodilation, hypotension

Central nervous system: Drowsiness, dizziness, sedation, CNS depression, increased intracranial pressure
Endocrine & metabolic: Antidiuretic hormone release
Gastrointestinal: Nausea, vomiting, constipation, biliary tract spasm
Genitourinary: Urinary tract spasm
Neuromuscular & skeletal: Skeletal muscle and chest will rigidity especially following rapid I.V. administration
Ocular: Miosis
Respiratory: Respiratory depression, apnea, respiratory arrest
Miscellaneous: Histamine release, physical and psychological dependence with prolonged use

Usual Dosage: Doses should be titrated to appropriate effects; wide range of doses is dependent upon desired degree of analgesia/anesthesia

Neonates, Infants, and Children <12 years: Dose not established; A high percent of newborn infants receiving alfentanil (prior to procedures) at doses of 9-15 mcg/kg (mean dose: 11.7 mcg/kg) developed chest wall rigidity; 9 out of 20 newborns (45%) developed mild or moderate rigidity that did not affect ventilation, while 4 out of 20 (20%) had severe rigidity interfering with respiration for ~5-10 minutes; use of a skeletal muscle relaxant to prevent chest wall rigidity is recommended; however, smaller alfentanil doses may be required in newborns. Further studies are needed to determine appropriate doses of alfentanil in pediatric patients.

Administration Parenteral:

I.V.: Inject slowly over 3-5 minutes or by I.V. continuous infusion

Monitoring Parameters:

Respiratory rate, blood pressure, heart rate, neurological status (for degree of analgesia/anesthesia)

Nursing Implications:

Alfentanil may produce more hypotension compared to fentanyl, therefore, be sure to administer slowly and ensure patient has adequate hydration

(Taketomo: Pediatric Dosage Handbook 1999-2000, pp.39-41)

<u>Alfentanil</u>

Alfentanil, a synthetic opioid chemically related to fentanyl, with a rapid onset and brief duration of action.

In a randomized, controlled, double blind, crossover trial,... each patient received saline as placebo and two different doses of alfentanil, 10 and 20 μg/kg intravenously, in random order... two minutes before three separate endotracheal suctions, at least six hours apart, to 10 infants.

Tracheal suction is a painful procedure. The dose of alfentanil required for pain relief (20 µg/kg) causes a high incidence of rigidity and thus should be used only with muscle relaxant.

(Saarenmaa: Alfentanil as procedural pain relief in newborn infants. Arch Dis child 1996;75:F103-F107)

Alfentanil

Indication: Sedation in ventilated preterm infants.

Dose: 20 µg/kg given by infusion over 30 minutes followed by 5 µg/kg/hour over a 48-hour period.

Comments: Above produced steady state median alfentanil concentrations of 54.5 ng/ml (range: 7-73 ng/ml) with no evidence of drug accumulation. [Single dose (20 µg/kg)] injection over two minutes was associated with a transient fall in blood pressure, heart rate, and arterial oxygen tension.

(Marlow: Alfentanil pharmacokinetics in preterm infants. Arch Dis Child 1990;80:304-307)

ALLOPURINOL (Zyloprim)

Supplied: Tablets 100mg, 300mg
Lyophilized powder: 500mg

Administration: PO, IV
Allopurinol is rarely indicated for use in children, except in those with hyperuricemia secondary to malignancy, or in cases of certain rare inborn errors of purine metabolism (1).

Extemporaneous Compounding (Recipe)

Dosage form: Oral suspension
Made from: Tablets
Concentration: 20mg/mL
Stability: 60 days
Store: Refrigerate
Label: Shake well

Ingredient	Strength	Quantity
Allopurinol tablets	300 mg	8
Ora-Sweet or Ora-Sweet SF		
Ora-plus		aa qs 120 mL

Instructions: Place the tablets in a mortar and reduce to a fine powder. Add approximately 20 mL of vehicle and mix to a uniform paste. Add vehicle in geometric portions to almost desired volume while mixing. Transfer to a graduate and qs to volume with vehicle. Mix well. (11)

Allopurinol (Zyloprim)

Dose & Route: Child: 10 mg/kg/24hr PO÷BID-QID

Max dose: 800mg/24h

Remarks: **Adjust dose in renal insufficiency**. Must maintain adequate urine output and alkaline urine.

Drug interaction: increases serum theophylline levels; may increase the incidence of rash with ampicillin and amoxicillin; and increase risk of hypersensitivity reactions with ACE inhibitors and thiazide diuretics.

Side Effects include rash, neuritis, hepatotoxicity, GI disturbance, bone marrow suppression, and drowsiness.

(Siberry: The Harriet Lane Handbook 2000, p.621)

<u>Allopurinol</u>

Indication: Birth Asphyxia

Administration: IV

Dosage: 20 mg/kg q12h x 2 doses, 1st dose at < 4 h of age

(Van Bel: Effects of Allopurinol on Postasphyxial Free Radical Formation, Cerebral Hemodynamics, and Electrical Brain Activity. Pediatrics 1998;101:185-193)

<u>Allopurinol</u>

Allopurinol was formulated by suspending 20 mg of allopurinol in mucilage in a concentration of 20 mg/ml and a single dose of 20 mg/kg was given daily by oesophageal-gastric tube for seven days. The daily dose of 20 mg/kg was diluted with an equal volume of water for injection to achieve an osmolality of 409 mOsm/kg...In this trial of prophylactic allopurinol for the prevention of PVL in preterm babies, no protective effect was apparent...The failure of allopurinol prophylaxis in this group of infants is probably related to the complex nature of the pathological processes and to the timing of treatment.

(Russell: Randomised controlled trial of allopurinol prophylaxis in very preterm infants. Arch Dis Child 1995;73:F27-F31)

<u>Allopurinol</u>

For Hypoplastic Left Heart Syndrome Patients:
Six patients received a single, intravenous infusion of 5 mg/kg of allopurinol. The other six patients received a single allopurinol dose of 10 mg/kg. Each dose was diluted in 5% dextrose to a final concentration of 5 mg/mL and infused over 20 minutes.

Sodium allopurinol was provided by the Burroughs Wellcome Company, Research Triangle Park, NC.

(McGaurn: The Pharmacokinetics of Injectable Allopurinol in Newborns With the Hypoplastic Left Heart Syndrome. Pediatrics 1994;94:820-823)

ALUMINUM HYDROXIDE (Alternagel, Amphojel)

Supplied: Suspension 320mg, 675mg/5ml
Liquid 600mg/5ml

Administration: PO

Aluminum Hydroxide

Dose & Route: Doses in ml are based on the 320 mg/5 ml suspension concentration:

Peptic Ulcer:
Child: 5-15 ml PO Q3-6hr or 1-3hr PC and HS.

Prophylaxis against GI Bleeding:
Neonates: 1 ml/kg/dose Q4hr PRN
Infant: 2-5 ml/PO Q1-2hr
Child: 5-15 ml/PO Q1-2hr

Hyperphosphatemia: 50-150 mg/kg/24hr÷Q4-6hr PO

Remarks: Use with **caution** in patients with renal failure and upper GI hemorrhage.

Interferes with the absorption of several orally administered medications, including digoxin, indomethacin, isoniazid, tetracyclines, and iron.

May cause constipation, decreased bowel motility, encephalopathy, and phosphorus depletion.

(Siberry: The Harriet Lane Handbook 2000, pp. 621-622)

Aluminum Hydroxide

Route: PO

Neonatal Dose: 2-5 mL/dose q3-4h

Pediatric Dose: Infant: 2-5 mL/dose

Children: 5-15 mL/dose.
Use every 1-2 h in critically ill and every 3-4 h to treat peptic ulcer

Discussion: For hyperphosphatemia use 50-150 mg/kg/24 h given every 4-6 h for all ages; doses used in critically ill patients are also those used for prophylaxis of GI bleeding.

(Rudolph: Rudolph's Pediatrics 1996, p.2171)

ALUMINUM HYDROXIDE/MAGNESIUM HYDROXIDE

(Mylanta, Maalox)

AH=Aluminum Hydroxide/MH=Magnesium Hydroxide

Supplied: Suspension per 5ml:
Maalox Suspension: 225mg AH and 200mg MH
Mylanta: 200mg AH and 200mg MH

Administration: PO

Aluminum Hydroxide with Magnesium Hydroxide

Dose & Route: Same as for aluminum hydroxide preparations. **Do not use** combination product for hyperphosphatemia.

Remarks: May have laxative effect. May cause hypokalemia. Use with **caution** in patients with renal insufficiency (magnesium), gastric outlet obstruction.

Interferes with the absorption of the benzodiazepines, chloroquine, digoxin, phenytoin, tetracyclines, and iron.
(Siberry: The Harriet Lane Handbook 2000, p.622)

AMIKACIN (Amikin)

Supplied: Injection 100mg, 500mg in 2ml vial; 1gm in 4ml vial

Administration: IM, IV

In pediatric patients, the amount of fluid used for diluting the drug should be sufficient to infuse the amikacin over a 30- to 60-minute period. Infants should receive a 1- to 2-hour infusion. Stable for 24 hours in D5W or NS at a concentration of 0.25mg/ml and 5.0mg/ml (1).

The recommended final concentration of administration is 5mg/ml. The usual duration of infusion is 30 minutes (6).

Compatible: Dextrose, furosemide, heparin (in low concentrations of 0.5 to 1 unit/ml used to maintain IV line patency), magnesium, parenteral nutrition,* morphine, sodium chloride, ranitidine, vancomycin.

* Drugs reported as being compatible with parenteral nutrition in published studies using test solutions may not be compatible with the particular formulation your infant is receiving. Components in neonatal parenteral nutrition are individualized based on the infant's body weight, serum electrolytes, fluid, and other nutrient requirements, making most solutions unique. Observe the solution and tubing carefully for signs of precipitation during the 24-hour infusion period when drugs are . Certain drugs may be admixed into the parenteral nutrition bag. See Driscoll, and associates' review of the use of parenteral nutrition as a drug vehicle (9).

Incompatible: Amphotericin B, ampicillin, chlorothiazide, heparin (in high concentrations of more than 1 unit/ml used for systemic anticoagulation and in some heparin flushes), phenytoin (9).

<u>Amikacin</u>

Antibacterial Drugs for Newborn Infants:
Dose (mg/kg or Units [U]/kg) and Frequency of Administration

Route: IV, IM

Dose: <u>Infants 0-4 wk</u>
BW <1200 g: 7.5 every 18-24 h

<u>Infants <1 week old</u>
BW ≤1200-2000 g: 7.5 every 12 h
BW >2000 g: 7.5-10 every 12 h

<u>Infants ≥1 wk old</u>
BW ≤2000-2000 g: 7.5-10 every 8 or 12 h
BW >2000 g: 10 every 8 h

Notes: Optimal dosage should be based on determination of serum concentrations, especially in low-birth-weight (<1500 g) infants. In very-low-birth-weight (<1200 g) every 18 to 24 hours dosing may be appropriate in the first week of life.

Dosage for the aminoglycosides may differ from those recommended by the manufacturer in the package insert.

Antibacterial Drugs for Pediatric Patients Beyond the Newborn Period: Dosage per kg/d

Route: IV, IM
Mild to Moderate Infections: Inappropriate

Severe Infections: 15-22.5 mg in 3 doses (daily adult dose, 15 mg/kg; maximum, 1.5 g)

Comment: 30 mg/kg/d in 3 doses is recommended by some consultants

Notes: Dosages for the aminoglycosides may differ from those recommended by the manufacturers (see package insert).

(American Academy of Pediatrics: Report of the committee on Infectious Diseases. Red Book 2000, pp.651-653, 662)

<u>Amikacin</u>

Suggested Dosage Schedules for Antibiotics Used in Newborns
Route: IV, IM
Dosage (mg/kg) and interval of administration:

<u>Weight <1200 g</u>
Age 0-4 WK: 7.5 q12h

<u>Weight 1200-2000 g</u>
Age 0-7 Days: 7.5 q12h
Age >7 Days: 7.5 q8h

<u>Weight >2000 g</u>
Age 0-7 Days: 10 q12h
Age >7 Days: 10 q8h

Note: Appropriate dosage schedule should be based on serum concentrations measurements.

(Remington: Infectious Diseases of the Fetus and Newborn Infant 2001, p.1454)

<u>Amikacin</u>

Route: IM, IV
Dosage (mg/kg/dose) by Gestational age plus weeks of life:

≤26 Wks: 7.5 q24h
27-34 Wks: 7.5 q18h
35-42 Wks: 10 q12h
≥43 Wks: 10 q8h

Comment: Desired serum concentrations: 20-30 µg/ml (peak), <10 µg/ml (trough)

(Nelson: Pocket Book of Pediatric Antimicrobial Therapy 2000-2001 p.17)

Amikacin Sulfate (Amikin)

Classification: Aminoglycoside.

Action and spectrum:

Primarily bactericidal against Gram-negative organisms by inhibiting protein synthesis. Active against Gram-negative bacteria, including most *Pseudomonas* and *Serratia* spp. No activity against anaerobic organisms.

Route: IM or IV (infuse over 30 min).

Dosage: Dosage should be monitored and adjusted by use of pharmacokinetics. Initial empiric dosing based on body weight:

<1.2 kg and 0-4 weeks postnatal age:
- 7.5 mg/kg/dose q18-24h

1.2-2 kg:
- 0-7 Days: 7.5 mg/kg/dose q12-18h
- >7 Days: 7.5 mg/kg/dose q8-12h

>2 kg:
- 0-7 Days: 10 mg/kg/dose q12h
- >7 Days: 10 mg/kg/dose q8h

Elimination: Renal (glomerular filtration); half-life is 4-8 h; volume of distribution is 0.6 L/kg.

Comments: Lowest overall resistance of all the aminoglycosides and thus should be reserved for infections with organisms resistant to other aminoglycosides. Adjust dosage according to serum peak and trough levels. Draw serum levels at about the fourth maintenance dose (draw a serum trough sample 30 min to just before the dose and a serum peak sample 30 min after infusion is complete). Therapeutic peak level is 25-35 mcg/mL, and trough level is 10 mcg/mL. Nephrotoxicity is associated with serum trough concentrations >10 mcg/mL; ototoxicity, with serum peak concentrations >35-40 mcg/mL (more cochlear damage than vestibular).

(Gomella: Neonatology 1999, p.552)

Amikacin

Usual Dosage: I.M., I.V., (dosage should be based on an estimate of ideal body weight except in neonates; neonatal dosage should be based on actual weight unless the patient has hydrocephalus or hydrops fetalis):

Neonates:

0-4 weeks, <1200 g: 7.5 mg/kg/dose every 18 hours

Postnatal age ≤7 days:
- 1200-2000 g: 7.5 mg/kg/dose every 12 hours
- >2000 g: 7.5-10 mg/kg/dose every 12 hours

Postnatal age >7 days:
- 1200-2000 g: 7.5-10 mg/kg/dose every 8-12 hours
- >2000 g: 10 mg/kg/dose every 8 hours

Infants and Children: 15-22.5 mg/kg/day divided every 8 hours. Treatment for nontuberculous mycobacterial infection: 15-30 mg/kg/day divided every 12-24 hours as part of a multiple drug regimen; maximum dose: 1.5 g/day

Monitoring Parameters:

Urinalysis, urine output, BUN, serum creatinine, peak and trough serum amikacin concentrations; be alert to ototoxicity

Not all infants and children who receive aminoglycosides require monitoring of serum aminoglycoside concentrations. Indications for use of aminoglycoside serum concentration monitoring include:

- treatment course >5 days
- patients with decreased or changing renal function
- patient with poor therapeutic response
- infants <3 months of age
- atypical body constituency (obesity, expanded extracellular fluid volume)
- clinical need for higher doses or shorter intervals (eg, cystic fibrosis, burns, endocarditis, meningitis, critically ill patients, relatively resistant organisms)
- patients on hemodialysis or chronic ambulatory peritoneal dialysis
- signs of nephrotoxicity or ototoxicity
- concomitant use of other nephrotoxic agents

Reference Range:

Peak: 20-30 µg/mL
Trough: <10 µg/mL

Nursing Implications:

Aminoglycoside levels measured from blood taken from Silastic central catheters can sometimes give falsely elevated readings; peak serum levels should be drawn 30 minutes after the end of a 30-minute infusion; trough levels are drawn within 30 minutes before the next dose; provided optimal patient hydration

(Taketomo: Pediatric dosage Handbook 1999-2000, pp.50-52)

AMINOCAPROIC ACID (Amicar)

Supplied: Syrup 250mg/ml
Injection 250mg/ml in 20ml, 96ml

Administration: IV, PO

Pharmacology: Inhibits fibrinolysis via inhibition of plasminogen activator substances and, to a lesser degree, through antiplasmin activity (1).
Injection contains benzyl alcohol which has been associated with toxicity in neonates. Toxicity appears to have resulted from administration of large amounts (100-400mg/kg/day) of benzyl alcohol in these neonates (3).

Aminocaproic Acid (Amicar)

Dose & Route: Loading dose: 100-200 mg/kg IV/PO
Maintenance: 100 mg/kg/dose Q4-6hr.
Max dose: 30 gm/24hr

Remarks: **Contraindications:** DIC, hematuria.
Dose should be reduced by 15-25% in oliguria or end stage renal disease. Hypercoagulation may be produced when given in conjunction with oral contraceptives.

May cause nausea, diarrhea, malaise, weakness, headache, decreased platelet function, and hypotension. Elevation of serum potassium may occur, especially in patients with renal impairment.

(Siberry: The Harriet Lane Handbook 2000, pp.6224-625)

Aminocaproic Acid

Indication: Patients thought to be at high risk for hemorrhagic complications on ECMO.

Amicar was administered as a 100 mg/kg IV bolus either just prior to or immediately following cannulation. It was then administered continuously at 30 mg/kg/h until decannulation. Administration was via either the patient or the ECMO circuit.

While on ECMO the activated clotting times (ACTs) were maintained between 180 and 200 seconds. In order to monitor the effect of Amicar, plasminogen activator times (PATs)[12] and D-Dimer titers were routinely measured prior to administration of Amicar, 1 hour after bolus infusion, and every third day thereafter until decannulation. Serum for Amicar levels was also obtained but due to long turnaround times, the results were not used clinically.

Amicar levels, although not utilized for patient management, varied from 39 to 433 μg/mL but in most instances were in the therapeutic range (110 to 350 μg/mL). In one patient with a renal and hepatic insufficiency, levels exceeded 1,000 μg/mL with neither patient nor circuit complications occurring.

At this dose, fibrinolysis was successfully inhibited in all patients treated with Amicar as evidenced by PATs prolonged beyond 2 hours. It is unknown whether a lower dose could achieve the same prolongation of PAT. In this study there was no evidence of progressive disseminated intravascular coagulation (DIC) even in septic patients as evidenced by stable D-Dimer titers.

We conclude: (1) Amicar is effective in decreasing the incidence of ICH and other hemorrhagic complications associated with ECMO; (2) Amicar appears to be safe and is associated with a low incidence of thrombotic complications; and (3) the use of Amicar should be considered for patients thought to be at high risk for hemorrhagic complications on ECMO.

(Wilson: Aminocaproic acid decreases in the incidence of intracranial hemorrhage and other hemorrhagic complications of ECMO. J Pediatr Surg 1993;28:536-541)

Epsilon-Aminocaproic Acid

Hemorrhagic complications are common in patients placed on extracorporeal life support (ECLS), especially in those who have additional risk factors. Several centers use epsilon-aminocaproic acid (EACA), (...A loading dose of 100 mg/kg was given, followed by a continuous infusion of 30 mg/kg/h....) in their high-risk ECLS patients in an attempt to decrease the incidence of such complications, despite the fact that no controlled trials have been performed examining the risks and benefits of its use. The authors report the case of a neonate who had fatal aortic thrombosis during EACA administration.

(Hocker: Fatal Aortic Thrombosis in a Neonate During Infusion of Epsilon-Aminocaproic Acid. J Pediatr Surg 1995;30:1490-1492)

AMINOPHYLLINE (Aminophylline, Somophyllin)

Supplied: Oral Liquid 105mg/5ml (= 90mg theophylline)
Injection 250mg and 500mg vials
(=19.7mg theophylline/ml)

Administration: IV, PO

For intermittent infusion, dilute with at least an equal volume of IV fluid (preferably D5W) and infuse over 20 to 30 minutes (2).

A rapid infusion has been associated with marked hypotension, syncope, and death (1).

Do not give continuous infusion to neonates (2).

IM injection produces intense local pain and sloughing of tissue.

Aminophylline

Dose/kg: Loading dose: 4-6 mg
Route & frequency: IV once

Dose/kg: Maintenance dose: 1-2 mg
Route & frequency: IV q8h-q12h
Give first maintenance dose 8-12 hr after the loading dose

Comments: Therapeutic levels:
Bronchospasm: 10-20 µ/mL
Neonatal apnea: 6-13 µg/mL
Signs of toxicity include irritability, GI upset and arrhythmias. When switching to theophylline, remember that aminophylline is 80% theophylline.

(Avery: Neonatology Pathophysiology and Management of the Newborn 1999, p.1551)

Theophylline (Aminophylline)

Dosage: Loading dose: 5 to 6 mg/kg by slow IV infusion

Maintenance dose: 1 to 2 mg/kg/dose every 8 to 12 hours IV or PO

Comments: Intravenous administration is as aminophylline which is 85% by weight theophylline; serum theophylline concentrations should be monitored and doses adjusted to achieve peak concentrations between 6 and 13 μg/ml for apnea or 10 to 20 μg/ml for bronchodilation; theophylline is metabolized in part to caffeine in infants, and these levels shoud be monitored as well as theophylline levels.

(Fanaroff: Neonatal-Perinatal Medicine 1997, p.1749)

<u>Aminophylline</u>

Dose & Route: IV Loading: 6 mg/kg IV over 20 min. (each 1.2 mg/kg/dose raises the serum theophylline concentration 2 mg/L)

IV Maintenance: Continuous IV drip:
Neonates: 0.2 mg/kg/hr
6wk-6mo: 0.5 mg/kg/hr
6mo-1 yr: 0.6-0.7 mg/kg/hr
The above total daily doses may also be administered IV ÷ Q4-6hr.

Neonatal Apnea:
Loading Dose: 5-6 mg/kg IV or PO
Maintenance Dose: 1-2 mg/kg/dose Q6-8hr, IV or PO

Remarks: Consider mg of theophyline available when dosing aminophylline.

Monitoring serum levels is essential especially in infants and young children. Intermittent dosing for infants and children 1-5 yr may require Q4 hr dosing regimen due to enhanced metabolism.

Side effects: restlessness, GI upset, headache, tachycardia, seizures (may occur in absence of other side effects with toxic levels).

Therapeutic level (theophyline): for asthma, 10-20 mg/L; for neonatal apnea, 6-13 mg/L.

Recommended Guidelines for obtaining levels:
IV bolus: 30 min after infusion
IV continuous: 12-24 hr after initiation of infusion
PO liquid, immediate-release tab:
  Peak: 1 hr post dose
  Trough: just before dose
PO sustained-release:
  Peak: 4 hr post dose
  Trough: just before dose
Ideally, obtain levels after steady state has been achieved (after at least one day of therapy). See Theophyline for drug interactions.

Use in breastfeeding may cause irritability in infant.

(Siberry: The Harriet Lane Handbook 2000, pp.625-626)

AMIODARONE HCL (Cordarone)

Supplied: Injection 50 mg/mL in 3 mL ampules
(has benzyl alcohol 20.2mg/ml)
Tablet 200mg

Administration: PO, IV

Comment: Each tablet contains 75 mg iodine (1), each ml of injection contains 18.7mg Iodine. Injection must be diluted before administration.

<u>Extemporaneous Compounding (Recipe)</u>

Dosage form: Oral suspension
Made from: Tablets
Concentration: 5 mg/mL
Stability: 91 d (4° C); 42 d (25° C)
Store: Refrigerate
Label: Shake well

Ingredient	Strength	Quantity
Amiodarone tablets	200 mg	3
Methylcellulose	1%	90 mL
Syrup		10 mL
Water		qs ad 120 mL

Instructions: Crush the tablets with a mortar and pestle. Add the methylcellulose/syrup mixture in small amounts. Triturate until uniform and qs with water. (11)

<u>Amiodarone</u>

Class: III Prolong repolarization

Uses: Life-threatening drug-resistant SVT (JET), AFL, VT; incessant drug-resistant SVT (WPW), IAH, ?PJRT, AET; drug of choice for congenital JET, postop JET

Dose (Level) PO: 10 mg/kg/day divided BID x 10 days, then 5 mg/kg QD; try to ↓ to <5 mg/kg or 5/7 days
IV: 1 mg/kg bolus q5min x 5, may repeat q12hr

Mode of Action: Mild local anesthetic; α-, β-, and Ca^{++} blockade; at rapid stimulation rates, depresses conduction; smooth muscle vasodilator, depresses automaticity; localized hypothyroidism in all cardiac cells

ECG/EP Changes: ↓↓HR if SSS; ↑ QRS, QT (effect at 0.53 sec);
↑ CSNRT, ↑ ERP in all cardiac tissues

Side Effects: Bradycardia, corneal microdeposits, rash, nausea, ataxia; effect – rT3>50; toxicity-rT3>90; hypotension (IV); ↑ level of dig., quinidine, procainamide; warfarin ↑ PT

(Garson: The science and practice of pediatric cardiology 1998, p.2953)

<u>Amiodarone</u>

Amiodarone is a potent agent for control of a wide spectrum of cardiac tachyarrhythmias. Amiodarone was released in the United States for intravenous therapy, and a body of literature for its safety and effectiveness in resistant arrhythmias in children has been published.

Dosing: PO: 10-15 mg/kg load. 2-5 mg/kg chronic
Warnings: Skin, liver, thyroid, pulmonary hypotension, bradycardia

Dosing: IV: 5 mg/kg load (in divided doses), 10-15 mg/kg/day infusion.
Warnings: Skin, liver, thyroid, pulmonary hypotension, bradycardia

Drug Action: It is a sodium channel blocker with voltage and frequency dependence, a noncompetitive alpha- and beta-adrenergic receptor blocker, and an inhibitor of presynaptic norepinephrine release.

Oral Administration, Kinetics, Metabolites:

Amiodarone is lipid soluble and absorbed more slowly than any other antiarrhythmic agent, a peak plasma concentration occurs 3 to 7 hours after an oral dose.

Levels of either drug can remain substantial up to 3 months after amiodarone is discontinued. Therapeutic plasma levels range from 1.0 to 2.5 µg/ml, but they correlate poorly with clinical efficacy, partly because of the actions of the metabolite and the peripheral storage of both drugs.

Although the drug is present in breast milk, its concentration there is low and should not be a contraindication to breast-feeding.

Intravenous Administration:

In a multicenter trail of intravenous amiodarone for resistant, life-threatening pediatric tachyarrhythmias, the drug showed a rapid onset of action: a clinical electrophysiologic effect often occurred during the initial bolus dose. The antiarrhythmic effect can persist for 1 to 6 hours. Amiodarone is mixed in 5% dextrose solution to prevent precipitation.

Dosing and Interactions:

An oral loading protocol of 10 to 15 mg/kg/day is often provided for 5 to 10 days. During loading this dosage is usually split in a twice-daily schedule to avoid gastrointestinal side effects. Some centers, particularly in Europe, advocate a higher dose loading for 3 to 5 days, using up to 50 mg/kg/day.

The goal of long-term oral therapy is to use the lowest possible effective daily dosage. This is generally 2 to 5 mg/kg as a once-a-day dose. Amiodarone is only available as a 200-mg tablet. Although it can be broken into halves or quarters or even given every other day, a suspension is often made at a concentration of 10 mg/ml. Anecdotal experience from a number of institutions indicates that the suspension is stable for up to 1 month.

In the largest studies of intravenous amiodarone to date in young patients, a 5-mg/kg bolus was used and divided into five 1-mg/kg aliquots. Each was given over 5 minutes. No adverse effect was seen in the first 1- to 3-mg/kg bolus, so the drug can probably be given as two 2.5-mg/kg boluses. The average successful load was 6 mg/kg. Infusions of amiodarone were administered predominantly in those with ventricular tachyarrhythmias at 10 to 15 mg/kg/day.

The most frequently cited example of amiodarone interaction is digoxin coadministration, when digoxin levels may rise 25 to 100%. Decreasing the digoxin dose by 33 to 50% is prudent. Coadministration of amiodarone with most other antiarrhythmic agents, particularly procainamide, flecainide, quinidine, and phenytoin, also causes increased levels of theses drugs.

Side Effects: The most commonly noted non-cardiac side effects with oral amiodarone administration in children are skin photosensitivity, chemical hepatitis, hypothyroidism, hyperthyroidism, and corneal microdeposits. All patients should be advised to apply high-grade sunblock. Liver and thyroid function tests should be performed periodically. Amiodarone has a high iodine content, likely responsible for its effects on thyroid function. Therapy with thyroid replacement hormones, if necessary, does not seem to interfere with antiarrhythmic effect.

Cardiac side effects include sinus bradycardia, AV node blocks, and proarrhythmia. Torsades de pointer occurs rarely (<1%). In adult patients on long-term oral amiodarone, serious and irreversible pulmonary fibrosis can occur. This phenomenon has not been reported in the pediatric population, possibly because patients have not been on the drug long enough or in high enough maintenance doses for pulmonary abnormalities to appear.

Side effects with intravenous therapy are predominantly related to hypotension. If intravenous amiodarone is given to a patient receiving high inspired oxygen concentrations, an adult respiratory distress syndrome may occur.

(Gillette: Clinical Pediatric Arrhythmias 1999, pp.231-248)

<u>Amiodarone</u>

Uses: VT, JET, resistant recurrent PSVT, AFI, very rapid AET

Dosing: 5 mg/kg/30 min up to 20 mg/kg as load: 10-15 mg/kg/24 hr as continuous infusion.

Acute Side Effects:
Hypotension; sinus bradycardia or Atrioventricular (AV) block if intrinsic disease

Other Considerations:
Increases level of digoxin, procainamide, quinidine

AET, atrial ectopic tachycardia; AFl, atrial flutter; JET, junctional ectopic tachycardia; PSVT, paroxysmal supraventricular tachycardia; VT, ventricular tachycardia.

(Gillette: Clinical Pediatric Arrhythmias 1999, p.152)

<u>Amiodarone HCl</u>

Route & Dose: Children PO:
<1 yr: 600-800 mg/1.73 m^2/24 hr ÷ Q12-24 hr then reduce to 200-400 mg/1.73 m^2/24 hr

≥1 yr: 10-15 mg/mg/24 hr ÷ Q12-24 hr x 4-14 days and/or until adequate control achieved then reduce to 5 mg/mg/24 hr ÷ Q12-24 hr if effective

Children IV (limited data):
5 mg/kg over 30 minutes followed by a continuous infusion starting at 5 micrograms (mcg)/kg/min; infusion may be increased up to a maximum of 10 mcg/kg/min or 20 mg/kg/24 hr

Comments: **Contraindicated** in severe sinus node dysfunction, marked sinus bradycardia, 2nd and 3rd degree AV block.

Long elimination half-life (40-55 days). Major metabolite is active.

Increases cyclosporin, digoxin, phenytoin, tacrolimus, warfarin, calcium channel blockers, theophylline, and quinidine levels.

Proposed therapeutic level with chronic oral use: 1-2.5 mg/L.

Asymptomatic corneal microdeposits should appear in all patients. Alters liver enzymes, thyroid function. Pulmonary fibrosis reported in adults. May cause worsening of preexisting arrhythmias with bradycardia and AV block. May also cause anorexia, nausea, vomiting, dizziness, paresthesias, ataxia, tremor, and hypo- or hyper-thyroidism.

Intravenous continuous infusion concentration for peripheral administration **should not exceed** 2 mg/ml and **must be** diluted with D5W. The preservative-free intravenous product is available as an orphan drug from Academic Pharmaceuticals. Inc. at (847) 735-1170.

(Siberry: The Harriet Lane Handbook 2000, pp.625-627)

AMMONIUM CHLORIDE

Supplied: Injection 26.75% (5mEq/ml) in 20ml
Administration: IV INFUSION
<u>MUST BE DILUTED BEFORE USE</u>. Administer by slow IV infusion. Do not exceed a concentration of 1% to 2%

ammonium chloride in NS (1). In the absence of edema or hyponatremia dosage may be calculated on the basis of chloride deficit by the following formula: mEq of Chloride ion (as ammonium chloride) = chloride deficit (in mEq/L) x 0.2 x body weight (in kg). Approximately one-half of the calculated volume of ammonium chloride should be administered; the carbon dioxide combining power should be rechecked and the necessity for further treatment determined. Calculated osmolarity of 10 mOsm/ml (3). IV solutions of ammonium chloride should be administered very slowly to avoid ammonia toxicity.

Ammonium chloride

Dose/kg: Metabolic alkalosis: 1-2 mEq
Route & frequency: PO, IV x 1

Dose/kg: Urinary acidification: 0.25-0.37 mEq
Route & frequency: PO, IV q6h

Comments: GI irritation. Hyperventilation. Pain at site of injection if infused too rapidly. Maximum concentration for injection = 0.4 mEq/mL. Infusion rate should not exceed 1 mEq/kg/h

(Avery: Neonatology Pathophysiology and Management of the Newborn 1999, p.1551)

Ammonium chloride

Dosage: 1 mEq/kg/hr IV up to 50 mg/kg/hr
75 mg/kg/dose PO divided every 6 hours

Comments: Dilute IV solution to <0.4 mEq/ml
May cause acidosis; titrate to desired serum Cl^- level

(Fanaroff: Neonatal-Perinatal Medicine 1997, p.1751)

Ammonium chloride

Urinary Acidification:
Dose and Route: Child: 75 mg/kg/24hr÷Q6h PO or IV.
Max dose: 6 g/24hr.
Injection: Dilute to concentration not >0.4mEq/ml. Infusion **not to exceed** 50 mg/kg/hr or 1 mEq/kg/hr.

Remarks: **Contraindicated** in hepatic or renal insufficiency; use with **caution** in infants.

May produce acidosis, hyperammonemia, and GI irritation. Monitor serum chloride level, acid/base status and ammonia.

Administer oral doses after meals.

(Siberry: The Harriet Lane Handbook 2000, p.629)

Ammonium chloride

Route: IV, PO

Neonatal Dose: None Established

Pediatric Dose: IV: 4 mEq/kg/dose
PO: 75 mg/kg/24h q6h with meals

Discussion: Avoid use with renal or hepatic impairment; dilute IV solutions to 2% solutions and give <2 mL/min. Use caution in infants because it may cause GI irritation.

(Rudolph: Rudolph's Pediatrics 1996, p.2171)

AMODIAQUINE

Amodiaquine

Disease/Organism: Malaria

CDC Malaria Hotline (24 hrs a day) 1-770-488-7788

Amodiaquine

Prophylaxis:

For areas without chloroquine-resistant P. falciparum:

Chloroquine 5 mg base/kg (max 300 mg) PO once weekly, beginning 1 week before arrival in malarial zone and continuing for 4 weeks after last exposure (drugs available in liquid form outside the USA); PLUS (optional) beginning with final 2 weeks of chloroquine Rx, primaquine 0.3mg base/kg PO daily x 14 days after departure from endemic area for individuals heavily exposed to mosquitoes

For areas where chloroquine-resistant P. falciparum exists:

Mefloquine for children >45 kg 250 mg PO once weekly starting 1 wk before travel and for 4 wks after leaving area; for children 5-9 kg, 1/8 tab; 10-19 kg, ¼ tab; 20-30 kg. ½ tab; 31-45 kg, ¾ tab OR doxycycline (patient > 7 yrs) 2 mg/kg (max 100 mg) PO daily

Treatment of disease:

Plasmodium vivax, P. ovale P malariae chloroquine-susceptible P. falciparum:

Chloroquine 10 mg base/kg (max 600 mg) PO stat, then 5 mg base/kg at 6 hrs, 24 hrs and 48 hrs after initial dose (alternative: at 6, 12, 24, and 36 hrs); For parenteral therapy, quinidine 10 mg/kg (max 600 mg) IV (1 hr infusion) followed by continuous infusion of 0.02 mg/kg/min until oral therapy can be given (3 days maximum); It's advisable to monitor patients receiving quinidine in an ICU setting. Prevention of relapse (P. vivax, P, ovale): primaquine 0.3 mg base/kg/day x 14 d

P. falciparum chloroquine-resistant

Quinine 25 mg/kg/day (max 2 g/day) PO div q8h x 3 days (or longer) AND doxycycline (patients > 7 yrs) 2 mg/kg daily x 7 OR Fansidar (pyrimethamine-sulfadoxine): < 1 yr, ¼ tab; 1-3 yrs, ½ tab; 4-8 yrs, 1 tab; 9-14 yrs, 2 tab; > 14 yrs, 3 tabs as a single dose on last day of quinine; NOTE: Several alternative regimens have been reported for Fansidar-resistant infections: Check with the CDC; For parenteral therapy, quinidine, as above; NOTE; Corticosteroids are contraindicated in cerebral malaria;

Iron chelation therapy may be beneficial in cerebral malaria.

(Nelson: Pocket Book of Pediatric Antimicrobial Therapy 2000-2001, pp.64-65)

AMOXICILLIN (Amoxil, Larotids, Trimox)

Supplied: Drops, powder for 50mg/ml in 15ml and 30ml
Suspension, powder for 125mg/5ml; 250mg/5ml in 80ml,100ml, 150ml, 200ml

Administration: PO
Following reconstitution, the suspensions should preferably be refrigerated, but refrigeration is not necessary. The suspensions are stable for 14 days at room temperature (3). Amoxicillin has the advantage of more complete absorption than ampicillin (1). May add required amount of suspension to formula, milk, fruit juice; take immediately and consume in entirety (1).

Amoxicillin

Antibacterial Drugs for Pediatric Patients Beyond the Newborn Period: Dosage per kg/d

Route: PO

Mild to Moderate Infections: 25-50 mg/kg/d in 3 doses

Severe Infections: Inappropriate

Comments: Larger dosage (80-90 mg in 2 doses) for otitis media caused by penicillin-resistant pneumococci

Note: In patients with history of allergy to penicillin or one of its many congeners, alternative drugs are recommended. In some circumstances, a cephalosporin or other β-lactam class drug may be acceptable. However, these drugs should not be used in patients with an immediate hypersensitivity (anaphylaxis) to penicillin because approximately 5% to 15% of penicillin-allergic patients will also be allergic to the cephalosporins.

(American Academy of Pediatrics: Report of the Committee on Infectious Diseases 2000, pp.658,662)

Amoxicillin

Dose/kg: 7-13 mg

Route and frequency: PO q8h

Comments: See comments for Ampicillin

(Avery: Neonatology Pathophysiology and Management of the Newborn 1999, p.1551)

AMOXICILLIN-CLAVULANATE POTASSIUM (Augmentin)

AMOX = Amoxicillin

CLA= Potassium Clavulanate

Supplied: Suspension, powder for "125"
(125mg AMOX & 31.25mg CLA/5ml)

Suspension, powder for "250"
(250mg AMOX & 62.5 mg CLA/5ml)
Both supplied in 75ml, 100ml, 150ml
Suspension "200" (200mg amoxicillin + 28.5mg CLA/5ml).
Suspension "400" (400mg amoxicillin + CLA 57mg/5ml
Both supplied as 50ml, 75ml, 100ml

Administration: PO

Each 31.25mg of potassium clavulanate has 0.16 mEq of K. Refrigerate reconstituted oral suspensions and discard after 10 days (3). Shake well before using.

The every 12-hour regimen is associated with significantly less diarrhea, however the 200mg and 400mg formulations contain aspartame and should not be used by phenyl ketonurics. (1)

<u>Amoxicillin-Clavulanate</u> (7:1 formulation)

Antibacterial Drugs for Pediatric Patients Beyond the Newborn Period
Dosage per kg/d

Route: PO

Mild to moderate infections: 45 mg of amoxicillin in 2-3 doses

Severe Infections: Inappropriate

Comments: A 14:1 amoxicillin:clavulanate formulation awaiting Food and Drug Administration approval
Dosage: 90 mg in 2 doses for multidrug-resistant pneumococcal otitis media

Note: In patients with history of allergy to penicillin or one of its many congeners, alternative drugs are recommended. In some circumstances, a cephalosporin or other β-lactam class drug may be acceptable. However, these drugs should not be used in patients with an immediate hypersensitivity (anaphylaxis) to penicillin because approximately 5% to 15% of penicillin-allergic patients will also be allergic to the cephalosporins

(American Academy of Pediatrics: Report of the Committee on Infectious Diseases. Red Book 2000, pp.658, 662)

<u>Amoxicillin</u>

Condition: Otitis Media, Newborn
Therapy: Few controlled treatment trials in newborns; Suggest using initial therapy as for older infants (see Nelson, Otitis Media Acute, p.24); If no response, obtain middle ear fluid for culture
Comment: Augmentin may have advantage because of activity vs. coliforms and staphylococcus (10-20% of cases)

Condition: Otitis Media, Coliform Bacteria
Therapy: Augmentin 30-40 mg/kg/day PO divided q8-12h x 10 days
Comment: Cefotaxime if parenteral therapy needed

Condition: Otitis Media, Haemophilus

Therapy: Augmentin 30-40 mg/kg/day PO div q8-12 OR Amoxicillin 30-40 mg/kg/day PO div q8-12h if susceptible

(Nelson: Pocket Book of Pediatric Antimicrobial Therapy 2000-2001, p.11)

Amoxicillin - Clavulanic Acid (Augmentin)

Dosage based on amoxicillin component.

Dose & Route: Children <3 months: 30 mg/kg/24hr ÷ BID PO (recommended dosage form is 125 mg/5 ml suspension)

Children 3 months and older:

TID dosing (see remarks):

20-40 mg/kg/24 hr ÷ TID PO

BID dosing (see remarks):

25-45 mg/kg/24 hr ÷ BID PO

Remarks: Clavulanic acid extends the activity of amoxicillin to include beta-lactamase producing strains of H. influenzae. M. catarrhalis, N. gonorrhoeae, some S. aureus. **Adjust dose in renal failure**

(Siberry: The Harriet Lane Handbook 2000, pp.630-631)

AMPHOTERICIN B (Fungizone)

Supplied: Topical Lotion, Cream, Ointment 3%
Injection, lyophilized cake 50mg/vial

Administration: IV, Topical

IV ADMINISTRATION:
Dilute the contents of the vial with SWFI only. Do not reconstitute with saline solutions. For initial concentration of 5mg/ml, rapidly inject 10ml SWFI directly into the lyophilized cake. Shake the vial immediately until the colloidal solution is clear. ADMINISTER by slow IV infusion over 6 hours at a concentration of 0.1mg/ml in D5W (1).

Reconstituted preparations should be protected from light and are stable for 24 hours at room temperature, or 1 week when refrigerated (3). Although infusion solutions of Amphotericin B are light-sensitive, loss of drug activity is reported to be negligible when solutions are exposed to light for 8 hours. Therefore, it is probably not necessary to cover infusion containers under normal administration conditions in the hospital (1).

The recommended final concentration for administration is 0.1mg/ml. The usual duration of infusion is 2 to 6 hours (6).

Do not mix with saline or electrolytes. The use of any solution other than those recommended or the presence of a bacteriostatic agent (eg; benzyl alcohol) may cause precipitation of amphotericin B (2). If administered through an existing IV line, flush with D5W prior to and following infusion; Otherwise administer via a separate line (1).

Amphotericin B

Amphotericin B is the most widely used antimicrobial agent for fungal infections, but alternative or adjunctive therapy has been employed successfully for specific fungi. Amphotericin B is a polyene antibiotic that reacts with sterols in cell membranes and results in cellular damage and lysis. The drug is effective topically for some cutaneous, mucocutaneous, and gastrointestinal fungal infections, but it is not absorbed from the gastrointestinal tract in quantities sufficient to give adequate serum levels in patients with disseminated or deep tissue fungal infections. In such instances, amphotericin B must be given intravenously. Serum levels in adults average 1.5 μg/ml 1 hour after intravenous injection of 0.6 t0 1 mg/kg; the half-life is approximately 24 hours, but levels of 0.14 μg/ml have been detected in serum for at least 3 weeks. Only one tenth to one twentieth of the serum level is distributed into CSF, and in some cases of fungal meningitis, it may be necessary to administer amphotericin B intrathecally.

The toxicity of amphotericin B in humans is significant, and adults frequently experience nausea, vomiting, headache, chills, and fever during infusion of the antibiotic. Patients may become tolerant to these side effects, but pretreatment with salicylates and phenothiazines is helpful in deducing these symptoms, as is administration of hydrocortisone hemisuccinate before or with the infusion (in adults, the usual dose of hydrocortisone semisuccinate is 25 to 50 mg). Convulsions or cardiac arrhythmias may occur during infusion, especially if the drug is administered too rapidly or if the concentration of amphotericin B exceeds 0.1 mg/ml of diluent. In adults and older children, phlebitis at the site of infusion is common but may be reduced by careful technique and frequent changing of intravenous site. Anemia occurs frequently and may require blood transfusions. Hypokalemia can be corrected with potassium replacement and must be carefully watched for. Nephrotoxicity is the most important kind of toxicity associated with administration of amphotericin B. Renal damage appears to correlate with total dose of amphotericin B and results from drug-induced renal vasoconstriction as well as form direct action of amphotericin B on renal tubules. There may be a rise in serum creatinine and blood urea nitrogen levels and a decrease in creatinine clearance, as well as cylindruria, renal tubular acidosis, tubular necrosis, and nephrocalcinosis.

In all but one infant, the toxicity was reversible when the drugs were discontinued. In addition, he found no difference in toxicity when the maximum daily dose of amphotericin B was 0.5 or 1 mg/kg. In contrast, Baley and co-workers found significant nephrotoxicity in very low birth weight infants when given amphotericin B at a dose of 1 mg/kg per day versus 0.5 mg/kg per day.

Minimal inhibitory concentrations of amphotericin B for fungi causing disease in infants and recommended total dose of amphotericin B are presented in Table. Others have indicated that lower doses of amphotericin B may be effective. Of importance are reports of resistance of some species of *Candida* to amphotericin B, necessitating species identification of *Candida* isolates as well as determination of minimal inhibitory concentrations to antifungal agents.

The initial intravenous dose of amphotericin B in adults usually does not exceed 0.1 mg/kg and is given in 5% dextrose and water in a concentration no greater than 0.1 mg/ml. Amphotericin B should not be diluted in normal saline because a precipitate forms. After the initial dose, the amount of amphotericin B may be increased gradually until the maximum daily dose of 1 to 1.5 mg/kg is achieved. The maximum daily dose and duration of therapy may depend on the focus and extent of fungal disease as well as on the minimal inhibitory concentration of the organism with amphotericin B. The speed at which maximum dosage can be reached is influenced by the side effects experienced by the infant. At that time, the antibiotic may be given daily or on alternate days. Many authors have suggested following serum levels of amphotericin B as a guide to therapy, although, because of the predictable pharmacokinetics of amphotericin B, obtaining levels may not be necessary. Rate of administration varies with tolerance to side effects, but the daily dose should be given slowly over at least 4 to 6 hours.

Intrathecal administration of amphotericin B may be necessary in patients with fungal meningitis, particularly if the fungus can be demonstrated in CSF after the maximum daily dose in intravenous therapy has been reached. The drug may be given into the lumbar sac, into the cisterna magna, or into the lateral ventricle either directly or by way of an indwelling intraventricular reservoir. If the later is to be employed alone, normal CSF circulation should be documented to ensure that amphotericin B will be distributed throughout the subarachnoid space. There are few data regarding the ideal intrathecal dose of amphotericin B in children with fungal meningitis. Klein and co-workers instilled 0.05 mg every third day for two administrations in an infant with *Candida* meningitis. The initial intrathecal dose in infants should be 0.01 mg, gradually increased over a period of 5 to 7 days to 0.1 mg given every other day or every third day. Amphotericin B for intrathecal administration should be diluted in sterile distilled water containing no bacteriostatic agents.

Concentration should not exceed 0.25 mg/ml diluent, and further dilution with CSF is recommended. Some infants with *Candida* meningitis have recovered with intravenous amphotericin B therapy alone. Complications of intrathecal amphotericin B administration include CSF pleocytosis (arachnoiditis), transient radiculitis, and sensory loss. Adults often complain of headache, and convulsions occur occasionally.

Administration of amphotericin B in other sites in infants has not been critically evaluated. Klein and co-workers employed intra-articular amphotericin B in the child they reported with septic arthritis caused by *Candida.* The dose used was 0.5 mg on a single occasion. Hill and colleagues reported instillation of 0.4 ml of a 0.01% solution of amphotericin B into the anterior chamber of the eye in an infant with *Candida* endophthalmitis.

TABLE
Minimal Inhibitory concentrations (MIC) of Amphotericin B and Recommended Total dose

FUNGUS	MIC (μ/ml)	TOTAL DOSE (mg/kg)
Candida species	0.09-3.12	25-30
Cryptococcus neoformans	0.2-1.0	15-30
Coccidioides immitis	0.78	70
Aspergillus species	1.9 - >4.0	15-45
Phycomycetes	3.0-6.0	Unknown

(Remington: Infectious Diseases of the Fetus and Newborn Infant 2001, pp.835-836)

Amphotericin B

Recommended Doses of Parenteral and Oral Antifungal Drugs (see Antifungal Drugs for Systemic Fungal Infections, for detailed information)

Route: IV

Dose (per day) 0.25-0.5 mg/kg initially, increase as tolerated to 0.5-1.5 mg/kg; infuse as single dose over 2-3 h; 0.5-1.0 mg/kg weekly for suppressive therapy in HIV-infected patients with cryptococcosis or histoplasmosis

Adverse Reactions:

Fever, chills, gastrointestinal tract symptoms, headache, hypotension, renal dysfunction, hypokalemia, anemia, cardiac arrhythmias, neurotoxicity, anaphylaxis

Route: IT

Dose (per day) 0.025 mg, increase to 0.5 mg twice a week

Adverse Reactions:

Headache, gastrointestinal tract symptoms, arachnoiditis/radiculitis

(American Academy of Pediatrics: Report of the committee on infectious Diseases. Red Book 2000, p.670)

Amphotericin B (Fungizone)

Classification: Antifungal agent

Action and spectrum:

Acts by binding to sterols and disrupting the fungal cell membranes. Broad spectrum of activity against Candida spp and other fungi.

Route: IV

Dosages: Initially: Test dose of 0.25 mg/kg IV over 4 h.. Use 0.1 mg/mL concentration in D_5W. Incompatible with NaCl.

Increment: Increase the daily dosage by 0.25 mg/kg/day qd-qod as tolerated to a maximum daily or alternate-day dosage of 0.75-1.5 mg/kg. A total dosage of 30-35 mg/kg should be given over 6 weeks or longer, although a lower dose may suffice. In general, infusions should be given over 2-6 h, although infusion over 1-2 h may be used if tolerated.

Intrathecal or intraventricular: Reconstitute with sterile water at 0.25 mg/mL; dilute with CSF fluid and reinfuse. Usual dose: 0.25-0.5 mg.

Liposomal amphotericin B: 5 mg/kg IV

Elimination and metabolism: Slow renal excretion.

Adverse effects: Few adverse effects in neonates as opposed to adults. May cause fever, chills, vomiting, thrombophlebitis at injection sites, renal tubular acidosis, renal failure, hypomagnesemia, hypokalemia, bone marrow suppression with reversible decline in hematocrit, hypotension, hypertension, wheezing, and hypoxemia. Fewer adverse effects with liposomal amphotericin B.

Comments: Irritation at infusion site may be reduced by addition of heparin (1 unit/mL). Protect solution from light. Monitor serum potassium, magnesium, urea nitrogen, creatinine, alkaline phosphatase, and AST (SGOT) qd-qod until the dosage is stabilized, then every week. Monitor complete blood cell count (CBC) every week. Discontinue if blood urea nitrogen (BUN) is >40 mg/dL, serum creatinine >3 mg/dL or liver function tests are abnormal.

(Gomella: Neonatology 1999, pp.552-553)

Amphotericin B

Suggested Dosage of Antifungal Agents for Infants with systemic or Severe Local Fungal Infection

Dosage (mg/kg per day): 0.5-1

(Remington: Infectious diseases of the Fetus and Newborn Infant, 2001, p.838)

Amphotericin B

Candidiasis, Disseminated infection

Therapy: Amphotericin B 1.0 mg/kg IV daily as 3-4 hour infusion in 5% dextrose solution (no saline); Total dosage 30-35 mg/kg given over period of 6 wks or longer; For patients with renal failure and those not tolerating or failing to

	respond, Abelcet 5 mg/kg IV, or AmBisome 3-5 mg/kg or Amphotec 3-5 mg/kg daily can be used; Itraconazole may be considered for indolent, non-CNS disease.
Comments:	Treat for tissue invasion, not colonization; Monitor K, Mg, HCO_3, Hgb, and renal function; Sodium loading may help azotemia; Total dosage and duration of therapy individualized.
Therapy:	Amphotericin B (as above) but daily dosage 0.5-0.75 mg/kg OR amphotericin B PLUS flucytosine 100 mg/kg/day PO div q6h or Albelcet AmBisome or Amphotec (as above); Fluconazole 6-12 mg/kg IV or PO daily for noncompromized host (some strains resistant to fluconazole).
Comments:	Hematologic toxicity and diarrhea with flucytosine; Keep serum concentration <100 μg/ml; Replace IV catheter in catheter-associated candidemia.

Candidiasis, urinary infection.

Therapy:	Fluconazole 3-6 mg/kg once daily OR flucytosine 50 mg/kg/day div q6h; Amphotericin B (50 μg/ml) bladder irrigation if catheter in place.
Comments:	Stopping antibiotic or removing Foley catheter sometimes leads to spontaneous cure in the normal host.

(Nelson: Pocket Book of Pediatric Antimicrobial Therapy 2000-2001, pp.56-57)

Amphotericin B

Amphotericin B deoxycholate or conventional amphotericin B is the drug of choice for most progressive, potentially life-threatening fungal infections. Amphotericin B is fungicidal against a broad array of fungal species excluding *Fusarium* and *Pseudallescheria boydii*. It may cause adverse reactions, particularly renal toxic effects, that limit its use in certain patients.

Amphotericin B is administered in 5% dextrose in water at a concentration of 0.1 mg/mL for delivery through a central or peripheral venous catheter. Amphotericin B is administered intravenously in a single daily dose of 0.5-1.5 mg/kg per day. Prolonged infusions were once recommended to avoid toxicity, but in adults and older children an infusion time of 1 hour is often well tolerated and theoretically increases blood-to-tissue gradient, thereby improving drug delivery. After completing 1 week of daily therapy, adequate serum concentrations of the drug usually can be maintained by administering double the daily dose (maximum, 1.5 mg/kg) on alternate days. The duration of therapy depends on the type and extent of the specific fungal infection.

Amphotericin B is eliminated by a renal mechanism for weeks after therapy is discontinued. No adjustment in dose is required for neonates or for children with impaired renal function because he serum concentration is not significantly increased in these patients. Hemodialysis and peritoneal dialysis do not significantly lower serum concentrations of the drug.

Infusion-related reactions to amphotericin B include fever, chills, and sometimes nausea, vomiting, headache, generalized malaise, hypotension, and arrhythmias. Onset usually is within 1 to 3 hours after starting the infusion; duration typically is less than an hour. Hypotension and arrhythmias are idiosyncratic reactions that are unlikely to occur if not observed after the initial dose, but also occur in association with rapid infusion. Multiple regimens have been used to attempt to prevent infusion-related reactions, but few have been studied in controlled clinical trials. Pretreatment with acetaminophen, alone or combined with diphenhydramine, may alleviate febrile reactions, although these reactions appear to be less common in children than in adults. Hydrocortisone (25 to 50 mg in adults and older children) also can be added to the infusion to deduce febrile and other systemic reactions. Tolerance to the febrile reactions develops with time, allowing tapering and eventual discontinuation of the hydrocortisone and often antipyretics.

(American Academy of Pediatrics: Report of the Committee on Infectious Diseases. Red Book 2000, pp.668-669)

Amphotericin B

Stability: Reconstitute only with sterile water without preservatives, not bacteriostatic water, benzyl alcohol, sodium chloride, or other electrolyte solutions may cause precipitation; can be diluted in D_5W, $D_{10}W$, up to $D_{20}W$; for I.V. infusion, an in-line filter (>1 micron mean pore diameter) may be used; irrigating solutions should be diluted in sterile water; short-term exposure (<24 hours) to light during I.V. infusion does **not** appreciably affect potency.

Usual Dosage Medication errors, including deaths, have resulted from confusion between lipid-based forms of amphotericin (Abelcet, Amphotec, AmBisome) and conventional amphotericin B for injection; conventional amphotericin B for injection doses should not exceed 1.5 mg/kg/day

Neonates, Infants, and Children:
I.V.: Test dose: 0.1 mg/kg/dose to a maximum of 1 mg; infuse over 20-60 minutes; an alternative method to the 0.1 mg/kg test dose is to initiate therapy with 0.25 mg/kg amphotericin administered over 6 hours; frequent observation of the patient and assessment of vital signs during the first several hours of the infusion is recommended.

Initial therapeutic dose: If the 0.1 mg/kg test dose is tolerated without the occurrence of serious adverse effects, a therapeutic dose of 0.4 mg/kg can be given the same day as the test dose.

The daily dose can then be gradually increased, usually in 0.25 mg/kg increments on each subsequent day until the desired daily dose is reached; in critically ill patients, more rapid dosage acceleration (up to 0.5 mg/kg increments on each subsequent day) may be warranted.

Maintenance dose: 0.25-1 mg/kg/day given once daily; infuse over 2-6 hours; rapidly progressing disease may require short-term use of doses to 1.5 mg/kg/day; once therapy has been established, amphotericin B can be administered on an every-other day basis at 1-1.5 mg/kg/dose.

Intrathecal, intraventricular, or intracisternal (preferably into the lateral ventricles through a cisternal Ommaya reservoir): 25-100 mcg every 48-72 hours; increase to 500 mcg as tolerated

Dosing adjustment in renal Impairment:

Dosage adjustments are not necessary with pre-existing renal impairment; if decreased renal function is due to amphotericin, the daily dose can be decreased by 50% of the dose can be given every other day. Therapy may be held until serum creatinine concentrations begin to decline.

Administration: Oral: Swish medication around in the mouth as long as possible before swallowing or use a nonabsorbent swab to apply the medication on the oral lesions; administer between meals to permit prolonged contact with oral lesions

Parenteral: Amphotericin is administered by I.V. infusion over 2-6 hours at a final concentration not to exceed 0.1 mg/mL through a peripheral venous catheter; in patients unable to tolerate a large fluid volume, amphotericin B at a final concentration not to exceed 0.5 mg/mL in D_5W or $D_{10}W$ may be administered through a central venous catheter

Monitoring Parameters:

BUN and serum creatinine levels should be determined every other day while therapy is increased and at least weekly thereafter; serum potassium and magnesium should be monitored closely; monitor electrolytes, liver function, hematocrit, CBC regularly; monitor input and output; monitor for signs of hypokalemia (muscle weakness, cramping, drowsiness, EKG changes, etc); blood pressure, temperature, pulse, respiration

Patient Information:

Amphotericin cream may slightly discolor skin and stain clothing; personal hygiene is very important to hep reduce the spread and recurrence of lesions; avoid covering topical applications with occlusive bandages; most skin lesions require 1-3 weeks of therapy

Nursing Implications:

Cardiovascular collapse has been reported after rapid amphotericin injection; may premedicate patients who experience mild adverse reactions with acetaminophen and diphenhydramine 30 minutes prior to the amphotericin infusion. Meperidine and ibuprofen may help to reduce fevers and chills.

(Taketomo: Pediatric Dosage Handbook 1999-2000, pp.65-68)

AMPHOTERICIN B CHOLESTERYL SULFATE COMPLEX

(Amphotec)

Supplied: Powder for injection 50 mg (as cholesteryl) in 20 ml single use vials, 100 mg (as cholesteryl), in 50 ml single use.

Administration: A test dose is advisable (e.g., 10 ml of final preparation containing 1.6 to 8.3 mg infused over 15-30 minutes). The recommended dose is 3-4 mg/kg/day prepared as a 0.6 mg/ml (range 0.16 to 0.83 mg/ml infusion delivered at a rate of 1 mg/kg/hr. Do not filter or use an in-line filter. Reconstitute with sterile water for injection. Do not use saline or dextrose for reconstitution. After further dilution with 5% Dextrose for injection, refrigerate (2°-8°C, 36°-46°F), and use within 24 hours. (1)

Amphotericin B cholesteryl sulfate complex (ABCD)

Recommended Doses of Parenteral and Oral Antifungal Drugs

Route: IV

Dose (per day): 3-6 mg/kg infused at a rate of 1 mg/kg per hour

Adverse Reactions:

Fever, Chills, other reactions associated with amphotericin B, but less nephrotoxicity; hepatotoxicity

Note: Experience with drug in children is limited.
Limited or no information about use in newborn infants is available.

(American Academy of Pediatrics: Report of the Committee on Infectious Diseases. Red Book 2000, pp.670-671)

Amphotericin B Cholesteryl Sulfate

Route & Dose: IV: Start at 3-4 mg/kg/24 hr QD, dose may be increased to 6 mg/kg/24 hr if necessary.

Mix with D_5W to concentration of 0.16-0.83 mg/ml.

Test dose: 10 ml of the diluted solution administered over 15-30 minutes has been recommended.

Infusion Rate: Give first dose at 1 mg/kg/hr, if well tolerated, infusion time can be gradually shortened to a minimum of 2 hr.

Comment: Monitor renal, hepatic, electrolyte, and hematologic status closely. Thrombocytopenia, tachycardia, hypokalemia, hypomagnesemia, hypocalcemia, hyperglycemia, diarrhea, dyspnea, back pain, and increases in aminotransferases and bilirubin may occur.

Common infusion-related reactions include fever, chills, rigors, nausea, vomiting, hypotension, and headache; may premedicate with acetaminophen, diphenhydramine and meperidine (see Amphotericin B remarks).

Doses as high as 7.5 mg/kg/24 hr have been used to treat invasive fungal infections in BMT patients.

(Siberry: The Harriet Lane Handbook 2000, p.632)

AMPHOTERICIN B LIPID COMPLEX (Abelcet)

Supplied: Suspension for injection 100 mg/20 ml in 10 and 20 ml single use vials with 5-microns filter needles.

Administration: IV

The recommended dose is 5 mg/kg/day prepared as a 1 mg/ml infusion and delivered at a rate of 2.5 mg/kg/hr. For pediatric patients and patients with cardiovascular disease, the drug may be diluted to a final concentration of 2 mg/ml. If the infusion exceeds 2 hours, mix the contents by shaking the infusion bag every 2 hours. Do not use an in-line filter. (1)

Preparation of infusion:

Do not dilute or reconstitute with saline solutions or mix with other drugs or electrolytes. The use of any solution other than those recommended or the presence of a bacteriostatic agent (e.g., benzl alcohol) may cause precipitation of amphotericin B. (1)

<u>Amphotericin B lipid complex</u> (Abelcet)

Lipid formulations of amphotericin B have a role in some children who are intolerant of or refractory to amphotericin B deoxycholate. None of these formulations have been demonstrated to have efficacy that is superior to that of conventional amphotericin B. Amphotericin B lipid complex (Abelcet) is approved by the Food and Drug Administration for treatment of invasive fungal infections in children and adults who are refractory to or intolerant of conventional amphotericin B therapy, which is defined as (1) renal dysfunction with a serum creatinine level of 1.5 mg/dL or greater that develops during therapy or (2) disease progression after a total dose of amphotericin B of at least 10 mg/kg. Amphotericin B cholesteryl sulfate complex (Amphotec) is a colloidal complex that is approved by the

Food and Drug Administration for treatment of invasive aspergillosis in adults who cannot tolerate or fail to respond to amphotericin B deoxycholate. The liposomal formulation of amphotericin B (AmBisome) is approved for adults who cannot tolerate or fail to respond to conventional amphotericin B therapy for aspergillosis, candidiasis, cryptococcosis, or febrile neutropenia. In recommended doses, these lipid formulations cost 10 to 65 times more per day than amphotericin B. These lipid formulations currently are undergoing clinical evaluation for treatment of other fungal infections and for use in children.

(American Academy of Pediatrics: Report of the Committee on Infectious Diseases. Red Book 2000, p.669)

<u>Amphotericin B Lipid Complex (ABLC)</u>

Recommended doses of Parenteral and Oral Antifungal Drugs

Route: IV

Dose (per day): 5 mg/kg infused over 2 h

Adverse Reactions: Fever, chills, other reactions associated with amphotericin B, but less nephrotoxicity; hepatotoxicity

Note: Experience with drug in children is limited. Limited or no information about use in newborn infants is available.

(American Academy of Pediatrics: Report of the Committee on Infectious Diseases. Red Book 2000, pp.670-671)

<u>Amphotericin B Lipid Complex</u>

Dose/kg: 1-5 mg (increase dose daily in 1 mg/kg increments)

Route & frequency: Infuse over 2 h

Comments: Use higher doses for meningitis, osteoarthritis, cryptococcal infections, and aspergillosis. Mix to a 1-2 m/mL dilution with D5W only. Do not mix with saline or any other drug. Flush line with D5W.

(Avery: Neonatology Pathophysiology and Management of the Newborn 1999, p.1552)

<u>Amphotericin B Lipid Complex</u>

Route & Dose: IV: 2.5-5 mg/kg/24 hr QD
Mix with D_5W to concentration 1 mg/ml or 2 mg/ml for fluid restricted patients.

Infusion Rate: 2.5 mg/mg/hr; shake the infusion bag every 2 hours if total infusion time exceeds 2 hours.

Comment: Monitor renal, hepatic, electrolyte, and hematologic status closely. Thrombocytopenia, anemia, leukopenia, hypokalemia, hypomagnesemia diarrhea, respiratory failure, skin rash, and increase in liver enzymes and bilirubin may occur.

Common infusion-related reactions include fever, chills, rigors, nausea, vomiting, hypotension, and headache; may premedicate with acetaminophen, diphenhydramine and meperidine (see Amphotericin B remarks).

(Siberry: The Harriet Lane Handbook 2000, pp.632-633)

AMPHOTERICIN B LIPOSOMAL (Ambisome)

Supplied: Powder for injection 50 mg (as liposomal) in single dose vials with 5-microm filter.

Administration: The recommended dose is 3-5 mg/kg/day prepared as a 1-2 mg/ml infusion delivered initially over 120 minutes, infusion time may be reduced to 60 minutes if well tolerated or increased if patient experiences discomfort. Lower infusion concentrations of 0.2-0.5 mg/ml may be appropriate for infants and small children to provide sufficient volume for infusion. An in-line membrane filter of ≥ 1 micron mean pore decimeter maybe used. (1)

Use within 6 hours of dilution with 5% Dextrose. (1)

Liposomal amphotericin B

Suggested Dosage of Antifungal Agents for Infants with systemic or Severe Local Fungal Infection

Dosage (mg/kg per day): 5

(Remington: Infectious Diseases of the Fetus and Newborn Infant 2001, p.838)

Liposomal Amphotericin B Lipid Complex (AmBisome)

Recommended Doses of Parenteral and Oral Antifungal Drugs

Route: IV

Dose (per day): 5 mg/kg infused over 1-2 h

Adverse Reactions:

Fever, chills, other reactions associated with amphotericin B, but less nephrotoxicity; hepatotoxicity

Notes: Experience with drug in children is limited

Limited or no information about use in newborn infants is available

(American Academy of Pediatrics: Report of the Committee on Infectious Diseases. Red Book 2000, pp.670-671)

Amphotericin B, Liposomal

Route & Dose: IV: 3-5 mg/kg 24 hr QD

Max with D_5W to concentration 1-2 mg/ml (0.2-0.5 mg/ml may be used for infants and small children).

Infusion Rate: Administer dose over 2 hours; infusion may be reduced to 1 hour if well tolerated.

Comment: Monitor renal, hepatic, electrolyte, and hematologic status closely. Thrombocytopenia, tachycardia, hypokalemia, hypomagnesemia, hypocalcemia, hyperglycemia, diarrhea, dyspnea, skin rash, low back pain, and increases in liver enzymes and bilirubin may occur.

Common infusion-related reactions include fever, chills, rigors, nausea, vomiting, hypotension, and headache; may premedicate with acetaminophen, diphenhydramine and meperidine (see Amphotericin B remarks).

(Siberry: The Harriet Lane Handbook 2000, p.633)

AMPICILLIN (Omnipen, Polycillin-N)

Supplied: Suspension, powder for 100mg/ml in 20ml
Suspension, powder for 125mg/5ml, 250mg/5ml (100ml, 150ml, 200ml)
Injection, powder for 125mg, 250mg, 500mg vials, 1gm (contains 2.9 to 3.1 mEq Na/gm)

Administration: IV, IM, PO
Ampicillin preparations for parenteral use should be reconstituted according to the manufacturer's instructions.

Following reconstitution with SWFI for IM or direct IV injection, the ampicillin solution should be used within 1 hour. Ampicillin solutions containing less than 30mg/ml are stable for 8 hours at room temperature, or 48 hours when refrigerated in SWFI or NS. DIRECT IV injections should be made over 10 to 15 minutes to avoid the possibility of seizures.

After reconstitution, oral suspensions are preferably refrigerated. They are stable for 7 days at room temperature or 14 days refrigerated (3).

Ampicillin

Antibacterial Drugs for Newborn Infants:
Dose (mg/kg or Units [U]/kg and Frequency of Administration

Route: IV, IM

Dose: Infants 0-4 wk
BW <1200 g: 25-50 every 12 h

Infants <1 wk old
BW ≤ 1200 g: 25-50 every 12 h
BW >2000 g: 25-50 every 8 h

Infants ≥1 wk old
BW ≤2000-2000 g: 25-50 every 8 h
BW >2000 g: 25-50 every 6 h

Notes: For meningitis, the larger dosage is recommended
Higher doses are recommended for the treatment of group B streptococcal meningitis

Antibacterial Drugs for Pediatric Patients Beyond the Newborn Period:
Dosage per kg/d

Route: IV, IM
Mild to moderate infections: 100-150 mg in 4 doses

Route: PO
Mild to Moderate Infections: 50-100 mg in 4 doses

Route: IV, IM
Severe infections: 200-400 mg in 4 doses.

Route: PO
Severe Infections: Inappropriate

Comment: Larger dosage recommended for treatment of meningitis
Diarrhea occurs in approximately 20% of recipients

Note: In patients with history of allergy to penicillin or one of its many congeners, alternative drugs are recommended. In some circumstances, a cephalosporin or other ß-lactam class drug may be acceptable. However, these drugs should not be used in patients with an immediate hypersensitivity (anaphylaxis) to penicillin because approximately 5% to 15% of penicillin-allergic patients will also be allergic to the cephalosporins.

(American Academy of Pediatrics: Report of the Committee on Infectious Diseases. Red Book 2000, pp.652,658,662)

Ampicillin

Suggested Dosage Schedules for Antibiotics Used in Newborns
Route: IV, IM

Dosage (mg/kg) and Interval of Administration:

Meningitis: Weight <1200 g
Age 0-4 WK: 50 q12h

Weight 1200-2000 g
Age 0-7 Days: 50 q12h
Age >7 Days: 50 q8h

Weight >2000 g
Age 0-7 Days: 50 q8h
Age >7 Days: 50 q6h

Other Infections: Weight <1200 g
Age 0-4 WK: 25 q12h

Weight 1200-2000 g
Age 0-7 Days: 25 q12h
Age >7 Days: 25 q8h

Weight >2000 g
Age 0-7 Days: 25 q8h
Age >7 Days: 25 q6h

(Remington: Infectious Diseases of the Fetus and Newborn Infant 2001, p.1454)

Ampicillin (Polycillin, Others)

Classification: Semisynthetic penicillinase-sensitive penicillin.

Action and spectrum:

The penicillins are bactericidal and act by inhibiting the late stages of cell wall synthesis. As effective as penicillin G in pneumococcal, streptococcal, and meningococcal infections and also is active against many strains of *Salmonella* spp, *Shigella* spp, *Proteus mirabilis*, *Escherichia coli*, and *Listeria* spp and most strains of *Haemophilus influenzae*. Inactivated by staphylococcal and *H influenzae* β-lactamases.

Route: PO, IM, IV.

Dosage: Meningitis:
Age 0-7 days: 100-200 mg/kg/day IV or IM divided q12h.
Age >7 days: 200-300 mg/kg/day IV or IM divided q6-8h; maximum: 400 mg/kg/day.

Other indications:
Age 0-7 days: 100 mg/kg/day PO, IV, or IM divided q12h.
Age >7 days: 100 mg/kg/day PO, IV, or IM divided 6-8h.

Elimination and metabolism:
90% excreted unchanged in urine. Half-life in neonates is 2 h.

Adverse effects: Hypersensitivity, rubella-like rash, abdominal discomfort, nausea, vomiting, diarrhea, eosinophilia. Very large doses may cause CNS excitation or convulsions.

Comments: The penicillin of choice in combination with an aminoglycoside in the prophylaxis and treatment of infections with group B streptococci, group D streptococci (enterococci), and *Listeria monocytogenes*. Contains 3 meq of sodium per gram.

(Gomella: Neonatology 1999, p.553)

Ampicillin

Indication: For meningitis

Initial treatment: The optimal initial treatment in a newborn with bacterial meningitis of unknown cause is a combination of ampicillin and an aminoglycoside. The choice of aminoglycoside among gentamicin, kanamycin, amikacin, and tobramycin depends particularly on the susceptibility of gram-negative bacteria likely to be found in a given nursery population, but gentamicin is used most commonly. Although more readily demonstrated in vitro than in vivo, the combination of ampicillin and an aminoglycoside has been shown to be synergistic versus several common gram-negative and gram-positive organisms. The *usual doses, prior to results of cultures*, are for ampicillin, 100 to 150 mg/kg/day in the first week of life and 200 mg/kg/day after the first week, and for gentamicin, 5 mg/kg/day in the first week and 7.5 mg/kg/day after the first week. The drugs can be administered intramuscularly, but intravenous administration is preferred.

(Volpe: Neurology of the Newborn 2001, p.796)

Ampicillin

Route & Dose: Neonate IM/IV:

<7 days:
<2 kg: 50-100 mg/kg/24 hr IM/IV ÷ Q12 hr
≥2 kg: 75-150 mg/kg/24 hr IM/IV ÷ Q8 hr

≥7 days:
<1.2 kg: 50-100 mg/kg/24 hr ÷ Q12 hr IM/IV
1.2-2 kg: 75-150 mg/kg/24 hr ÷ Q8 hr IM/IV
>2 kg: 100-200 mg/kg/24 hr ÷ Q6 hr IM/IV

Comment: Use higher doses to treat CNS disease. CSF penetration occurs only with inflamed meninges.

Adjust dose in renal failure

Produces the same side effects as penicillin, with cross-reactivity. Rash commonly seen at 5-10 days. May cause interstitial nephritis, diarrhea, and pseudomembranous enterocolitis.

(Siberry: The Harriet Lane Handbook 2000, p.634)

AMPICILLIN/SULBACTUM (Unasyn)

Supplied: Injection, power for 1.5gm (1gm ampicillin/0.5gm sulbactam)
Injection, power for 3.0gm (2gm ampicillin/1.0gm sulbactam)

Administration: IV, IM
IV Administration: Add 3.2ml, 6.4ml SWFI to 1.5gm, 3.0gm vial respectively for a concentration of 375mg/ml (250mg ampicillin/125 sulbactam). Stable for 1 hour. Further dilute (NS, D5W) to yield solutions of 3 to 45mg/ml. Give by slow injection over at least 10 to 15 minutes, or infuse greater dilutions over 15 to 30 minutes (1).

Ampicillin-sulbactam (Unasyn)

Antibacterial Drugs for Pediatric patients Beyond the Newborn Period
Dosage per kg/d

Route: IV

Mild to Moderate Infections: 100-150 mg of ampicillin in 4 doses

Severe Infections: 200-400 mg of ampicillin in 4 doses

Comments: Not approved for infants and children

Note: In patients with history of allergy to penicillin or one of its many congeners, alternative drugs are recommended. In some circumstances, a cephalosporin or other ß-lactam class drug may be acceptable. However, these drugs should not be used in patients with an immediate hypersensitivity (anaphylaxis) to penicillin because approximately 5% to 15% of penicillin-allergic patients will also be allergic to the cephalosporins

Patients with a history of allergy to penicillin G or V should be considered for subsequent skin testing. Many such patients can be treated safely with penicillin, since only 10% of children with such history are proven allergic when skin-tested.

(American Academy of pediatrics: Report of the Committee on Infectious Diseases. Red Book 2000, pp.658,662)

<u>Ampicillin Sodium/Sulbactam Sodium</u> (Unasyn)

Classification: Combination ß-lactamase inhibitor and ß-lactam agent.

Action and spectrum:

The bactericidal spectrum of ampicillin is extended by the addition of sulbactam, a ß-lactamase inhibitor, to include ß-lactamase-producing strains of *Staphylococcus aureus*, *Staphylococcus epidermidis*, enterococcus, *Haemophilus influenzae*, *Branhamella catarrhalis*, and *Klebsiella* spp, including *K pneumoniae*. Also has good activity against *Bacteroides fragilis*, making it a suitable choice for single drug treatment of intra-abdominal and pelvic infections caused by susceptible organisms.

Route: IV, IM

Dosage: Meningitis:

Age 0-7 days: 100-200 mg/kg/day IV q12h.
Age > 7 days: 200-300 mg/kg/day IV or IM q 6-8h.

Other indications:

Age 0-7 days: 100 mg/kg/day IV or IM q 12h.
Age >7days: 100 mg/kg/day IV or IM q 6-8h.

Elimination: See Ampicillin, above.

Adverse effects: See Ampicillin, above.

Comments: See Ampicillin, above

(Gomella: Neonatology 1999, p.553)

AMRINONE LACTATE (Inocor)

Supplied: Injection 5 mg/ml in 20 ml

Administration: IV

Administer as supplied, or dilute in normal or one-half normal saline to a concentration of 1 to 3 mg/ml. Use diluted solutions within 24 hours.

DO NOT DILUTE with dextrose solutions prior to injection. A chemical interaction occurs slowly over 24 hrs when amrinone is mixed directly with dextrose – containing solution.

It may be injected into a running infusion through a y-connector or directly into the tubing where preferable. Do not administer furosemide in IV lines containing amrinone, or a precipitate will form immediately (1).

Amrinone

THERAPY FOR AUCTE CONGESTIVE CARDIAC FAILURE

Dose and Route of Administration:

Load with 0.75 mg/kg/dose x 2-3 doses over 15 minutes each. Maintain on 5-10 µg/kg/minute

Hemodynamic Effects:

Increases cardiac output if preload is normal or increased.

Complications and Comments Regarding Use:

Hypotension: hemodynamic monitoring required

Note: Milrinone is considered 10 to 30 times more potent than its parent drug, amrinone. After intravenous injection, the serum half-lives of amrinone and milrinone are 2.6 to 3.6 and 0.8 hours, respectively, in patients with congestive heart failure. Amrinone is primarily metabolized by the liver, but also is partially excreted unchanged in the urine to a variable degree. Milrinone is largely excreted by the kidneys.

When used acutely, amrinone and milrinone improve cardiac output, decrease right and left ventricular filling pressures, and decrease systemic vascular resistance. There typically are minimal effects on heart rate or blood pressure in patients with congestive heart failure and following cardiac surgery. Early concern was raised that amrinone achieved its effects solely as a function of its vasodilating action, but recent studies show that amrinone also increases left ventricular contractility.

Loading the patient with amrinone appears to be more difficult than loading with milrinone. Although the package insert calls for a loading dose of 0.75 mg/kg intravenously given over several minutes, we have found that two or sometimes three of these loading doses is preferable. The maintenance infusion rate is 5 to 10 µg/kg/minute. However, we generally prefer milrinone, which we have found to have fewer hemodynamic side effects than amrinone. We load patients with 50 µg/kg of intravenous milrinone over several minutes. The maintenance dose is 0.35 to 0.75 µg/kg/minute. Serous adverse side effects from intravenous amrinone and milrinone are not common, and consist of significant hypotension, reversible thrombocytopenia, and ventricular ectopy. Because of the vasodilating effect of the drug, blood pressure and cardiac output should be monitored carefully and intravascular volume must be adequate before intravenous loading. Amrinone may increase hepatic enzyme levels in the serum and may cause gastrointestinal symptoms.

(Garson: The science and practice of pediatric cardiology 1998, pp.2329-2341)

Amrinone

Dose: 3-10 µg/kg/min

Mode of Action: Phosphodiesterase inhibition, positive inotrope, peripheral vasodilator

Adverse Effects: Arrhythmia, hypotension, thrombocytopenia, GI upset

Comments: Questionable efficacy in newborns, young children

(Garson: The science and practice of pediatric cardiology 1998, p.2950)

Amrinone

Dose: Loading dose = 1-3 mg/kg IV over 30 min.
Continuous infusions = 5-10 μg/kg/min.

Comments: Cannot be mixed with dextrose solutions.

(Allen: Moss and Adams' Heart Disease in Infants, Children, and Adolescents 2001, pp.1460-1468)

Amrinone

Dosage: Loading dose: 3 mg/kg IV
Maintenance dose: 5-20 μg/kg/min

Comments: May also have positive inotropic properties; loading dose should be repeated with each increase in infusion rate; thrombocytopenia may occur.

(Fanaroff: Neonatal-Perinatal Medicine 1997, p.1753)

Amrinone Lactate

Neonate: 0.75 mg/kg IV bolus over 2-3 min, followed by maintenance infusion of 3-5 mcg/kg/min
Children and Adults: 0.75 mg/kg IV bolus over 2-3 min, followed by maintenance infusion of 5-10 mcg/kg/min.
(IV bolus may need to be repeated in 30 min in neonates and children)
Max dose: 10 mg/kg/24 hr

Remarks: Onset of action: 2-5 minutes with peak effects in 10 minutes.

Monitor for hypotension (which can be controlled with NS fluid boluses), arrhythmias, thrombocytopenia, hepatotoxicity, and GI effects; monitor fluid and electrolytes. Diuresis may result from improvement in cardiac output and may require dosage reduction of diuretics.

(Siberry: The Harriet Lane Handbook 2000, p.635)

ANTACIDS

Antacids

Therapy for Reflux

Common doses: 0.5-1 mL/kg/dose, 3-8 times a day; 1-2 hr PC, HS

Partial list of side effects:
diarrhea, constipation, rickets, aluminum or magnesium toxicity

(Wyllie: Pediatric Gastrointestinal Disease 1999m, p.180)

Antacids

Indication: Adjunct to the treatment of gastric and duodenal ulcer disease and for prophylaxis against other ulceration in severely ill patients.

Dose: The smallest dose necessary should be used, e.g. 0.5 to 1 mL/kg liquid antacid for infants...to achieve a predetermined target pH of gastric fluid.... Antacids should be administered 1 hour postprandially. Chronic administration of an oral antacid for more than 2 weeks should be done cautiously with appropriate monitoring for possible local and systemic adverse effects.

(Reed: Drug therapy and the gastrointestinal tract. Semin Perinatol 1992;16:21-31)

SEE ALSO: ALUMINUM HYDROXIDE/MAGNESIUM HYDROXIDE AND ALUMINUM HYDROXIDE

AQUAPHOR

Aquaphor

In addition to this routine skin care, the treatment groups received 1.5 ml of Aquaphor applied to the entire body except the face and scalp. Treatment began within the first 24 hours of life; thereafter, ointment was applied twice daily (at 8:00 PM) for 14 days. All but two infants were placed in double-walled incubators by the fourth day of life.

Conclusion: Aquaphor ointment, used during the first two postnatal weeks, improved skin condition in infants of 26 to 30 weeks' gestation without changing skin bacterial flora. We speculate that improved skin condition may limit transepidermal water loss and decrease portals of entry for pathogens, thereby potentially decreasing fluid and electrolyte imbalances and sepsis in very low birth weight infants.

(Pabst: The Effects of Application of Aquaphor on Skin Condition, Fluid Requirements, and Bacterial Colonization in Very Low Birth Weight Infants. J Perinatol 1999;9(4):278-283)

Aquaphor

Preservative-free ointment (Aquaphor Ointment, Beiersdoff Inc., Norwalk, Conn.) therapy decreased TEWL (Transepidermal Water Loss) for 6 hours after application, decreased the severity of dermatitis and decreased bacterial colonization of axillary skin. Infants treated with ointment had fewer blood and cerebrospinal fluid cultures positive for microorganisms. These data support the use of topical ointment therapy in very premature infants during the first weeks after birth.

(Nopper: Topical ointment therapy benefits premature infants. J Pediatr 1996;128:660-669)

ARGININE HCL (R-Gene 10)

Supplied: 10% Arginine HCL in 500ml (950mOsm/L)
Administration: IV
With 47.5 mEq chloride ion per 100ml (1)

Arginine hydrochloride

Dosage: 0.3 to 1 mEq/kg/hr IV
Comments: In high doses may stimulate growth hormone release
(Fanaroff: Neonatal-Perinatal Medicine 1997, p.1751)

Arginine

Recommendation:
High-dose arginine is very effective in reducing plasma levels of ammonia in patients with citrullinemia and argininosuccinic aciduria. Arginine-HCL should preferably be given through a central line and may require simultaneous administration of sodium bicarbonate.

Rational: In these disorders arginine promotes incorporation of ammonia into the amino acids citrulline and argininosuccinate, providing an alternative pathway for waste nitrogen excretion. High-dose arginine-HCL may cause metabolic acidosis, and it can cause tissue necrosis if extravasation occurs.

Recommendation:
Where available, plasma levels of ammonia scavenging drugs should be monitored to avoid toxicity.

Rationale: Variable drug excretion may cause toxicity. In the absence of drug levels, a serum anion gap of >15 mEq/L and an anion gap that has risen >6 mEq/L could indicate drug accumulation and increased risk for toxicity.
(The Urea Cycle Disorders Conference Group: Consensus statement from a conference for the Management of Patients with Urea cycle Disorders. J Pediatr 2001;138:S1-S5)

Arginine

Therapeutic Category:
Diagnostic Agent, Growth Hormone Function; Metabolic Alkalosis Agent

Usual Dosage: IV:
Inborn errors of urea synthesis: Infants and Children: 0.8 g/kg initially, then 0.2-0.8 g/kg/day as a continuous infusion

Metabolic alkalosis:
Infants, Children: Arginine hydrochloride dose (g) = weight (kg) x 0.1 x [HCO_3 – 24] where HCO_3 = the patient's serum bicarbonate concentration in mEq/L; give ½ to 2/3 of calculated dose and re-evaluate

Note: Arginine hydrochloride is a fourth-line treatment for uncompensated metabolic alkalosis after sodium chloride, potassium chloride, and ammonium chloride supplementation has been optimized.

To correct hypochloremia:
Infants, Children: Arginine hydrochloride dose (mEq) = 0.2 x weight (kg) [103 – Cl] where Cl = the patient's serum chloride concentration in mEq/L; give ½ to 2/3 of calculated dose and re-evaluate

Note: Arginine hydrochloride should never be used as initial therapy for chloride supplementation but as an alternative in the patient who is unresponsive to sodium chloride or potassium chloride supplementation.

Administration: Parenteral: May be infused without further dilution; maximum rate of I.V. infusion: 1 g/kg/hour (4.75 mEq/kg/hour) (maximum dose: 60 g/hour = 285 mEq over 1 hour)

Monitoring Parameters:
Acid-base status (arterial or capillary blood gases), serum electrolytes, BUN, glucose, plasma growth hormone concentrations (when evaluating growth hormone reserve)

Reference Range:
If intact pituitary function, human growth hormone levels should rise after arginine administration to 10-30 ng/mL (control range: 0-6 ng/mL)

Nursing Implications:
I.V. infiltration of arginine hydrochloride may cause necrosis and phlebitis; prolongation of the infusion may diminish the stimulus to the pituitary gland and nullify the test.

(Taketomo: Pediatric Dosage Handbook 2000-2001; pp.95-96)

ASPIRIN (Acetylsalicylic acid, ASA)

Supplied: Tablet, chewable 81mg
Suppositories, 120mg (refrigerate)
Administration: PO, PR
Comment: Do not use in children or teenagers with chickenpox or flu symptoms due to the possibility of Reye's syndrome.

Aspirin (ASA, various trade names)

Dose & Route: Analgesic/antipyretic: 10-15 mg/kg/dose PO Q4-6 hr up to total 60-80 mg/kg/24 hr.

Max dose: 4 g/24hr

Anti-inflammatory: 60-100 mg/kg/24hr PO÷Q6-8hr

Kawasaki disease: 80-100 mg/kg/hr PO÷QID during febrile phase until defervesce then decrease to 3-5 mg/kg/24hr PO QAM. Continue for at least 8 weeks or until both platelet count and ESR normal.

Remarks: **Do not use** in children <16 yr for treatment of chicken pox or flu-like symptoms (risk of Reye's syndrome), in combination with other non-steroidal anti-inflammatory drugs, or in severe renal failure. Use with **caution** in bleeding disorders, renal dysfunction, gastritis, and gout. May cause GI upset, allergic reactions, liver toxicity, and decreased platelet aggregation.

Drug Interactions: may increase effects of methotrexate, valproic acid, and warfarin which may lead to toxicity (protein displacement). Buffered dosage forms may decrease absorption of ketoconazole, tetracycline.

Therapeutic levels: antipyretic/analgesic: 30-50 mg/L, antiinflammatory: 150-300 mg/L, Tinnitus may occur at levels of 200-400 mg/L. Recommended serum sampling time at steady state: obtain trough level just prior to dose following 1-2 days of continuous dosing. Peak levels obtained 2 hours (for non-sustained release dosage forms) after a dose may be useful for monitoring toxicity.

Pregnancy category changes to "D" if full-dose aspirin is used during the 3rd trimester. **Adjust dose in renal failure.**

(Siberry: The Harriet Lane Handbook 2000, pp.636-637)

Aspirin

Route: PO, PR

Neonatal Dose: 5 mg/kg/dose Q4-6H

Pediatric Dose: 65-100 mg/kg/24hr. or 10-20 mg/kg/dose Q4-6H

Discussion: Because of toxicity use cautiously in <2 yr-olds; because of Reyes syndrome do not use during viral illnesses especially flu or with varicella; higher doses are used as antirheumatic and keep serum level at 15-30 mg/dl; adjust dose for renal failure.

(Rudolph: Rudolph's Pediatrics 1996, p.2172)

ATENOLOL (Tenormin)

Supplied: Tablets 25mg, 50mg, 100mg
Injection 5mg in 10ml amps.

Comment: In patients with impaired renal function, doses an/or frequency of administration of atenolol must be modified in response to the degree of renal impairment. (3)

Atenolol

Atenolol is a common, long-acting beta blocker in pediatrics.

Dosing: PO: 1-3 mg/kg/day

Warnings: Postural hypotension, cool extremities

Dosing and Interactions:

The starting dosage of atenolol is 1 to 2 mg/kg/day, up to as high as 3 mg/kg/day. Because of the sustained-release nature of the agent, it can be given once a day or twice daily. There are no reported significant drug interactions.

Side Effects: Because atenolol does not cross the blood-brain barrier, the side effect profile is considerable reduced compared with propranolol. Cardiovascular effects are similar to propranolol, and postural hypotension may occur. Although atenolol is a selective beta agent, the risk of bronchospasm is not eliminated completely. Cool extremities can be a common complaint.

(Gillette: Clinical Pediatric Arrhythmias 1999, pp.231-248)

Atenolol

Class: II β-Blockers

Uses: Hypertension, prolonged QTc, exercise-induced VT

Dose (Level) 12.5-50 mg PO QD approx 1 mg/kg

Mode of Action: More β_1 selective, no local anesthetic effect, central reduction of sympathetic output

ECG/EP Changes: Slow HR, may ↓ QT

Side Effects: Fewer CNS effects than propranolol; postural hypotension, CHF, diarrhea, nausea; may ↑ TG, VLDL; contraindicated with verapamil

(Garson: The science and practice of pediatric cardiology 1998, p.2953)

Atenolol

Dose & Route: Children: 1-1.2 mg/kg/dose PO QD
Max dose: 2 mg/kg/24 hr

Remarks: **Contraindicated** in pulmonary edema, cardiogenic shock, May cause bradycardia, hypotension, second or third degree AV block, dizziness, fatigue, lethargy, headache. Wheezing and dyspnea have occurred when daily dosage exceeds 100 mg/24hr. **Avoid** abrupt withdrawal of the drug. Does not cross the blood-brain barrier; lower incidence of CNS side effects compared to propranolol. **Adjust doe in renal impairment**. IV administration rate **not to exceed** 1 mg/min.

(Siberry: The Harriet Lane Handbook 2000, p.638)

Atenolol

Dose: 1-2 mg/kg/day p.o. (single daily dose).

(Allen: Moss and Adams' Heart Disease in Infants, Children, and Adolescents 2001, pp.1460-1468)

ATRACURIUM BESYLATE (Tracrium)

Supplied: Injection 10mg/ml in 5ml, 10ml units (benzyl alcohol contained in MDV)

Administration: IV

Administer IV. Atracurium Besylate should not be administered by IM injection, since there are no clinical data to support this route of administration and tissue irritation may result. At concentrations of 0.2mg/ml or 0.5mg/ml, Atracurium is stable for 24 hours when stored at room temperature or when refrigerated in the following IV solutions: D5W, NS, D5NS (3). Do not use lactated ringers.

Compatible: Cimetidine, dobutamine, dopamine, epinephrine, fentanyl, gentamicin, heparin, hydrocortisone, isoproterenol, lorazepam, midazolam, morphine, nitroglycerin, vancomycin (9).

Incompatible: Diazepam (9), aminophylline.

Comment: DO NOT administer in the same syringe or through the same needle as an alkaline solution (5).

Atracurium

Dose/kg: Initial dose: 0.3-0.5 mg

Route & frequency: IV, once

Dose/kg Maintenance dose: 0.08-0.1 mg

Route & frequency: Every 20-45 min to maintain paralysis

Comments: Hypertension associated with histamine release. Ventilatory rate may need to be adjusted to compensate for loss of spontaneous ventilation. Aminoglycoside antibiotics prolong duration of action. Contains 9 mg benzyl alcohol/mL. Elimination not substantially altered by renal or hepatic dysfunction.

(Avery: Neonatology Pathophysiology and Management of the Newborn 1999, p.1552)

Atracurium

Dosage: Loading dose: 0.2-0.4 mg/kg IV. Dose may be repeated as needed or use:
Maintenance infusion: 2-10 μg/kg/min

Comments: Drug is eliminated by Hofmann degradation so that no dosage adjustment required in hepatic or renal disease. May cause histamine release; duration of paralysis 20 to 45 minutes after a single dose.

(Fanaroff: Neonatal-Perinatal Medicine 1997, p.1752)

Atracurium

Route: IV

Neonatal Dose: 0.3 mg/kg/dose. Maintenance: 0.05-0.06 mg/kg every 15 min. or sooner if needed.

Pediatric Dose: 0.3 mg/kg/dose. Maintenance: 0.08-0.1 mg/kg; >2 y: give every 15-25 min.

Discussion: To reverse effects use neostigmine plus atropine (see Neostigmine); do not use IM; may cause histamine release and bradycardia.

(Rudolph: Rudolph's Pediatrics 1996, p.2172)

Atracurium

Initial dose: 0.3 to 0.5 mg/kg/ IV; repeat dose 0.125 mg/kg.

By Infusion: During halothane or isoflurane anesthesia: loading dose of 0.3 mg/kg, and infusion of 5 to 6 mcg/kg/min.

During balanced anesthesia with fentanyl: loading dose of 0.4 mg/kg, and infusion of 9 to 10 mcg/kg/min.

Atracurium is a non-depolarizing neuromuscular blocking agent with a shorter duration of action (± 30 minutes) than d-tubocurarine or pancuronium. It decomposes at physiologic pH to inactive compounds (Hoffmann elimination) and hence has a predictable rate of elimination even in the presence of severe hepatic or renal disease. The shorter duration of action and constant rate of metabolism make this drug ideal for administration by continuous infusion.

Atracurium usually has little effect on the CVS. It dose release histamine, especially if large doses are given rapidly, and should not be given to patients with asthma.

An anaphylactoid reaction has been described in an infant following induction with thiopental and atracurium. In pediatric practice, atracurium is especially useful in the short case (eg. pyloric stenosis) and in the patient with hepatic or renal impairment.

(Steward: Manual of Pediatric Anesthesia 1995, pp.62,511)

ATROPINE

Supplied: Injection 0.05mg/ml in 5ml Syringes
Injection 0.1 mg/ml in 5ml, 10ml Syringes
Injection 0.3mg, 0.4mg, 0.5mg, 0.8mg, 1.0mg in 1ml

Administration: IV, ET, Intraosseous, SQ, IM
Although at least one manufacturer recommends that atropine sulfate be given slowly and with caution, the drug is generally given IV rapidly, since slow injection of the drug may cause a paradoxical slowing of the heart rate (3).
Minimum Pediatric Dose: 0.1 mg (3).

Atropine Sulfate

Indications and use:
Sinus bradycardia, cardiopulmonary resuscitation, reversal of neuromuscular blockade. Used preoperatively to inhibit salivation and reduce excessive secretions of the respiratory tract.

Actions: A competitive antagonist of acetylcholine at smooth muscle, cardiac muscle, and various glandular cells, leading to increased heart rate, reduced GI motility and tone, urinary retention, cycloplegia, and decreased salivation and sweating.

Route: IV, IM, SC, PO, Intratracheal.

Dosage: Bradycardia in infants and children: 0.02-0.03 mg/kg/dose q5 min prn. Maximum 1 mg.

Preanesthetic: 0.03 mg/kg/dose.

Adverse effects: Xerostomia, blurred vision, mydriasis, tachycardia, palpitations, constipation, urinary retention, ataxia, tremor, hyperthermia. Toxic effects are especially likely in children receiving low doses.

Comments: Contraindicated in thyrotoxicosis, tachycardia secondary to cardiac insufficiency, and obstructive GI disease. In low doses, may cause paradoxical bradycardia secondary to its central actions.

(Gomella: Neonatology 1999, p.554)

Atropine

Aerosol Therapy in Neonates

0.03-0.05 mg/kg.
Dilute with NS to 2.5 mL.
Dose: every 6-8 h.

Side Effects:
Tachycardia
Arrhythmia
Hypotension
Ileus
Airway dryness
Thick secretions
Suggest use in combination with albuterol

(Gomella: Neonatology: Management, Procedures, On-call Problems, Diseases and Drugs 1999, p.56)

Atropine

Bradycardia:
Dose/kg: 0.02 mg
Route and frequency:
IV over 1 min; min single dose 0.1 mg, max single dose 0.5 mg

May repeat every 5 min to a maximum *total* dose of 1 mg or 0.04 mg/kg

Comments: May cause hyperthermia, urinary retention, tachycardia, and elevated WBC count

Antidote: physostigmine

Bronchospasm:
Dose/kg: 0.03-0.05 mg
Route and frequency:
Via inhalation q8h-q6h; min single dose 0.25 mg, max single dose 1 mg

(Avery: Neonatology Pathophysiology and Management of the Newborn 1999, p.1552)

Atropine

Usual Dosage Note:
Doses <0.1 mg have been associated with paradoxical bradycardia

Neonates, Infants and Children:
Preanesthetic: Oral, I.M., I.V., S.C.:
<5 kg: 0.02 mg/kg/dose 30-60 minutes preop then every 4-6 hours as needed; use of a minimum dosage of 0.1 mg in neonates <5 kg will result in dosages >0.02 mg/kg; there is no documented minimum dosage in this age group

>5 kg: 0.01-0.02 mg/kg/dose to a maximum 0.4 mg/dose 30-60 minutes preop; minimum dose: 0.1 mg

Bradycardia: I.V., intratracheal: 0.02 mg/kg, minimum dose 0.1 mg, maximum single dose: 0.5 mg in children and 1 mg in adolescents; may repeat in 5-minute intervals to a maximum total dose of 1 mg in children or 2 mg in adolescents. (**Note**: For intratracheal administration, must be diluted; see Administration.) When treating bradycardia in neonates, reserve use for those patients unresponsive to improved oxygenation and epinephrine.

(Taketomo: Pediatric dosage Handbook 1999-2000, pp.98-99)

Atropine Sulfate

Dose & Route: Pre-anesthesia dose:
Child: 0.01 mg/kg/dose SC/IV/IM, **max dose**: 0.4 mg/dose; min dose: 0.1 mg/dose; may repeat Q4-6 hr

Cardiopulmonary Resuscitation:
Child: 0.02 mg/kg/dose IV Q5 min X 2-3 doses PRN; **min dose**: 0.1 mg; **max single dose**: 0.5 mg in children

Bronchospasm: 0.05 mg/kg/dose in 2.5 ml NS; min dose: 0.25 mg; **max dose**: 1 mg Q6-8 hr via nebulizer.

Ophthalmic:
Child: (0.5% solution) 1-2 drops in each eye QD-TID

Remarks: **Contraindicated** in glaucoma, obstructive uropathy, tachycardia, thyrotoxicosis, **Caution** in patients sensitive to sulfites.

Doses <0.1 mg have been associated with paradoxical bradycardia. Side effects include: dry mouth, blurred vision, fever, tachycardia, constipation, urinary retention, CNS signs (dizziness, hallucinations, restlessness, fatigue, headache).

In case of bradycardia, may give via endotracheal tube (dilute with NS to volume of 1-2 ml). Use injectable solution for nebulized use; can be mixed with albuterol for simultaneous administration.

(Siberry: The Harriet Lane Handbook 2000, pp.638-639

AZATHIOPRINE (Imuran)

Supplied: Tablets 50mg
Injection: 100mg/vial, in 20 ml vials

Administration: IV, PO

IV: For IV use only. Add 10ml SWFI to vial. Use within 24 hours. Further dilution into NS or dextrose is usually made for infusion. The final volume depends on the infusion time. It is usually 30 to 60 minutes, but ranges from 5 minutes to 8 hours for daily dose (1).

Azathioprine

Dose & Route: Immunosuppression:
Initial: 3-5 mg/kg/24 hr IV/PO QD
Maintenance: 1-3 mg/kg/24 hr IV/PO QD

Remarks: Toxicity: bone marrow suppression, rash, stomatitis, hepatotoxicity, alopecia, arthralgias, and GI disturbances. Use 1/4-1/3 dose when given with allopurinol. Monitor CBC, platelets, total bilirubin, alkaline phosphatase, BUN, creatinine. **Adjust dose in renal failure**.

(Siberry: The Harriet Lane Handbook 2000, p.640)

SEE ALSO: IMMUNOSUPPRESSION AGENTS

AZITHROMYCIN (Zithromax)

Supplied: Powder for oral suspension:
100mg/5ml, in 300mg bottles
300mg/15ml, in bottle with dropper
600mg/15ml, in bottle with dropper
900mg/22.5ml, in bottle with dropper
Capsules 250mg, 500mg powder for injection

Administration: PO

Comment: Azithromycin is an azalide antibiotic, a subclass of the macrolides. Administer at least 1 hour before or 2 hours after a meal. (1)

Injections should be infused over a period >60 minutes. Do not use azithromycin as a bolus or IM. (2)

Azithromycin (Zithromax)

Antibacterial Drugs for Pediatric Patients Beyond the Newborn Period: Dosage per kg/d

Route: PO

Mild to moderate infections: 5-12 mg/kg once daily

Severe infection: Inappropriate

Comments: Otitis: 10 mg/kg on first day, 5 mg/kg per day for an additional 4 d
Pharyngitis: 12 mg/kg per day for 5 days

(American Academy of Pediatrics: Report of the Committee on Infectious Diseases. Red Book 2000, p.657)

AZTREONAM (Azactam)

Supplied: Injection, powder for 500mg, 1gm, 2gm vial
Administration: IV, IM

For DIRECT intermittent IV injection, the contents of a vial should be reconstituted by adding 6 to 10 ml SWFI. The appropriate dose of reconstituted solution may then be injected slowly over a period of 3 to 5 minutes either directly into a vein or into the tubing of a compatible IV solution.

For INTERMITTENT IV infusion, further dilute the initial reconstituted solution to a final concentration not exceeding 20mg/ml. Intermittent infusions should be infused over 20 to 60 minutes.

The recommended final concentration for infusion is 20mg/ml. The duration of infusion is >6 mg/kg/min (6).

Aztreonam is stable in D5W, NS, D10W in a concentration < 20mg/ml for 7 days refrigerated, or 2 days at room temperature. For concentrations >20mg/ml, the solutions should be used promptly if they are not prepared with SWFI or NS (2).

For IM administration, reconstitute vials with at least 3ml of SWFI or NS per gram of Aztreonam (1).

Aztreonam

Antibacterial Drugs for Newborn Infants:
Dose (mg/kg or Units [U]/kg) and Frequency of Administration

Route: IV, IM

Dose: Infants 0-4 wk
BW <1200 g: 30 every 12 h

Infants <1 wk old
BW ≤1200-2000 g: 30 every 12 h
BW >2,000 g: 30 every 8 h

Infants ≥1 wk old
BW ≤2000-2000 g: 30 every 8 h
BW >2000 g: 30 every 6 h

Antibacterial Drugs for Pediatric Patients Beyond the Newborn Period
Dosage per kg/d
Route: IV, IM
Mild to Moderate Infections: 90 mg in 3 doses
Severe Infections: 120 mg in 4 doses

Note: In patients with history of allergy to penicillin or one of its many congeners, alternative drugs are recommended. In some circumstances, a cephalosporin or other ß-lactam class drug may be acceptable. However, these drugs should not be used in patients with an immediate hypersensitivity (anaphylaxis) to penicillin because approximately 5% to 15% of penicillin-allergic patients will also be allergic to the cephalosporins
(American Academy of Pediatrics: Report of the Committee on Infectious Diseases. Red Book 2000, pp.651,653,662)

Aztreonam

Administered: IV

Dosages (mg/kg/day) and Intervals of Administration:

Body weight < 2000 g
0-7 days old: 60 div q12h
8-28 days old: 90 div q8h

Body weight > 2000 g
0-7 days old: 90 div q8h
8-28 days old: 120 div q6h

> 28 days old: 120 div q6h

(Nelson: Pocket Book of Pediatric Antimicrobial Therapy 2000-2001, p.16)

Aztreonam

Suggested Dosage Schedules for Antibiotics Used in Newborns

Route: IV, IM

Dosage (mg/kg) and Interval of Administration:

Weight <1200 g
Age 0-4 WK: 30 q12h

Weight 1200-2000 g
Age 0-7 Days: 30 q12h
Age >7 Days: 30 q8h

Weight >2000 g
Age 0-7 Days: 30 q8h
Age >7 Days: 30 q6h

(Remington: Infectious Diseases of the Fetus and Newborn Infant 2001, p.1454)

Aztreonam (Azactam)

Classification: Monobactam antibiotic.

Action and spectrum:
Antibacterial activity due to inhibition of mucopeptide synthesis in the cell wall. Bactericidal against most Enterobacteriaceae and *Pseudomonas aeruginosa* but little or no activity against Gram-positive aerobic or anaerobic bacteria.

Route: IV

Dosage: Premature infants: 50 mg/kg/dose q12h
Term infants: 50 mg/kg/dose q8h

Elimination: Renal (glomerular filtration and secretion). Half-life is approximately ~6-10 h. Volume of distribution 0.26-0.36 L/kg.

Adverse effects: Diarrhea, nausea, vomiting, rash irritation at infusion site, increased prothrombin time, transient eosinophilia.

Comments: Used primarily for *Pseudomonas infections.*

(Gomella: Neonatology 1999, p.554)

Aztreonam

Dose & Route: Neonate:

30 mg/kg/dose:

<1.2 kg and 0-4 wk age: Q12 hr IV/IM

1.2-2 kg and 0-7 days: Q12 hr IV/IM

1.2-2 kg and >7 days: Q8 hr IV/IM

>2 kg and 0-7 days: Q8 hr IV/IM

>2 kg and >7 days: Q6 hr IV/IM

Children:

90-120 mg/kg/24 hr ÷ Q6-8 hr IV/IM

Cystic fibrosis:

150-200 mg/kg/24 hr ÷ Q6-8 hr IV/IM

Maximum Dose: 8 g/24 hr

Remarks: Well-absorbed IM. Low cross-allergenicity between aztreonam and other beta-lactams. Adverse reactions: thrombophlebitis, eosinophilia, leukopenia, neutropenia, thrombocytopenia, elevation of liver enzymes, hypotension, seizures, confusion. Good CNS penetration. **Adjust dose in renal failure**.

(Siberry: The Harriet Lane Handbook 2000, pp.641-642)

BACITRACIN

Supplied: Ophthalmic Ointment 500 Units/gm
Topical Ointment 500 Units/gm
Administration: Topical, ophthalmic

Bacitracin

Route & Dose: Top: as ointment (500 units/gm), q 4-8 h
(Taeusch: Avery's Diseases of the Newborn 1998, p.1343)

BECLOMETHASONE DIPROPIONATE

(Beclovent, Vanceril - Respiratory inhalants)
(Beconase, Beconase AQ, Vancenase, Vancenase AQ - Intranasal steroid)

Supplied: Aerosol 42mcg/actuation
Administration: Inhalation (note: not product used in LaForce article)

Beclomethasone

Infants were selected based on inclusion criteria of birth weight ≤1250 g, gestational age <33 weeks, postnatal age 3 to 14 days, and requirement for mechanical ventilation. Calculation of the total daily actuations delivered to the infant was based on the desired beclomethasone dose to be delivered beyond the endotracheal tube (40 µg/kg/d, tapered weekly to 5 µg/kg/d over a 28-day period), the infant's weight, and the amount of beclomethasone exiting the endotracheal tube (1.7 µg/actuation [unpublished data]).

... we conclude that this specific regimen of inhaled beclomethasone therapy in premature infants at risk for BPD was associated with mild decreases in basal plasma cortisol levels, but there was no evidence of adrenal suppression in response to 3.5 µg/kg cosyntropin stimulation. Future studies of other inhaled glucocorticoid formulations, regimens, or delivery systems should continue to evaluate the effect of inhaled glucocorticoid therapy on the neonatal HPA axis and adrenal function.

(Cole: Adrenal function in premature infants during inhaled beclomethasone therapy. J Pediatr 1999;135:65-70)

Beclomethasone Dipropionate

Dose & Route: Oral Inhalation (1 inhalation = 42 mcg):
6-12 yr: 1-2 inhalations TID-QID or 2-4 inhalations BID; **max** 10 inhalations/24 hr.

6-12 yr: 2 inhalations BID; **max** 5 inhalations/24 hr

Oral Inhalation (NIH-National Heart Lung and Blood Institute recommendations):

Nasal Inhalation:
6-12 yr: 1 spray each nostril TID
Aqueous nasal spray:
>6 yr: 1-2 sprays each nostril BID

Remarks: Not recommended for children <6 yr. Dose should be titrated to lowest effective dose. **Avoid** using higher than recommended doses, since hypothalamic, pituitary, or adrenal suppression may occur.

Rinse mouth and gargle with water after oral inhalation; may cause thrush. Consider using with spacers for oral inhalation.

(Siberry: The Harriet Lane Handbook 2000, p.643)

Beclomethasone

We studied 15 infants (birth weight, 720 to 1740 gm) who were recovering from respiratory distress syndrome, who required mechanical ventilation at 7 to 14 days of age, and in whom the attending neonatologist diagnosed early chronic lung disease on the basis of clinical status and the progression of changes on chest radiographs. The infants received three or four puffs of beclomethasone twice a day for 7 days .... Beclomethasone was delivered through an Aerochamber spacer (Monaghan Medical Corp., Plattsburgh, N.Y.) designed for in-line use with a ventilator circuit....We found significantly more episodes of desaturation to less than 85% before administration than after administration ($p < 0.05$). The transcutaneous carbon dioxide values increased 4 to 10 mm Hg during delivery ($p < 0.02$) but returned to baseline by 30 minutes.

(Liu: A trial of the safety of inhaled beclomethasone in ventilator-treated neonates. J Pediatr 1996;129:154-156)

Beclomethasone Nebulization

For brochopulmonary dysplasia:

The treatment consisted of nebulization of 50 mcg of beclomethasone (Vancenase AQ Nasal; Schering) in 2 ml saline solution, or nebulization of 2 ml saline solution, every 8 hours for 28 days. Authors found no striking increase in the incidence of infection, which is serious side effects of systemic therapy.

(LaForce: Controlled trial of beclomethasone dipropionate by nebulization in oxygen- and ventilator-dependent infants. J Pediatr 1993;122:285-288)

BETHANECOL CHLORIDE (Urecholine)

Supplied: Injection 5mg/ml, 1 ml vial
Tablets 5mg, 10mg, 25mg, 50mg

Administration: PO (Freely soluble in water)

Bethanechol

Bethanechol (β-methylcholine carbanmate) is the most commonly used cholinergic agonist.

Side effects of bethanechol have significantly limited its use. Although the above studies in infants and children reported no major side effects, general experience in both children and adults suggest that incidence of side effects is quite high. Cholinergic side effects are reported to occur in up to 15 to 20 percent of adults using the drug. These side effects are the result of over stimulation of the parasympathetic nervous system, and include abdominal cramps, diarrhea...

The usual recommended oral dosage for bethanechol in infants and children is 0.6 mg/kg in three divided doses.

(Walker: Pediatric Gastrointestinal Disease 2000, p.1814)

<u>Bethanechol</u>

Therapy for Reflux

Common doses: 0.1-0.3 mg/kg/dose tid or qid: AC, HS

Partial list of side effects:

Cholinergic: hypotension, flushing, headache, bronchospasm, salivation, abdominal cramping

Partial list of contraindications:

Urinary or gastrointestinal obstruction, perforation, hemorrhage, recent surgery, peritonitis, hypotension, bradycardia, epilepsy, asthma, hyperthyroidism, peptic ulcer

(Wyllie: Pediatric Gastrointestinal Disease 1999, p.180)

<u>Bethanechol Chloride</u>

Dose & Route: Abdominal distention/urinary retention
PO: 0.6 mg/kg/24hr÷Q6-8 hr
SC: 0.12-0.2 mg/kg/24hr÷Q6-8hr

Gastroesophageal reflux:
0.1-0.2 mg/kg dose 30 min-1hr AC and HS;
max: 4 doses/24 hr

Remarks: **Contraindicated** in asthma, mechanical GI or GU obstruction, peptic ulcer disease, hyperthyroidism, cardiac disease, seizure disorder. May cause hypotension, nausea, bronchospasm, salivation, flushing, abdominal cramps. **Warning: severe hypotension may occur when given with ganglionic blockers (trimethaphan). Do not give IV or IM**. Atropine is the antidote.

(Siberry: The Harriet Lane Handbook 2000, p.644)

<u>Bethanecol</u>

Route & Dose: PO: 0.1-0.2 mg/kg/dose q 6-8 h or 3mg/m^2 dose q 8 h
20 min before feeding

Adverse Effects, Cautions:

Diarrhea, jitteriness, tremors, sleeplessness, bronchoconstriction, increased tracheobronchial secretions.

(Taeusch: Avery's Diseases of the Newborn 1998, p.1343)

BLOOD COMPONENTS

RED BLOOD CELL TRANSFUSION

Red Blood Cell Transfusion

Transfusion Guidelines for Preterm Infants

Hematocrit / Hemoglobin:*	Ventilator Requirement and/or Symptoms:	Transfusion Volume:
Hct≤35/Hgb≤11	Infants requiring moderate or significant mechanical ventilation (MAP >8 cm H_2O and Fio_2>40%)	15 mL/kg PRBCs over 2-4 h
Hct≤30/Hgb≤10	Infants requiring minimal mechanical ventilation (any mechanical ventilation, or CPAP >6 cm H_2O and Fio_2≤40%)	15 mL/kg PRBCs over 2-4 h
Hct≤25/Hgb≤8	Infants on supplemental oxygen who are not requiring mechanical ventilation and one or more of the following is present: • ≤24 hours of tachycardia (HR >180) or tachypnea (RR >80) • An increased oxygen requirement from the previous 48 hours, defined as ≤four-fold increase in nasal canula flow (i.e., ¼ L/min to 1 L/min) or an increase in nasal CPAP ≤20% from the previous 48 hours (i.e. 10 cm to 12 cm H_2O) • An elevated lactated concentration (≤2.5 mEq/L) • Weight gain <10 g/kg/d over the previous 4 days while receiving ≤100 kcal/kg/d • An increase in the episodes of apnea and bradycardia (>9 episodes in 24 h or ≤2 episodes in 24 h requiring bag-mask ventilation) while receiving therapeutic doses of methylxanthines • Undergoing surgery	
Hct≤20/Hgb≤7	Infant without any symptoms and an absolute reticulocyte count <100,000 cells/μL (RBC x % uncorrected retics)	20 mL/kg PRBCs over 2-4 h (divide into two 10 mL/kg volumes if fluid sensitive)

CPAP, continuous positive airway pressure; Fio_2, fractional inspired oxygen; HR, heart rate; MAP, mean airway pressure; PRVCs, packed red blood cells; RBC, red blood cells; RR, respiratory rate.

*Hematocrit values are percentages; hemoglobin values are given in units of grams per deciliter.

(Christensen: Hematologic Problems of the Neonate 2000, p.161)

Erythrocyte Transfusion (Blood Transfusion, Packed RBC, PRBC)

A consistent Approach to Erythrocyte Transfusions in the NICU

Transfusion Product:

In general, we administer erythrocytes as packed erythrocytes from cytomegalovirus-negative donors, 15 mL/kg body weight, over 2 to 4 hours. Irradiation is performed when immune deficiency is suspected, organ transplantation is anticipated, or intrauterine transfusions have been given. An attempt is made to use directed-donor blood on parental request. Patients on extracorporeal membrane oxygenation or with certain types of congenital heart disease are not included in this approach.

(Calhoun: consistent approaches to procedures and practices in neonatal hematology. Clinics in Perinatology 2000,27:733-753)

Red Blood Cell Transfusion

Guidelines for Red Blood Cell Transfusions

Most RBC transfusions given to neonatal patients are small in volume (10 to 15 mL/kg) and are repeated frequently to replace blood drawn for laboratory studies. There is no proven benefit to routinely replacing phlebotomy blood losses milliliter for milliliter.

(Christensen: Hematologic Problems of the Neonate 2000, p.407)

Packed RBC (PRBC)

Blood Component Replacement

Packed RBC (PRBC) transfusion: concentrated RBCs, with HCT of 55-70%. Typed, crossmatched product preferred where possible; O-negative or O-positive blood may be used if transfusion cannot be delayed. O-negative is preferred for females of or below child-bearing age to reduce risks of Rh sensitization.

Unless rapid replacement is required for acute blood loss or shock, infuse no faster than 2-3 mL/kg per hour (generally 10 mL/kg aliquots over 4 hours) to avoid congestive heart failure.

(Siberry: The Harriet Lane Handbook 2000, p.319)

RBC transfusion

Very low birth weight (VLBW) infants frequently require small volume (10-20 ml/kg) RBC transfusions.

(Lilleyman: Pediatric Hematology 1999, p.720)

FRESH FROZEN PLASMA

Fresh Frozen Plasma (FFP)

The dose of FFP depends on the clinical situation and the underlying disease process. When FFP is given for coagulation factor replacement, the dose is 10-20 ml/kg. This dose will usually raise the level of coagulation factors by 20% immediately after infusion.

(Lilleyman: Pediatric Hematology 1999, p.727)

PLATELETS

Platelets

A Consistent Approach to Prophylactic Platelet Transfusions in the NICU

Platelet Transfusion Protocol:

Transfusion Product. Patients qualifying for a platelet transfusion should receive 10 to 15 mL/kg of a cytomegalovirus-negative standard platelet suspension, prepared from a fresh unit of whole blood or by platelet pheresis. This should be sufficient to increase the platelet count of a thrombocytopenic infant by approximately 100,000/μL. No volume-reducing processing is routinely recommended, because of the risk of platelet loss, clumping, and dysfunction caused by the additional handling.

(Calhoun: consistent approaches to procedures and practices in neonatal hematology. Clinics in Perinatology 2000,27:733-753)

Platelet Transfusions

Guidelines for Platelet Transfusions

The goal of most platelet transfusions is to raise the count to above $100x10^9/L$. This goal can be achieved consistently by the infusion of 5 to 10 mL/kg of standard platelet suspensions prepared from fresh units of whole blood or by automated platelet pheresis. Platelet suspensions should be transfused as rapidly as the baby's overall condition permits, certainly within 2 hours.

(Christensen: Hematologic Problems of the Neonate 2000, pp.412-413)

Platelets

Usually give 4 units/m^2, or approximately 10 mL/kg of normally concentrated platelet product. The platelet count is raised by 10,000-15,000/mm^3 by giving 1 unit/m^2. For infants and children, 10 mL/kg will increase the platelet count by approximately 50,000/mm^3. Hemorrhagic complications are rare with platelet counts >10,000/mm^3. Platelet count 50,000/mm^3 is advisable for minor procedures such as lumbar puncture; >100,000/mm^3 is advisable for major surgery or intracranial operation. Peak posttransfusion concentration is reached 45-60 minutes after transfusion.

Note: Platelet products should not be refrigerated because this promotes premature platelet activation and clumping.

(Siberry: The Harriet Lane Handbook 2000, pp:320-321)

GRANULOCYTES

Granulocyte Transfusions

A consistent approach to Granulocyte Transfusions in the NICU

Patients: The typical recipient of a neutrophil transfusion in our NICU has early onset sepsis and shock, is receiving mechanical ventilation and infusions of pressors, has a blood neutrophil concentration well below 1000/μL with a left shift, and has already received intravenous immune globulin (IVIG). For patients in this situation, we estimate that the likelihood of survival is very low. We have no evidence that rG-CSF is useful for patients in this condition. We administer 15 mL/kg of apheresis-collected irradiated cells over a period of 1 hour. We also measure a leukocyte count and differential on the bag of cells so that the exact dose of neutrophils delivered can be calculated. We aim to deliver a quantity of neutrophil of at least one normal total blood granulocyte pool, circulating plus marginated cells, which is 0.3 to 0.7 x 10^9/cells/kg body weight.

(Calhoun: Consistent approaches to procedures and practices in neonatal hematology. Clinics in Perinatology 2000, 27:733-753)

BRETYLIUM TOSYLATE (Bretylol)

Supplied: Injection 50mg/ml in 10ml

Administration: IV, IM

Safety and efficacy of this drug in children have not been established. Bretylol has been administered to a limited number of pediatric patients, but such use has been inadequate to fully define the proper dosage and limitations for use (1).

For IMMEDIATELY LIFE THREATENING VENTRICULAR ARRHYTHMIAS: Administer undiluted by rapid IV injection. For continuous suppression, administer as a constant infusion. An alternative maintenance schedule is to infuse the dose every 6 hours over 10-30 minutes. More rapid infusion may cause nausea and vomiting.

For OTHER VENTRICULAR ARRHYTHMIAS, administer the diluted solution over 10-30 minutes. For maintenance therapy, the same dose may be administered every 6 hours, or a constant infusion may be started (1). Physically compatible in D5W or NS (1).

For ventricular arrhythmias which are not immediately life-threatening, administer diluted solution over a period of 10 to 30 minutes (1).

IM administration: Vary injection site. Repeated injections into the same site may cause atrophy and necrosis of muscle tissue, fibrosis vascular degeneration and inflammatory changes (1).

Bretylium

Class: III

Uses: VF (dig. toxicity)
VT

Doses (Level): 5 mg/kg IV 1 min

Mode of Action: Inhibits NE release, Epi reuptake; weak cholinergic effects and local anesthetic; increase VF threshold

ECG/EP Changes: NO ECG changes

Side Effects: Transient ↑ BP and ↑ arrhythmia (if dig.-induced); later ↓ BP from vasodilation; quinidine antagonizes bretylium

(Garson: The science and practice of pediatric cardiology 1998, p.2953)

<u>Bretylium</u>

Bretylium has limited applications in the pediatric patient. It is mostly utilized in resuscitative settings for polymorphic ventricular tachycardias or monomorphic ventricular tachycardias resistant to other standard forms of therapy.

Dosing: IV: 5 mg/kg push

Warnings: Hypotension

Dosing: The intravenous dose of bretylium is 5 mg/kg as a rapid push during ventricular fibrillation. There are hypotensive effects such that in patients with hemodynamically table ventricular tachycardia, it should be diluted in 5% dextrose and given more slowly. The total dose should not exceed 30 mg/kg. A continuous infusion can be used at 15 to 30 µg/kg/min.

Bretylium may reverse the local anesthetic effect of quinidine and other sodium channel-blocking agents. This factor explains, to some degree, its application in quinidine-induced torsades de pointes. Although bretylium is given for digoxin-induced arrhythmias, the drug may worsen these rhythms initially because of the early release of norepinephrine. Tricyclic antidepressants block bretylium's synaptic effects.

Side Effects: The predominant adverse effect is hypotension, but during resuscitative measures this is rarely a concern if the rhythm being treated is ventricular fibrillation. The hypotensive effect is due to bretylium's peripheral adrenergic blocking properties.

(Gillette: Clinical Pediatric Arrhythmias 1999,pp.231-248)

<u>Bretylium</u>

Uses: VF (especially with digoxin toxicity), VT

Dosing: 5 mg/kg over 1 min; may be doubled

Acute Side Effects: Hypotension

Other Considerations: Quinidine antagonizes effect

VT, ventricular tachycardia; VF, ventricular fibrillation.

(Gillette: Clinical Pediatric Arrhythmias 1999, p.152)

<u>Bretylium</u>

Guidelines for Dosage: Antidysrhythmics

Dosage: 5 mg/kg i.v.; may repeat every 15-20 min to a maximum total of 30 mg/kg

Maintenance = 5 mg/kg every 6-8 h

(Allen: Moss and Adams' Heart Disease in Infants, Children, and Adolescents 2001, pp.1460-1468)

Bretylium Tosylate

Dose & Route: IV: 5-10 mg/kg/dose; may repeat Q10-20 min for **total dose** of 30 mg/kg.

IM: 2-5 mg/kg x 1
Maintenance dose (IM, IV): 5 mg/kg/dose Q6-8 hr

Remarks: **Contraindicated** in arrhythmias induced by digoxin toxicity. May cause initial hypertension followed by hypotension. May cause PVCs and increased sensitivity to digitalis and catecholamines.
Reduce dose in renal failure.

(Siberry: The Harriet Lane Handbook 2000, p.646)

BUMETANIDE (Bumex)

Supplied: Tablets: 0.5 mg, 1 mg, 2 mg.
Injection: 0.25 mg/ml in 2ml, 4ml, 10ml vials

Administration: IV, IM, PO.
Administer IV over a period of 1 to 2 minutes. It is stable with D5W, NS, LR in glass and viaflex containers. There are no significant absorption effects or loss due to drug degradation. Freshly prepare solutions and use within 24 hours.

Cross-sensitivity with furosemide is rare. Bumetanide can be substituted at about a 1:40 ratio of bumetanide to furosemide in patients allergic to furosemide (1).

Bumetanide (Bumex)

Indications and use:
Management of edema associated with congenital heart disease, congestive heart failure, hepatic or renal disease.

Actions: Inhibition of the active chloride and, possibly, sodium transport systems of the loop of Henle. Urinary excretion of sodium, chloride, potassium, hydrogen, calcium, magnesium, ammonium, phosphate, and bicarbonate increases with bumetanide-induced diuresis. Renal blood flow increases substantially due to renovascular dilation.

Route: PO, IV, IM.

Dosage: 0.015 mg/kg/dose up to 0.1 mg/kg/d.

Adverse effects: Hypokalemia, hypochloremia, hyponatremia, metabolic alkalosis, and hypotension.

Comments: Patients refractory to furosemide may respond to bumetanide for diuretic therapy. Although patient may respond differently, bumetanide is ~40 times more potent on a milligram per milligram basis than furosemide.

(Gomella: Neonatology 1999, p.555)

Bumetanide

Dosage: 0.1 mg/kg/dose IV to start. Increase as needed in 0.1 mg/kg increments. Oral dosing is identical to IV.

Comments: This is a loop diuretic that is more potent than furosemide as a diuretic but is equipotent in causing ototoxicity and liver damage; thus it is safer; it may be used at the same dose orally and intravenously because of excellent bioavailability.

(Fanaroff: Neonatal-Perinatal Medicine 1997, p.1749)

Bumetanide

Use: Management of edema secondary to congestive heart failure or hepatic or renal disease including nephrotic syndrome; may also be used alone or in combination with antihypertensives in the treatment of hypertension

Contraindications: Hypersensitivity to bumetanide or any component; in anuria or increasing azotemia

Warnings: Loop diuretics are potent diuretics; excess amounts can lead to profound diuresis with fluid and electrolyte loss; close medical supervision and dose evaluation is required; in vitro studies using pooled sera from critically ill neonates have shown bumetanide to be a potent displacer of bilirubin; avoid use in neonates at risk for kernicterus.

Usual Dosage: Oral, I.M., I.V.:

Neonates (see Warnings): 0.01-0.05 mg/kg/dose every 24-48 hours

Infants and Children: 0.015-0.1 mg/kg/dose every 6-24 hours (maximum dose: 10 mg/day)

Administration: Oral: Administer with food to decrease GI irritation
Parenteral: Administer without additional dilution by direct I.V. injection over 1-2 minutes

Monitoring Parameters: Blood pressure, serum electrolytes, renal function

Additional Information: Patients with impaired hepatic function must be monitored carefully, often requiring reduced doses; larger doses may be necessary in patients with impaired renal function to obtain the same therapeutic response

(Taketomo: Pediatric Dosage Handbook 1999-2000, pp.135-136)

Bumetanide (Bumex)

Dose: 1 mg PO is approx. equal to 40 mg PO furosemide

Mode of Action: Potent loop diuretic

Adverse Effects: Hypokalemia, hyponatremia, alkalosis

Comments: Very limited experience in young children

(Garson: The science and practice of pediatric cardiology 1998, p.2951)

CAFFEINE CITRATE

Supplied: Oral solution 20mg/ml 3 ml
Powder 125gm, 500gm

Administration: PO

Caution: The sodium benzoate component in caffeine and sodium benzoate injection reportedly produces kernicterus in neonates by uncoupling albumin-bilirubin binding (1).

Orphan drug status [Caffeine (Neocaf)]. Sponsor O.P.R. Development, L.P. Contact office Orphan Products Development (HF-35). (301) 443-2043 (1).

Extemporaneous Compounding (Recipe)

Dosage form: Injection
Made from: Powder
Concentration: 10 mg/mL
Stability: 3 months
Store: Refrigerate

Ingredient	Strength	Quantity
Caffeine powder		1 g
Bacteriostatic water for injection USP		qs ad 100 mL

Instructions: Dissolve the caffeine powder in the bacteriostatic water for injection in a clean glass graduate. Draw this solution into a plastic syringe, attach a sterile 0.22-µ filter, and filter into an empty sterile vial. (11)

Caffeine Citrate

Indications and use: Apnea of prematurity.

Actions: Similar to those of other methylxanthine drugs (eg, theobromine and theophylline). Caffeine appears to be more active on and less toxic to the CNS and the respiratory system. Proposed mechanisms of action include increased production of cAMP and alterations of intracellular calcium concentrations. Stimulates the CNS and exerts a positive inotropic effect on the myocardium. Stimulates voluntary skeletal muscle and gastric acid secretion. Increases renal blood flow and glomerular filtration rate. Stimulates glycogenolysis and lipolysis.

Route: IV, (not IM), PO.

Dosage: Loading dose: 20 mg caffeine citrate (10 mg caffeine base) IV or PO.
Maintenance dose (caffeine base): 2.5-5.0 mg/kg/day as a single daily dose.

Adverse effects: Nausea, vomiting, gastric irritation, agitation, tachycardia, and diuresis. Symptoms of overdosage include arrhythmias and tonic-clonic seizures.

Comments: Contraindicated in hypersensitivity to the drug. Therapeutic levels are 5-25 mcg/mL; severe toxicity is associated with levels >50 mcg/mL. Initial half-life in neonates is 90-100 h, decreasing to 6 h at ~60 weeks' postconceptual age. Serum levels should be monitored.

(Gomella: Neonatology 1999, p.555)

<u>Caffeine</u>

Route & Dose: PO, IV: loading dose = 10 mg/kg; maintenance dose = 2.5 mg/kg/dose q 24 h (doses are for the nonsalt form of drug-caffeine base).

Adverse Effects and Cautions:
Restlessness, emesis, tachycardia; therapeutic plasma concentration = 5-20 µg/ml free base

(Taeusch: Avery's Diseases of the Newborn 1998, p.1343)

<u>Caffeine</u> (Caffeine citrate)

Dose & Route: **Doses expressed in mg of caffeine citrate. To convert to mg of caffeine base divide citrate dose by 2**.
Neonatal apnea:
Loading dose: 10-20 mg/kg IV/PO x 1
Maintenance dose: 5-10 mg/kg/dose
PO/IV QD, to begin 24 hr after loading dose.

Remarks: **Avoid use** in symptomatic cardiac arrhythmias. Caffeine benzoate formulation has been associated with causation of kernicterus in neonates.

Therapeutic levels: 5-25 mg/L.

Cardiovascular, neurologic, or GI toxicity reported at serum levels >50 mg/L.

Recommended serum sampling time: obtain trough level within 30 minutes prior to an oral dose. Steady-state is typically achieved 3 weeks following the initiation of therapy. Levels obtained prior to steady-state are useful for preventing toxicity.

(Siberry: The Harriet Lane Handbook 2000, pp.649-650)

CALCITRIOL (Rocaltrol cap, Calcijex inj)

Supplied: Capsules 0.25mcg and 0.5mcg
Injection 1mcg, 2mcg/ml

Administration: PO, IV
Unlabeled usage: To manage hypocalcemia in premature infants, 1 mcg of oral calcitriol daily has been used during the first five days of life. To control hypocalcemia tetany in infants, some clinicians have used an IV calcitriol dosage of 0.05 mcg/kg for 5 to 12 days (3).

<u>Calcitriol</u> (1,25-dihydroxycholecalciferol, Rocaltrol)

Dose & Route: Renal failure: Children:
Oral: Suggested dose range 0.01-0.05 mcg/kg/24hr.
Titrate in 0.005-0.01 mcg/kg/24hr increments Q4-8 wk based on clinical response.
IV: 0.01-0.05 mcg/kg/dose given 3 x/week

Remarks: Most potent vitamin D metabolite available. Monitor serum calcium and phosphorus. **Avoid** concomitant use of Mg^{++}-containing antacids. IV dosing applies if patient under going hemodialysis.

Contraindicated in patients with hypercalcemia, vitamin D toxicity. Side effects include; weakness, headache, vomiting, constipation, hypotonia, polydipsia, polyuria, myalgia, metastatic calcification, etc.

Pregnancy category changes to "D" if used in doses above the recommended daily allowance.

(Siberry: The Harriet Lane Handbook 2000, p.651)

Calcitriol

Route: PO, IV
Neonatal Dose: 0.05 mcg/kg/24 hr.
Pediatric Dose: 0.01-0.05 mcg/kg/24 hr. Titrate increments Q2-4 wk.

Discussion: Most potent vitamin D available; monitor for hypercalcemia; do not use magnesium antacids.

(Rudolph: Rudolph's Pediatrics 1996, p.2174)

CALCIUM

Calcium Equivalents

Calcium salt	Calcium (mg/gram)	Calcium (mEq/gram)	% Calcium
Calcium acetate	253	12.7	25.3
Calcium carbonate	400	20	40
Calcium chloride	270	13.5	27
Calcium citrate	211	10.6	21.1
Calcium glubionate	64	3.2	6.5
Calcium gluceptate	82	4.1	8.2
Calcium gluconate	90	4.5	9
Calcium lactate	130	6.5	13
Calcium phosphate			
Dibasic	230	11.5	23
Tribasic	400	20	40

(1)

CALCIUM CARBONATE

(Calcium Carbonate, Titralac, Ro kare)

Supplied: Suspension 500mg/5ml (1.25 gm Calcium Cabonate/5mL)
400mg/5ml (1 gm Calcium Cabonate/5mL)

Comment: Contains 40% Calcium, 20mEq Calcium/g.

Calcium Carbonate

Doses expressed in mg of elemental Calcium. To convert to mg of salt, divide elemental dose by 0.4

Dose & Route: Hypocalcemia:
Neonates: 50-150 mg/kg/24 hr ÷ Q4-6 hr PO;
max dose: 1 g/24 hr

Children: 45-65 mg/kg/24 hr PO ÷ QID

Remarks: Side effects: constipation, hypercalcemia, hypophosphatemia, hypomagnesemia, nausea, vomiting, headache, confusion. May reduce absorption of tetracycline, iron, and effectiveness of polystrene sulfonate. May potentiate effects of digoxin. Some products may contain trace amounts of Na. Administer each dose with meals or with lots of fluid.

(Siberry: The Harriet Lane Handbook 2000, p.651)

Calcium carbonate

Route: PO

Neonatal Dose: Prophylaxis of GI bleeding:
100-250 mg/dose (2-5 mL/dose at concentration of 250 mg/5mL) q1-2h as needed

Calcium replacement:
RDA is 900 mg/d (360 mg/d of elemental calcium)

Pediatric Dose: Prophylaxis of GI bleeding or ulcer treatment:
250-750 mg/dose (5-15 mL/dose at concentration of 250 mg/mL) q1-2h

Calcium replacement:
RDA is 1250-2000 mg/d (500-800 mg/d of elemental calcium)

Discussion: There is 4.5 mEq of calcium per g of calcium carbonate; for ulcer treatment use the hourly dose only for the first 2 wk of treatment, then dose it every 3-6 h after meals and at bedtime until healed

(Rudolph: Rudolph's Pediatrics 1996, p.2174)

CALCIUM CHLORIDE

Supplied: Injection 10% Solution 1gm/10ml

Administration: IV
1 gram calcium chloride contains 270mg (13.6mEq) calcium FOR IV USE ONLY (1). Osmolarity is approximately 1765 Mosm/L (5). Calcium Chloride, by any route of administration, produces more irritation than the other calcium salts and has been reported to cause GI hemorrhage when taken orally (3).

Compatible: Alprostadil, dopamine, epinephrine, morphine (9).

Incompatible: Sodium bicarbonate (9).

Calcium Chloride (10%)

Dosage (pediatric) 20 mg/kg per dose

Remarks: Give slowly

Therapeutic Considerations

Calcium is essential to excitation-contraction coupling. when cardiac muscle cells are excited, calcium ions enter the cytoplasm and induce the coupling of action and myosin. This event is terminated when calcium ions are actively pumped out of the cytoplasm. In normal hearts calcium increases myocardial contractile function. In the presence of myocardial ischemia, energy sources are depleted and this pumping mechanism may be compromised, allowing calcium to accumulate in the cytoplasm. This hypercalcemia may have toxic consequence.

Approximately half of intravascular calcium is ionized. This physiologically active portion must be considered when evaluating the child's calcium balance. The plasma ionized calcium is affected by pH and serum albumin concentration because these factors affect calcium binding to protein. Acidosis increases the plasma ionized calcium., and alkalosis the plasma ionized calcium. Although a fall in serum albumin concentration is associated with a decrease in total calcium, the ionized calcium concentration may remain normal because a smaller amount of calcium is bound to protein. conversely, although a rise in serum albumin is associated with a rise in total calcium concentration, the ionized calcium concentration may be inadequate because more calcium is bound to protein.

Septic shock and blood transfusions have also been linked with alterations in serum ionized calcium. Children with septic shock may demonstrate a decrease in serum ionized calcium despite a normal total serum calcium. The serum ionized calcium may also fall after administration of blood preserved with citrate-phosphate-dextran.

Inotropic effects of calcium following cardiac arrest were initially documented in cardiovascular surgical patients after cardiopulmonary bypass. However, studies have shown that calcium entry into the cell cytoplasm is the final common pathway of cell death, and calcium administration during cardiac arrest may actually cause injury. The deleterious effects of calcium are also suggested by the salutary effects of calcium channel blockers in myocardial preservation during cardiopulmonary bypass.

Indications:

Calcium is not recommended for the treatment of either asystole or electromechanical dissociation. NO evidence supports its use in asystole, and its value in the treatment of electromechanical dissociation is questionable. Evidence also suggests that administration of an adrenergic drug is much more effective than calcium in the treatment of electromechanical dissociation.

Calcium therapy is indicated for treatment of documented or suspected hypocalcemia, hyperkalemia, hypermagnesemia, and calcium channel blocker overdose.

Dose: Calcium is available as three different salts. Calcium chloride or calcium gluconate will effectively correct hypocalcemia, provided that each delivers an equivalent dose of elemental calcium. Calcium gluconate (10%) contains approximately 9 mg/mL of elemental calcium, and calcium chloride (10%) contains approximately 27.2 mg/mL of elemental calcium. the dose and volume of calcium gluconate must be three times the dose and volume of calcium chloride to provide an equivalent dose of elemental calcium. Calcium chloride is most commonly used in critically ill children and adults and appears to produce consistently higher and more predictable levels of elemental calcium when administered to correct hypocalcemia.

The current recommended dose of 5 to 7 mg/kg of elemental calcium for treatment of hypocalcemia is extrapolated from adult data and limited pediatric data. Calcium chloride is a 10% solution (100 mg/mL of the calcium salt) that contains 1.36 mEq/mL elemental calcium (27.2 mg/mL elemental calcium). Therefore, a dose of 0.2 to 0.25 mL/kg calcium chloride will deliver 5 to 7 mg/kg elemental calcium (20 to 25 mg/kg calcium salt). The first dose of calcium should be infused *slowly* (no faster than 100 mg/min) and repeated once after 10 minutes, if required. Since repeated doses of calcium increase the risk of morbidity, the dose should be repeated only if *measured* calcium deficiency, particularly plasma ionized calcium deficiency, is present.

Precautions: Rapid calcium administration may induce significant bradycardia and even cardiac asystole, especially if the patient is receiving digoxin. Calcium forms an insoluble precipitate in the presence of sodium bicarbonate. It can sclerose peripheral veins and produce a severe chemical burn if the medication infiltrates into surrounding tissue.

(American Academy of Pediatrics. American Heart Association. Pediatric Advance Life Support. 1997, pp.6-10, 6-11, 6-14)

<u>Calcium Chloride</u>

Indications and use:

Symptomatic hypocalcemia such as neonatal tetany. Last-resort agent in cardiac arrest when other agents have failed to improve myocardial contraction. Overdose of calcium channel blocker.

Actions: Calcium is essential for the functional integrity of the nervous, muscular, skeletal, and cardiac systems and for clotting function.

Route: IV, PO.

Dosage: Cardiac arrest (as last resort): 20-30 mg/kg/dose (10% solution) IV q10min prn.
Maintenance in infants: 70 mg/kg/day IV divided q6h or as infusion.

Adverse effects: Arrhythmias (eg, bradycardia) and deterioration of cardiovascular function. Extravasation may cause skin sloughing. May potentiate digoxin-related arrhythmias.

Comments: Contraindicated in ventricular fibrillation or hypercalcemia. Use with caution in digitalized patients. Chloride salt is preferred to gluconate form (see Calcium Gluconate) during cardiac arrest because the calcium in the chloride is already ionized and the gluconate requires metabolism to release the calcium ion. Precipitates when mixed with sodium bicarbonate.

(Gomella: Neonatology 1999, pp.555-556)

Calcium Chloride (27% Elemental Calcium)

Dose & Route: Doses expressed in mg of CaCl
Cardiac arrest:
Infant/Child: 20 mg/kg/dose IV (0.2 ml/kg/dose) Q10 min.

MAXIMUM IV ADMINISTRATION RATES:
IV push: **Do not exceed** 100 mg/min
IV infusion: **Do not exceed** 45-90 mg/kg/hr with a **maximum concentration** of 20 mg/ml.

Remarks: Use IV with extreme caution. Extravasation may lead to necrosis. Hyaluronidase may be helpful for extravasation. Central-line administration is preferred IV route of administration. **Do not administer IM or SC route.**

Rapid IV infusion associated with bradycardia, hypotension, and peripheral vasodilation. May cause hyperchloremic acidosis.

(Siberry: The Harriet Lane Handbook 2000, p.652)

Calcium

Indication: For Neonatal Seizures

I do not administer calcium routinely to all newborns during the initial seizure, except in the unusual instance of a classic presentation for later-onset hypocalcemia. If hypocalcemia is present, 5% calcium gluconate is given intravenously in a dose of 4 ml/kg (200 mg/kg). electrocardiogram, or at least cardiac rhythm by auscultation, should be monitored during administration. It si important to recognize that phenobarbital can suppress the seizures of hypocalcemia, and, thus, a decrease in seizures after phenobarbital administration does not rule out hypocalcemia as cause. If hypomagnesemia is present, magnesium sulfate is best given intramuscularly as a 50% solution in a dose of 0.2 ml/kg. In this regard it should be recalled that approximately one half of newborns with seizures secondary to later-onset hypocalcemia also have hypomagnesemia. The importance of treating these hypocalcemic infants with magnesium is emphasized by the following facts: (1) the administration of calcium to such infants may increase renal excretion of magnesium, aggravate the hypomagnesemia, and maintain the convulsive state; and (2) the administration of magnesium has been shown to correct *both* the hypocalcemia and the hypomagnesemia, perhaps by increasing movement of calcium from bone to plasma. However, magnesium cannot be administered with abandon because magnesium can produce a neuromuscular blockade. Transient weakness and hypotonia (without concentrations of plasma magnesium out of the normal range) are often noted in infants given magnesium. Moreover, it should be recalled that the maintenance doses of magnesium and calcium shown in Table 5-30 should be administered only as long as needed to avoid hypomagnesemia or hypocalcemia.

(Volpe: Neurology of the Newborn 2001, p.208)

SEE ALSO: THERAPY FOR NEONATAL SEIZURES p.657

Calcium chloride (10%)

Dose: 1 mL IV <7 kg

Comments: Increases contractility, systemic vascular resistance; may cause bradycardia; may cause skin slough

(Garson: The science and practice of pediatric cardiology 1998, p.2956)

CALCIUM GLUBIONATE (NeoCalglucon)

Supplied: Syrup 1.8gm Calcium Glubionate/5ml 480ml (supplies 115mg Calcium/5ml)

Administration: PO

1gm calcium glubionate contains 64mg (3.2mEq) calcium (3).

Calcium Glubionate (Neo-Calglucon)

Dose/kg: Hypocalcemia: 10-20 mg elemental Ca

Route & Frequency: PO; q6h

Comments: Give prior to feeds for best absorption. High osmotic load; large dose may cause diarrhea. Dilute 1:1 with sterile water to halve osmolarity. Monitor serum Ca levels.

(Avery: Neonatology Pathophysiology and Management of the Newborn, 1999, p.1553)

Calcium glubionate

Route & Dose: PO: treatment = 500-1000 mg/kg/day q 3-4 h; supplement = 150 mg/kg/day q 3-4 h

Adverse Effects and Cautions:

High osmotic load of syrup may cause diarrhea

Comment: 23mg Elemental Ca^{2+}/ml

(Taeusch: Avery's Diseases of the Newborn 1998, p.1343)

Calcium Glubionate*

Dosage: 500 mg/kg/day divided every 4-8hr PO.

Comments: High osmotic load.

(* Corrected following communication with author)

(Fanaroff: Neonatal-Perinatal Medicine 1997, p.1751)

Calcium Glubionate (Neocalglucon, 6.4% Elemental calcium)

Dose & Route: **Doses expressed in mg Calcium glubionate**
Neonatal hypocalcemia: 1200 mg/kg/24hr PO÷Q4-6hr
Maintenance:
Infant/Child: 600-2000 mg/kg/24hr PO÷QID; **max dose**: 9 g/24hr

Remarks: Side effects include GI irritation, dizziness, and headache. Best absorbed when given before meals. Absorption inhibited by high phosphate load. High osmotic load of syrup (20% sucrose) may cause diarrhea.

(Siberry: The Harriet Lane Handbook 2000, p.652)

CALCIUM GLUCEPTATE

Supplied: Injection 1.1gm/5ml in 5ml amps
Administration: IM, IV
1.1gm Calcium Gluceptate contains 90mg (4.5mEq) Calcium.

For IM administration inject into the lateral thigh in infants (1). For IV administration, inject undiluted at a rate not exceeding 1 to 2 ml/minute. For intermittent infusion, infuse at a rate not exceeding 200mg/minute (2).

Calcium Gluceptate

Route: IV, IM

Neonatal Dose: Cardiac arrest: 110 Mg/kg/dose given slowly and repeated q10 min if needed.
Maintenance: 200-700 mg/kg/24h by infusion or in divided doses.

Pediatric Dose: Cardiac arrest: 110 mg/kg/dose given slowly and repeated q10min if needed.
Maintenance: 200-500 mg/kg/24 h by infusion or in divided doses.

Discussion: Has 4.5 mEq of calcium per 1 g of calcium gluceptate; give IV doses at a rate of no more than 50 mg/min; for exchange transfusions give 100 mg/kg/dose after each 100 mL of blood exchanged.

(Rudolph: Rudolph's Pediatrics 1996, p.2174)

CALCIUM GLUCONATE

Supplied: Injection 10% Solution (1gm/10ml)
Administration: IV
1 gram calcium gluconate contains 93mg (4.65mEq) calcium.

For IV use only, either by direct IV injection at a rate not greater than 0.5mL to 2mL/minute or by intermittent IV infusion. SC or IM injection may cause severe tissue necrosis and/or sloughing (1).

See hyaluronidase for calcium extravasation (author)

Calculated osmolarity is 700 mOsm/L(5).

Compatible: Amikacin, aminophylline, dobutamine, epinephrine, erythromycin, famotidine, heparin with hydrocortisone, labetalol, lidocaine, magnesium, methicillin, penicillin G, phenobarbital, potassium chloride, tobramycin, vancomycin, tolazoline.

Note: Compatibility of calcium with phosphate in parenteral nutrition depends on a number of factors (discussed in text) (9).

Incompatible: Amphotericin B, indomethacin, methylprednisolone, metoclopramide, sodium bicarbonate (9).

Calcium Gluconate10%
(9.4 10% mg elemental Ca^{2+}/mL)

Dose/kg: Hypocalcemia: 10-20 mg elemental Ca
Route & frequency: IV, PO q6-q12h

Dose/kg: Cardiac arrest: 10 mg elemental CA
Route & frequency: IV may repeat every 10 min

Comments: May cause bradycardia and potentiation of digitalis.

Extravasation causes necrosis of subcutaneous tissues. Do not use scalp veins. Precipitates with NaBicard and Phosphate slats. Monitor serum Ca levels.

(Avery: Neonatology Pathophysiology and Management of the Newborn 1999, p.1552)

Calcium Gluconate (9.4% calcium)

Dose & Route: **Doses expressed in mg Calcium gluconate**
Maintenance/hypocalcemia:
Neonates: IV: 200-800 mg/kg/24hr÷Q6hr.
Infants: IV: 200-500 mg/kg/24hr÷Q6hr.
PO: 400-800 mg/kg/24hr÷Q6hr

For cardiac arrest:
Infants and children: 100 mg/kg/dose (1 ml/kg/dose) IV Q10 min.

MAXIMUM IV ADMINISTRATIN RATES:
IV push: **Do not exceed** 100 mg/min
IV infusion: **Do not exceed** 120-240 mg/kg/hr with a **maximum concentration** of 50 mg/ml

Remarks: **Avoid** peripheral infusion as extravasation may cause tissue necrosis. IV infusion associated with hypotension and bradycardia. Also associated with arrhythmias in digitalized patients. May precipitate when used with bicarbonate. **Do not use scalp veins! Do not administer IM or SC**.

(Siberry: The Harriet Lane Handbook 2000, p.653)

Calcium Gluconate

Acute Treatment of Neonatal Seizures

Dose: 5% solution: 4 mL/kg IV

(Hill: Neonatal Seizures Pediatrics in Review 2000;21:117-121)

Calcium gluconate (10%)

Dose: 0.3-0.6 mL/kg IV

Comments: Increased contractility, systemic vascular resistance; may cause bradycardia; may cause skin slough

(Garson: The science and practice of pediatric cardiology 1998, p.2956)

Calcium Gluconate

The citrate buffer binds calcium and transiently lowers ionized calcium levels. Treatment of suspected hypocalcemia in patients receiving transfusions is *controversial*. Some physicians routinely administer 1-2 mL of 10% calcium gluconate by slow infusion after 100-200 mL of exchange donor blood. Others maintain that this treatment has no therapeutic effect unless hypocalcemia is documented by electrocardiogram showing a change in the Q-T interval.

(Gomella: Neonatology: Management, Procedures, On-call Problems, Diseases and Drugs 1999, p.168)

CALCIUM LACTATE

Supplied: Tablets 325 and 650mg

Administration: PO

1 gm Calcium Lactate contains 130mg (6.5mEq) calcium (1).

Calcium lactate 13%

Route & Dose: PO: 0.5 gm/kg/day in divided doses q 6-8 h

Adverse Effects and Cautions:

See Calcium gluconate; gastrointestinal irritation

(Taeusch: Avery's Diseases of the Newborn 1998, p.1343)

Calcium Lactate (13% Ca^{++})

Dosage: 500 mg/kg/day divided every 4-8 hr PO

(Fanaroff: Neonatal-Perinatal Medicine 1997, p.1751)

Calcium Lactate (13% calcium)

Dose & Route: **Doses expressed in mg of Calcium lactate.**

Infants: 400-500 mg/kg/24 hr PO ÷ Q4-6hr.

Children: 500 mg/kg/24 hr PO ÷ Q6-8 hr.

Remarks: Give with meals. Do not dissolve tablets in milk.

(Siberry: The Harriet Lane Handbook 2000, p.654)

CAPTOPRIL (Capoten)

Supplied: Tablets 12.5 mg, 25mg, 50mg, 100mg

Administration: PO

Solution - the tablets may be used. In one study, the stability of Captopril in various solutions (stored in glass bottles) was tested. The results are as follows:

Syrup, 7 days at 4° and 22°C, 39° and 72°F;
Distilled water, 7 days at 22° and 14 days at 4°C;
Distilled water plus sodium ascorbate 14 days at 22°C and 56 days at 4°C (1).

Extemporaneous Compounding (Recipe)

Dosage form: Oral suspension
Made from: Tablets
Concentration: 1 mg/mL
Stability: 56 days
Store: Refrigerate
Label: Shake well

Ingredient	Strength	Quantity
Captopril tablets	50 mg	2
Sodium ascorbate injection or ascorbic acid tablets		500 mg
Distilled water		qs add 100 mL

Instructions: Allow 2 tablets of captopril 50 mg to dissolve in 50 mL of water in a graduate. Add the contents of a 500-mg ampul of sodium ascorbate or a 500-mg ascorbic acid tablet to the mixture and qs with distilled water. Shake well to disperse. Do not filter.

Note: A sulfur-like odor is not indicative of captopril degradation. (11)

Captopril (Capoten)

THERAPY FOR ACUTE CONGESTIVE CARDIAC FAILURE

Dose and Route of Administration:

Neonates and children: begin at 0.3 mg/kg/dose p.o. q8h; titrate to hemodynamic effect.
Older children and adolescents: 12.5 to 25.0 mg/dose q8h (maximum = 75 mg/dose).

Hemodynamic Effects:

Mixed vasodilation. Lowers systemic vascular resistance and preload.

Complications and Comments Regarding Use:

Proteinuria, Neutropenia, Hyperkalemia

Note: We begin captopril orally or by nasogastric administration at 0.3 mg/kg/day divided in three doses, and increase the dosage according to the desired hemodynamic effects as determined by the physical exam. The drug is best absorbed during fasting, as absorption is reduced by one-third if taken after meals. Peak blood levels occur in 30 to 90 minutes. The plasma clearance rate is about 2 hours, and the drug is rapidly excreted in the urine. About 50% of an orally administered dose appears in the urine within 4 hours. The elimination of captopril closely follows the creatinine clearance, so the dose must be decreased for patients with renal dysfunction. Serious side effects and toxicities are unusual, but proteinuria, nephrotic syndrome, glomerulonephritis, and neutropenia have been reported. It is very important to keep in mind that captopril spares potassium at the renal level, which is important in these patients, who often simultaneously receive diuretics along with supplemental potassium.

(Garson: The science and practice of pediatric cardiology 1998, pp.2329-2341)

Captopril (Capoten)

Indications and use: Congestive heart failure and hypertension.

Actions: Competitive inhibitor of angiotensin-converting enzyme. Causes fall in angiotensin II and aldosterone levels, decrease in systemic vascular resistance, and augmentation of cardiac output.

Route: PO

Dosage: Neonates: Initial: 0.05 mg/kg/dose, then 0.1-0.4 mg/kg/dose 1-4 times daily.
Infants: 0.05 mg/kg/dose, then 0.5-6.0 mg/kg/day divided q6-24h.

Adverse effects: Hypotension, rash, fever, eosinophilia, neutropenia, GI disturbances. A low initial dose is used because some infants have experienced a dramatic drop in blood pressure

Comments: Use with caution in patients with low renal perfusion pressure. Reduce dose with renal impairment. and in sodium- and water-depleted patients.

(Gomella: Neonatology 1999, p.556)

Captopril

Vasodilator Therapy in Children with CHF

Dose/Route of Administration:

Infants: 0.1-0.5 mg/kg/dose PO q 8-12 hr,
4 mg/kg/day max

Disadvantages: May cause neutropenia or proteinuria, mild GI distress, taste impairment, or rashes

Clinical Use of Orally Available Vasodilators

Captopril is the first and best-known ACE inhibitor. It is generally given before meals and enters the circulation rapidly, with peak plasma concentrations observed approximately 60 minutes after a single dose. The plasma half-life is only about 2 hours, but the duration of effect is about 8 hours. The drug is generally well tolerated. Mild side effects include rashes, taste impairment, and mild gastrointestinal disturbance. Neutropenia can occur and may require cessation of therapy. Potassium supplementation or potasium-sparing diuretics are not necessary in using captopril and, in face, should be avoided to prevent possible hyperkalemia. Enalapril is a newer drug with a mechanism of action similar to captopril's. Its use is gaining popularity in children. It has the advantage of a less frequent dosing schedule, which may increase patient compliance.

(Garson: The science and practice of pediatric cardiology 1998, pp.2321-2322)

Captopril (Capoten)

Dose: 0.1-0.5 mg/kg/dose PO q8-12hr in infants, max. 4 mg/kg/day
0.1-2 mg/kg/dose PO q8-12hr older children

Mode of Action: Competitive inhibition of angiotensin-converting enzyme, some aldosterone inhibition

Adverse Effects: Hypotension if volume-depleted, rash taste impairment, GI upset, neutropenia, proteinuria

Comments: Avoid potassium-sparing diuretics and K^+ supplements

(Garson: The science and practice of pediatric cardiology 1998, p.2951)

Captopril

Route & Dose: PO: 0.05-0.1 mg/kg/dose q 6-24 h; increase dose up to 0.5 mg/kg/dose to control blood pressure

Adverse Effects and Cautions:
High initial doses may cause hypotension and renal insufficiency

(Taeusch: Avery's Diseases of the Newborn 1998, p.1343)

Captopril

Dose/kg: 0.05-0.1 mg; may titrate up to 0.5 mg

Route & frequency: PO q6h-q24h

Comments: Give 1 h prior to feeds. Adjust dose in renal dysfunction Monitor blood pressure; severe hypotension may occur in patients who are Na^+ or volume depleted. May cause rash, proteinuria, neutropenia.

(Avery: Neonatology Pathophysiology and Management of the Newborn 1999, p.1552)

Captopril

Dose & Route: Neonates: 0.1-0.4 mg/kg/24 hr PO ÷ Q6-8 hr
Infants: Initially 0.15-0.3 mg/kg/dose; titrate upward if needed; **max dose**: 6 mg/kg/24 hr ÷ QD-QID
Children: Initially 0.3-0.5 mg/kg/dose Q8 hr; titrate upward if needed; **max dose**: 6 mg/kg/24 hr ÷ BID-QID

Remarks: Onset within 15-30 min of administration. Peak effect within 1-2 hr. **Adjust dose with renal failure**. Should be administered on an empty stomach 1 hr before or 2 hr after meals. Titrate to minimal effective dose.

Use with **caution** in collagen vascular disease. May cause rash, proteinuria, neutropenia, cough, angioedema, hyperkalemia, hypotension, or diminution of taste perception (with long0term use). Known to decrease aldosterone and increase renin production.

Pregnancy category is a "C" during the first trimester but changes to a "D" for the second and third trimester.
(Siberry: The Harriet Lane Handbook 2000, p.654)

<u>Captopril</u>

Two infants with biopsy-proven microcystic Finnish congenital nephrotic syndrome (onset at birth) were treated with a combination of captopril and indomethacin for 2 1/2 and 2 years, respectively; they had a marked reduction of urinary protein excretion without further need for albumin infusions......At 2 months of age, combined therapy with captopril (gradually increasing dosage to a maximum of 5 mg/kg body weight) and indomethacin (maximum dosage 4 mg/kg) was begun.
(Pomeranz: Successful treatment of Finnish congenital nephrotic syndrome with captopril and indomethacin. J Pediatr 1995;126:140-142)

CARBAMAZEPINE (Tegretol)

Supplied: Tablets, Chewable 100mg
Tablets 200mg
Oral Suspension 100mg/5ml

Administration: PO

Administration of phenobarbital, phenytoin, or primidone, or a combination of these may lower serum levels of carbamazepine. Erythromycin and cimetidine may inhibit the metabolism of carbamazepine.
The pharmacologic effect of both drugs may be decreased (1).

Shake suspension well before using. DO NOT administer suspension simultaneously with other liquid medicinal agents or diluents (1).

<u>Carbamazepine</u>

Indication: For Neonatal Seizures

Carbamazepine has been reported to be effective as an initial agent in the treatment of neonatal seizures in a study of 10 full-term infants with hypoxic-ischemic encephalopathy. All patients showed an "excellent" clinical response. Therapeutic levels were achieved within 2 to 4 hours after a loading dose of 10 mg/kg administered by nasogastric tube. However, variability in blood levels suggests that more data are needed to determine the value of this agent.
(Volpe: Neurology of the Newborn 2001, p.206)

<u>Carbamazepine</u> (Tegretol)

Indications and use:

Anticonvulsant. Prophylaxis against partial (especially complex partial), primary generalized tonic-clonic seizures and mixed seizures, including the above. Not effective for absence (petit mal) seizures.

Actions: Acts by reducing polysynaptic responses and blocking the posttetanic potentiation.

Pharmacokinetics:

Absorbed slowly from the GI tact. Protein binding is 76%. Metabolized in the liver to active epoxide by cytochrome P450 3A4. Induces liver enzymes and increases its own metabolism. Eliminated 72% in urine and 28% in feces. Half-life in neonates is 8-28 h. Therapeutic range is 4-12 mcg/mL. *Interactions*: Erythromycin, isoniazid, and cimetidine may inhibit hepatic metabolism of carbamazepine, resulting in increased carbamazepine serum concentrations. Concurrent phenobarbital may lower carbamazepine serum levels. Carbamazepine may induce metabolism of warfarin, phenytoin, theophylline, benzodiazepines, and corticosteroids. Thyroid function tests may show decreased values with carbamazepine.

Route: PO. No parenteral form available.

Dosage: 5 mg/kg/day PO initially. May increase weekly to 10 mg/kg/day, then to a maximum of 20 mg/kg/day if needed. Administer the daily dose in 3-4 divided doses. Administer with feedings.

Adverse effects: GI: Nausea and vomiting. Hematologic: Leukopenia, thrombocytopenia, aplastic anemia, and agranulocytosis. Cardiovascular: Congestive heart failure, heart block, and cardiovascular collapse. CNS: Dystonia, drowsiness, and behavioral changes. Ophthalmic: Eyes: scattered punctate cortical lens opacities. Endocrine/metabolic: Syndrome of inappropriate antidiuretic hormone (SIADH). Hepatic: Hepatitis and cholestasis. Dermatologic: Rash and Stevens-Johnson syndrome. Genitourinary: Urine retention, azotemia, oliguria, and anuria. Monitor CBC, liver function, and urinalysis; perform periodic eye exam. Do not discontinue abruptly, as seizures may result in epileptic patients.

Comments: Avoid switching between Tegretol and generic carbamazepine if possible, because changes in carbamazepine serum concentration and seizure activity may result; monitor serum concentrations.

(Gomella: Neonatology 1999, pp. 556-557)

<u>Carbamazepine</u> (Tegretol)

Dose & Route: <6yr:

Initial: 10-20 mg/kg/24 hr PO ÷ BID-TID (QID for suspension)

Increment: q5-7 days up to 35 mg/kg/24 hr PO

Remarks: **Contraindicated** for patients taking MAO inhibitors or who are sensitive to tricyclic antidepressants. Erythromycin, verapamil, cimetidine, and INH may increase serum levels.

Carbamazepine may decrease activity of warfarin, doxycycline, oral contraceptives, cyclosporin, theophyline, phenytoin, benzodiazepines, ethosuximide, and valproic acid. Carbamazepine is a substrate and inducer of CYP 450 3A3-4

Suggested dosing intervals for specific dosages forms: Extended release tabs or caps (BID); chewable and immediate release tablets (BID-TID); suspension (QID). Doses may be administered with food. Do not crash or chew extended release dosage forms. Do not administer the oral suspension simultaneously with other liquid medicines or diluents.

Drug metabolism typically increases after the first month of therapy due to hepatic autoconduction. $T_{1/2}$ = 25-65 hrs, initially. $T_{1/2}$ for children = 8-14 hrs.

Therapeutic blood levels: 4-12 mg/L.
Recommended serum sampling time: obtain trough level within 30 minutes prior to an oral dose. Steady-state is typically achieved one month following the initiation of therapy (following enzymatic autoinduction). Levels obtained prior to steady-state are useful for preventing toxicity.

Side effects include sedation, dizziness, diplopia, aplastic anemia, neutropenia, urinary retention, nausea, SIADH, and Stevens-Johnson syndrome. Pretreatment CBCs and LFTs is suggested. Patient should be monitored for hematologic and hepatic toxicity. **Adjust dose in renal impairment**.

(Siberry: The Harriet Lane Handbook 2000, p.655)

CARDIOVERSION (Defibrillation)

Cardioversion (Defibrillation)

DC Counter Shock: SVT: 0.25-1.0 J/kg
VT: 1.0-2.0 J/kg

(Allen: Moss and Adams' Heart Disease in Infants, Children, and Adolescents 2001, pp.1460-1468)

Cardioversion (Defibrillation)

DC Shock: 1-2 J/kg

Comments: Use 0.5-1 J/kg for cardioversion. For defibrillation, may require 2-4 J/kg

(Allen: Moss and Adams' Heart Disease in Infants, Children, and Adolescents 2001, pp.1460-1468)

Cardioversion

Ventricular Fibrillation

Defibrillation: The definitive treatment for VF or pulseless VT is prompt defibrillation, but defibrillation is not indicated for treatment of asystole. Ventilation with 100% oxygen and chest compressions should be continued until the moment of defibrillation. Ideally, vascular access is secured, but defibrillation should not be delayed to achieve this access.

Defibrillation is the untimed (asynchronous) depolarization of a critical mass of myocardial cells to allow spontaneous organized myocardial depolarization to resume. If organized depolarization does not resume, VF will continue or will progress to electrical silence. At this point restoration of spontaneous cardiac activity may be impossible. Synchronized cardioversion also results in depolarization of the myocardium, but cardioversion provides depolarization that is timed (synchronous) with the patient's intrinsic electrical activity. Since the patient with VF has no organized cardiac electrical activity, defibrillation must be provided.

Successful defibrillation requires the passage of sufficient electric current (amperes) through the heart. This current flow depends on the energy (joules) provided and the transthoracic impedance (ohms), which is the resistance to current flow. If transthoracic impedance is high, more energy is required to achieve sufficient current for successful defibrillation or cardioversion. Factors that determine transthoracic impedance include energy selected, electrode size, paddle-skin coupling material, number of shocks, time intervals between shocks, phase of ventilation, size of chest, and paddle electrode pressure.

Energy Dose: The optimal energy dose for defibrillation in infants and children has not been established. Although available information does not demonstrate a relation between energy dose and weight, a starting dose of 2 J/kg for defibrillation is recommended until further data are available. To minimize transthoracic impedance, the operator should press firmly on the electrode paddles during defibrillation. If VF continues after defibrillation with 2 J/kg, the energy level should be doubled (4 J/kg), since the initial energy level may have been too small. If the second attempt at defibrillation is delivered rapidly after the first, the current delivered to the heart will be increased because the initial attempt reduces transthoracic impedance. The third attempt, if it is necessary, should again use an energy level of 4 J/kg. When three shocks are required, they should be delivered rapidly and consecutively. Time between shocks should be just brief enough to check the rhythm with the electrode paddles in place. If VF continues, the second and third attempts at defibrillation should be made without pausing to perform

CPR or check the pulse. If VF continues despite the tree defibrillation attempts, energy levels may need to be increased further, but ventilation with 100% oxygen, chest compressions, and epinephrine administration should precede further defibrillation attempts. Continued VF may necessitate additional therapy with epinephrine, lidocaine, or bretylium. Whenever epinephrine, lidocaine, or bretylium is administered to the patient with VF, *each* dose should be followed within 30 to 60 seconds by defibrillation (4 J/kg). If VF is terminated but then recurs, defibrillation should be repeated at the energy level that previously resulted in successful defibrillation.

Paddle Size: Paddle size is one determinant of transthoracic impedance – the larger the size, the lower the impedance. The paddle selected should be the largest size that allows good chest contact over the entire paddle surface area and good separation between the two paddles. "Infant" paddles (4.5 cm) should generally be used for infants up to approximately 1 year of age or 10 kg. "Adult" paddles (8 to 13 cm) should generally be used for patients older than 1 year or weighing more than 10 kg.

Electrode Interface: Since the skin acts as a resistor between the electrode paddles and the heart, a low-impedance interface medium (such as electrode cream or paste, saline-soaked gauze pads, or self-adhesive defibrillation pads) is recommended. Sonographic gels are unacceptable, alcohol pads represent a fire hazard and can produce serious chest burns, and bare paddles result in very high chest impedance. The interface medium under one electrode paddle (eg, saline from a saline-soaked pad) must not come in contact with the medium under the other electrode, or bridging will occur. If bridging occurs, a short circuit will be created and an inadequate amount of current will traverse the heart.

Electrode Position: Electrode paddles must be placed so that the heart is between them. Anterior-posterior electrode position, with one electrode on the anterior chest over the heart and the other on the back, is theoretically superior but impractical during CPR. In standard electrode position, one paddle is placed on the upper right chest below the clavicle and the other to the left of the left nipple in the anterior axillary line. A mirror-image electrode placement is used if dextrocardia is present. Anterior-posterior paddle placement may be necessary for an infant if only adult paddles are available.

Defibrillation Sequence: If VF is observed on the ECG monitor:

1. Continue ventilation with 100% oxygen and chest compressions without interruption (except during defibrillation).

2. Apply conductive medium to infant paddles (patient younger than approximately 1 year) or adult paddles (patient older than 1 year).
3. Turn on the defibrillator power; the synchronous mode should *not* be activated.
4. Select the energy dose and charge the capacitor.
5. Stop chest compressions and place paddles in the proper position on the chest.
6. Recheck the rhythm on the monitor.
7. Clear the area to ensure that no personnel are in contact with the patient, the bed, or the equipment ("one – I am clear; two – your are clear; three – everybody is clear").
8. Apply firm pressure to the paddles while simultaneously depressing the discharge buttons.
9. Evaluate ECG.

(American Academy of Pediatrics. American Heart Association. Pediatric Advance Life Support 1997, pp.7-12,7-13,7-14)

<u>Synchronized Cardioversion</u>

Synchronized cardioversion is the treatment of choice for patients with tachyarrhythmias (SVT, VT, atrial fibrillation, atrial flutter) who show evidence of cardiovascular compromise. Synchronization of delivered energy with the GCG reduces the possibility of inducing VF, which can occur if an electrical impulse is delivered during the relative refractory period of the ventricle. The initial energy dose is 0.5 J/kg, and if the tachyarrhythmia persists, the dose is doubled. If conversion to sinus rhythm still dose not occur, the diagnosis if SVT should be reconsidered; sinus tachycardia may actually be present. The procedure for synchronized cardioversion is the same as that outlined for defibrillation (see below), with the following exceptions:

1. If the paddles are not of the monitoring type, the ECG must be joined to the defibrillator.
2. The synchronizer circuit must be activated (a light blinks, and an indicator flashes on the monitor with each QRS). On some older models, the QRS must be upright for proper activation.
3. The discharge buttons must be pressed and held until the countershock is delivered (often several QRS complexes).

Ideally infants and children should be intubated and ventilated with 100% oxygen before cardioversion, and secure vascular access (venous or intraosseous) should be achieved. Administration of a sedative and an analgesic should also be considered. However, if shock is present, cardioversion should not be delayed while these therapies are instituted.

(American Academy of Pediatrics. American Heart Association. Pediatric Advance Life Support 1997, p.7-7)

Cardioversion

Indications: Symptomatic supraventricular tachycardia or ventricular tachycardia accompanied by cardiovascular instability.

Dosage/Dosage Interval:

Initial dose is 0.5 J/kg; double dose each time for a total of three attempts (range, 0.25-2 wt-s/kg). If IV access is available, administer adenosine before cardioversion, but do not delay cardioversion while attempting to obtain IV access. Correct acidosis, hypoxemia, and hypothermia before, during, and after cardioversion attempts.

Adverse Reactions:

Energy doses of 5-6 J/kg can result in severe myocardial burns, congestive cardiomyopathy secondary to reduced contractility, and death.

(Cloherty: Manual of Neonatal Care 1998, p.687)

CARNITINE (Carnitor, VitaCarn, L-carnitine)

Supplied: Tablet 330mg, capsule 250mg
Solution 100mg/ml
Injectable 1 gm/5mL

Administration: PO

Comment: May be given alone or dissolve in drinks or liquid food (1).

Carnitine (Carnitor, Vitacam)

Dosage/Dosage Interval (oral DL carnitine doses)

Indications: Carnitine deficiency

Dosage/route/frequency: 50-100 mg/kg/day, PO.
Initial dose: 50 mg/kg/day, slowly increase to 100 mg/kg/day. Max. dose 3 g/day

Indications: Cardiomyopathy: load

Dosage/route/frequency: 100 mg/kg/dose, PO

Indications: Cardiomyopathy: maintenance

Dosage/route/frequency: 200 mg/kg/day, PO

Monitoring: Blood chemistries and serum carnitine level. Normal serum carnitine levels are 22.6-33.9 µmol/L. Normal cord blood levels are 30-50 nmol/ml.

Clinical Considerations:

The recommended dose of L-carnitine enteral liquid is 50-100 mg/kg/day. Administer higher doses with caution and only if clinical and biochemical considerations make it likely that they will be of benefit.

Adverse Reactions: Transient diarrhea.

(Cloherty: Manual of Neonatal Care 1998, p.687)

Carnitine

L-Carnitine Treatment:

Patients were treated with intravenous L-carnitine and/or oral L-carnitine. Intravenous L-carnitine was generally given to inpatients (eg, for treatment of acute catabolic episodes at the time of hospitalization) and oral L-carnitine was provided to outpatients.

The mean dose of carnitine administered was 96 mg/kg and ranged from 14 mg/kg/day to 455 mg/kg/day.

Conclusion: Results suggest that L-carnitine provides clinical benefit in treating pediatric cardiomyopathy. There is a need for further exploration of potential explanatory factors for the higher mortality observed in the population of patients treated with ACE inhibitors.

(Helton: Metabolic Aspects of Myocardial Disease and a Role for L-Carnitine in the Treatment of Childhood Cardiomyopathy: Pediatrics 2000;105:1260-1270)

Carnitine

Dose: 50-100 mg/kg/day p.o. divided bid or tid; maximum daily dose 3 g.

(Allen: Moss and Adams' Heart Disease in Infants, Children, and Adolescents 2001, pp1460-1468)

Carnitine

Carnitine supplementation (controversial)

Carnitine synthesis and storage are not well developed in infants <34 weeks' gestation. Carnitine is a carrier molecule necessary for oxidation of long-chain fatty acids. An exogenous source of carnitine is available from human milk and infant formulas; however, studies have shown that infants on TPN become deficient in 6-10 days. Carnitine can be added to TPN solutions at a safe initial dose of 10 mg/kg/day.

(Gomella: Neonatology: Management, Procedures, On-call Problems, Diseases and Drugs 1999, p.91)

Carnitine

Dose & Route: Oral:

Children: 50-100 mg/kg/24 hr PO ÷ Q8-12 hr; increase slowly as needed and tolerated to **max dose** of 3g/24 hr

IV:

Children: 50 mg/kg as loading dose; may follow with 50 mg/kg/24 hr IV infusion; maintenance: 50 mg/kg/24 hr ÷ Q4-6 hr; increase to **maximum** of 300 mg/kg/24 hr if needed.

Remarks: May cause nausea, vomiting, abdominal cramps, diarrhea, body odor. Give bolus IV infusion over 2-3 minutes.

(Siberry: The Harriet Lane Handbook 2000, p.656)

Carnitine

For Treatment of Glutaric Aciduria Type II

After confirming the diagnosis of GA II and implementing therapy with IV carnitine (200 to 300 mg/kg per day) and oral riboflavin (100 mg/kg per day), the patient was weaned off the ventilator within 3 days. His atelectasis disappeared. His blood glucose, lactate, bilirubin, prothrombin time and partial thromboplastin time, platelet count, and liver and muscle enzymes normalized after 6 days of therapy. He regained his strength gradually and his seizures and apneic episodes resolved. After 4 weeks, the hepatosplenomegaly and ascites had completely resolved. Repeated chest x-ray and echocardiography indicated normal heart size and function and complete disappearance of the inferior vena cava thrombus. He was discharge from the hospital at 2 months of age in good condition on high-caloric formula low in fat and protein, oral riboflavin, and high-dose oral carnitine.

The patient's adhered to the treatment. However, between 2 and 4 months of age, the patient's clinical condition deteriorated due to repeated acidotic hypoglycemia attacks, vomiting associated with poor weight gain, and worsening hypotonia. At 4 months of age, a repeated MS/MS study showed a low free carnitine level and slightly increased acylcarnitines species typical of GA II. Because of his clinical deterioration and low plasma carnitine level, a central venous line (Infuse-A-Port, distributed by Horizon Medical Products, Manchester, GA) was inserted and IV carnitine (200 mg/kg three times per week) was started and maintained for 6 months. After IV carnitine therapy, the patient's condition stabilized; he started babbling, socially interacting, rolling over, had relatively good head control, and could maintain sitting balance for 3 seconds. His follow-up developmental assessment at the age of 6 months showed a playful child with good social interaction who could sit with support; apart from mild hypotonia, his neurologic examination was essentially normal. Brain magnetic resonance imaging (MRI) showed mild brain atrophy and delayed myelination. Repeated electroencephalography, visual-evoked potentials, brainstem evoked potentials, electromyography, and nerve conduction studies were normal. At 10 months of age, a repeated MS/MS showed a normal acylcarnitine profile; however, free carnitine was significantly elevated, so he was switched from an IV to an oral carnitine preparation. Later on, however, his clinical condition deteriorated with increased hypotonia and loss of previously acquired milestones. The Port-A-Cath was reinserted, and IV carnitine therapy was resumed at 12 months of age. Meanwhile, his blood free carnitine level was maintained in the high range, which was closely monitored through repeated MS/MS testing.

(Al-Essa: Glutaric Aciduria Type II: Observations in Seven Patients With Neonatal- and Late-Onset Disease. J Perinatol 2000;2:120-128)

CARVEDILOL (Coreg)

Supplied: Tablets: 3.125mg, 6.25mg, 12.5mg, 25mg
Administration: PO

Carvedilol

Dosage: Initial dose = 0.05 mg/kg given b.i.d. (maximum 3.125 mg b.i.d.).

May titrate upward weekly to 0.4-0.5 mg/kg/dose given b.i.d.; Do not exceed maximum adult dose of 25-50 mg p.o. b.i.d.

Comments: Recently approved for congestive heart failure in adults; may cause decompensation initially; use in children not yet established

(Allen: Moss Adam's Heart Disease in Infants, Children, and Adolescents 2001, pp.1460-1468)

CEFACLOR (Ceclor)

Supplied: Suspension, powder for 125mg/5ml; 187mg/5ml, 250mg/5ml, 375mg/5ml
Administration: PO
Refrigerate suspension after reconstitution, discard after 14 days (1)

Cefaclor (Ceclor)

Antibacterial Drugs for Pediatric Patients Beyond the Newborn Period: dosage per kg/d

Route: PO
Mild to Moderate Infections: 20-40 mg in 2 or 3 doses

Severe Infections: Inappropriate.

Comments: A twice daily regimen as been demonstrated to be effective for treatment of acute otitis media

Notes: In patients with history of allergy to penicillin or one of its many congeners, alternative drugs are recommended. In some circumstances, a cephalosporin or other beta-lactam class drug may be acceptable. However, these drugs should not be used in patients with an immediate hypersensitivity (anaphylaxis) to penicillin because approximately 5% to 15% of penicillin-allergic patients will also be allergic to the cephalosporins.

(American Academy of Pediatrics: Report of the Committee on Infectious Diseases. Red Book 2000, pp.653,662)

CEFAZOLIN (Ancef, Kefzol)

Supplied: Injection, powder for 500mg, 1gm vials (contains 2.1mEq Na/gm)

Administration: IV, IM

IM injection: Initial reconstitution add 2ml and 2.5ml to vials containing 500mg, 1gm cefazolin to provide solutions containing concentrations approximately 225mg, or 330mg/ml. Stable at room temperature for 24 hours, or 96 hours when refrigerated.

For DIRECT IV INJECTION, these solutions should be further diluted in approximately 5ml SWFI (Ancef) or at least l0ml SWFI (Kefzol). The appropriate dose should then be injected over 3 to 5 minutes directly into a vein or the tubing of a freely flowing compatible IV solution (3).

For INTERMITTENT INFUSION, dilute to a final concentration of 10 to 20mg/ml (1). This route is preferred. Infuse over 30 to 60 minutes (2). Stable in D5W, D10W, NS for 96 hours at this concentration when refrigerated (3).

Cefazolin (Ancef)

Antibacterial Drugs for Pediatric Patients Beyond the Newborn Period
Dosage per kg/d

Route: IV, IM

Mild to Moderate Infection: 25-50 mg in 3 doses

Severe Infections: 50-100 mg in 3 doses

Notes: In patients with history of allergy to penicillin or one of its many congeners, alternative drugs are recommended. In some circumstances, a cephalosporin or other beta-lactam class drug may be acceptable. However, these drugs should not be used in patients with an immediate hypersensitivity (anaphylaxis) to penicillin because approximately 5% to 15% of penicillin-allergic patients will also be allergic to the cephalosporins.

(American Academy of Pediatrics: Report of the Committee on Infectious Diseases. Red Book 2000, pp.654,662)

Cefazolin

Suggested Dosage Schedules for Antibiotics Used in Newborns
Route: IV, IM
Dosage (mg/kg) and Interval of Administration:

Weight <1200 g
Age 0-4 WK: 20 q12h

Weight 1200-2000 g
Age 0-7 Days: 20 q12h
Age >7 Days: 20 q12h

Weight >2000 g
Age 0-7 Days: 20 q12h
Age >7 Days: 20 q8h

(Remington: Infectious Diseases of the Fetus and Newborn Infant 2001, p.1454)

Cefazolin

Routes: IV, IM.

Dosages (mg/kg/day) and Intervals of Administration:

Body weight < 2000g
0-7 days old: 40 div q12h
8-28 days old: 40 div q12h

Body weight >2000 g
0-7 days old: 40 div q12h
8-28 days old: 60 div q8h
> 28 days old: 60 div q8h

(Nelson: Pocket Book of Pediatric Antimicrobial Therapy 2000-2001, p.16)

Cefazolin Sodium (Ancef, Kefzol)

Classification: First-generation cephalosporin.

Action and spectrum:
A broad-spectrum semisynthetic β-lactam antibiotic bactericidal by virtue of its inhibition of cell wall synthesis. Good activity against Gram-positive cocci (except enterococci), including penicillinase-producing staphylococci. Gram-negative coverage includes *Escherichia coli*, most Klebsiella spp, many strains of *Haemophilus influenzae*, and indole-positive *Proteus* spp. Organism resistance is primarily due to elaboration of β-lactamases, which inactivate the antibiotic through hydrolysis.

Route: IM, IV (infuse over 20-30 minutes).

Dosage: Newborn and premature infants:
<2000 g: 40 mg/kg/day divided q12h.
>2000 g and age >7 days: 60 mg/kg/day divided q12h.

Age 1 month and older: 25-100 mg/kg/day divided q6-8h.

Elimination and metabolism:
100% excreted unchanged in urine.
Half-life is 1.5-4 hours.

Adverse effects: Infrequent except for allergic reactions, including fever, rash and urticaria. May cause leukopenia, thrombocytopenia, and a positive Coombs test reaction. Excessive dosage (especially in renal impairment) may result in CNS irritation with seizure activity.

Comments: Use with caution in patients with a history of severe allergic reactions to penicillins. Dosage reduction is required in moderate to severe renal failure. Contains 2 meq sodium per gram.

(Gomella: Neonatology 1999, p.557)

CEFIXIME (Suprax)

Supplied: Suspension, powder for 100mg/5ml in 50, 100ml

Administration: PO
The incidence of adverse GI effects including diarrhea and loose stools, in children receiving cefixime oral suspension is comparable as to that seen in adults. Safety and

effectiveness of Suprax in children aged less than six months have not been established (3).

After mixing, the suspension may be kept for 14 days at room temperature or may be refrigerated (3).

Cefixime may be given without regards to meals (3).

Cefixime (Suprax)

Antibacterial Drugs for Pediatric patients Beyond the Newborn Period: Dosage per kg/d

Route: PO

Mild to moderate infections: 8 mg in 1 or 2 doses

Severe infections: Inappropriate

Comments: Diarrhea occurs in 10%-15% of patients; inadequate activity against penicillin nonsusceptible pneumococci

Notes: In patients with history of allergy to penicillin or one of its many congeners, alternative drugs are recommended. In some circumstances, a cephalosporin or other beta-lactam class drug may be acceptable. However, these drugs should not be used in patients with an immediate hypersensitivity (anaphylaxis) to penicillin because approximately 5% to 15% of penicillin-allergic patients will also be allergic to the cephalosporins.

(American Academy of Pediatrics: Report of the Committee on Infectious Diseases. Red Book 2000, pp.654,662)

CEFOPERAZONE (Cefobid)

Supplied: Injection, powder for: 1gm and 2gm vials (contains 1.5mEq Na/gm)

Administration: IV, IM

Direct rapid IV injection of the drug is not recommended by the manufacturer. (3)

For IV administration, reconstitute the vials by adding 3.8ml and 7.2ml SWFI to the 1gm and 2gm vials respectively for a concentration of 250mg/ml. For intermittent infusion, further dilute to a concentration of 2mg to 50mg/ml. Stable at this concentration for 24 hours at room temperature in D5W, NS, and D10W. It is stable for 5 days refrigerated at these concentrations in D5W and NS.

Maximum solubility of cefoperazone is ≈ 475mg/ml compatible diluent (1).

DO NOT mix cefoperazone directly with an aminoglycoside. If concomitant therapy is necessary use sequential intermittent IV infusion provided that separate secondary IV tubing is used and the primary IV tubing is irrigated between doses. Administer cefoperazone prior to the aminoglycoside (1).

INTERMITTENT INFUSIONS should be administered over 15 to 30 minutes (3).

Safety and effectiveness in children has not been established (3).

<u>Cefoperazone</u> (Cefobid)

Antibacterial Drugs for Pediatric Patients Beyond the Newborn Period: Dosage per kg/d

Route: IV, IM

Mild to Moderate Infections: 100-150 mg in 2 or 3 doses

Severe infections: No data available

Comments: Not approved for children

Notes: In patients with history of allergy to penicillin or one of its many congeners, alternative drugs are recommended. In some circumstances, a cephalosporin or other beta-lactam class drug may be acceptable. However, these drugs should not be used in patients with an immediate hypersensitivity (anaphylaxis) to penicillin because approximately 5% to 15% of penicillin-allergic patients will also be allergic to the cephalosporins.

(American Academy of Pediatrics: Report of the Committee on Infectious Diseases. Red Book 2000, pp.654,662)

<u>Cefoperazone</u> (Cefobid)

Dose & Route: <u>Infant & Child</u>: 100-200 mg/kg/24hr ÷Q8-12hr IV/IM

Remarks: Use with **caution** in penicillin allergic patients or in patients with hepatic failure, or biliary obstruction. Drug is extensively excreted in bile. May cause disulfiram-like reaction with ethanol. Bleeding and bruising may occur especially in patients with vitamin K deficiency. Does not penetrate well into cerebrospinal fluid.

(Siberry: The Harriet Lane Handbook 2000, p.659j)

<u>Cefoperazone</u>

Route: IV, IM

Neonatal Dose: <1 wk: IV: 25 mg/kg/24 h once daily
1-4 wk: IV: 25-50 mg/kg/24 h q12-24h

Pediatric Dose: IV, IM: 50-200 mg/kg/24 h q8-12h
Max: 12 g/d

Discussion: Do not use if allergic to penicillin; may give vitamin K for prevention of hypoprothrombinemia.

(Rudolph: Rudolph's Pediatrics 1996, p.2175)

CEFOTAXIME (Claforan)

Supplied: Injection, powder for 500mg, 1gm and 2gm vials (contains 2.2mEq Na/gm)

Administration: IV, IM
A solution of 1 gm Cefotaxime in 14 ml SWFI is isotonic.

For DIRECT IV INJECTION, add 10ml SWFI to 1gm or 2gm vial for a concentration of 95mg or 180mg/ml respectively. The appropriate dose may then be injected directly into the vein over a 3- to 5- minute period, or slowly into the tubing of a freely flowing compatible IV solution.

INTERMITTENT IV INFUSIONS of cefotaxime are generally infused over 20 to 30 minutes in a concentration of 20mg to 40mg/ml in a compatible solution (3).

Cefotaxime concentrations of 50mg to 330mg/ml in SWFI are stable for 24 hours at room temperature, or 10 days under refrigeration (3).
Cefotaxime concentrations of 10mg to 40mg/ml for intermittent infusion in D5W, NS, D10W are stable for 24 hours at room temperature or 5 days under refrigeration (3).

Cefotaxime

Antibacterial Drugs for Newborn Infants:
Dose (mg/kg or Units [U]/kg) and Frequency of Administration:

Route: IV, IM

Dose:

Infants 0-4 wk
BW <1200 g: 50 every 12 h

Infants <1 wk old
BW ≤1200-2000 g: 50 every 12 h
BW >2000 g: 50 every 8 or 12 h

Infants ≥1 wk old
BW ≤2000-2000 g: 50 every 8 h
BW >2000 g: 50 every 6 or 8 h

Antibacterial Drugs for Pediatric Patients Beyond the Newborn Period:
Dosage per kg/d

Route: IV, IM
Mild to Moderate Infections: 75-100 mg in 3 or 4 doses

Severe Infections: 150-200 mg in 3 or 4 doses

Comments: A regimen of 300 mg in 3 or 4 doses can be used for therapy of meningitis

Infants Born to Mothers With Gonococcal Infections.
When prophylaxis is administered correctly, infants born to mothers with gonococcal infections infrequently develop gonococcal ophthalmia. However, since gonococcal ophthalmia or disseminated infection occasionally can occur in this situation, infants born to mothers with gonorrhea should receive a single dose of ceftriaxone, 125 mg intravenously or intramuscularly; for premature and low-birth-weight infants, the dose is 25 to 50 mg/kg to a maximum of 125 mg Cefotaxime in a single dose (100 mg/kg given intravenously or intramuscularly) is an alternative.

Note: In patients with history of allergy to penicillin or one of its many congeners, alternative drugs are recommended. In some circumstances, a cephalosporin or other ß-lactam class drug may be acceptable. However, these drugs should not be used in patients with an immediate hypersensitivity (anaphylaxis) to penicillin because approximately 5% to 15% of penicillin-allergic patients will also be allergic to the cephalosporins

(American Academy of Pediatrics: Report of the Committee on Infectious Diseases: Red Book 2000, pp.651,654,260,662)

Cefotaxime

Suggested Dosage Schedules for Antibiotics Used in Newborns

Route: IV, IM

Dosage (mg/kg) and Interval of Administration:

Weight <1200 g
Age 0-4 WK: 50 q12h

Weight 1200-2000 g
Age 0-7 Days: 50 q12h
Age >7 Days: 50 q8h

Weight >2000 g
Age 0-7 Days: 50 q12h
Age >7 Days: 50 q8h

(Remington: Infectious Diseases of the Fetus and Newborn Infant 2001, p.1454)

Cefotaxime Sodium (Claforan)

Classification: Third-generation cephalosporin.

Action & spectrum:

Mechanism of action is identical to that of other β-lactam antibiotics and is bactericidal. Active chiefly against Gram-negative organisms (except *Pseudomonas* spp), including *Escherichia coli, Enterobacter* spp, *Klebsiella* spp., *Haemophilus influenzae* (including ampicillin-resistant strains), *Proteus mirabilis* and indole-positive *Proteus* spp, *Serratia marcescens, Neisseria gonorrhoeae,* and, Ne*isseria meningitidis*. Generally poor activity against Gram-positive aerobic organisms.

Route: IM, IV (infuse over 30 minutes).

Dosage: Meningitis: 200 mg/kg/day divided q6h
Other indications:
<7 days old: 100 mg/kg/day divided q12h
>7 days old: 150 mg/kg/day divided q8h

Elimination and metabolism:

Excreted principally unchanged in the urine.
Half-life in neonates is 1-4 hours.

Adverse effects: Hypersensitivity reactions, thrombophlebitis, serum sickness-like reaction with prolonged administration, diarrhea, and, rarely, blood dyscrasias, hepatic dysfunction, or renal damage.

Comment: should be reserved for suspected or documented Gram-negative meningitis or sepsis. When used as empiric therapy, combine with ampicillin or aqueous penicillin G to provide Gram-positive coverage (ie, group B streptococci, pneumococci, and *Listeria monocytogenes*). High degree of stability to β-lactamases. Third-generation cephalosporins have been proven to induce the emergence of multi-drug-resistant bacteria when used excessively and without proper clinical indications. Contains 2.2 meq of sodium per gram.

(Gomella: Neonatology 1999, pp.557-558)

Cefotaxime

Routes: IV, IM

Dosages (mg/kg/day) and Intervals of Administration:

Body weight < 2000g
0-7 days old: 100 div q12h
8-28 days old: 150 div q8h

Body weight >2000g
0-7 days old: 100 div q12h
8-28 days old: 150 div q8h

> 28 days old: 200 div q6h

(Nelson: Pocket Book of Pediatric Antimicrobial Therapy 2000-2001, p.16)

Cefotaxime

Condition: Sepsis and Meningitis, Gonococcal
Therapy: Ceftriaxone 25-50 mg/kg IV, IM once daily OR Cefotaxime 100 mg/kg/day IV, IM div q12h

Comment: Duration of therapy uncertain (? 5 days)

(Nelson: Pocket Book of Pediatric Antimicrobial Therapy 2000-2001, p.10)

Cefotaxime

Condition: Conjunctivitis - Gonococcal
Therapy: Ceftriaxone 25-50 mg/kg (max. 125mg) IV, IM OR cefotaxime 100 mg/kg IV, IM as a single dose; (More than 1 day of therapy may be used for severe cases)

Comment: Saline irrigation of eyes; Treat mother and her sexual partner; Evaluate for chlamydial infection

(Nelson: Pocket Book of Pediatric Antimicrobial Therapy 2000-2001, p.9)

CEFOXITIN (Mefoxin)

Supplied: 1gm, 2gm vial
(Contains 2.3mEq Na/gm)

Administration: IV, IM
For IV administration, add 10cc SWFI to 1gm vial for concentration of 95mg/ml. Add 10ml or 20ml SWFI to 2gm vial for concentration of 180mg/ml or 95mg/ml. Stable for 24 hours at room temperature, or 7 days when refrigerated.

Direct IV injection: Administer dose IVP over 3 to 5 minutes.

Intermittent IV injection: If diluted to a concentration of 1-20mg/ml in D5W, D10W, NS stable for 24 hours at room temperature or 48 hours refrigerated (1, 3).

Compatible: Parenteral nutrition*.

* Drugs reported as being compatible with parenteral nutrition in published studies using test solutions may not be compatible with the particular formulation your infant is receiving. Components in neonatal parenteral nutrition are individualized based on the infant's body weight, serum electrolytes, fluid, and other nutrient requirements, making most solutions unique. Observe the solution and tubing carefully for signs of precipitation during the 24-hour infusion period when drugs are co-infused. Certain drugs may be admixed into the parenteral nutrition bag. See Driscoll, and associates' review of the use of parenteral nutrition as a drug vehicle (9).

DO NOT add solutions of cefoxitin to aminoglycoside solutions because of potential interaction, administer separately to the same patient.

<u>Cefoxitin</u> (Mefoxin)

Antibacterial Drugs for Pediatric Patients Beyond the Newborn Period: Dosage per kg/d

Route: IV, IM

Mild to Moderate Infections: 80-100 mg in 3-4 doses

Severe Infections: 80-160 mg in 4-6 doses

Note: In patients with history of allergy to penicillin or one of its many congeners, alternative drugs are recommended. In some circumstances, a cephalosporin or other ß-lactam class drug may be acceptable. However, these drugs should not be used in patients with an immediate hypersensitivity (anaphylaxis) to penicillin because approximately 5% to 15% of penicillin-allergic patients will also be allergic to the cephalosporins

(American Academy of Pediatrics: Report of the Committee on Infectious Diseases. Red Book 2000, pp.654,662)

<u>Cefoxitin</u> (Mefoxin)

Indications and use:

Treatment of infectious from Gram-negative enteric organisms, ampicillin-resistant *Haemophilus influenzae*, and anaerobic bacteria, including *Bacteroides fragilis* spp.

Actions: A second-generation cephalosporin. A β-lactam antibiotic bactericidal by inhibiting cell wall synthesis.

Route: IV, IM

Dosage: <2 kg and >7 days old: 90 mg/kg/day divided q8h
≥3 months old: 80-160 mg/kg/day divided q4-6h

Adverse effects: Usually well tolerated. May cause rash, thrombophlebitis, a
positive direct Coombs' test, eosinophilia, and increase in liver enzymes.
(Gomella: Neonatology 1999, p.558)

Cefoxitin (Mefoxin)

Dose & Route: Infant & Child: 80-160 mg/kg/24hr÷Q4-8hr IM/IV

Remarks: Use with **caution** in penicillin allergic patients or in presence of renal impairment. Has good anaerobic activity. CSF penetration is poor. **Adjust dose in renal failure**.
(Siberry: The Harriet Lane Handbook 2000, p.661)

CEFTAZIDIME (Fortaz, Tazicef)

Supplied: Injection, powder for 500mg, 1gm, 2gm vial (Contains 2.3mEq Na/gm)

Administration: IV, IM
Carbon dioxide is released as ceftazidime dissolves, generating pressure within the container. A vent needle should be inserted AFTER the drug has dissolved (3).

For IV administration, add 10ml SWFI to 1gm or 2gm vials for a concentration of 100mg/ml, and 170mg/ml to 180 mg/ml respectively (1).

For DIRECT IV INJECTION, the appropriate dose should be injected over 3 to 5 minutes into a vein or into the tubing of a compatible IV solution.

For INTERMITTENT IV INFUSION, further dilute to a concentration of 10mg/ml to 40mg/ml and infuse over 15 to 30 minutes. Stable in D5W, NS, D10W at these concentrations for 18-24 hours at room temperature, or 7 days when refrigerated at these concentrations (1).

Compatible: Parenteral nutrition,* metronidazole
* Drugs reported as being compatible with parenteral nutrition in published studies using test solutions may not be compatible with the particular formulation your infant is receiving. Components in neonatal parenteral nutrition are individualized based on the infant's body weight, serum electrolytes, fluid, and other nutrient requirements, making most solutions unique. Observe the solution and tubing carefully for signs of precipitation during the 24-hour infusion period when drugs are co-infused. Certain drugs may be admixed into the parenteral nutrition bag. See Driscoll, and associates' review of the use of parenteral nutrition as a drug vehicle (9).

Incompatible: Ranitidine, Aminophylline. DO NOT add aminoglycoside antibiotics to ceftazidine. Give separately (1).

Ceftazidime (Fortaz)

Antibacterial Drugs for Newborn Infants:
Dose (mg/kg or Units [U]/kg) and Frequency of Administration

Dose: Infants 0-4 wk
BW <1200 g: 50 every 12 h

Infants <1 wk old
BW ≤1200-2000 g: 50 every 12 h
BW >2000 g: 50 every 8 or 12 h

Infants ≥1 wk old
BW ≤2000-2000 g: 50 every 8 h
BW >2000 g: 50 every 8 h

Antibacterial Drugs for Pediatric Patients Beyond the Newborn Period: Dosage per kg/d

Route: IV, IM

Mild to Moderate Infections: 75-100 mg in 3 doses

Severe Infections: 125-150 mg in 3 doses

Comments: Only cephalosporin with anti-Pseudomonas activity that has been approved for use in children

Notes: In patients with history of allergy to penicillin or one of its many congeners, alternative drugs are recommended. In some circumstances, a cephalosporin or other beta-lactam class drug may be acceptable. However, these drugs should not be used in patients with an immediate hypersensitivity (anaphylaxis) to penicillin because approximately 5% to 15% of penicillin-allergic patients will also be allergic to the cephalosporins

(American Academy of Pediatrics: Report of the Committee on Infectious Diseases. Red Book 200, pp.651,654,662)

Ceftazidime

Suggested Dosage Schedules for Antibiotics Used in Newborns

Route: IV, IM

Dosage (mg/kg) and Interval of Administration:

Weight <1200 g
Age 0-4 Wk: 50 q12h

Weight 1200-2000 g
Age 0-7 Days: 50 q12h
Age >7 Days: 50 q8h

Weight >2000 g
Age 0-7 Days: 50 q8h
Age >7 Days: 50 q8h

(Remington: Infectious Diseases of the Fetus and Newborn Infant 2001, p.1454)

Ceftazidime

Routes: IV, IM

Dosages (mg/kg/day) and Intervals of Administration:

Body weight < 2000g
0-7 days old: 100 div q12h
8-28 days old: 150 div q8h

Body weight >2000g
0-7 days old: 100 div q12h
8-28 days old: 150 div q8h

> 28 days old: 150 div q8h

(Nelson: Pocket Book of Pediatric Antimicrobial Therapy 2000-2001, p.16)

Ceftazidime (Fortaz, Tazidime)

Classification: Third-generation cephalosporin

Action and spectrum:

A broad-spectrum Gram-negative semisynthetic β-lactam antibiotic bactericidal by virtue of its inhibition of cell wall synthesis. Has poor Gram-positive activity as compared to first-generation cephalosporins but has good activity against Gram-negative aerobic bacteria including *Neisseria meningitidis*, *Haemophilus influenzae*, and most of the Enterobacteriaceae. Has excellent activity against *Pseudomonas aeruginosa* (the best of all third-generation cephalosporins). Little activity against *Listeria monocytogenes* and enterococci.

Route: IM, IV (infuse over 20-30 min).

Dosage:
<2000 g <7 days 30 mg/kg/dose IV q12h
>2000 g <7 days 30 mg/kg/dose IV q8h
>2000 g >7 days 30 mg/kg/dose IV q8h

Elimination: Renal (glomerular filtration) 100% excreted unchanged. Half-life 2.2-4.7 h.

Adverse effects: Infrequent except for allergic reactions including fever, rash and urticaria. May cause transient leukopenia, neutropenia, and thrombocytopenia, direct positive Coombs' test, and transient elevation in liver function test.

Comments: Penetrates well into CSF; concentrations approximate 25-50% of serum concentrations. In combination with ampicillin (for Listeria spp.) can be used to treat suspected Gram-negative meningitis in the neonate. Also an alternative to aminoglycosides for *P aeruginosa* therapy, particularly in patients with renal failure.

(Gomella: Neonatology 1999, p.558)

CEFTIZOXIME (Cefizox)

Supplied: Injection, powder for 500mg, 1gm, 2gm vial (contain 2.6 mEq Na/gm)

Administration: IV, IM

For IV administration, add 10ml, 20ml SWFI to 1gm, 2gm vial respectively for a concentration of 95mg/ml.

For DIRECT IV INJECTION, the appropriate dose should be injected over 3-5 minutes directly or into the tubing of a compatible IV solution.

For INTERMITTENT INFUSION, dilute to a final concentration of 20mg/ml to 40mg/ml in NS, D5W, D10W (1). Intermittent IV infusions are generally infused over 15-30 minutes (3).

After reconstitution or dilution in IV fluids above, Ceftizoxime is stable for 24 hours at room temperature or 96 hours refrigerated (1).

1gm Ceftizoxime in 13ml SWFI is Isotonic

Ceftizoxime (Cefizox)

Antibacterial Drugs for pediatric Patients Beyond the Newborn Period: Dosage per kg/d

Route: IV, IM

Mild to Moderate Infections: 100-150 mg in 3 doses

Severe Infections: 150-200 mg in 3 or 4 doses

Notes: In patients with history of allergy to penicillin or one of its many congeners, alternative drugs are recommended. In some circumstances, a cephalosporin or other beta-lactam class drug may be acceptable. However, these drugs should not be used in patients with an immediate hypersensitivity (anaphylaxis) to penicillin because approximately 5% to 15% of penicillin-allergic patients will also be allergic to the cephalosporins

(American Academy of Pediatrics: Report of the Committee on Infectious Diseases. Red Book 2000, pp.655,662)

Ceftizoxime (Cefizox)

Dose & Route: Infant & Child: 150-200 mg/kg/24hr÷Q6-8hr IV/IM

Remarks: Use with **caution** in penicillin allergic patients or in presence of renal impairment. Good CNS penetration. **Adjust dose in renal failure**.

(Siberry: The Harriet Lane Handbook 2000, p.663)

Ceftizoxime

Dosage: 50 mg/kg/dose every 12 hours IV if <2 weeks of age and every 8 hours IV if >2 weeks of age.

(Fanaroff: Neonatal-Perinatal Medicine 1997, p.1745)

CEFTRIAXONE (Rocephin)

Supplied: Injection, powder for 250mg, 500mg, 1gm vials (contains 3.6mEq Na/gm)

Administration: IV, IM

IM ADMINISTRATION: Add 0.9ml, 1.8ml, 3.6ml diluent (SWFI, NS, D5W, 1% lidocaine injection) to 250mg, 500mg, 1gm vials respectively for a concentration of 250mg/ml. Stable for 3 days when refrigerated. When lidocaine injection is used, it is for IM USE ONLY.

IV ADMINISTRATION: BY INTERMITTENT INFUSIONS over 10-30 minutes by a constant infusion. Add 2.4ml, 4.8ml, 9.6ml diluent (SWFI, NS, D5W) to the 250mg,

500mg, 1gm vials respectively for a concentration of 100mg/ml. Intermittent infusions should be diluted to a concentration of 10 to 40mg/ml. Stable in D5W, NS, D10W for 3 days at room temperature or 10 days refrigerated (3).

Intermittent IV infusions of ceftriaxone have generally been infused over 15-30 minutes in adults or over 10-30 minutes in neonates or children. Although intermittent IV injection (use is not currently approved by FDA) is achieved by injecting the appropriate dose directly into the vein over 2-4 minutes (5).

<u>Ceftriaxone</u> (Rocephin)

Antibacterial Drugs for Newborn Infants:
Dose (mg/kg or Units [U]/kg) and Frequency of Administration

Route: IV, IM

Dose:

<u>Infants 0-4 wk</u>
BW <1200 g: 50 every 24 h

<u>Infants <1 wk old</u>
BW ≤1200-2000 g: 50 every 24 h
BW >2000 g: 50 every 24 h

<u>Infants ≥1 wk old</u>
BW ≤2000-2000 g: 50 every 24 h
BW >2000 g: 50-75 every 24 h

Note: Drug should not be administered to hyperbilirubinemic neonates, especially those born prematurely.

Antibacterial Drugs for Pediatric Patients Beyond the Newborn Period
Dosage per kg/d

Route: IV, IM
Mild to Moderate Infections: 50-75 mg in 1 or 2 doses

Severe Infections: 80-100 mg in 1 or 2 doses

Comments: Larger dosage appropriate for penicillin-resistant pneumococcal meningitis

Note: In patients with history of allergy to penicillin or one of its many congeners, alternative drugs are recommended. In some circumstances, a cephalosporin or other beta-lactam class drug may be acceptable. However, these drugs should not be used in patients with an immediate hypersensitivity (anaphylaxis) to penicillin because approximately 5% to 15% of penicillin-allergic patients will also be allergic to the cephalosporins

(American Academy of Pediatrics: Report of the Committee on Infectious Diseases. Red Book 2000, pp.651,655,662)

<u>Ceftriaxone</u>

Infants Born to Mothers With Gonococcal Infections.

When prophylaxis is administered correctly, infants born to mothers with gonococcal infections infrequently develop gonococcal ophthalmia. However, since gonococcal ophthalmia or disseminated infection occasionally can occur in this situation, infants born to mothers with gonorrhea should receive a single dose of ceftriaxone, 125 mg intravenously or intramuscularly; for premature and low-birth-weight infants, the dose is 25 to 50 mg/kg to a maximum of 125 mg Cefotaxime in a single dose (100 mg/kg given intravenously or intramuscularly) is an alternative.

(American Academy of Pediatrics: Report of the Committee on Infectious Diseases. Red Book 2000, p.260)

Ceftriaxone

Suggested Dosage Schedules for Antibiotics Used in Newborns
Route: IV, IM

Dosage (mg/kg) and Interval of Administration:

Weight <1200 g
Age 0-4 WK: 50 q24h

Weight 1200-2000 g
Age 0-7 Days: 50 q24h
Age >7 Days: 50 q24h

Weight >2000 g
Age 0-7 Days: 50 q24h
Age >7 Days: 75 q24h

(Remington: Infectious Diseases of the Fetus and Newborn Infant 2001, p.1454)

Ceftriaxone

Routes: IV, IM

Dosages (mg/kg/day) and Intervals of Administration:

Body weight < 2000g
0-7 days old: 50 once daily
8-28 days old: 50 once daily

Body weight >2000g
0-7 days old: 50 once daily
8-28 days old: 75 once daily

>28 days old: 100 once daily

(Nelson: Pocket Book of Pediatric Antimicrobial Therapy 2000-2001, p.16)

Ceftriaxone

Condition: Conjunctivitis – Gonococcal

Therapy: Ceftriaxone 25-50 mg/kg (max. 125mg) IV, IM OR cefotaxime 100 mg/kg IV, IM as a single dose; (More than 1 day of therapy may be used for severe cases)

Comment: Saline irrigation of eyes; Treat mother and her sexual partner; Evaluate for chlamydial infection

(Nelson: Pocket Book of Pediatric Antimicrobial Therapy 2000-2001, p.9)

Ceftriaxone Sodium (Rocephin)

Classification: Third-generation cephalosporin.

Action & spectrum:
Mechanism of action identical to that of other β-lactam antibiotics. High degree of stability to β-lactamases and good activity against both Gram-negative and gram-positive organisms except for *Pseudomonas* spp, enterococci, methicillin-resistant staphylococci, and *Listeria monocytogenes*. Has longest serum half-life of all currently available cephalosporins.

Route: IM, IV (infuse over 30 minutes).

Dosage: Meningitis: 100 mg/kg/day divided q12h
Other infections: 50 mg/kg/day divided q12-24h.

Elimination and metabolism:
Both biliary and renal excretion.
Half-life is 5.2-8.4 hours.

Adverse effects: Mild diarrhea and eosinophilia are most common. May also cause neutropenia, rash, thrombophlebitis, and bacterial (GI) or fungal overgrowth. Rare reports of increased prothrombin times. Increases free and erythrocyte-bound bilirubin in premature infants with hyperbilirubinemia; use with caution in infants with hyperbilirubinemia.

Comments: Many clinical studies support once-a-day dosing. Do not use as sole drug in infections due to staphylococci or pseudomonas. Combine with ampicillin for initial empiric therapy of meningitis (ceftriaxone has poor activity against *Listeria*). Generally no dosage reduction is required in renal or hepatic dysfunction. Contains 2.4 meq sodium per gram.

(Gomella: Neonatology 1999, pp.558-559)

Ceftriaxone

Dose & Route: Neonate:
Gonococcal ophthalmia or prophylaxis: 25-50 mg/kg/dose IM/IV x 1; **max dose**: 125 mg/dose

Infant and child: 50-75 mg/kg/24 hr ÷ Q12-24 hr IM/IV (see remarks)

Meningitis (including penicillin resistant pneumococci): 100 mg/kg/24 hr IM/IV ÷ Q12 hr; **max dose**: 4 g/24 hr

Acute otitis media: 50 mg/kg IM x 1; **max dose**: 1g

Remarks: Use with **caution** in penicillin-allergic patients or in presence of renal impairment. May cause reversible cholelithiasis, sludging in gallbladder, and jaundice.

Use with **caution in neonates** and continuous dosing because of risk for hyperbilirubinemia. Consider using an alternative 3rd generation cephalosporin with similar activity.

80-100 mg/kg/24 hr ÷ Q12-24 hr has been recommended for infections outside the CSF due to penicillin-resistant pneumococci.

(Siberry: The Harriet Lane Handbook 2000, pp.663-664)

CEFUROXIME (Zinacef, Kefurox)

Supplied: Oral suspension 125mg/5ml, 250mg/5ml (as axetil), in 50ml, 100ml bottles.
Injection, powder for 750mg, 1.5gm vials (contains 2.4mEq/Na gm)

Administration: IV, IM
IV administration
For Zinacef add 8ml, 16ml SWFI to 750mg, 1.5gm vial respectively for a concentration of 90mg/ml.
For Kefurox add 9ml, 14ml to 750mg, 1.5gm vial respectively for a concentration of 100 mg/ml (1).

The appropriate dose should then be injected directly into a vein over 3 to 5 minutes or injected into the tubing of a freely flowing compatible IV solution. Stable for 24 hours at room temperature, or 7 days if refrigerated.

For INTERMITTENT INFUSION, further dilute to a final concentration of 7.5mg to 15mg/ml in NS, D5W, and DIOW infuse over 15 to 60 minutes. These dilutions are stable for 24 hours at room temperature, or 7 days refrigerated (3).

Oral suspension: shake well before each use. Store reconstituted suspension between 2°-25°C (36-77°F), either in the refrigerator or at room temperature. Discard after 10 days.

Cefuroxime

Antibacterial Drugs for Pediatric patients Beyond the Newborn Period: Dosage per kg/d

Route: IV, IM
Mild to Moderate Infections: 75-100 mg in 3 doses

Severe Infections: 100-150 mg in 3 doses

Note: In patients with history of allergy to penicillin or one of its may congeners, alternative drugs are recommended. In some circumstances, a cephalosporin or other β-lactam class drug may be acceptable. However, theses drugs should not be used inpatients with an immediate hypersensitivity (anaphylaxis) to penicillin because approximately 5% to 15% of penicillin-allergic patients will also be allergic to the cephalosporins.

(American Academy of Pediatrics: Report of the Committee on Infectious Diseases. Red Book 2000, pp.655,662)

Cefuroxime Sodium (Kefurox, Zinacef)

Classification: Second-generation cephalosporin.

Action & spectrum:

Mechanism of action identical to that of other β-lactam antibiotics. Active against both Gram-positive and Gram-negative organisms, including streptococci (except enterococci), both penicillinase-producing and non-penicillinase-producing staphylococci (not including methicillin-resistant staphylococci), *Escherichia coli*, *Haemophilus influenzae* (including ampicillin-resistant strains), *Klebsiella* spp, *Neisseria gonorrhoeae*, *Neisseria meningitidis*, *Proteus mirabilis*, *Salmonella* spp, *Shigella* spp, and *Enterobacter* spp.

Route: IM, IV (IV preferred; infuse over 30 minutes).

Dosage: 100 mg/kg/day divided q12h.

Elimination and metabolism:

Primarily excreted unchanged in the urine.
Half-life is 5-8 h in infants <4 days and 1.6-3.8 h in infants >8 days.

Adverse effects: Generally free of adverse effects but may cause hypersensitivity reactions, thrombophlebitis, elevated serum transaminases, mildly elevated BUN, diarrhea, and, rarely, blood dyscrasias (transient neutropenia, leukopenia, thrombocytopenia).

Comments: The only first- or second-generation cephalosporin that crosses the blood-brain barrier. Provides no activity against *Listeria* spp. so ampicillin should be added in initial empiric therapy. Has added Gram-negative coverage over first-generation cephalosporins while retaining very good Gram-positive coverage. Decrease dosage in renal failure. Contains 2.4 meq sodium per gram. Limited experience in neonates.

(Gomella: Neonatology 1999, p.559)

Cefuroxime (Zinacef, Kefurox)

Dose & Route: IM/IV:
Neonates: 20-60 mg/kg/24 hr ÷ Q12 hr
Infant/Child: 75-150 mg/kg/24 hr ÷ Q8 hr;
Max dose: 6 g/24 hr

Remarks: Use with **caution** in penicillin allergic patients or in Presence of renal impairment. May cause thrombophlebitis at infusion site. Not recommended for meningitis.

(Siberry: The Harriet Lane Handbook 2000, p.664)

CEPHALEXIN (Keflex)

Supplied: Suspension, powder for 125mg/5ml in 60, 100, 200ml
Suspension, powder for 250mg/5ml in 100, 200ml

Administration: PO
Refrigerate suspension after reconstitution and discard after 14 days (1).

Cephalexin

Antibacterial Drugs for Pediatric Patients Beyond the Newborn Period:
Dosage per kg/d:
Route: PO
Mild to Moderate Infections: 25-50 mg in 3-4 doses

Severe Infections: Inappropriate

Notes: In patients with history of allergy to penicillin or one of its may congeners, alternative drugs are recommended. In some circumstances, a cephalosporin or other β-lactam class drug may be acceptable. However, theses drugs should not be used inpatients with an immediate hypersensitivity (anaphylaxis) to penicillin because approximately 5% to 15% of penicillin-allergic patients will also be allergic to the cephalosporins.

(American Academy of Pediatrics: Report of the Committee on Infectious Diseases. Red Book 2000, pp.655,662)

Cephalexin

Condition: Skin and Soft Tissues, Impetigo neonatorum
Therapy: Cleansing alone OR oxacillin IV, IM OR cephalexin 50 mg/kg/day PO div q6-8h, OR mupirocin topically; x 5 days

Comment: No antibiotic for superficial impetigo; Chlorhexidine baths; Break lesions with alcohol swab.

(Nelson: Pocket Book of Pediatric Antimicrobial Therapy 2000-2001, p.12)

CEPHALOSPORINS

Cephalosporins

There is one report of cefotaxime use for empiric therapy of suspected sepsis in a neonatal intensive care unit for 5 years without major problems of resistance, but it has been a more common experience that pathogens resistant to multiple cephalosporins emerge rapidly. For this reason, expanded spectrum cephalosporins should be used selectively for documented bacterial infections and not used extensively for empiric antibiotic therapy of suspected sepsis.

(Nelson: Therapy for Neonatal Sepsis. Seminars in Pediatric Infectious Diseases 1994;5:15-19)

Cephalosporins

Initial empiric treatment of a neonate with suspected bacterial septicemia or meningitis is ampicillin and an aminoglycoside. An alternative regimen of ampicillin and a cephalosporin (such as cefotaxime) active against most gram-negative bacilli can be used, but rapid emergence of cephalosporin-resistant strains, especially *Enterobacter cloacae, Klebsiella* species, and *Serratia* species, can occur as a result of routine use of expanded-spectrum cephalosporins in a nursery. Hence, routine use of expanded-spectrum is not recommended unless gram-negative bacterial meningitis is strongly suspected.

(American Academy of Pediatrics: Report of the Committee on Infectious Diseases. Red Book 2000, p.242)

Cephalosporin

The risks and benefits should be considered thoroughly before routine use of third-generation cephalosporins. One disadvantage is an increased risk for developing gastrointestinal colonization and perhaps subsequent infection with fungi and drug-resistant bacteria. On the other hand, these cephalosporins are safe and effective against many of the common neonatal pathogens, and there is extensive experience with cefotaxime use during neonatal period. Because the third-generation cephalosporins do not cause the dose-related toxicities seen with previous agents, such as aminoglycosides and chloramphenicol, monitoring of serum concentrations is not necessary.

(Fanaroff: Neonatal Perinatal Medicine 1997,p.727)

CEPHAPIRIN (Cefadyl)

Supplied: 1gm (contains 2.36mEq Na/gm)

Administration: IV

Cephapirin

Route: IV, IM

Neonatal Dose: <1 wk: 40 mg/kg/24 h given q12h
1-4 wk: 40-80 mg/kg/24 h given q6-8h

Pediatric Dose: Severe infections: 150-200 mg/kg/24 h
Moderate infections: 100-150 mg/kg/24 h, in divided doses given q6h
Max dose: 12 g/24 h

Discussion: Reduce dose with renal impairment; with a GFR of 25-50 mL/min max dose is 1.5g q6h; with GFR 10-25 mL/min use max dose of 1 g q6h; and for a GFR <10 mL/min use max dose of 12 g/24 h

(Rudolph: Rudolph's Pediatrics 1996, p.2176)

CEPHRADINE (Velosef)

Supplied: Powder for suspension:
125 mg/5ml, 250 mg/5ml (in 100 ml, (contains Na 6 mEq/gm).

Administration: PO, IV, IM
May be given without regard to meals.
After reconstitution the oral suspensions retain their potency for 7 days at room temperature and 14 days if refrigerated (1).

Cephradine

Antibacterial Drugs for Pediatric Patients Beyond the Newborn Period: Dosage per kg/d

Cephradine (Anspor)
Route: PO
Mild to Moderate Infections: 25-50 mg in 2-4 doses
Severe Infections: Inappropriate

Cephradine (Velosef)
Route: IV, IM
Mild to Moderate Infections: 50-100 mg in 4 doses
Severe Infections: 100 mg in 4 doses

Notes: In patients with history of allergy to penicillin or one of its may congeners, alternative drugs are recommended. In some circumstances, a cephalosporin or other β-lactam class drug may be acceptable. However, theses drugs should not be used inpatients with an immediate hypersensitivity (anaphylaxis) to penicillin because approximately 5% to 15% of penicillin-allergic patients will also be allergic to the cephalosporins.

(American Academy of Pediatrics: Report of the Committee on Infectious Diseases. Red Book 2000, pp.655,662)

CHLORAL HYDRATE (Noctec)

Supplied: Syrup 250mg/5ml and 500mg/5ml
Suppositories 324mg, 500mg, 648mg

Administration: PO
For oral use dilute syrup with water, infant formula, or fruit juice.
Dilute syrup in water before PR use (1,3).

Comment: May cause irritation of skin and mucous membranes.
Osmolality of 500mg/5ml syrup is 3500 mOsm/kg.

Chloral Hydrate (Aquachloral Supprettes, Noctec)

Indications and use: Sedation

Actions: CNS depressant. Mechanism of action not completely understood. Usual doses produce mild CNS depression and quiet, deep sleep; higher doses can result in general anesthesia with concurrent respiratory depression.

Route: PO, PR

Dosage: 20-40 mg/kg/dose PO or rectally divided q6-8h prn.

Sedation prior to electroencephalography and other procedures: 30-75 mg/kg/dose once PO, PR. Usually 50 mg/kg/dose once, with orders to repeat 25 mg/kg/dose once if needed. Use the lowest effective dose.

Adverse effects: GI irritation resulting in nausea, vomiting, and diarrhea, paradoxical excitation, respiratory depression, particularly if administered with opiates and barbiturates. Direct hyperbilirubinemia with chronic use. Overdose can be lethal.

Comments: Contraindicated with marked renal or hepatic impairment.

(Gomella: Neonatology 1999, p.559-560)

Chloral Hydrate

Dose/kg: Sedative: 10-15 mg

Route & Frequency: PO, PR q6-q8h prn

Dose/kg: Hypnotic: 25-50 mg

Route & Frequency: PO, PR; once

Comments: May cause paradoxical excitement and accumulation of toxic metabolites. Use with caution in hepatic and/or renal failure. May cause GI distress and indirect hyperbilirubinemia.

(Avery: Neonatology Pathophysiology and Management of the Newborn 1999, p.1553)

Chloral Hydrate

Usual Dosage: Oral, rectal:

Neonates: 25 mg/kg/dose for sedation prior to a procedure; **Note**: Repeat doses should be used with great caution, as drug and metabolites accumulate with repeated use; toxicity has been reported after 3 days in a preterm neonate and after 7 days in a term neonate receiving chloral hydrate 40-50 mg/kg every 6 hours.

Infants and Children:

Sedation, anxiety: 25-50 mg/kg/day divided every 6-8 hours, maximum dose: 500 mg/dose

Prior to EEG: 25-50 mg/kg/dose 30-60 minutes prior to EEG; may repeat in 30 minutes to a total maximum of 100 mg/kg or 1 g total for infants and 2 g for children

Hypnotic: 50 mg/kg; maximum dose: 2 g/dose/day

Sedation, nonpainful procedure: 50-75 mg/kg/dose 30-60 minutes prior to procedure; may repeat 30 minutes after initial dose if needed, to a total maximum dose of 120 mg/kg or 1 g total for infants and 2 g total for children.

Administration: Oral: Minimize unpleasant taste and gastric irritation by administering with water, infant formula, fruit juice, or ginger ale; do not crush capsule, contains drug in liquid form with unpleasant taste

Monitoring Parameters:

Level of sedation; vital signs and O_2 saturation with doses used for sedation prior to procedure

Nursing Implications:

May cause irritation of skin and mucous membranes

Additional Information:

Not an analgesic; osmolality of 500 mg/5 mL syrup is approximately 3500 mOsm/kg

(Taketomo: Pediatric Dosage Handbook 1999-2000, pp.190-192)

Chloral hydrate

Dose: 30-100 mg/kg PO, PR

Mode of Action: Hypnotic sedative

Adverse Effects: Idiosyncratic and allergic reactions
(Garson: The science and practice of pediatric cardiology 1998, p.2955)

Chloral Hydrate

Dose & Route: Children:
Sedative: 25-50 mg/kg/24 hr PO/PR ÷ Q6-8 hr;
max dose: 500 mg/dose
Sedation for procedures: 25-100 mg/kg/dose PO/PR;
max dose: 1 g/dose (infants); 2 g/dose (children)

Remarks: **Contraindicated** in patients with hepatic or renal disease. May cause GI irritation, paradoxical excitement, hypotension, and myocardial/respiratory depression. Chronic administration in neonates can lead to accumulation of active metabolites. Requires same monitoring as other sedatives.

Not analgesic. Peak effects occur within 30-60 minutes. Do not exceed 2 weeks of chronic use. **Avoid** use in severe renal failure. Sudden withdrawal may cause delirium tremens.
(Siberry: The Harriet Lane Handbook 2000, p.667)

CHLORAMPHENICOL (Chloromycetin)

Supplied: 250mg capsules
Injection, powder for 1 gm vial (contains 2.3mEq Na/gm)

Administration: IV, PO
For DIRECT IV INJECTION, add 10ml SWFI to 1 gm vial to provide a concentration of 100mg Chloramphenicol/ml. The appropriate dose is then administered over a period of at least one minute. It must be hydrolyzed to its active form and there is a lag in achieving adequate blood levels following infusion. This dilution is stable for 30 days at room temperature (3).

Chloramphenicol sodium succinate is intended for IV use only, it is ineffective when given IM (1).

Chloramphenicol

Antibacterial Drugs for Pediatric Patients Beyond the Newborn Period: Dosage per kg/d

Chloramphenicol palmitate
Route: PO, (not available in the United States)
Mild to Moderate Infections: Inappropriate

Severe Infections: 50-100 mg in 4 doses

Comments: Optimal dosage is determined by measurement of serum concentrations with resulting modifications to achieve therapeutic concentrations

Chloramphenicol succinate
Route: IV
Mild to Moderate Infections: Inappropriate

Severe Infections: 50-100 mg in 4 doses

Comments: Use only for serious infections because of the rare occurrence of aplastic anemia after administration
(American Academy of Pediatrics: Report of the Committee on Infectious Disease. Red Book 2000, p656

Chloramphenicol
Suggested Dosage Schedules for Antibiotics Used in Newborns
Route: IV, PO
Dosage (mg/kg) and Interval of Administration:

Weight <1200 g
Age 0-4 WK: 25 q24h

Weight 1200-2000 g
Age 0-7 Days: 25 q24h
Age >7 Days: 25 q24h

Weight >2000 g
Age 0-7 Days: 25 q24h
Age >7 Days: 25 q12h

Note: Appropriate dosage schedule should be based on serum concentration measurements
(Remington: Infectious Diseases of the Fetus and Newborn Infant 2001, p.1454)

CHLORHEXIDINE GLUCONATE (Hibiclens, Peridex)

Supplied: Topical liquid 2%
Cleanser 4% in 4oz, 8oz, others
Oral rinse 0.12% in 480ml
Administration: Topical, oral

Chlorhexidine
Condition: Skin and Soft Tissues, Impetigo neonatorum

Therapy: Cleansing alone OR oxacillin IV, IM OR cephalexin 50 mg/kg/day PO div q6-8h, OR mupirocin topically; x 5 days

Comment: No antibiotic for superficial impetigo; Chlorhexidine baths; Break lesions with alcohol swab.
(Nelson: Pocket Book of Pediatric Antimicrobial Therapy 2000-2001, p.12)

SEE ALSO: SKIN and CORD CARE

SEE ALSO: POVIDONE-IODINE
(Garland: Comparison of 10% povidone-iodine and 0.5% chlorhexidine gluconate for the prevention of peripheral intravenous catheter colonization in neonates: a prospective trail. Pediatr Infect Dis J 1995;14:510-516)

CHLOROQUINE (Aralen)

CHLOROQUINE PHOSPHATE

Supplied: Tablet 250 mg (equiv. to 150 mg base)
Tablet 500 mg (equiv. to 300 mg base)
Administration: PO

CHLOROQUINE HCL

Supplied: Injection 50 mg (equiv. to 40 mg base)/ml in 5 ml
Administration: IM
The WHO and some experts state that chloroquine should not be administered parenterally to children. However, data in a limited number of pediatric patients suggest that CAUTIOUS use of parenteral therapy administered by methods intended to reduce the risk of high, potentially toxic peak concentrations of the drug (i.e. by continuous IV infusion or by IM or SC injection in small, frequent doses) may be considered for the treatment of severe chloroquine sensitive malaria in children. Such methods of administration appear to reduce the risk of severe toxicity (3).

Chloroquine Phosphate (Aralen PO_4)

Administered: PO
Dosage: 10 mg base/kg/day q24h
Comment: 500 mg tablet (equivalent to 300 mg base).
NON-NEWBORN SECTION

(Nelson: Pocket Book of Pediatric Antimicrobial Therapy 2000-2001, p.73)

Chloroquine HCL (Aralen HCL)

Administered: IM
Dosage: 5 mg base/kg 1 or 2 doses.
Comment: 250 mg amp (equivalent to 200 mg base).
NON-NEWBORN SECTION

(Nelson: Pocket Book of Pediatric Antimicrobial Therapy 2000-2001, p.73)

Chloroquine

There are several types of antimalarial drugs that act at different stages of the plasmodium life cycle.

Blood schizonticides such as chloroquine, quinine and quinidine act only on parasites in erythrocytic phase.

Chloroquine given in a initial dose of 10mg of chloroquine base/kg body weight administered orally, followed by doses of 5mg base/kg at 6, 24, and 48 hours after the initial dose, is frequently used.

(Fanaroff: Neonatal Perinatal Medicine 1997, p.765)

Chloroquine

Disease/Organism: Malaria
CDC Malaria Hotline (24 hrs a day) 1-770-488-7788 and online information at www.cdc.gov.

It is advisable for physicians who are not familiar with treating malaria to consult with CDC physicians. The following suggestions do not cover all situations.

Prophylaxis:

For areas without chloroquine-resistant P. falciparum:

Chloroquine 5 mg base/kg (max 300 mg) PO once weekly, beginning 1 week before arrival in malarial zone and continuing for 4 weeks after last exposure (drugs available in liquid form outside the USA); PLUS (optional) beginning with final 2 weeks of chloroquine Rx, primaquine 0.3mg base/kg PO daily x 14 days after departure from endemic area for individuals heavily exposed to mosquitoes

Treatment of disease:

Plasmodium vivax, P. ovale P malariae chloroquine-susceptible

P. falciparum:

Chloroquine 10 mg base/kg (max 600 mg) PO stat, then 5 mg base/kg at 6 hrs, 24 hrs and 48 hrs after initial dose (alternative: at 6, 12, 24, and 36 hrs); For parenteral therapy, quinidine 10 mg/kg (max 600 mg) IV (1 hr infusion) followed by continuous infusion of 0.02 mg/kg/min until oral therapy can be given (3 days maximum); It's advisable to monitor patients receiving quinidine in an ICU setting. Prevention of relapse (P. vivax, P, ovale): primaquine 0.3 mg base/kg/day x 14 d

P. falciparum chloroquine-resistant

Quinine 25 mg/kg/day (max 2 g/day) PO div q8h x 3 days (or longer) AND doxycycline (patients > 7 yrs) 2 mg/kg daily x 7 OR Fansidar (pyrimethamine-sulfadoxine): < 1 yr, ¼ tab; 1-3 yrs, ½ tab; 4-8 yrs, 1 tab; 9-14 yrs, 2 tab; > 14 yrs, 3 tabs as a single dose on last day of quinine; NOTE: Several alternative regimens have been reported for Fansidar-resistant infections: Check with the CDC; For parenteral therapy, quinidine, as above; NOTE; Corticosteroids are contraindicated in cerebral malaria; Iron chelation therapy may be beneficial in cerebral malaria.

(Nelson: Pocket Book of Pediatric Antimicrobial Therapy 2000-2001, pp.64-65)

CHLOROTHIAZIDE (Diuril)

Supplied: Injection, powder for 500mg vial (contains 2.5mEq Na/500mg)
Oral Suspension 250mg/5ml

Administration: IV, PO

For IV administration, reconstitute vial with 18ml SWFI to yield a concentration of 27.8mg/ml (3). Discard unused solution after 24 hours. The solution is compatible with dextrose or sodium chloride infusion solutions (1).

An isotonic solution is made when 18ml SWFI is added to the 500mg vial (1).

DO NOT give SQ or IM.
Extravsation must be rigidly avoided (2).

<u>Chlorothiazide</u> (Diuril)

Indications and use: Fluid overload, pulmonary edema, and hypertension.

Actions: The thiazide diuretics enhance the excretion of NaCl and water by interfacing with transport of sodium ions across the renal tubular epithelium in the cortical nephron. Potassium, bicarbonate, magnesium, phosphate, and iodide excretion are also enhanced, whereas calcium excretion is decreased. Duration of action of chlorothiazide and hydrochlorothiazide is 6-12 h; onset of action is within 2 h, and peak action is at 3-6 h.

Route: PO, IV
Dosage: 10-30 mg/kg/day divided q12h.

Adverse effects: Hypokalemia, hypochloremic alkalosis, prerenal azotemia, hyperuricemia, hyperglycemia, hypermagnesemia, volume depletion, and dilutional hyponatremia may occur in situations of excessive fluid intake.

Comments: Do not use in patients with anuria or hepatic dysfunction.

(Gomella: Neonatology 1999, p.560)

<u>Chlorothiazide</u> (Diuril)

Dose: 20-40 mg/kg/day PO divided BID (2 mg/day [sic] max)

Mode of Action: Distal renal tubular inhibition

Adverse Effects: Hypokalemia, hyperbilirubinemia, hyperglycemia

Comments: Rare hypersensitivity reaction with rash, pancytopenia; use caution with coadministration with proarrhythmic drugs

(Garson: The science and practice of pediatric cardiology 1998, p.2951)

<u>Chlorothiazide</u>

Dosage: 20-30 mg/kg/day divided every 12 hr PO or IV.
Comments: May cause hypokalemia, alkalosis, hyperglycemia; effective in the treatment of nephrocalcinosis secondary to loop diuretics; poor oral bioavailability necessitating increased oral doses.

(Fanaroff: Neonatal-Perinatal Medicine 1997, p.1749)

CHLORPROMAZINE (Thorazine)

Supplied: Injection 25mg/ml in 2ml (some parenteral products contain benzyl alcohol)
Syrup 10mg/5ml

Administration: IV, IM, PO
For direct IV injection, chlorpromazine should be diluted with 0.9% NACL to a concentration NOT exceeding 1mg/ml. This diluted product is administered at a rate of 0.5mg/min in children. The manufacturer recommends that

the drug generally not be used in children .... "younger than 6 months of age" .... unless the condition to be treated is potentially life-threatening (3).

Chlorpromazine

Indication: Drug therapy for withdrawal syndrome in infants

Chlorpromazine therapy has been satisfactory in several series. It was used exclusively in the largest series reported, involving 178 treated infants. The drug is effective in treating both the central nevous system and gastrointestinal phenomena. The currently recommended dose is 2 to 3 mg/kg/day, administered in divided doses every 6 hours. The drug may be given orally. Marked improvement usually occurs within 24 hours, and the duration of therapy is 2 to 3 weeks. This drug carries the uncommon risks of causing extrapyramidal phenomena in the newborn and of lowering the seizure threshold.

(Volpe: Neurology of the Newborn 2001, p.882)

Chlorpromazine

Route & Dose: PO, IM, IV: 0.2-0.5 mg/kg doses prn withdrawal symptoms

Adverse Effects and Cautions:

Extrapyramidal symptoms; potentiates hypnotics and narcotics; hypotension

(Taeusch: Avery's Diseases of the Newborn 1998, p.1344)

Chlorpromazine

Route: IV, IM
Neonatal Dose: 2-3 mg/kg/24 h q6h for 4 d
Pediatric Dose: 0.5-1.0 mg/kg/dose

Route: PO
Neonatal Dose: >4 d: decrease above dose over 2-3 wk
Pediatric Dose: 2 mg/kg/24 h q4-6h

Route: PR
Pediatric Dose: 1-2 mg/kg/dose q6-8h

Discussion: Neonatal dosing is for withdrawal from maternal heroin use; children are more susceptible to extrapyramidal reactions, orthostatic hypotension, and atropine-like effects; much higher doses used for psychiatric indications.

(Rudolph: Rudolph's Pediatrics 1996, p.2177)

CHOLECYSTOKININ

Cholecystokinin

The authors investigated whether parenteral nutrition-associated cholestasis (PNAC) in surgical neonates could be alleviated by the administration of cholecystokinin-octapeptide (CCK). Two groups of infants were studied, after major abdominal or cardiac surgery in the newborn period. The low-dose group consisted of three infants with PNAC who received cholecystokinin-octapeptide (Sincalide) at a dose of 0.02 μg/kg intravenously (IV), twice daily. The high-dose group comprised eight infants with PNAC who received an initial dose of 0.02 μg/kg IV or intramuscularly, three times daily on the first day, followed by daily doubling of the dose up to as high as 0.32 μg/kg. In the low-dose group, direct bilirubin levels declined a mean of 50.2 ± 14.5%. ...By excluding these patients (...overt liver failure) from the high-dose group, the decline in bilirubin levels increased to 49.6 ± 10.9%....despite some dramatic declines in bilirubin levels, it has not been established that such treatment will prevent progressive liver injury in such infants. Clearly, a randomized study of CCK compared with placebo may begin to answer such questions.

(Teitelbaum: Treatment of Parenteral Nutrition-Associated Cholestasis With Cholecystokinin-Octapeptide. J Pediatr Surg 1995;30:1082-1085)

CHOLESTYRAMINE (Questran, Questran Light)

Supplied: Powder 4gm anhydrous cholestyramine resin per 9 gm in 9gm packets and 378gm can.
Powder for Oral suspension 4gm anhydrous cholestyramine resin per 5gm powder in 210 gm can and 5 gm packets. Contains Aspartame.

Administration: PO

Comment: To avoid esophageal irritation or blockage or intestinal blockage, the powder should not be taken in dry form.

Cholestyramine Resin (Questran)

Classification: Resin-binding agent.

Indications and use:
For use as a resin-binding agent in patients with chronic diarrhea and short gut syndrome to decrease fecal output.

Action: Cholestyramine resin releases chloride ion and absorbs bile acid in the intestine, forming a nonabsorbable complex preventing enterohepatic recirculation of bile salts.

Route: PO

Dosage: 1-2 g/dose bid to qid.

Elimination: Not absorbed, excreted in the feces.

Adverse effects: Constipation. High doses can cause hyperchloremic acidosis and increased urinary calcium excretion.

Comments: May bind concurrent oral medications.

(Gomella: Neonatology 1999, pp.560-561)

Cholestyramine (Questran)

Dose/kg: 80 mg of the active resin

Route & Frequency: PO; tid with feeds

Comment: May cause constipation, diarrhea, malabsorption of fat soluble vitamins and metabolic acidosis. Alters absorption of drugs when given concurrently. Give oral meds 1 h prior to, or 4-6 h after, cholestyramine.

(Avery: Neonatology pathophysiology and Management of the Newborn 1999, p.1553)

Cholestyramine (Questran, Cholybar)

Dose & Route: **All doses based in terms of anhydrous resin.** Children: 240 mg/kg/24hr ÷ TID. Give PO as slurry in water, juice or milk before meals.

Remarks: May cause constipation, abdominal distension, diarrhea, vomiting, vitamin deficiencies (A,D,E,K), and rash. Hyperchloremic acidosis may occur with prolonged use. Give other oral medications 4-6 hr after cholestyramine or 1 hr before dose to avoid decreased absorption.

(Siberry: The Harriet Lane Handbook 2000, p.671)

CICLOPIROX OLAMINE (Loprox)

Supplied: Cream 1% in 15gm, 30gm, 90gm
Lotion 1% in 30ml

Comment: A broad spectrum antifungal agent that inhibits the growth of pathogenic dermatophytes, yeasts and Malassezia furfur. It exhibits fungicidal activity in vitro against isolates of Trichophyton rubrum, T. mentagrophytes, Epidermophyton floccosum, Microsporum canis and Candida albicans (1).

Ciclopirox

Route: Topical

Neonatal Dose: Massage into affected area twice daily in the morning and evening.

Pediatric Dose: Massage into affected area twice daily in the morning and evening.

Discussion: Diaper rash is treated for 2 wk, while most other fungal infections are treated for 4 wk.

(Rudolph: Rudolph's Pediatrics 1996, p.2177)

CIMETIDINE (Tagamet)

Supplied: Oral solution 300mg/5ml
Injection 150mg/ml in 2ml, 8ml

Administration: PO, IM, IV
For intermittent IV infusion, dilute to a concentration of 6mg/ml and infuse over a period of 15 to 20 minutes (1,3). Stable for 48 hours in NS, D5W, D10W (1).

Cimetidine (Tagamet)

Indications & Dose: Duodenal and gastric ulcers, hypersecretory conditions (eg. Zollinger-Ellison syndrome).

Actions: A histamine (H_2) receptor antagonist; competitively inhibits the action of histamine on the parietal cells, decreasing gastric acid.

Route: IV, PO

Dosage: Neonates: 5-10 mg/kg/day IV or PO divided q8-12h.
Infants: 20 mg/kg/day IV or PO divided q6h.

Adverse effects: CNS toxicity such as alterations in consciousness, antiandrogenic effects, cholestatic jaundice, increased serum concentrations of hepatic-metabolized drugs. Reduce the theophylline dose 50% if used concurrently.

Comments: Limited use in neonates. May add daily dose to the parenteral nutrition regimen and infuse over 24 h to avoid the need for q6-8h administration.

(Gomella: Neonatology 1999, p.561)

Cimetidine

Therapy for Reflux

Common doses: 5-10 mg/kg/dose qid AC, HS

Partial list of side effects:
headache, confusion, pancytopenia, gynecomastia, cholestasis

(Wyllie: Pediatric Gastrointestinal Disease 1999, p.180)

Cimetidine

Dose/kg: 2.5-5 mg

Route & Frequency: IV, IM PO Q6h

Comments: May cause diarrhea, rash, neutropenia, and gynecomastia. Increases blood levels of theophylline, phenytoin, and other drugs. Decrease dose in renal dysfunction.

(Avery: Neonatology Pathophysiology and Management of the Newborn 1999, p.1553)

Cimetidine (Tagamet)

Dose & Route: Neonates: 5-20 mg/kg/24 hr IM/PO/IV Q6-12 hr
Infants: 10-20 mg/kg/24 hr IM/PO/IV ÷ Q6-12 hr.
Children: 20-40 mg/kg/24 hr IM/PO/IV ÷ Q6 hr.

Remarks: Diarrhea, rash, myalgia, confusion, neutropenia, gynecomastia, elevated liver function tests, or dizziness may occur. Inhibits cytochrome P-450 oxidase system, therefore increases levels of hepatically metabolized drugs (i.e. theophylline, phenytoin, lidocaine, diazepam, warfarin). Cimetidine may decrease the absorption of iron, ketoconazole, and tetracyclines. **Adjust dose in renal failure**.

(Siberry: The Harriet Lane Handbook 2000, p.672)

CIPROFLOXACIN (Cipro)

Supplied: Ophthalmic solution 3.5mg/ml in 2.5, 5ml dropper containers.
Tablets: 100mg, 250mg, 500mg, and 750mg
Inj 1% vial 100mg/20ml, 200mg/40ml
Infusion in D5W 100ml, 400mg/200ml, 200mg/100ml

Administration: IV infusion over 60 minutes.
Preferred time of ciprofloxacin dosing is 2 hours after a meal (1).

Dilute vials before use with a suitable IV solution to a final concentration of 1-2mg/ml
Stable up to 14 days at refrigerated or room temperature when diluted with N.S. or D5W (1).

Incompatibilities: aminophylline, amoxicillin, clindamycin, mezlocillin (1).

Ciprofloxacin (Cipro)

Antibacterial Drugs for Pediatric Patients Beyond the Newborn Period: Dosage per kg/d

Route: PO
Mild to Moderate Infections: 20-30 mg in 2 doses
Severe Infections: 30 mg in 2 doses
Comments: Not approved for patients younger than 18 years of age

Route: IV
Mild to Moderate Infections: Inappropriate
Severe Infections: 20-30 mg in 2 doses

Note: In patients with history of allergy to penicillin or one of its may congeners, alternative drugs are recommended. In some circumstances, a cephalosporin or other β-lactam class drug may be acceptable. However, theses drugs should not be used inpatients with an immediate hypersensitivity (anaphylaxis) to penicillin because approximately 5% to 15% of penicillin-allergic patients will also be allergic to the cephalosporins.
(American Academy of Pediatrics: Report of the Committee on Infectious Disease. Red Book 2000, pp.656,662)

Ciprofloxacin

Suggested Dosage Schedules for Antibiotics Used in Newborns
Route: IV
Dosage (mg/kg) and Interval of Administration:
Weight 1200-2000 g
Age >7 Days: 10-20 q24h

Weight >2000 g
Age >7 Days: 20-30 q12h

Note: Doses suggested based on anecdotic clinical experience
(Remington: Infectious Diseases of the Fetus and Newborn Infant 2001, p.1454)

Ciprofloxacin

The infant received intravenous ciprofloxacin, 10 mg/kg per dose every 12 hours, in combination with gentamicin for 25 days.

Conclusion: Ciprofloxacin should be considered in the treatment of neonatal infection caused by multidrug-resistant Gram-negative organisms. Although the published experience with this drug suggests that it is effective and that significant toxicity is not common, its use should be restricted to the treatment of serious infections for which an alternative antibiotic is not available.

(Khaneja: Successful Treatment of Late-Onset Infection due to Resistant Klebsiella pneumoniae in an Extremely Low Birth Weight Infant Using Ciprofloxacin. J Perinatol 1999;19:311-314)

CISAPRIDE (Propulsid)

Supplied: Tablets 10, 20 mg
Suspension 1mg/ml

Contraindications: Concomitant administration of Ketoconazole, intraconazole, miconazole IV or troleandomycin.

Warnings: Cardiac effects - Rare cases of serious cardiac arrhythmias, including ventricular arrhythmias and torsades de pointes associated with QT prolongation, have been observed in patients taking cisapride with other drugs that inhibit cytochrome P450 IIIA4. Some of these events have been fatal (1).

Cisapride

Conclusions. Cisapride treatment of premature infants of <36 weeks' gestation and <3 months of age in NICUs appears to be widespread in the United States. Complications and adverse events were seen when cisapride was administered in excessive dosages or in combination with a drug that inhibits its metabolism and leads to increased serum concentrations. Severe toxicities such as arrhythmias were reported with a frequency of <1/11,000 NICU admissions.

However, in a retrospective survey, episodes of toxicity, including mortality, attributable to cisapride may not have been recognized or reported.

(Ward: Cisapride: A survey of the Frequency of Use and Adverse Events in Premature Newborns. Pediatrics 1999;103:469-472)

Cisapride

Side Effects: Side effects of cisapride generally appear to be minimal and directly related to its effect on the GI tract. Rarely there are reports of abdominal cramps and borborygmi. Occasionally diarrhea may occur, but in a review of 1500 patients treated with cisapride, diarrhea occurred in 4 percent of cisapride-treated patients and 3 percent of placebo-treated patients. Even with long-term use, cisapride has no effect on biochemical or hematological parameters. As with other drugs that alter GI motility and thus transit time, absorption of certain drugs may be altered with the use of cisapride. In a study using healthy volunteers, serum levels of digoxin were reduced, but the difference before and after cisapride was not significant. Cisapride may increase absorption of cimetidine and ranitidine, acenocoumarol, and diazepam.

The most concerning side effect and significant risk factor associated with the use of cisapride is its proarrhythmic effects. Cisapride appears to have a dose-dependent effect on certain myocardial K^+ channels and there are now numerous reports of sinus or supraventricular tachycardia. Despite these reports, the epidemiologic data has not confirmed that the use of cisapride alone at appropriate doses leads to a significantly increased risk of serious ventricular arrhythmias. Bernardini, in a prospective trial, demonstrated that QTc intervals were significantly increased in a group of infants (25 to 41 week gestation) when given cisapride 0.42-1.6 mg/kg per day. Even those with prolongation above 450 milliseconds remained clinically asymptomatic. Ward surveyed neonatal centers across the United States. Of the 58,000 premature newborns (<36 weeks gestation), approximately 19 percent were receiving cisapride. Arrhythmias were reported in three patients, two of whom received a 10-fold overdose of cisapride, and one other infant was receiving erythromycin. Other side effects attributed to cisapride were diarrhea and gagging. Thus severe toxicity reported to the authors was only 1:11,000 patients, but this is a retrospective study. The author readily admits episodes of toxicity may have been under-reported or unrecognized. Cisapride should still be used with caution in young infants.

Both the European Society for Paediatric Gastroenterology, Hepatology, and Nutrition and the North American Society for Pediatric Gastroenterology and Nutrition have published medical position papers which provide appropriate guidelines for prescribing cisapride. Concomitant use of cisapride with drugs that block P450 3A4 metabolism (erythromycin, clarithromycin, azole fungals, the antidepressant nefazodone, and protease inhibitors) is contraindicated. Due to concern about the risk of cardiac arrhythmias the prescribing of cisapride in some countries, such as United States, has become restricted. Dosing which generally should not exceed 0.8 mg/kg per day may be divided in to three or four doses a day up to the recommended adult dosage of 10 mg qid, or 20 mg bid. doses up to 20 mg qid have been used in adults with gastroparesis. Twenty mg at bedtime has been used for maintenance therapy for gastroesophageal reflux.

(Walker: Pediatric Gastrointestinal Disease 2000, pp.1811-1813)

<u>Cisapride</u> (Propulsid)

Indications and use:

GI motility disorders, such as delayed gastric emptying, gastroesophageal reflux, excessive regurgitation, and vomiting.

Actions: Stimulates GI motility by increasing the release of acetylcholine from the myenteric plexus. Improves transit in both the small and large intestine, increases lower esophageal sphincter pressure, and accelerates gastric emptying.

Route: PO

Dosage: 0.15-0.3 mg/kg/dose given q6-8h 15-30 min prior to feedings.

Adverse effects: Diarrhea and drowsiness. Avoid using in situations where GI motility stimulation would be dangerous (eg, mechanical obstruction).

Comments: Anticholinergic drugs may antagonize effects. Concurrent ketoconazole raises cisapride serum concentrations and has caused prolonged Q-T intervals on the electrocardiogram and ventricular arrhythmias (may also occur with itraconazole, miconazole, and fluconazole).

(Gomella: Neonatology 1999, p.561)

<u>Cisapride</u>

Therapy for Reflux

Common doses: 0.2 mg/kg/dose qid AC, HS

Partial list of side effects:

Cramping, arrhythmias

Partial list of contraindications:

Concurrent use of macrolide or antifungal antibiotics: ketoconazole, itraconazole, miconazole, troleandomycin, erythromycin, clarithromycin

(Wyllie: Pediatric Gastrointestinal Disease 1999, p.180)

<u>Cisapride</u>

Dose/kg: 0.15-0.3 mg

Route & frequency: tid-qid, 15-30 min prior to feeds

Comments: May cause diarrhea, nausea, and vomiting

Do not administer with ketoconazole, itraconazole, miconazole, and troleandomycin due to possible occurrence of cardiac arrhythmias.

(Avery: Neonatology Pathophysiology and Management of the Newborn 1999, p.1554)

<u>Cisapride</u>

Dose & Route: Neonates: 0.1-0.2 mg/kg/dose Q6-12 hr PO

Infants and Children: 0.2-0.3 mg/kg/dose TID-QID PO; **max dose**: 10 mg/dose

Remarks: **Contraindicated** in patients taking medications that inhibit cytochrome P-450 3A4 to increase serum cisapride serum levels (substrate); potentially resulting in fatal cardiac arrhythmias. These medications include: ketoconazole, itraconazole, miconazole, fluconazole, erythromycin, clarithromycin, troleandomycin, nefazodone, indinavir, and ritonavir. Do not use inpatients with cardiac disease (especially, torsades de pointes, long QT syndrome, sinus node dysfunction, and 2nd and 3rd degree AV block). **Avoid concomitant use of drugs known to prolong the QT**

interval (i.e. quinidine, procainamide, sotalol, tricyclic antidepressants, maprotiline, phenothiazines, astemizole, and sparfloxacin).
(Siberry: The Harriet Lane Handbook 2000, p.673)

CITRATE

Inquiries can be made to: National Information Center for Orphan Drugs and Rare Diseases (800)456-3505. (1) www.rarediseases.org

Citrate

For therapy in argininosuccinate lyase deficiency. Maintenance therapy consisted of intravenous citrate supplementation 8.64 mmol/kg/24 hr throughout the last 19 days of the patient's hospital course. A case report.
(Iafolla: Citrate therapy in argininosuccinate lyase deficiency. J Pediatr 1990;117:102-105)

Citrate Mixtures, Oral

Indications: Metabolic acidosis
Content (mEq) in each ml of citrate mixture

	Na	K	Citrate
Polycitra	1	1	2
Polycitra-K	0	2	2
Bicitra	1	0	1
Oracit	1	0	1

Dosage/Dosage Interval:
5-15 ml/kg/dose q6-8h, PO or 2-3 mEq/kg/day divided q6-8h. Adjust dose to maintain desired urine pH; 1 mEq citrate equivalent to 1 mEq HCO_3.

Precautions: Use with caution in infants receiving potassium supplements.

Adverse Reactions: Laxative effect.
(Cloherty: Manual of Neonatal Care 1998, p.693)

CITRULLINE (L-Citrulline)

Supplied: Powder; in 25 grams
Obtain from a chemical supply house.

Citrulline

Definitions: CPS = Carbamyl phosphate synthetase I
OTC = Ornithine transcarbamylase

Recommendation:
L-citrulline, given by nasogastric tube during the initial phase of intravenous therapy, may be useful in the treatment of CPS and OTC deficiency.

Rationale: This recommendation is based on consensus clinical experience. Citrulline is not available intravenous form.

Given (orally) in CPS and OTC deficiency, it has the advantage of removing one nitrogen atom while being converted to arginine.

Recommendation:

Where available, plasma levels of ammonia scavenging drugs should be monitored to avoid toxicity.

Rationale: Variable drug excretion may cause toxicity. In the absence of drug levels, a serum anion gap of >15 mEq/L and an anion gap that has risen >6 mEq/L could indicate drug accumulation and increased risk for toxicity.

(The Urea Cycle Disorders Conference Group: Consensus statement from a conference for the Management of Patients with Urea cycle Disorders. J Pediatr 2001;138:S1-S5)

CLARITHROMYCIN (Biaxin)

Supplied: Suspension, Granules for:
125mg/5ml in 50, 100ml, fruit punch flavor
250mg/5ml in 50ml, 100ml fruit punch flavor

Administration: PO
Shake suspension well before each use
Do not refrigerate and use within 14 days (1).
May be given with or without food.

Clarithromycin

Clinical Diagnosis: Otitis media, acute. Infants and Children (pneumococcus, Haemophilus, Moraxella most common)

Therapy: Usual therapy: amoxicillin 80-90 mg/kg/day PO div q8h

For failures or recurrences: amoxicillin-clavulanate 80-90 mg of amoxicillin component/kg/day PO div q8h OR cefuroxime axetil 30 mg/kg/day PO div q12h OR ceftriaxone 50 mg/kg/day IM q24h; x 1-3 doses

Other approved drugs: azithromycin, cefaclor, cefdinir, cefixime, cefpodoxime, cefprozil, ceftibuten, clarithromycin, erythromycin-sulfisoxazole, loracarbrf, trimethoprim-sulfamethoxazole

Comment: Recommendations based on CDC Working Group report (Pediatr Infect Dis J, January 1999;18:1-9); Gram's stain and cultures of pus, if available; If compromised host, suspect unusual infection (Tympanocentesis for culture may be necessary)

A Note on Acute Otitis Media with Effusion:

Several antibiotic regimens are effective for acute otitis media (AOM). Customarily, amoxicillin is used initially and other drugs are given for amoxicillin failures or relapses. The physician should consider advantages and disadvantages regarding antibacterial spectrum, palatability of suspensions, and cost. TMP/SMX is not effective for group A streptococcal infection. When prophylaxis is indicated, use amoxicillin or sulfa drug in one-half the therapeutic dose once or twice daily. How penicillin resistance in pneumococci affects empiric therapy is an unresolved issue.

(Nelson: Pocket Book of Pediatric Antimicrobial Therapy 2000-2001, pp.24-25)

CLINDAMYCIN (Cleocin)

Supplied: Solution, granules for 75mg/5ml in 100ml
Injection 150mg/ml in 2ml, 4ml, 6ml
(contains benzyl alcohol)

Administration: IV, PO, IM
Oral administration: Reconstitute by adding 75ml water to the 100ml bottle in two portions. Shake well. DO NOT refrigerate the solution; it may thicken and be difficult to pour(1). It is stable for two weeks at room temperature (1).

For IV administration, dilute to a concentration NOT exceeding 18mg/ml. For intermittent IV infusion, the diluted solution should be infused over a period of at least 10 to 60 minutes (1).

The recommended final concentration for administration is 18mg/ml. Duration of infusion 15-30 minutes (6).

Stable for 16 days at room temperature in a concentration of 6mg, 9mg, 12mg/ml in D5W or NS, or 32 days refrigerated (3).

Compatible: Alprostadil, magnesium sulfate, meperidine, morphine, parenteral nutrition*.

* Drugs reported as being compatible with parenteral nutrition in published studies using test solutions may not be compatible with the particular formulation your infant is receiving. Components in neonatal parenteral nutrition are individualized based on the infant's body weight, serum electrolytes, fluid, and other nutrient requirements, making most solutions unique. Observe the solution and tubing carefully for signs of precipitation during the 24-hour infusion period when drugs are co-infused. Certain drugs may be admixed into the parenteral nutrition bag. See Driscoll, and associates' review of the use of parenteral nutrition as a drug vehicle (9).

Incompatible: Gentamicin, ranitidine, tobramycin (9).

Clindamycin (Cleocin)

Antibacterial Drugs for Newborn Infants:
Dose (mg/kg or Units [U]/kg) and Frequency of Administration

Route: IV, IM, PO

Dose: Infants 0-4 wk
BW <1200 g: 5 every 12 h

Infants <1 wk old
BW ≤1200-2000 g: 5 every 12 h
BW >2000 g: 5 every 8 h

Infants ≥1 wk old
BW ≤2000-2000 g: 5 every 8 h
BW >2000 g: 5-7.5 every 6 h

Antibacterial Drugs for Pediatric Patients Beyond the Newborn Period
Dosage per kg/d

Route: IM. IV
Mild to Moderate Infections: 15-25 mg in 3-4 doses
Severe Infections: 25-40 mg in 3-4 doses

Comments: Active against anaerobes, especially *Bacteroides* species; active against many multidrug-resistant pneumococci

Route: PO
Mild to Moderate Infections: 10-20 mg in 3-4 doses
Severe Infections: Inappropriate

Comments: Effective for otitis media caused by many multidrug-resistant pneumococci

(American Academy of Pediatrics: Report of the Committee on Infectious Disease. Red Book 2000, pp.651, 656)

Clindamycin

Suggested Dosage Schedules for Antibiotics Used in Newborns
Route: IV, IM, PO
Dosage (mg/kg) and Interval of Administration:

Weight <1200 g
Age 0-4 WK: 5 q12h

Weight 1200-2000 g
Age 0-7 Days: 5 q12h
Age >7 Days: 5 q8h

Weight >2000 g
Age 0-7 Days: 5 q8h
Age >7 Days: 5 q6h

(Remington: Infectious Diseases of the Fetus and Newborn Infant 2001, p.1454)

Clindamycin

Routes: IV, IM, PO
Dosages (mg/kg/day) and Intervals of Administration:

Body weight < 2000g
0-7 days old: 10 div q12h
8-28 days old: 15 div q8h

Body weight > 2000 g
0-7 days old: 15 div q8h
8-28 days old: 20 div q6h

>28 days old: 30 div q6h

(Nelson: Pocket Book of Pediatric Antimicrobial Therapy 2000-2001, p.16)

Clindamycin (Cleocin)

Action & spectrum: Bactericidal activity by inhibiting protein synthesis. Active against both aerobic and anaerobic streptococci (except enterococci), most staphylococci (except methicillin-resistant strains), Bacteroides spp (except *Bacteroides melaninogenicus*), *Fusobacterium varium*, *Actinomyces israelii*, *Clostridium perfringens*, and *Clostridium tetani*. Chiefly used against the above anaerobes. Not effective against Gram-negatives or many clostridial species.

Route: PO, IM, IV (infuse over 10-20 min).

Dosage:
<1200 g: 10 mg/kg/day divided q12h
<2000 g and 0-7 days old: 10 mg/kg/day divided q12h.
<2000 g and >7 days old: 15 mg/kg/day divided q8h.
>2000 g and 0-7 days old: 15 mg/kg/day divided q8h.
>2000 g and >7 days old: 20 mg/kg/day divided q6h.

Elimination and metabolism: Primarily hepatic metabolism.

Adverse effects: Sterile abscess formation at IM injection site. Vomiting and diarrhea occur frequently. Pseudomembranous colitis due to suppression of normal flora and overgrowth of *Clostridium difficile* is uncommon but potentially fatal (treated with oral vancomycin or metronidazole). Rash, glossitis, and pruritus occur occasionally. Serum sickness, anaphylaxis, hematologic (granulocytopenia, thrombocytopenia), and hepatic abnormalities occur rarely.

Comments: Does not cross the blood-brain barrier; therefore, do not use to treat meningitis.

(Gomella: Neonatology 1999, pp.561-562)

CLOTRIMAZOLE (Lotrimin, Mycelex)

Supplied:
Cream 1% in 15gm, 30gm, 45mg
Solution 1% in 10ml, 30ml
Lotion 1% in 30ml

Comment: A broad spectrum antifungal agent that inhibits the growth of pathogenic dermatophytes, yeasts and Malassezia furfur. In vitro activity same as Ciclopirox (1).

Clotrimazole (Desenex, Lotrimin, Mycelex, Fungoid)

Topical Drugs for Superficial Fungal Infections:

Strength: 1%
Formulation: Cream, Lotion, Solution, Suppositories
Applications per day 2
Adverse Reactions/Notes:
Irritant dermatitis; hives
Notes: Nonprescription drug.

(American Academy of Pediatrics: Report of the Committee on Infectious Diseases. Red Book 2000, pp.673-674)

<u>Clotrimazole</u>

Clotrimazole is another imidazole derivative that has been used as a topical agent in infants with mucocutaneous candidiasis. Cohen and co-workers found clotrimazole to be as effective as nystatin in infants with thrush. Montello and associates also reported an infant with thrush who was successfully treated with clotrimazole applied to the mouth and thumb. Milne also found it to be effective in oral candidiasis, and although a longer course with it was necessary to cure the infection than with nystatin, there were fewer relapses. Clotrimazole has been reported to increase myeloperoxidase activity within leukocytes, which may account for some of the drug's effectiveness.

(Remington: Infectious Diseases of the Fetus and Newborn Infant 2001, p.837)

<u>Clotrimazole</u> (Lotrimin, Mycelex)

Dose & Route: Topical: apply to skin BID x 4-8 wks

Remarks: May cause erythema, blistering or urticaria with topical use. Liver enzyme elevation, nausea and vomiting may occur with troches.

(Siberry: The Harriet Lane Handbook 2000, p.678)

CLOXACILLIN (Tegopen)

Supplied: Suspension, powder for 125mg/5ml in 100, 200ml

Administration: PO

Oral solutions are stable for 14 days refrigerated. Stored at room temperature, they are stable for 3 days (3).

Since food interferes with GI absorption of cloxacillin, the drug should be administered at least 1 hour before or 2 hours after meals (1).

<u>Cloxacillin</u> (Tegopen, Cloxapen)

Antibacterial Drugs for Pediatric Patients Beyond the Newborn Period:
Dosage per kg/d
Route: PO
Mild to Moderate Infections: 50-100 mg in 4 doses
Severe Infections: Inappropriate

Note: In patients with history of allergy to penicillin or one of its may congeners, alternative drugs are recommended. In some circumstances, a cephalosporin or other β-lactam class drug may be acceptable. However, theses drugs should not be used inpatients with an immediate hypersensitivity (anaphylaxis) to penicillin because approximately 5% to 15% of penicillin-allergic patients will also be allergic to the cephalosporins.

(American Academy of Pediatrics: Report of the Committee on Infectious Diseases. Red Book 2000, pp.660, 662)

<u>Cloxacillin</u>

Condition: Otitis Media, Staphylococcus Aureus

Therapy: Cloxacillin or cephalexin 50 mg/kg/day PO div q6-8h x 10 days

Comment: Oxacillin if unable to treat PO
(Nelson: Pocket Book of Pediatric Antimicrobial Therapy 2000-2001, p.11)

CODEINE

Supplied: Injection 30mg, 60mg/ml
Tablets 15mg, 30mg, 60mg
Soluble Tablets 15mg, 30mg, 60mg

Administration: IM, SQ, PO

DO NOT use IV in children (1).

Codeine (Various Brands)

Dose & Route: Analgesic:
Children: 0.5-1.0 mg/kg/dose Q4-6h IM, SC or PO
Max dose: 60 mg/dose

Remarks: **Do not use in children <2 yr old as antitussive.** Not intended for IV use, due to large histamine release and cardiovascular effects. Side effects: CNS and respiratory depression, constipation, cramping, hypotension, pruritus. May be habit forming.

For analgesia, use with acetaminophen orally. **Adjust dose in renal failure**.
(Siberry: The Harriet Lane Handbook 2000, pp. 679-680)

Codeine

Route: IM, SC, PO

Neonatal Dose: 1-3 mg/kg/24 h q4-6h

Pediatric Dose: 1-4 mg/kg/24 h q4-6h Max: 60 mg/dose.

Discussion: Effective antitussive alone but poor analgesic alone and should be combined with aspirin or acetaminophen for oral analgesic use.
(Rudolph: Rudolph's Pediatrics 1996, p.2178)

COLESTIPOL (Colestid)

Supplied: Tablets 1gm
Granules, 300gm, 500gm bottles, 5gm packets

Administration: PO
Granules: mix in liquids, soups, cereals or pulpy fruits. DO NOT take dry. Stir until completely mixed. Colestipol will not dissolve (1).
Tablets: Swallow tablets whole one at a time; do not cut, chew, or crush (1).

Colestipol (Colestid)

Indication: Infants with short bowel syndrome... anion exchange resin that can bind excessive bile acids, ameliorating bile acid induced diarrhoea.

Dose: 250 mg/kg/day in three to four divided doses.

Comments: These medications are useful in patients with limited ileal resections; in extensive resections. They can cause further depletion of the bile acid pool and exacerbate steatorrhoea. Hyperchloremic acidosis may result from excessive doses. Serum electrolytes must be carefully monitored during initial therapy and periodically thereafter.

(Hay: Neonatal Nutrition & Metabolism 1991, pp.444, 2000)

COLISTIN SULFATE (Coly Mycin S Suspension, Polymixin E)

Supplied: Oral suspension, powder for: 25mg (colistin)/5ml in 60mL bottles.

Administration: PO

Reconstitute with 37ml distilled water in two portions. SHAKE WELL. The suspension is stable for two weeks below 59 F (1).

Colistin Sulfate

For Newborns with EPEC gastroenteritis

On the basis of these data, there appears to be sufficient evidence to recommend oral administration of nonabsorbable antibiotics in the treatment of severely or moderately ill newborns with EPEC gastroenteritis. The drug most frequently used for initial therapy is neomycin sulfate in a dosage of 100 mg/kg per day administered PO every 8 hours in three divided doses. In communities in which neomycin-resistant EPEC has been prevalent, treatment should be started with colistin sulfate or polymyxin B in a dosage of 15 to 20 mg/kg PO daily, divided into three equal doses. However, it is rarely necessary to use this approach.

(Remington: Infectious Diseases of the Fetus and Newborn Infant 2001 p.1264)

COPPER

Supplied: Copper injection: 0.4mg/mL (as 1.07mg cupric Cl)
Cupric sulfate injection: 0.4mg/mL (as 1.57mg sulfate)
2mg/mL (as 7.85mg sulfate)

Administration: Supplement to IV solutions given for TPN

Copper Sulfate

Indication: Copper deficiency in premature infants.

Preparation: 1% solution of copper sulfate

Dose: PO 200 to 600 μg Cu/day
IV 20 μg/kg/day

Caution: IV copper should be reduced or withheld in the presence of cholestatic disease.

Toxicity: Acute ingestion of quantities of copper that are 1,000 time the daily requirement can have a fatal outcome.

Acute copper poisoning has toxic effects on the liver, kidneys, heart and central nervous system, and causes intravascular hemolysis.

Chronic copper toxicity may cause cirrhosis.
(Hay: Neonatal Nutrition & Metabolism 1991, pp.217-218)

SEE ALSO: TRACE MINERALS

CORTICOTROPIN (ACTH, ACTHAR)

Supplied: Injection, powder for 25 unit and 40 unit vials
Injection, repository 40 and 80 units/mL in 1mL, 5mL

Administration: Injection, powder: After reconstitution, it is administered IM, SC. May be given IV for diagnostic purposes.
Injection, repository: IM or SC, NOT FOR IV use (1).

Corticotropin (ACTH)

Dosage: 1.6 units/kg/day divided every 6-8 hr. IV, IM, SC.
(Fanaroff: Neonatal-Perinatal Medicine 1997, p.1750)

ACTH (Corticotropin, Acthar)

Dose & Route: Antiinflammatory:
Aqueous: 1.6 U/kg/24hr IV, IM, or SC÷Q6-8hr
Gel: 0.8 U/kg/24hr÷Q12-24hr IM

Infantile Spasms: Many regimens exist.
Gel: 20-40 U/24hr IM QD x 6 weeks or 150 U/m^2/24 hr IM ÷ BID for 2 weeks; followed by a gradual taper.

Remarks: **Contraindicated** in acute psychoses, CHF, Cushing's disease, TB, peptic ulcer, ocular herpes, fungal infections, recent surgery, sensitivity to porcine products; IV administration for diagnostic purposes only. **Gel dosage form is only for the IM route.**

Can have hypersensitivity reaction. Similar adverse effects as corticosteroids.
(Siberry: Harriet Lane Handbook 2000 p.617)

Corticotropin (ACTH)

Treatment lasted for 2 weeks (Table 1). ACTH (ACTHARGEL, Rhõne-Poulenc-Rorer, Collegeville, PA; 150 U/m^2/day) was given intramuscularly in two divided doses. Prednisone (2 mg/kg/day was given orally in two divided doses.

Tapering schedules:
ACTH: For 3 days 30 U/M^2 in the morning.
For 3 days 15 U/m^2 in the morning.
For 3 days 10 U/m^2 in the morning.
For 6 days 10 U/m^2 every other morning.

Prednisone: For 3 days the morning dose (1 mg/kg) only.
For 6 days half the morning dose (0.5 mg/kg) only.
For 6 days 0.5 mg/kg every other morning.

Using a prospective, randomized approach, a 2-week course of high-dose ACTH is superior to 2 weeks of prednisone for treatment of IS, as assessed by both clinical and EEG criteria.

(Baram: High-dose Corticotropin (ACTH) Versus Prednisone for Infantile Spasms: A Prospective, Randomized, Blinded Study. Pediatrics 1996;97:375-379)

Corticotropin (ACTH)

Infants were randomly assigned to receive either ACTH (Cortrosyn), 0.1 μg/kg, or saline placebo. Subsequently a dose comparison trial was initiated, with a higher dose of ACTH (0.2 μg/kg) substituted for the placebo group. In VLBW infants, these doses closely approximate 1 and 2 μg/m^2, respectively. In all infants a baseline blood sample of 1.2 ml was taken on the second morning of life for measurements of cortisol....ACTH or saline placebo was then infused for 5 minutes. After 60 minutes, 0.8 ml of blood was collected for determinations of cortisol, ...Infants with spontaneous morning cortisol values 414 nmol/L or greater ≥15.0 μg/dl) were considered to have adrenocortical insufficiency. A normal adrenal response to ACTH stimulation was defined as a 60-minute postinfusion cortisol level of 414 nmol/L or more (≥15.0 μg/dl)....Most infants (76%) had baseline cortisol concentrations <14 nmol/L (15.0 μg/dl), and of those, only 36% responded to stimulation with ACTH, 0.1 μg/kg. Raising the ACTH dose to 0.2 μg/kg resulted in a response rate of 67% (p=0.09) but decreased the sensitivity of the test.

(Korte: Adrenocortical function in the very low birth weight infant: Improved testing sensitivity and association with neonatal outcome. J Pediatr 1996;128:257-263)

Corticotropin (ACTH)

An ACTH stimulation test was performed during the afternoon of day 5,6,or 7 of life (day of birth = day 0) ...A blood sample was drawn for baseline cortisol concentration, after which cosyntropin (α 1-24 corticotropin), a synthetic analog of ACTH, was administered intravenously or intramuscularly, at a dose of 3.5 μg/kg....we prospectively defined a positive response to be a rise in plasma cortisol of ≥9 μg/dL (248nM/L)....84% of patients who recovered without BPD, but only 26% of BPD patients, achieved a prospectively defined positive cortisol response to ACTH (≥9 μg/dL; P<.005).

(Watterberg: Evidence of Early Adrenal Insufficiency in Babies Who Develop Bronchopulmonary Dysplasia. Pediatrics 1995;95:120-125)

Corticotropin (ACTH)

High- or low-dose therapy with corticotropin (adrenocorticotropic hormone; ACTH). Twenty-six patients receiving the high-dose therapy were treated as follows: 150 U/m^2 per day for 3 weeks, 80 U/m^2 per day for 2 weeks, 80 U/m^2 every other day for 3 weeks, and 50 U/m^2 per day every other day for 1 week, with the dosage then tapered to zero during a 3-week period. The 24 patients assigned to the low-dose therapy group received 20 to 30 U/day for 2 to 6 weeks; the dosage was then tapered to zero during a 1-week period....no major difference in the effectiveness of these two regimens in the treatment of infantile spasms with respect to spasm cessation and improvement in the patients' electroencephalographic findings.

(Hrachovy: High-dose, long-duration versus low-dose, short-duration corticotropin therapy for infantile spasms. J Pediatr 1994;124:803-806)

CORTISONE
CORTISONE ACETATE (Cortone Acetate, Cortisone)

Supplied: Tablets 5, 10mg, 25mg.
Injection, suspension 50mg/ml

Administration: IM, PO
FOR IM ADMINISTRATION ONLY. Do not inject IV.
Parenteral dosages contains benzyl alcohol 9 mg/ml (3).

Cortisone

Dosage: 25 mg/m^2/day divided every 8 hr.
12 mg/m^2/day single dose IM.

Comments: Physiologic replacement.

(Fanaroff: Neonatal-Perinatal Medicine 1997, p.1750)

Cortisone

Dose/kg: Physiologic replacement: 0.25 mg
Route & Frequency: IM; q24h

Dose/kg: Antiinflammatory: 1-2.5 mg
Route & Frequency: IM; q12-24h

Dose/kg: Stress: 0.5-1 mg
Route & Frequency: IM during illness or perioperatively

Comments: Slow IM absorption. Risk of infection. Hypertension. Salt retention. Adrenal suppression. Hyperglycemia. Leukocytosis.

(Avery: Neonatology 1994, p.1440)

SEE ALSO: PREDNISONE

COSYNTROPIN (Cortrosyn)

Supplied: Injection 0.25mg/vial with diluent

Administration: IV, IM

Each 0.25 mg of Cosyntropin is equivalent to 25 units of corticotropin. (3)
May be given IM or by direct IV injection over a 2-minute period (3).

Cosyntropin (Cortrosyn)

Indications and use: Aid in diagnosis of adrenocortical insufficiency.

Actions: Stimulates the adrenal cortex to secrete cortisol (hydrocortisone) and other substances.

Dosage: 0.015 mg/kg (1 dose only).

Route: IM, IV (infuse initial dilution over 2 min).

Comments: For rapid diagnostic screening of adrenocortical insufficiency, plasma cortisol concentrations should be measured prior to and 60 min after administration of cosyntropin; 0.25 mg = 25 USP units of corticotropin.

(Gomella: Neonatology 1999, p.562)

CROMOLYN (Intal)

Supplied: Opthalmic solution: 4%, in 2.5, 10ml bottles
Inhalation: 20mg/2mL in UD plastic vials
Solution for nebulization: 20mg vial
Solution (for nebulizer only) 20mg/amp
Aerosol spray: delivers 800 mcg/actuation
Opthalmic nasal solutions: 40mg/ml. Each actuation delivers 5.2mg.
Capsule (oral): 100mg

Administration: Inhalation
Opthalmic
Oral

Cromolyn (Intal)

Dose: 20 mg. Dilute with NS to 3 mL. Dose: every 6-8 h

Side Effects: Anaphylaxis
Caution in patients with liver or renal disease
Bronchospasm from inflammatory response
Upper airway irritation

(Gomella: Neonatology: Management, Procedures, On-call Problems, Diseases and Drugs 1999, p.56)

Cromolyn

Dose/kg: 20 mg/dose

Route & frequency: Inhalation q6h-q8h

Comments: Bronchospasm, cough, nasal congestion, and pharyngeal irritation have been reported.

(Avery: Neonatology Pathophysiology and Management of the Newborn, 1999, p.1554)

Cromolyn

Dose & Route: Nebulization: 20 mg Q6-8 hr
Nasal: 1 spray each nostril TID-QID

Remarks: May cause rash, cough, bronchospasm, nasal congestion. May cause headache, diarrhea with oral use. Use with

caution in patients with renal or hepatic dysfunction. Bronchospasm and pharyngeal irritation may occur when using spinhaler product.

Therapeutic response often occurs within 2 weeks, however, a 4-6 week trial may be needed to determine maximum benefit. For exercise induced asthma, give no longer than 1 hour before activity. Oral concentrate and contents of capsule can only be diluted in water. Nebulized solution can be mixed with albuterol nebs.

(Siberry: The Harriet Lane Handbook 2000, p.681)

CYCLOMYDRIL (0.2% cyclopentolate / 1% phenylephrine)

Supplied: 2ml, 5ml drop-tainers
Administration: Ophthalmic drops

Cyclomydril

For ROP Exam: Each infant was then given 1 drop of Cyclomydril in each eye, followed by application of punctile pressure; this procedure was repeated 5 minutes later. The screening examination for ROP was performed approximately 1 hour later.

Conclusion: Current doses of mydriatics inhibit duodenal motor activity and delay gastric emptying, and these gastrointestinal effects of mydriatics may underlie the feeding difficulties seen in preterm infants on the day of screening examinations for ROP.

(Bonthala: Mydriatics slow gastric emptying in preterm infants. J Pediatr 2000;137:327-30)

CYCLOPENTOLATE (Cyclogyl, Ak-Pentolate)

Supplied: Solution 0.5%, 1%, 2% in 2ml, 5ml, 15ml

Cyclopentolate (Cyclogyl)

Dose & Route: Infant: 1 drop of 0.5% OU 5-10 min before exam.

Remarks: Do not use in narrow-angle glaucoma. May cause a burning sensation, behavioral disturbance, tachycardia, loss of visual accommodation. To minimize absorption, apply pressure over nasolacrimal sac for at least 2 min. CNS and cardiovascular side effects are common with the 2% solution in children.
Onset of action: 15-60 minutes.
Observe patient closely for at least 30 min after dose.

(Siberry: The Harriet Lane Handbook 2000. pp.681-682)

Cyclopentolate

In a prospective study of 26 premature infants, 5 μl microdrops were compared with standard 26 μl eye drops of cyclopentolate 0.5% and phenylephrine 2.5%. There was no statistical difference in pupil dilation. The 5 μl microdrops have potentially fewer adverse effects in premature infants.

(Wheatcroft: Reduction in mydriatic drop size in premature infants. Br J Ophthalmol 1993;77:364-365)

CYCLOPENTOLATE/PHENYLEPHRINE (Cyclomydril)

Supplied: Solution 0.2% cyclopentolate and 1% phenylephrine in 2ml, 5ml.

Cyclopentolate/phenylephrine (Cyclomydril)

Dose & Route: 1 drop OU Q5-10 min; **max dose**: 3 drops per eye.

Remarks: Used to induce mydriasis. See cyclopentolate for comments.

(Siberry: The Harriet Lane Handbook 2000, p.682)

CYCLOPHOSPHAMIDE (Cytoxan, Neosar)

Supplied: Tablets 25mg, 50mg
Injection 100mg, 200mg, 500mg, 1gm and 2gm vials.

Administration: IV, PO, intraperitoneally or intrapleurally; IM (1)

Preparation of oral solution:
Dissolve injectable cyclophosphamide in Aromatic Elixir. Store under refrigeration in glass containers and use within 14 days (1).

Cyclophosphamide

Indication: Life-threatening vascular tumor

Dose: IV cyclophosphamide 10mg/kg/day for 3 days.
A second course followed one month later for patient #2.

Conclusion: Cyclophosphamide appears to be an effective and well-tolerated therapy. This treatment should be considered when other therapeutic modalities are not feasible or seem less desirable.

(Hurvitz: Cyclophosphamide therapy in life-threatening vascular tumors. J Pediatr 1986;109:360-363)

CYCLOSPORINE (Sandimmune, Neoral)

Supplied: Capsules; soft gelatin: 25, 50, 100mg
Oral solution 100mg/mL in 50mL bottles w/graduated pipette (contains 12.5% alcohol)
Oral solution for Microemulsion 100mg/mL in 50mL (contains 9.5% alcohol)
IV solution: 50mg/ml, 5ml amps. (contains 32.9% alcohol)

Administration: IV, PO
Use oral solution within 2 months of opening.
IV diluted in NS, D5W-administered over 2-6 hours (1).

Cyclosporine (Sandimmune)

Neoral manufacturer recommends a 1:1 conversion ratio with Sandimmune. Due to its better absorption, however, lower doses of Neoral may be required.

Dose & Route: Oral: 15 mg/kg as a single dose given 4-12 hrs pre-transplant; give the same dose daily x 1-2 weeks post transplant then reduce by 5% per wk to 5-10 mg/kg/24hr ÷ Q12-24 hr.

IV: 5-6 mg/kg as a single dose given 4-12 hrs pre-transplant: administer over 2-6 hrs; give the same dose daily post-transplant until the patient able to tolerate the oral form.

Remarks: May cause nephrotoxicity, hepatotoxicity, hypomagnesemia, hyperkalemia, hyperuricemia, hypertension, hirsutism, acne, GI symptoms, tremor, leukopenia, sinusitis, gingival hyperplasia, headache. Use **caution** with concomitant use of other nephrotoxic drugs such as amphotericin b and aminioglycosides.

Plasma concentrations increased with the use of fluconazole, ketoconazole, erythromycin, verapamil, and corticosteroids. Plasma concentrations decreased with the use of carbamazepine, rifampin, phenobarbital, and phenytoin. Cyclosporine is a substrate for CYP450 3A4

Children may require dosages 2-3 times higher than adults. T-tube clamping may increase absorption. Plasma half-life 6-24 hrs.

Monitor trough levels (just prior to a dose at steady-state). Steady-state is generally achieved after 3-5 days of continuous dosing. Interpretation will vary based on treatment protocol and assay methodology (RIA monoclonal vs. RIA polyclonal vs. HPLC) as well as whole blood vs. serum sample.

(Siberry: The Harriet Lane Handbook 2000, pp.682-683)

SEE ALSO: IMMUNOSUPPRESSION AGENTS

CYSTEINE HCL

Supplied: Injection 50mg/5ml in 10ml

Administration: IV

Cysteine is a sulfur-containing amino acid. It is synthesized from methionine via the trans-sulfuration pathway in the adult, but newborn infants lack the enzyme necessary to effect this conversion. Therefore, cysteine is generally considered an essential amino acid in infants (1). Cysteine is relatively unstable over time in premixed solutions of crystalline amino acids, eventually converting to insoluble cysteine. To avoid such precipitation, cysteine is provided as an additive for use with crystalline amino acid solutions immediately prior to administration (1).

Cysteine HCL

Cysteine hydrochloride is often added to TPN solutions, because cysteine is unstable over time and is omitted from amino acid solutions. The premature infant lacks the ability to convert methionine to cysteine, so it is thus conditionally essential. The recommended dose is 40 mg of cysteine per gram of protein.

(Gomella: Neonatology: Management, Procedures, On-call Problems, Diseases and Drugs 1999, p.90)

Cysteine HCL

Dose: 60-120 mg/kg/day IV (= 0.5-1 mmol/kg/day)
May also be calculated as 100 mg cysteine for every 2.5 gm crystalline amino acids.

Use: An amino acid used as a component of PN.

An essential amino acid for infants, particularly preterm infants, because of an immaturity in the transsulfuration pathway of methionine to cysteine and taurine . Removal of cysteine from an otherwise adequate diet in 2- to 4-month-old preterm infants has resulted in lower rates of weight gain and nitrogen retention as well as lower plasma cysteine concentrations.

Addition of cysteine to neonatal PN lowers the pH of the solution and increases calcium and phosphorus solubility. This allows a larger amount of these minerals to be added.

Adverse Effects: Usually very well tolerated.

Metabolic Acidosis: Because it is available as the hydrochloride salt, cysteine adds to the chloride load of the infants. The risk of metabolic acidosis is greater in infants <1,250 mg. Metabolic acidosis may be managed by using the lower end of the dosage range and/or by use of acetate salts.

Comments: When infants have reached about 1 year of age, they can adequately metabolize methionine to cysteine, so cysteine no longer needs to be added to the PN solution.

(Zenk: Neonatal Medications & Nutrition. A Comprehensive Guide 2000. pp.144-145)

Cysteine (L-Cysteine HCL)

Route: IV

Neonatal Dose: 0.5-1 mmol/kg/24 h or 60-120 mg/kg/24 h daily diluted in parenteral nutrition solution.

Pediatric Dose: 0.5 g daily diluted in parenteral nutrition solution.

Discussion: This is to be added to a parenteral nutrition solution as an essential amino acid in preterm infants.

(Rudolph: Rudolph's Pediatrics 1996, p.2179)

DANTROLENE SODIUM (Dantrium)

Supplied: Capsules 25, 50, 100 mg
Powder for injection: 20 mg vial

Administration: IV, PO
Preparation of solution: Add 60 ml SWFI to vial (approx. conc 0.32 mg/ml). Use within 6 hours. Store at room temperature (1).

Dantrolene

Dose & Route: **Malignant Hyperthermia:**
Prevention:
PO: 4-8 mg/kg/24 hr ÷ Q6 hr x 1-3 days before surgery
IV: 2.5 mg/kg over 1 hr beginning 1.25 hr before anesthesia, additional doses PRN

Treatment: 1 mg/kg IV, repeat PRN to **max cumulative dose** of 10 mg/kg, then continue 4-8 mg/kg/24 hr PO ÷ Q6 hr for 1-3 days.

Remarks: **Contraindicated** in active hepatic disease. Monitor transaminases for hepatotoxicity. Use with **caution** in children with cardiac or pulmonary impairment. May cause change in sensorium, weakness, diarrhea, constipation, incontinence, and enuresis. **Avoid unnecessary exposure to sunlight. Avoid extravasation into tissues**. A decrease in spasticity sufficient to allow daily function should be therapeutic goal. Discontinue if benefits are not evident in 45 days.

(Siberry: The Harriet Lane Handbook 2000, p.684)

Dantrolene

Initial dose 2.5 mg/kg IV. If necessary continue to infuse IV at 1 mg/kg/min (up to 10 mg/kg) until the heart rate begins to slow and become regular, decreased muscle tone becomes evident, and the patient's temperature starts to fall. Then withhold the dantrolene and observe the heart rate, muscle tone, and temperature. If these deteriorate again, the infusion can be repeated at intervals of not less than 15 minutes until clinical improvement is apparent. Malignant hyperthermia may recur within the first 24 hours.

Steward: Manual of Pediatric Anesthesia 1995, pp.166-167)

DAPSONE (DDS)

Supplied: Tablets 25mg, 100mg
Administration: PO

Extemporaneous Compounding (Recipe)

Dosage form: Oral suspension
Made from: Tablets
Concentration: 2mg/mL
Stability: 21 days
Store: Refrigerate in amber glass
Label: Shake well

Ingredient	Strength	Quantity
Dapsone tablets	25 mg	8
Citric acid crystals		0.5 g
Purified water USP		25 mL
Syrup		qs 100 mL

Instructions: Crush the tablets in mortar. Dissolve citric acid crystals in water. Add citric acid solution to the dapsone tablet powder and mix until uniform. Then qs with syrup and store in amber glass bottle. (11)

Dapsone

Drug Regimens for *Pneumocystis carinii* Pneumonia Prophylaxis for Children 4 Weeks of Age or Older:
Alternative regimens if trimethoprim-sulfamethoxazole is not tolerated:

Dapsone (children ≥1 mo of age)
2 mg/kg (maximum 100 mg) administered orally once a day or 4 mg/kg (maximum 200 mg) orally every week
(American Academy of Pediatrics: Report of the Committee on Infectious Diseases. Red Book 2000, pp.463-465)

Dapsone

Route: PO
Dosage: 1 mg/kg/day
Interval: q24h
NON-NEWBORN SECTION
(Nelson: Pocket Book of Pediatric Antimicrobial Therapy 2000-2001, p.74)

Dapsone

Dose & Route: Pneumocystis carinii Prophylaxis:
Children ≥month: 2 mg/kg/24 hr PO QD;
max dose 100 mg/24 hr

Remarks: May cause hemolysis in G6PD deficiency, or methemoglobin reductase deficiency (primarily results in methemoglobinemia), or hemoglobin M. Side effects include: hemolytic anemia (dose related), agranulocytosis, aplastic anemia, nausea, vomiting, hyperbilirubinemia, headache, nephrotic syndrome, and hypersensitivity reaction (sulfone syndrome).

Suspension may not be absorbed as well as tablets.

2 mg/ml suspension product is also available via an IND for PCP prophylaxis from Jacobus Pharmaceutical Company (609) 921-7447
(Siberry: The Harriet Lane Handbook 2000, pp. 684-685)

DESMOPRESSIN ACETATE (DDAVP)

Supplied: Tablets: 0.1mg, 0.2mg
Injection 4mcg/mL

	Intranasal solution: 0.1mg/ml (0.1mg equals 400 IU arginine vasopressin), nasal spray pump, (50 doses of 10mcg) rhinal tube delivery system (1).
Administration:	IV Infusion over 15 to 30 minutes

<u>Intranasal dDAVP</u>

Indication: For Diabetes Insipidus

Despite conservative management, clinical symptoms persisted over the next 4 weeks, and treatment with continuous intravenous desmopressin was initiated at a dose of 1.5 mU/kg per hour. Over the next several weeks, the desmopressin infusion was titrated to maintain serum sodiums and urine output within a normal range. The patient responded well to this therapy, with serum sodium decreasing to the mid 140 range and urine output decreasing to 3 ml/kg per hour. During this time, he manifested good weight gain on full enteral feeds of fortified human milk at 150 ml/kg per day. On day 105 of life, therapy was converted to intranasal dDAVP at 0.5µg/day. The dDAVP was concentrated at 100 µg/10 ml and dosed as 0.025 ml every 12 hours. Over the next month, the dose was increased to 0.05 ml twice a day (1.0 µg/day). Serum sodiums remained stable at 141 to 148 meq/dl, with serum osmolarity at 289 to 291 U and urine output at 2 to 3 ml/kg per day. Therapy was well tolerated without any noted adverse events.

At 4 months of age, the patient was sent home on intranasal dDAVP following a relatively uneventful remaining hospital course. A magnetic resonance imaging scan performed shortly after discharge was within normal limits and without evidence of hypothalamic-pituitary abnormalities. At 24 months of age, he is continuing to develop normally. Attempts to wean him off therapy at this time were unsuccessful, and he remains on intranasal dDAVP at a dose of 1.0 µg/day divided every 12 hours.

In summary, we have presented the case of a very low birth weight premature infant with onset of idiopathic central DI in the first several weeks of life who was successfully managed with intranasal dDAVP. The diagnosis of idiopathic central DI should be considered in the neonate, including extremely premature infants, with onset of unexplained hypernatremia and polyuria. Families should be counseled that these symptoms may not be transient and may require long-term treatment. We recommend that intravenous desmopressin initially be administered at a dose of 1 to 3 mU/kg per hour once the diagnosis of central DI has been established. Once a clinical response has been established, the patient can be transitioned to intranasal dDAVP at a dose of 0.5 µg/day divided every 12 hours. This dose may then be subsequently titrated to achieve the desired clinical effect.

(Stapleton: Persistent Central Diabetes Insipidus Presenting in a Very Low Birth Weight Infant Successfully Managed With Intranasal dDAVP. J Perinatol 2000; 2:132-134)

DEXAMETHASONE (Decadron, Hexadrol)

Supplied: Tablets: 0.25mg, 0.5mg, 0.75mg, 1mg, 1.5mg, 2mg, 4mg, 6mg
Elixir 0.5mg/5ml (contains 5% alcohol)
Oral solution 0.5mg/5ml
Oral Intensol solution 0.5mg/0.5ml (contains 30% alcohol)
Injection-Na Phosphate 4mg/ml, in 1ml, 5ml, 10ml, 30ml vials

Administration: IV, IM, PO
For direct IV injection, use sodium phosphate salt in a concentration of 4mg/ml and inject over 3 to 5 minutes.

For intermittent infusion, dilute in at least an equal volume and infuse over a minimum of 10 minutes. Stable in D5W or NS (2).

Dexamethasone (Decadron)

Indications: Resistant neonatal hypoglycemia and airway edema. Used in weaning infants with BPD from the ventilator.

Actions: Primarily used as an antiinflammatory or immunosuppressive agent. Due to its minimal mineralocorticoid activity, not indicated for replacement therapy in adrenocortical insufficiency. A long-acting, potent glucocorticoid lacking sodium-retaining activity with low to moderate doses. Increases urinary calcium excretion.

Route: IV, IM, PO, inhalation.

Dosage: BPD: (Dosage not well established): 0.5 mg/kg/day IV divided q12h x 3 days; then 0.3 mg/kg/day divided q12h x 72h. Decrease dose by 0.1 mg/kg/day q72h until 0.1mg/kg/day is reached, then give on alternate days for 1 week and discontinue.

Neonatal hypoglycemia: (dosage not well established): 0.25 mg/kg/dose repeated q12h prn.

Airway edema: 0.25 mg/kg/dose q12h, generally beginning 24 h before planned extubation and continued for 2-4 doses after.

Adverse effects: With long-term use: increased susceptibility to infection, osteoporosis, growth retardation, hyperglycemia, fluid and electrolyte disturbances, cataracts, myopathy, and acute adrenal insufficiency.

(Gomella: Neonatology 1999, p.562)

Dexamethasone

Dose/kg: Antiinflammatory: 0.025-0.05 mg
Route & frequency: IV, IM, PO q6-q12h

Dose/kg: Airway edema: 0.25mg
Route & frequency: IV, IM, PO q6h pm
For extubation: Give first dose 4 h prior to extubation. Then repeat 4 and 12 h after extubation

Dose/kg: BPD
Route & frequency: IV, IM, PO
Taper:

Day	Daily dose	Frequency
1-3	0.5 mg/kg	+q12h
4-6	0.3 mg/kg	+q12h
7-9	0.27 mg/kg	+q12h
10-12	0.24 mg/kg	+q12h
13-15	0.22 mg/kg	+q12h
16-18	0.2 mg/kg	+q12h
19-21	0.18 mg/kg	+q12h
22-24	0.16 mg/kg	+q12h
25-27	0.14 mg/kg	+q12h
28-30	0.12 mg/kg	+q12h
31-38	0.1 mg/kg	qd
40, 42	0.1 mg/kg	qd

Comments: May increase risk of infection. May cause hypertension, salt retention, adrenal suppression, hyperglycemia, and leukocytosis. Consider steroid coverage for periods of stress after therapy for BPD, and in intercurrent illness (see BPD section). Give hydrocortisone stress doses for surgery up to 6 mo after stopping taper. See Hydrocortisone for stress dosing guidelines. All calculations must use the same body weight.

(Avery: Neonatology Pathophysiology and Management of the Newborn 1999, p.1554)

Dexamethasone

Dexamethasone is recommended for treatment of infants and children with Hib meningitis

(American Academy of Pediatrics: Report of the Committee on Infectious Disease. Red Book 2000, p.263)

Dexamethasone

Conclusions. The data suggest an impairment in brain growth, principally affecting cerebral cortical gray matter, secondary to systemic dexamethasone therapy. Although the premature infants who received dexamethasone were smaller with more severe respiratory disease, these findings are consistent with growing evidence of a potential deleterious effect of dexamethasone on neonatal brain and subsequent neurodevelopmental outcome. This apparent deleterious effect should be taken into consideration by clinicians when weighing the potential risks and benefits of this therapy for low birth weight infants with neonatal chronic lung disease.

(Murphy: Impaired Cerebral Cortical Gray Matter Growth After Treatment With Dexamethasone for Neonatal Chronic Lung Disease. Pediatrics 2001;107:217-221)

Dexamethasone

In conclusion, steroids have shown benefit in reducing BPD, but DXM has been associated with an unacceptable adverse effect profile. Therefore, there is an urgent need for alternatives to the present exclusive use of DXM. Together with a better knowledge about the pharmacologic effects of steroids, which may have theraputic impact is selecting the right molecule, we urgently need both additional basic research to understand which factors regulate alveolarization in the immature lung and new clinical trials to identify the "good" steroids (or at least better ones), to avoid the "bad" (DXM?), and to eliminate the "ugly" (early DXM?).

(Thébaud: Postnatal Glucocorticoid in Very Preterm Infants: "The Good, the Bad, and the Ugly'? Pediatrics 2001;107:413-415)

Dexamethasone

Early dexamethasone prophylaxis (EDP) and focal small bowel perforation (FSBP).

The EDP protocol used at the UWMC NICU consisted of 12 days of dexamethasone administration starting within 24 hours of birth. The initial dosage was 0.25 mg/kg twice a day of intravenous (i.v.) dexamethasone for the first 3 days; then a fixed taper was implemented over the next 9 days.

Indomethacin therapy consisted of four doses of 0.1 mg/kg i.v. given at 12, 24, 48, and 72 hours.

Infants who received EDP had a relative risk of perforation that was 12.3 times that of untreated infants. Those treated with indomethacin had a risk that was comparable with that for infants who did not receive indomethacin. Infants who received both EDP and indomethacin tended to have higher rates of pneumoperitoneum that infants who received EDP alone but comprised a cohort too small for valid analysis. The pathology of surgical specimens revealed FSBP with segmental loss of the muscularis externa. There was no evidence of fungal or bacterial infection in any of the surgical specimens.

Conclusion: These findings implicate EDP, but not indomethacin, as a significant risk factor for FSBP.

(Gordon: Early Postnatal Dexamethasone Increases the Risk of Focal Small Bowel Perforation in Extremely Low Birth Weight Infants. J Perinatol 1999;19(8)1:573-577)

Dexamethasone

Concurrently with the start of epinephrine infusion, infants received a single intravenous dose of either 0.25 mg/kg DXM or the corresponding volume of isotonic saline solution.

Conclusions: DXM was effective for the management of severe arterial hypotension in preterm infants not responding to standardized treatment.

(Gaissmaier: Single-dose dexamethasone treatment of hypotension in preterm infants. J Pediatr 1999;134:701-5)

Dexamethasone

Methods: In a prospective, blinded, placebo-controlled study, we randomly assigned 70 infants <28 weeks' gestation who were born in the hospital to receive dexamethasone (0.2 mg/kg) (n = 37) or normal saline solution (n = 33) within 2 hours of delivery. After an interim analysis showed that the incidence of intraventricular hemorrhage was much lower than expected...

Conclusion: Dexamethasone given within 2 hours of delivery to preterm infants <28 weeks' gestation resulted in lower ventilator settings and higher mean blood pressures during the first 7 days. Fewer infants required indomethacin to treat a patent ductus arteriosus.

(Kopelman: A single very early dexamethasone dose improves respiratory and cardiovascular adaptation in preterm infants. J Pediatr 1999;135:345-50)

Dexamethasone

Indication: Treatment of BPD

Dexamethasone Treatment:

A dexamethasone preparation (Decadron, Merck, West Point, PA) containing .4 mg/mL dexamethasone-sodium-phosphate was used. The dosage of dexamethasone included .5 mg/kg/d on days 1 and 2 of treatment, .25 mg/kg/d on days 3 and 4, and .1 mg/kg/d on days 5,6, and 7. Each daily dose of dexamethasone was administered by bolus intravenous infusion in 2 equally divided doses at 12-hour intervals. This dosage regimen was patterned after the study by Durand et al, in which both short-term and long-term pulmonary benefits and minimal side effect were shown in response to dexamethasone treatment.

Vitamin A Intake:

The vitamin A concentration of human milk was estimated to be 300 IU/dL, and that of preterm infant formula ws estimated to be 970 IU/dL. In addition, before the initiation of dexamethasone treatment, each infant received supplemental vitamin A in the form of retinyl palmitate (Aquasol A, Astra, Wastboro, MA) by either intramuscular injection or orogastric administration beginning shortly after birth. The dosage of supplemental vitamin A by intramuscular route was 2000 IU/kg/dose administered every other day, and that by orogastric route was 4000 IU/kg/dose administered daily. This supplemental vitamin A was withheld during the week of dexamethasone treatment and also during the following week.

Conclusion: In summary, we examined the changes in plasma vitamin A and RBP concentrations in response to postnatal dexamethasone treatment, and correlated these changes with the pulmonary outcome in a cohort of VLBW neonates with BPD. Postnatal dexamethasone treatment induced a significant, yet short-term, increase in plasma concentrations of both vitamin A and RBP. This increase was independent of the total intake of vitamin A and probably resulted from endogenous mobilization of vitamin A from the liver. Our data suggest that the beneficial pulmonary response to dexamethasone in infants with BPD is influenced, at least in part, by the vitamin A status, and that gender plays a role in this response. Additional studies are needed to determine the optimal usage of dexamethasone and vitamin A nutrition in these infants.

(Shenai: Vitamin A Status and Postnatal Dexamethasone Treatment in Bronchopulmonary Dysplasia. Pediatrics 2000;106:547-553)

<u>Dexamethasone</u>

Dexamethasone was administered intravenously over 10 minutes at a starting dose of 0.2 mg/kg per day divided every 12 hours and then was weaned off over 1 to 2 weeks.

Conclusions: Glucocorticoids improved pressure and stabilized clinical conditions of a group of newborns with refractory hypotension. Serum cortisol levels of these infants were relatively low. We speculate that a subset of critically ill term infants has relative adrenal insufficiency and glucocorticoid therapy may be essential.

(Tantivit: Low Serum Cortisol in Term Newborns With Refractory Hypotension. J Perinatol 1999;19:352-357)

<u>Dexamethasone</u>

Infants <30 weeks' gestation were eligible if they had RDS diagnosed by clinical and radiographic signs, required mechanical ventilation at 12 to 18 hours of age, and had received at least 1 dose of exogenous surfactant.

Syringes labeled dexamethasone study drug were sent to the nursery containing either the appropriate dose of dexamethasone (.5 mg/kg birth weight) or normal saline placebo, with the first dose administered between 12 and 18 hours of age and the second dose 12 hours later.

Conclusion: We conclude that the course of early dexamethasone in this report did not reduce the requirement for oxygen at 36 weeks' CGA, and survival was not improved. However, our regimen of early dexamethasone reduced the use of later prolonged dexamethasone therapy, and among survivors, reduced the median days on oxygen and ventilation. This course of early dexamethasone is safe and probably represents a near minimum dose for instituting a prophylactic regimen against BPD. Additional study is necessary to find the optimal dosing schedule in neonates, perhaps focusing on those predicted to be at high risk for developing CLD.

(Sinkin: Early Dexamethasone-Attempting to prevent Chronic Lung Disease. Pediatrics 2000;105:542-548)

Dexamethasone

Infants were randomized within six strata, defined in terms of birth weight (500-800 g, 801-1100 g, and 1101-1500 g) and gender, with a block size of 8. Infants randomized to dexamethasone were treated according to the following schedule: 0.25 mg/kg bid for 3 days, then 0.15 mg/kg bid for 3 days, then a 10% reduction in the dose every 3 days until the 0.1 mg/kg dose was reached on day 34. After 3 days on this dose, 0.1 mg/kg qod was given until 42 days after entry. Infants randomized to placebo were treated with an equivalent volume of vehicle. Dexamethasone and placebo were prepared by Merck, Sharpe, and Dohme (Whitehouse Station, NJ). Study drug or placebo was given intravenously as long as an intravenous line was necessary for standard clinical care; after this time, study drug was given enterally.

Conclusion. A 42-day tapering course of dexamethasone decreases the duration of ventilator and oxygen dependency in very low birth weight infants and is not associated with an increased risk of short-term adverse effects.

(Kothadia: Randomized Placebo-controlled Trial of a 42-Day Tapering Course of Dexamethasone to Reduce the Duration of Ventilator Dependency in Very Low Birth Weight Infants. Pediatrics 1999;104:22-27.)

Dexamethasone

Infants randomized to dexamethasone were treated according to the following schedule: 0.25 mg/kg bid for 3 days, then 0.15 mg/kg bid for 3 days, then a 10% reduction in the dose every 3 days until the dose of 0.1 mg/kg was reached on day 34. After 3 days on this dose, 0.1 mg/kg qod was given until 42 days after entry.

Conclusions: A 42-day tapering course of dexamethasone was associated with an increased risk of cerebral palsy. Possible explanations include an adverse effect of this therapy on brain development and/or improved survival of infants who either already have neurologic injury or who are at increased risk for such injury.

(O'Shea: Randomized Placebo-controlled Trial of a 42-Day Tapering Course of Dexamethasone to Reduce the Duration of Ventilator Dependency in Very Low Birth Weight Infants: Outcome of Study Participants at 1-Year Adjusted Age. Pediatrics 1999;104:15-21.)

Dexamethasone

Conclusion. We conclude that an early 3-day course of dexamethasone therapy increases survival without CLD, reduces CLD, and reduces late dexamethasone therapy in high-risk, low birth weight infants who receive surfactant therapy for respiratory distress syndrome.

Potential benefits of early dexamethasone therapy at the dosing schedule used in this trial need to be weighed against the risk for early intestinal perforation.

(Garland: Three-day Course of Dexamethasone Therapy to Prevent Chronic Lung Disease in Ventilated Neonates: A Randomized Trial. Pediatrics 1999;104:91-99.)

Dexamethasone (Decadron)

Dose & Route: Cerebral Edema:
Loading dose: 1-2 mg/kg/dose PO, IV, IM x 1
Maintenance: 1-1.5 mg/kg/24 hr ÷ Q4-6hr;
max dose: 16 mg/24 hr

Airway Edema:
0.5-2 mg/kg/24 hr PO, IV, IM ÷ Q6 hr (begin 24 hr before extubation and continue for 4-6 doses after extubation)
Croup: 0.6 mg/kg/dose IV, IM x 1 (use sodium phosphate injection)

Antiemetic:
Initial: 10 mg/m^2/dose IV; max: 20 mg
Subsequent: 5 mg/m^2/dose Q6 hr IV

Anti-inflammatory:
Children: 0.08-0.3 mg/kg/24hr PO, IV, IM ÷ Q6-12 hr

Meningitis:
>6 weeks old: 0.6 mg/kg/24 hr IV ÷ Q6 hr x 2 days; initiate prior to or with the first dose of antibiotic

Remarks: Toxicity: same as for prednisone. Use in meningitis (other than Haemophilus influenzae type b) remains controversial. Consult ID specialist or latest edition of Red Book.

Oral peak serum levels occur 1-2 hr and within 8 hr following IM administration. For other uses, doses based on body surface area, and dose equivalence to other steroids.

(Siberry: The Harriet Lane Handbook 2000, p.687)

Dexamethasone

Usual Dosage: Neonates:
Airway edema or extubation: I.V.: Usual: 0.25 mg/kg/dose given ~4 hours prior to scheduled extubation and then every 8 hours for 3 doses total; range: 0.25-1 mg/kg/dose for 1-3 doses; maximum dose: 1 mg/kg/day. **Note**: A longer duration of therapy may be needed with more severe cases.

Bronchopulmonary dysplasia (to facilitate ventilator weaning): Oral, I.V.: Numerous dosing schedules have been proposed; range 0.5-0.6 mg/kg/day given in divided doses every 12 hours for 3-7 days, then taper over 1-6 weeks

(Taketomo: Pediatric dosage Handbook 1999-2000, pp.277-278)

DIAZEPAM (Valium)

Supplied: Injection 5mg/ml in 2ml
Oral solution 5mg/5ml in 500ml
Oral Intensol solution 5mg/ml in 30ml

Administration: IV, PO
Direct IV administration is preferred, undiluted over a minimum of 3 minutes unless patient is on a ventilator. Intermittent infusion is not recommended. Do not mix with other drugs, solutions or IV fluids (other than D5W, NS) (2).
Safety and efficacy of parenteral diazepam has not been established in the neonate (1). Prolonged CNS depression has been observed in neonates, apparently due to inability to bio-transform diazepam into inactive metabolites.

Diazepam

Indication: For Neonatal Seizures
Although diazepam, like lorazepam, is an effective anticonvulsant in the newborn, we do not use this agent for several reasons. First, diazepam is a poor drug for maintenance because of extremely rapid clearance from brain (minutes after intravenous administration), and barbiturate usually must be used. Second, when used with barbiturate, diazepam carries an increased risk of severe circulatory collapse with respiratory failure. Third, the therapeutic dose is extremely variable and is not necessarily less than the toxic dose (0.30 and 0.36 mg/kg have led to respiratory arrest). Fourth, the vehicle for intravenous diazepam, in many preparations, contains sodium benzoate, which is a very effective uncoupler of the bilirubin-albumin complex and theoretically could increase the risk of kernicterus. Results of studies in Gunn rats suggested that the amount of benzoate in the usual diazepam preparation is not high enough to be a serious risk, but the work did not include intravenous administration or measurement of levels of bilirubin in brain. Fifth, although lorazepam shares the previous potential problem, this benzodiazepine appears to be at least as effective, has a longer duration of action, and exhibits less risk of serious side effects (see previous section).

Diazepam has been most effective as a continuous intravenous infusion. Thus one report describes the complete control of seizures in eight term newborns with severe perinatal asphyxia by continuous intravenous infusion of diazepam. Doses of approximately 0.3 mg/kg/hr were required. No patient was said to require assisted ventilation, although stupor and need for gavage feeding were present consistently.

(Volpe: Neurology of the Newborn 2001, p.205)

Diazepam

Indication: Drug therapy for withdrawal syndrome in infants.

Diazepam (Valium) has been used in the treatment of narcotic withdrawal and is apparently effective in the control of most of the central nervous system phenomena. Its advantage, if any, has been claimed to be a decrease in the time needed for treatment to approximately 1 week. However, this conclusion is based on a single small series. Although there are no controlled data from comparisons of diazepam and phenobarbital or chlorpromazine, available information suggests that diazepam is not as effective as paregoric. The dosage of diazepam needed for a beneficial response is not completely clear from published reports, but it appears to be approximately 0.5 to 1 mg intramuscularly every 8 hours.

(Volpe: Neurology of the Newborn 2001, p.882)

Diazepam (Valium)

Indications and use: Status epilepticus, convulsions refractory to other combined anticonvulsant agents; hyperglycinemia.

Actions: Exact mechanism is unknown; appears to act at the CNS to produce sedative, hypnotic, skeletal muscle relaxant, and anticonvulsant effects.

Dosage: Status epilepticus: 0.1-0.3 mg/kg/dose IV q15-30 min to maximum total dose of 2-5 mg.

Continuous refractory convulsions: 0.1-0.3 mg/kg/dose IV bolus followed by 0.3 mg/kg/h as continuous IV infusion (dilute in saline to 0.1 mg/mL).

Hyperglycinemia: 1.5-3.0 mg/kg/day PO divided q6-8h (in combination with sodium benzoate, 125-200 mg/kg/day PO divided q6-8h).

Adverse effects: May cause drowsiness, ataxia, rash, vasodilation, respiratory arrest, and hypotension.

Comments: **Observe for and be prepared to manage respiratory arrest**.

(Gomella: Neonatology 1999, p.562)

Diazepam

Has been used to treat withdrawal from narcotics. In one study there was a greater incidence of seizures following methadone withdrawal when babies were treated with diazepam rather than paregoric. When used to treat methadone withdrawal, it also impairs nutritive sucking more than does methadone alone. It may produce apnea

	when used with phenobarbital. It may be used for treatment of withdrawal from benzodiazepines and possibly also for the hyperexcitable phase following cocaine exposure.
Dosage:	0.5-2 mg every 6-8 h.

(Gomella: Neonatology 1999, p.406

Diazepam

Dosage:	0.1-3.0 mg/kg/dose IV, PR, PO, never IM, may repeat as needed For refractory seizures Loading dose: 0.1 mg/kg Maintenance infusion: 0.3-5 mg/kg/hr
Comments:	May displace bilirubin. Several active metabolites may accumulate with continued use; infants tend to be resistant to the sedative effects and require higher doses than older patients; IV and PR administration may be particularly effective for acute termination of seizures; rapid IV infusion may cause apnea. Titrate dose to effect; with each incremental increase in dose a bolus must be given

(Fanaroff: Neonatal-Perinatal Medicine 1997, p.1752)

Diazepam

Dose & Route:	Sedative/muscle relaxant: Children: IM or IV: 0.04-0.2 mg/kg/dose Q2-4 hr; **max dose**: 0.6 mg/kg within an 8-hr period. PO: 0.12-0.8 mg/kg/24 hr ÷ Q6-8 hr Status epilepticus: Neonate: 0.3-0.75 mg/kg/dose IV Q15-30 min x 2-3 doses >1 mo: 0.2-0.5 mg/kg/dose IV Q15-30 min; **max total dose**: <5 yr: 5 mg Rectal dose (using IV dosage form): 0.5 mg/kg/dose followed by 0.25 mg/kg/dose in 10 minutes PRN Rectal Gel: all doses rounded to the nearest available dosage strength; repeat dose in 4-12 hrs PRN 2-5 yr: 0.5 mg/kg/dose Diazepam IV Emulsion: Status Epilepticus & Severe Recurrent Seizures: >30 days old-5 yr: 0.2-0.5 mg slow IV Q2-5 min PRN **up to a total max** of 5 mg Tetanus Spasms (Respiratory assistance should be available): Infants >30 days old: 1-2 mg slow IV Q3-4 hr PRN ≥5 yr: 5-10 mg slow IV Q3-4 hr PRN
Remarks:	Hypotension and respiratory depression may occur. Use with **caution** in glaucoma, shock, and depression. Do not

use in combination with protease inhibitors. Concurrent use with CNS depressants, cimetidine, erythromycin, and valproic acid may enhance the effects of diazepam.

Administer the conventional IV product undiluted no faster than 2 mg/min. Do not mix with IV fluids.

The injectable emulsion product must always be handled with strict aspectic technique because it is an excellent growth media for microorganisms. Doses of this product must be injected slowly (no faster than 5 mg/min) and must not be administered through filters with pore sizes <5 microns or via polyvinyl chloride infusion sets.

In status epilepticus, diazepam must be followed by long-acting anticonvulsants. Onset of anticonvulsant effect: 1-3 min with IV route; 2-10 min with rectal route.

(Siberry: The Harriet Lane Handbook 2000, pp.688-689)

Diazepam

Usual Dosage: Children:
Status epilepticus: I.V.:
Neonates: (Not recommended as a first-line agent; conventional injection contains sodium benzoate and benzoic acid) 0.1-0.3 mg/kg/dose given over 3-5 minutes, every 15-30 minutes to a maximum total dose of 2 mg

Infants >30 days and Children <5 years: 0.05-0.3 mg/kg/dose given over 3-5 minutes, every 15-30 minutes to a maximum total dose of 5 mg **or** 0.2-0.5 mg/dose every 2-5 minutes to a maximum total dose of 5 mg; repeat in 2-4 hours as needed

Administration: Oral: Administer with food or water; do not chew extended release capsules; oral concentrate solution (5 mg/mL) should be diluted or mixed with water, juice, soda, applesauce, or pudding before use.

Parenteral: I.V.: Infants and children: Do not exceed 1-2 mg/minute I.V. push; adult maximum infusion rate: 5 mg/minute; rapid injection may cause respiratory depression or hypotension; emulsified diazepam injection is for I.V. use only; do not add emulsified diazepam injection to infusion sets containing polyvinyl chloride

(Taketomo: Pediatric dosage Handbook 1999-2000, pp.286-288)

DIAZOXIDE (Hyperstat, Proglycem)

Supplied: Oral suspension 50mg/ml in 30ml
Injection 15mg/ml in 20ml

Administration: IV, PO
Oral diazoxide produces a prompt, dose-related increase in blood glucose by inhibiting pancreatic insulin release, and also by an extrahepatic effect. The hyperglycemic effect begins within an hour, and generally lasts no more

than 8 hours with normal renal function. Insulin reverses diazoxide-induced hyperglycemia (1).

IV administration is used for hypertensive emergencies. The dose is administered by DIRECT IV INJECTION in 30 seconds or less. During and immediately following injection, the patient should remain supine (1).

Diazoxide (Hyperstat IV, Proglycem)

Indications and use: Hypertension and persistent neonatal hypoglycemia

Actions: Nondiuretic thiazide with antihypertensive and hyperglycemic effects. Reduces total peripheral vascular resistance by direct relaxation of arteriolar smooth muscle. Inhibits pancreatic insulin release.

Route: IV, PO

Dosage: IV: 3-5 mg/kg/dose; repeat in 20 min if no effect.
PO: 8-15 mg/kg/day in 2 - 3 divided doses q8-12h.

Adverse effects: When given for short periods, adverse effects rare. May cause bilirubin displacement from albumin, hypotension, hyperglycemia, hyperuricemia, rash, fever, leukopenia, thrombocytopenia, and ketosis.

(Gomella: Neonatology 1999, p.563)

Diazoxide

Dose/kg: Hypertension: 1-3 mg

Route & Frequency:
IV push every 5-15 min until blood pressure is controlled, then q4h-q24h

Dose/kg: Hypoglycemia: 2-5 mg

Route & Frequency: PO q8h-q12h

Comments: May cause hyperglycemia, ketoacidosis, GI irritation, salt and water retention, hypotension.

(Avery: Neonatology Pathophysiology and Management of the Newborn 1999, p.1554)

Diazoxide (Hyperstat)

Dose: 2-5 mg/kg IV push

Mode of Action: Direct vasodilator; may inhibit calcium current

Adverse Effects: Hypotension, hyperglycemia

Comments: Rapid IV push

(Garson: The science and practice of pediatric cardiology 1998, p.2951)

Diazoxide

Dose: 5 mg/kg slow IV over 30 min (does not require rapid bolus infusion).

Comments: Monitor BP continuously and discontinue infusion when BP reaches target level. May repeat 5 mg/kg slow IV x 2 (total 15 mg/kg over 90 min).

(Allen: Moss and Adams' Heart Disease in Infants, Children, and Adolescents 2001, pp.1460-1468)

Diazoxide

Dose & Route: Hypertensive Crisis:
1-3 mg/kg IV **up to a maximum** 150 mg/dose; repeat Q5-15 min PRN, then Q4-24hr.

Hyperinsulinemic Hypoglycemia (due to insulin-producing tumors):
Newborns and Infants: 8-15 mg/kg/24hr÷Q8-12hr PO

Remarks: May cause hyponatremia, salt and water retention, GI disturbances, ketoacidosis, rash, hyperuricemia, weakness, hypertrichosis and arrhythmias. Monitor BP closely for hypotension. Hyperglycemia occurs in majority of patients. Hypoglycemia should be treated initially with IV glucose; diazoxide should be introduced only if refractory to glucose infusion.

Peak antihypertensive effect with IV administration occurs within 5 minutes with a duration of 3-12 hours. Hyperglycemic effect with PO administration occurs within 1 hour with a duration of 8 hours.

(Siberry: The Harriet Lane Handbook 2000, p.690)

DICLOXACILLIN (Dynapen, Pathocil)

Supplied: Suspension, powder for 62.5mg/5ml in 100, 200ml

Administration: PO

Following reconstitution, oral suspensions are stable for 7 days at room temperature or 14 days refrigerated (1).

Dicloxacillin (Dynapen, Pathocil)

Antibacterial Drugs for Pediatric Patients Beyond the Newborn Period:
Dosage par kg/d
Route: PO
Mild to Moderate Infections: 25-50 mg in 4 doses
Severe Infections: Inappropriate
Comments: Excellent serum concentrations after oral administration
Note: In patients with history of allergy to penicillin or one of its may congeners, alternative drugs are recommended. In some circumstances, a cephalosporin or other β-lactam class drug may be acceptable. However, theses drugs should not be used inpatients with an immediate hypersensitivity (anaphylaxis) to penicillin because approximately 5% to 15% of penicillin-allergic patients will also be allergic to the cephalosporins.

(American Academy of Pediatrics: Report of the Committee on Infectious Disease. Red Book 2000, pp.660, 662)

Dicloxacillin, Sodium

Route: PO
Dosage: 12-25 mg/kg/day
Interval: q 6 hours.
NON-NEWBORN SECTION

(Nelson: Pocket Book of Pediatric Antimicrobial Therapy 2000-2001, p.74)

DIDANOSINE (Videx, DDI)

Supplied: Powder for oral solution, Pediatric 2g, 4g. Prior to dispensing, the pharmacist must constitute dry powder with purified water, USP, to an initial concentration of 20mg/ml and immediately mix the resulting solution with antacid to a final concentration of 10mg/ml (1).
Chewable/Dispersible Tablets 25, 50, 100, 150mg

Administration: PO

Didanosine (ddl)/Videx

Preparations: Pediatric powder for oral solution (must be mixed with antacid): 10 mg/mL

Dosage: Usual pediatric: In combination with other antiretrovirals: 90 mg/m^2 q 12 h

Pediatric range: 90 to 150 mg/m^2 q 12 h (Note: May need higher dosage for patients with central nervous system disease).

Neonatal (<90 d of age): Based on pharmacokinetic data from PACTG 239: 50 mg/m^2 q 12 h

Major Toxic Effects: Most frequent: diarrhea, abdominal pain, nausea, vomiting

Unusual (more severe): Peripheral neuropathy (dose-related), electrolyte abnormalities, hyperuricemia

Uncommon: Pancreatitis (dose-related) seems less common in children than adults; increased liver enzyme levels, retinal depigmentation (asymptomatic, reported with pediatric administration)

Drug Interactions: Possible decrease in absorption of ketoconazole, itraconazole, tetracycline; administer at least 2 h before or 2 h after ddl.

Ciprofloxacin absorption significantly decreased (chelation of drug by antacid); administer 2 h before or 6 h after ddl. Concomitant administration of ddl and delavirdine may decrease the absorption of these drugs; separate dosing by at least 2 h.

Ganciclovir may increase the AUC and peak levels of ddl and predispose to toxic effects.
Administration with protease inhibitors: indinavir should be administered at least 1 h apart from ddl on an empty stomach. Ritonavir should be administered at least 2.5 h apart from ddl.

TMP-SMX increases 3 TC blood levels (possibly competes for renal tubular secretion); unknown significance.

Special Instructions: ddl formulation contains buffering agents or antacids. Food decreases absorption; administer ddl on an empty stomach (1 h before or 2 h after meal). Further evaluation in children regarding administration with meals is under study.

For oral solution: Shake well, and keep refrigerated; admixture stable for 30 d.

(American Academy of Pediatrics: Report of the Committee on Infectious Diseases. Red Book 2000, p.679)

Didanosine (ddl)

Route: PO
Dosage: 180 mg/m^2/day
Interval: q12h
NON-NEWBORN SECTION

(Nelson: Pocket Book of Pediatric Antimicrobial Therapy 2000-2001, p.75)

Didanosine

Dose & Route: Neonates and Infants <3 months: 100 mg/m^2/24 hr ÷ Q12 hr PO
Children <13 yr:
Usual dose (in combination with other antiretrovirals): 180 mg/m^2/24 hr ÷ Q12 hr PO
Dose range: 180-300 mg/ m^2/24 hr ÷ Q12 hr ; higher dose may be required for CNS disease
Alternative Pediatric dosing based on 200 mg/m^2/24 hr, see the table below.

ALTERNATIVE PEDIATRIC DOSING

BSA	*Chewable tablets	Peds powder dose
<0.4	25mgQ12hr	31mgQ12hr
0.5-0.7	50mgQ12hr	62mgQ12hr
0.8-1	75mgQ12hr	94mgQ12hr
1.1-1.4	100mgQ12hr	125mgQ12hr

*Use at least two tablets to ensure adequate buffering capacity (e.g., give two 25mg tablets for 50mg dose).

Remarks: Side effects include: headaches, diarrhea, abdominal pain, nausea, vomiting, peripheral neuropathy (dose related), electrolyte abnormalities, hyperuricemia, increased liver enzymes, retinal depigmentation, CNS depression, rash/pruritis, myalgia, and pancreatitis (dose related, more in adults). Use with caution in patients on sodium restriction (264.5 mg Na/buffered tablet, 1380 mg Na/single dose packet).

Administer all doses on empty stomach. Impairs absorption of drugs requiring an acidic environment and drugs that have impaired absorption impaired in the presence of divalent ions,. (e.g., ketoconazole and fluoroquinolones, respectively). Separate dosing when used in combination with the following drugs: 1 hr before or after ddl (indinavir); 2 hr before or after ddl (delavirdine, ritonavir, fluoroquinolones, ketoconazole, itraconazole, tetracyclines, and dapsone). Consult package insert for additional details.

(Siberry: The Harriet Lane Handbook, 2000, p.691)

DIGOXIN (Lanoxin)

Supplied: Elixir, pediatric 50mcg (0.05mg)/ml in 50ml, 60ml
Injection, pediatric 100mcg (0.1mg)/ml in 1ml
Injection, (adult use) 0.25mg/ml in 2ml

Administration: PO, IV
FOR IV ADMINISTRATION, USE 100mcg/ml PEDIATRIC DOSAGE FORM (author).

Administration by DIRECT IV INJECTION over 5 minutes. It may be administered diluted or undiluted with a 4 fold or greater volume of SWFI, NS, or D5W and given least 5 minutes or longer. The use of less diluent could lead to precipitation of the digoxin. Use diluted product immediately (1).

If tuberculin syringes are used to measure very small doses, one must be aware of the problem of inadvertent over administration of digoxin. The syringe should NOT be flushed with the parenteral solution (3).

Compatible: Cimetidine,dextrose, famotidine, heparin, hydrocortisone, lidocaine, potassium chloride, parenteral nutrition,* sodium chloride, ranitidine.

Note: Even when it is compatible with other drugs being used, it is best to infuse this potent and important medication alone, if possible, to assure accurate delivery to the patient. Administer over five minutes.

* Drugs reported as being compatible with parenteral nutrition in published studies using test solutions may not be compatible with the particular formulation your infant is receiving. Components in neonatal parenteral nutrition are individualized based on the infant's body weight, serum electrolytes, fluid, and other nutrient requirements, making most solutions unique. Observe the solution and tubing carefully for signs of precipitation during the 24-hour infusion period when drugs are coinfused. Certain drugs may be admixed into the parenteral nutrition bag. See Driscoll, and associates' review of the use of parenteral nutrition as a drug vehicle (9).

Incompatible: Dobutamine, doxapram (9).

<u>Digoxin</u> (Lanoxin)

Indications and use:
Congestive heart failure, atrial fibrillation or flutter, and paroxysmal AV nodal tachycardia.

Actions: Exerts a positive inotropic effect on the myocardium. Antiarrhythmic actions are due to an increase in AV nodal refractory period produced by increased vagal activity and by a sympatholytic effect.

Route: IV, PO, IM

Dosage: TDD (total digitalizing dose) to be divided 1/2, 1/4, 1/4 q8h.

Note: Oral doses (elixir) are ~20% higher than IV doses listed below.

Premature infants (up to 2.5 kg)-- TDD 10-20 mcg/kg IV; maintenance: 2.5 mcg/kg/dose q12h IV.

Term infants—TDD: 30 mcg/kg IV; maintenance: 4 mcg/kg/dose q12h IV.

Infants 1-12 months—TDD: 35 mcg/kg IV; maintenance: 4-5 mcg/kg/dose q12h IV.
Reduce dose in renal dysfunction.

Therapeutic levels: 0.5-2.0 ng/mL, up to 3 ng/mL in infants. Considerable overlap exists between toxic and therapeutic serum levels.

Adverse effects: Persistent vomiting is usually the most common sign of digoxin toxicity in infants. Other adverse effects are anorexia, nausea, dysrhythmias (paroxysmal ventricular contractions, blocks, tachycardia, and other), and delirium. Toxicity is markedly enhanced by hypokalemia.

Management of toxicity:
Give Fab fraction of specific digoxin antibody (digoxin immune fab [ovine] **[Digibind]**) IV in equimolar amounts (ie, 60 mg Fab/1 mg of digoxin). Give KCl if hypokalemic.

Comments: Contraindicated in second- and third-degree block, idiopathic hypertrophic subaortic stenosis, and atrial flutter or fibrillation with slow ventricular rates.

(Gomella: Neonatology 1999, p.563)

<u>Digoxin</u>

Dose/kg: Total digitalizing dose (TDD) oral:
Premie: 20-30 μg
Term: 3-3.75 μg [sic]
1-24 mo: 35-60 μg

Route & Frequency:
Give 1/2 of the TDD initially, then 1/4 of the TDD q8h-q24h x 2 doses

Dose/kg: Oral maintenance dose (25% TDD):
Premie: 2.5-3.75 μg
Term: 3-3.75 μg
1-24 mo: 4-7.5 μg

Route & Frequency:
q12h

Dose/kg: TDD injectable:
Premie: 15-25 μg
Term: 20-30 μg
1-24 mo: 30-50 μg

Route & Frequency:
IV, IM follow same guidelines as for oral administration.

Dose/kg: IV, IM maintenance dose (25% TDD):
Premie: 2-3 μg
Term: 2.5-3.75 μg
1-24 mo: 3.75-6 μg

Route & Frequency:
IV, IM q12h

Comments: May cause bradycardia, PVCs, vomiting, poor feeding, and arrhythmias. Check ECG trace during digitalization and periodically adjust dose per clinical response and renal function. Bioavailability of elixir is 70%-85% of the injectable preparation.

(Avery: Neonatology Pathophysiology and Management of the Newborn 1999, p.1554)

Digoxin

Class: IV Digitalis glycosides

Uses: SVT (non-WPW) AV block in AF and AFL; ↓ rate AET, JET; inotropic PACs

Dose (Level) Total loading dose
Premature, 20 μg/kg PO

NB-6 mo, 30 μg/kg PO

>6 mo, 50 μg/kg PO

TLD is given as follows:
½ TLD, followed by ¼ TLD q8hr x 2;

Maintenance dose is 5-10 μg/kg/day divided q12hr
*IV dose = ¾ PO dose
(1-2 ng/mL >6 mo)
(1.5-3 ng/mL <6 mo)

Mode of Action: Na-K ATPase inhibition, positive inotrope, vagotonic

ECG/EP Changes: Increases PR; depresses ST; decreased QT; SAN = ↓ HR, ↑ SACT; Atr = ↓ ERP, ↑ auto; AVN = ↑ ERP, ↑ AH; Vent = ↓ ERP

Toxicity: ↓ conduction, ↑ auto, delayed after depolarizations; May ↑, no Δ or ↓ ERP of Kent bundle

Side Effects: AV block, SVT, PVCs (treat dig.-induced arrhythmias with phenytoin)
Nausea, vomiting,
FIT, lethargy, visual changes; quinidine, amiodarone, verapamil- ↑ dig. levels; worse with ↓ K^+, ↓ Ca^{++}, warfarin: ↑ PT

(Garson: The science and practice of pediatric cardiology 1998, p.2954)

Digitalis

Digoxin Dosage Schedule		
	Total Digitalizing Dose (µg/kg)	Maintenance Dose (µg/kg/day)
Premature infant	20-25	5
Full-term infant	30	8-10
Infant (< 2 years)	30-40	8-10
Child (>2 years)	30-40	8-10
Maximum dose	1 mg total	0.025 mg total

Intravenous dose = 75% of oral dose

Several preparations of digitalis are available for pediatric use; digoxin is the most commonly used digitalis glycoside. Digoxin is available in both oral and parenteral forms. Gastrointestinal absorption of digoxin varies from patient to patient and results in a lower serum concentration than does parenteral administration. The parenteral dose is therefore generally calculated to be 25% less than the oral dose. In addition, individual response to the drug varies, making it necessary to adjust the dosage of the medication according to the patient's response. Patients with inflammatory disease of the myocardium or in the post-operative state often have an enhanced sensitivity to the drug, which requires reducing the administered dose.

Intravenous digoxin therapy is available and can be used in instances of acute, severe heart failure. However, other forms of parenteral inotropic support are now available that may be more efficacious and safer to use. These therapies are described in detail in Chapter 109. Digoxin therapy is perhaps best used when the medication can be given orally to less seriously ill infants or children with congestive cardiac failure. A loading or "digitalizing" dose is often given over the first 24 hours, with one-half of the total digitalizing dose (TDD) being given initially and two one-quarter doses of the TDD given at 6- to 8-hour intervals following the previous dose. Oral maintenance therapy is usually begun 12 hours after the last "digitalizing" dose. When early signs of heart failure are present, the maintenance dosage may be started without the "digitalizing" dose, although the full therapeutic effect will not be realized for 4 to 7 days. The advantage of this approach is that it requires only one dosage calculation and decreases the likelihood of dosage errors or acute toxicity. A digoxin dosage schedule based on the patient's age is outlined in Table.

Although digitalis remains an important drug in the management of congestive cardiac failure, a relatively narrow gap exists between its optimal therapeutic dose and its toxicity. For this reason, when digitalis is prescribed, explicit instructions regarding dosing must be given to avoid errors that could prove fatal. The type of digitalis preparation to be used and its route of administration should be clearly specified. As indicated earlier, we use digoxin nearly exclusively. If a total digitalizing dose is to be used, the total amount of this dose should be listed along with the basis (i.e., the microgram per kilogram dose) for arriving at the determined amount. All calculated doses should be written in micrograms as well as the number of milliliters of the chosen preparation containing this amount. If at all possible, calculations should be checked independently by a second physician. When patients are discharged home on digoxin, parents should be shown how to administer the proper dose using a calibrated dropper, and parents should be familiar with the signs of digitalis toxicity (most often nausea and vomiting). The digoxin preparation must be stored at home out of the reach of other children because accidental ingestion of digitalis may prove fatal. The medicine is discarded soon after it is discontinued for the same reasons.

Occasionally, the use of digoxin requires monitoring of the serum concentration. Serum digoxin levels are most useful in the evaluation of patients in whom accidental ingestion has taken place or in any patient for whom the possibility of digoxin toxicity exists. It may also be useful to measure serum concentration as a measure of patient compliance with the prescribed medication. Therapeutic levels of digoxin are difficult to interpret because they tend to very with the clinical setting and from patient to patient. Sixty-five percent of infants on generally agreed-upon "standard" doses achieve levels greater than 2-0 ng/mL, which would be considered a level of toxicity in adults. The toxic range for infants appears to be in the range of 4 to 5 ng/mL, while in children it is on the order of 3 ng/mL. The best gauge is by monitoring the electrocardiogram for toxicity (second-degree atrioventricular block, PVCs) and by monitoring patient symptoms. Some children develop nausea and vomiting at a serum concentration below 1.5 ng/mL, a level that is normally considered nontoxic.

(Garson: The science and practice of pediatric cardiology 1998, pp.2320-2321)

<u>Digoxin</u>

Uses: PSVT; AFl or Afib for ventricular rate control; postoperative JET; AET

Dosing: Total PO load (½ / ¼ / ¼ q 8 hr):
- premature, 20 µg/kg;
- term-6 mo, 30 µg/kg;
- >6 mos, 40 µg/kg;
- maximum, 1.0 mg

Total IV load: (as above, but ¾ PO doses)

Acute Side Effects:

Sinus bradycardia; atrioventricular (AV) block; atrial tachy; accelerated junctional; premature atrial contractions (PACs); premature ventricular contractions (PVCs); nausea; lethargy; visual changes

Other Considerations:

Quinidine, amiodarone, verapamil ↑ digoxin level; toxicity more likely if low K^+ or high Ca^{+2}

AET, atrial ectopic tachycardia; AFib, atrial fibrillation; AFl, atrial flutter; JET, junctional ectopic tachycardia; PSVT, paroxysmal supraventricular tachycardia.

(Gillette: Clinical Pediatric Arrhythmias 1999, p.152)

Digoxin

Dosing:	PO: 30-50 mcg/kg load, divided (see text)
Warnings:	Gastrointestinal, gynecomastia, proarrhythmia
Dosing:	IV: 2/3-3/4 of oral dose, divided (see text)
Warnings:	Proarrhythmia

Oral Administration:

Peak plasma levels occur in 1 to 2 hours, and the elimination $t_{1/2}$ is long: 1.5 to 2 days.

The drug is excreted unchanged in the urine.

Therapeutic plasma digoxin concentrations are in the range of 0.7 to 2.0 ng/ml. The need for routine screening of digoxin levels is somewhat controversial. In infants, the presence of a digoxin-like immunoreactive substance may complicate the assay. Digoxin crosses the placenta readily; fetal levels approximate maternal levels.

Digoxin remains an important drug for therapy of fetal SVT.

Intravenous Administration:

The onset of electrophysiologic effect is obviously more rapid, on the order of 5 to 10 minutes.

Dosing an Interactions:

A loading protocol is generally followed for both oral and intravenous preparations. Usually, a TLD of 30 to 50 µg/kg is acceptable, with a slight decrease to 20 to 25 µg/kg for premature infants. This dose is divided as follows: 50% of the TLD initially, followed by two doses at 6-hour intervals of 25% of the TLD each. For intravenous loading, two thirds to three fourths of the TLD is used, divided in similar fashion. Oral liquid digoxin preparations are available in a 50-µg/ml concentration, and intravenous preparations are available as 100µg/ml. For this reason, and because digoxin remains one of the most common drugs prone to prescription error, both the total dose and the volume of dose, whether oral or intravenous, should be written on all orders. Maintenance dosages of digoxin are 7 to 10 µg/kg/day. The dose of digoxin needs to be decreased in patients with renal dysfunction and in congestive heart failure.

Side Effects and Interactions:

Side effects obviously include proarrhythmic effects, but also include gastrointestinal upset, visual changes, and drowsiness in small patients. Gynecomastia is a potential side effect with long-term use. Digoxin toxicity can occur at plasma levels as low as 2.0 ng/ml, but is more likely to occur at levels above 3.0 ng/ml. The cardiac manifestations of digoxin toxicity are somewhat age dependent. Younger patients tend to have more supraventricular arrhythmias and conduction disturbances, whereas adult patients are prone to ventricular arrhythmias, junctional tachycardia, AV block, and premature ventricular contractions.

Any coadministered antiarrhythmic agent generally will require a reduction in the dose of digoxin, and levels should be monitored periodically.

(Gillette: Clinical Pediatric Arrhythmias 1999,pp.231-248)

Digoxin

Dose & Route: Digitalizing: Total digitalizing dose (TDD) and maintenance doses in mcg/kg/24 hr (see table below).

Initial: ½ TDD, then ¼ TDD Q8-18 hr x 2 doses; obtain ECG 6 hr after dose to assess for toxicity

Maintenance (see table below):
<10 yr: Give maintenance dose ÷ BID
≥10 yr: Give Maintenance dose QD

Remarks: **Contraindicated** in patients with ventricular dysrhythmias. Use with caution in renal failure. May cause AV block or dysrhythmias. In the patient treated with digoxin, cardioversion or calcium infusion may lead to ventricular fibrillation (pretreatment with lidocaine may prevent this).

Excreted via the kidney; **adjust dose in renal failure**. Therapeutic concentration: 0.8-2 ng/ml. Higher doses may be required for supraventricular tachycardia. Neonates, pregnant women, and patients with renal, hepatic, or heart failure may have falsely elevated digoxin levels, due to the presence of digoxin-like substances.

$T_{1/2}$: premature infants, 61-170 hrs; full-term neonates, 35-45 hr; infants, 18-25 hr; and children, 35 hr.

Recommended serum sampling at steady-state: obtain a single level from 6 hours post dose to just before the next scheduled dose following 5-8 days of continuous dosing. Levels obtained prior to steady-state may be useful in preventing toxicity.

DIGOXN DIGITALIZING AND MAINTENANCE DOSES

	TDD		Maintenance	
Age	PO	IV / IM	PO	IV / IM
Premature	20	15	5	3-4
Full term	30	20	8-10	6-8
<2 yr	40-50	30-40	10-12	7.5-9
2-10 yr	30-40	20-30	8-10	6-8
>10yr and <100kg	10-15	8-12	2.5-5	2-3

TDD, total digitalizing dose.

(Siberry: The Harriet Lane Handbook 2000, p.692)

DIGOXIN IMMUNE FAB (Digibind)

Supplied: Injection, lyophylized powder 38mg/vial

Administration: IV

Each vial will bind approximately 0.5mg of digoxin or digitoxin. Add 4ml SWFI to vial for a concentration of 10mg/ml. MIX GENTLY. Since infants can have much smaller dosage requirements, administer with a tuberculin syringe. For very small doses, dilute a reconstituted vial with 34ml sterile isotonic saline (0.9% NaCl) to achieve a 1mg/ml concentration. Doses of 2mg or less, this dilution may be desirable (1).

Digoxin immune fab is administered IV over 15-30 minutes and infused through a 0.22 micron membrane filter. If cardiac arrest is imminent, give as bolus injection (1).

Solutions are stable for 4 hours if refrigerated (1).

Digoxin Immune FAB (Ovine)

Dose & Route: First, determine total body digoxin load (TBL):
TBL (mg) = serum digoxin level (ng/ml) x 5.6 x wt (kg) ÷ 1000, OR TBL (mg) = mg digoxin ingested x 0.8
Then, calculate digoxin immune Fab dose:
Dose in number of digoxin immune Fab vials: # vials = TBL ÷ 0.5
Infuse IV over 15-30 min (through 0.22 micron filter).

Remarks: **Contraindicated** if hypersensitivity to sheep products, or if renal or cardiac failure. May cause rapidly developing severe hypokalemia, decreased cardiac output, rash, edema. Digoxin therapy may be reinstituted in 3-7 days, when toxicity has been corrected.

(Siberry: The Harriet Lane Handbook 2000, p.693)

Digoxin Immune Fab

Guidlines for Dosage: Antidysrhythmics

Dose: Fab dose (mg) = (serum digoxin concentration in ng/ml x 5.6 x body weight in kg/1000 x 64. If the steady-state serum digoxin concentration is unknown, but reliable information is available on the amount ingested, the dose of Fab can be based on the fact that 40 mg (one vial) of Fab binds approximately 0.66 mg of digoxin.

Comments: Infuse i.v. over 15-30 min; monitor serum potassium; consider intradermal skin testing prior to infusion in individuals at increased risk for hypersensitivity reaction.

(Allen: Moss and Adams' Heart Disease in Infants, Children, and Adolescents 2001, pp.1460-1468)

Digoxin Immune Fab

Infants and Children Dose Estimates of Digibind (in mg) From Serum Digoxin Concentration

Patient Weight Kg	Serum Digoxin Concentration (ng/mL)						
	1	2	4	8	12	16	20
1	0.4 mg*	1 mg*	1.5mg*	3 mg	5 mg	6 mg	8 mg
3	1 mg*	2 mg*	5 mg	9 mg	14 mg	18 mg	23 mg
5	2 mg*	4 mg	8 mg	15 mg	23 mg	30 mg	38 mg
10	4 mg	8 mg	15 mg	30 mg	46 mg	61 mg	76 mg

*Dilution of reconstituted vial to 1mg/mL may be desirable.

Usual Dosage: To determine the dose of digoxin immune Fab, first determine the total body load of digoxin (TBL) or digitoxin (depending upon which product was ingested) as follows (using either an approximation of the amount ingested or a postdistribution serum digoxin/digitoxin concentration (C):

TBL of **digoxin** (in mg) = C (in ng/mL) x 5.6 x body weight (in kg)/1000
or
TBL = mg of **digoxin** ingested (as tablets or elixir) x 0.8

TBL of **digitoxin** (in mg) = C (in ng/mL) x 0.56 x body weight (in kg)/1000
or
TBL of **digitoxin** (in mg) = mg digitoxin ingested
Dose of digoxin immune Fab (**in mg**) I.V. = TBL x 76
Dose of digoxin immune Fab (**# vials**) I.V. = TBL/0.5
See table

Administration: Parenteral: I.V.: digoxin immune Fab is reconstituted by adding 4 mL sterile water, resulting in a 9.5 mg/mL concentration for I.V. infusion; the reconstituted solution may be further diluted with NS to a convenient volume (eg. 1 mg/mL); infuse over 15-30 minutes; to remove protein aggregates, 0.22 micron in-line filter is needed

Monitoring Parameters:
Serum potassium; serum digoxin/digitoxin level prior to first dose of digoxin immune Fab; (digoxin levels will greatly increase with Digibind use and are not an accurate determination of body stores); continuous EKG monitoring

(Taketomo: Pediatric Dosage Handbook 1999-2000, pp.298-300)

Digoxin Immune Fab

A 3-day-old newborn with digoxin overdose and acute renal failure was treated with digoxin immune Fab and peritoneal dialysis. Low levels of total digoxin were measured in the dialyzate, indicating poor elimination of the digoxin-Fab complex through peritoneal dialysis.

(Berkovitch: Acute Digoxin Overdose in a Newborn with Renal Failure: Use of Digoxin Immune Fab and Peritoneal Dialysis. Ther Drug Monit 1994;16:531-533)

DIHYDROTACHYSTEROL (Hytakerol, DHT)

Supplied: DHT Intensol solution, 0.2 mg/ml in 30ml (contains 20% alcohol)
HYTAKEROL solution, 0.25 mg/ml in OIL 15ml

Administration: PO
DIHYDROTACHYSTEROL 1mg is approximately equivalent to 3mg (120,000 IU) of Vitamin D-2 (1).

Dihydrotachysterol USP (DHT, Hytakerol)

Dose & Route: Hypoparathyroidism:
Neonates: 0.05-0.1 mg/24h PO

Infants/Young Children: Initial, 1-5 mg/24 hr PO x 4 days, then 0.5-1.5 mg/24 hr PO

Nutritional rickets: 0.5 mg X 1 PO or 13-50 mcg/24 hr PO QD until healing.

Remarks: Use with **caution** in patients with renal stones, renal failure, and heart disease. Monitor serum Ca^{++} and PO_4. Toxicities include hypercalcemia or hypervitaminosis D. May cause nausea, vomiting, anorexia, and renal damage.

Activated by 25-hydroxylation in liver; does not require 1-hydroxylation in kidney. More potent than Vit. D_2, but more rapidly inactivated (half life is hours v. weeks). Titrate dose with patient response. Oral Ca^{++} supplementation may be required.

(Siberry: The Harriet Lane Handbook 2000, p.693)

Dihydrotachysterol

Route: PO

Neonatal Dose: Hypoparathyroidism: 0.05 - 0.1 mg/24h

Pediatric Dose: Hypoparathyroidism: 1-6 yr: 0.1-0.5 mg/24 h

Hypophosphatemic vitamin D-resistant rickets: 0.25-1 mg/24 h

Nutritional rickets: 1 dose of 5 mg

Renal osteodystrophy: 0.6-6 mg/24 h until desired effect

Maintenance: 0.25-0.6 mg/24 h

Discussion: Works faster than vitamin D; monitor calcium and phosphorus which may need supplementation.

(Rudolph: Rudolph's Pediatrics 1996, p.2181)

DILTIAZEM HCL (Cardizem)

Supplied: Tablets 30mg, 60mg, 90mg, 120mg
25mg (5mg/mL); 50mg (5mg/mL)

Administration: PO
For continuous IV infusion stable in NS, D5W. Use within 24hours (1).

IV Compatibility: D5W, N.S.

Extemporaneous Compounding (Recipe)

Dosage form: Oral suspension
Made from: Tablets
Concentration: 12 mg/mL
Stability: 60 days
Store: Refrigerate
Label: Shake well

Ingredient	Strength	Quantity
Diltiazem hydrochloride tablets	90 mg	16
Ora-Sweet or Ora-Sweet SF Ora-plus	1:1 mixture	qs 120 mL

Instructions: Crush the tablets with a mortar and pestle and reduce to a fine powder. Add approximately 10 mL of the vehicle and mix until uniform. Add geometric amounts of vehicle to almost desired volume. Transfer to a graduate and qs to final volume with vehicle. (11)

Diltiazem

Diltiazem for pediatric patients has been confined predominantly to control of hypertension. The drug is available in both an oral and intravenous preparation, but no data are available from children, and few data are available from adults to extrapolate to children.

Dosing: PO: 30-120 mg tid (adult)
Warnings: Headache

Dosing: IV: 0.15-0.45 mg/kg load, 3 mcg/kg/min infusion
Warnings: Hypotension, AV block

Dosing: There are no clear guidelines on the oral dose of diltiazem in children. Adult doses are in the range of 30 to 120 mg three times a day. Intravenous doses are bolus doses of 0.15 to 0.45 mg/kg followed by an infusion rate of 0.003 mg/kg/min.

Side Effects: Therapy with diltiazem results in frequent but mild side effects, including headache and postural hypotension. Bradycardia and increased levels of AV block should be anticipated.

(Gillette: Clinical Pediatric Arrhythmias 1999,pp.231-248)

Diltiazem

Uses: PSVT; ventricular rate control for Afib/Fl

Dosing: 0.25 mg/kg up to 20 mg bolus over 2 min; repeat at 0.35 mg/kg up to 25 mg 15 min later, if necessary; 0.1-0.3 mg/kg/hr up to 15 mg/hr as infusion

Acute Side Effects:

Hypotension; sinus bradycardia; atrioventricular (AV) block

Other Considerations:

Use with caution if oral digoxin or beta blocker in use

AFib, atrial fibrillation; AFI, atrial flutter; PSVT, paroxysmal supraventricular tachycardia.

(Gillette: Clinical Pediatric Arrhythmias 1999, p.152)

DIPHENHYDRAMINE (Benadryl)

Supplied: Elixir, Syrup 12.5mg/5ml

Diphenhydramine

Route & Dose: PO: 5 mg/kg/day q 6 h

Adverse Effects and Cautions:

Somnolence

(Taeusch: Avery's Diseases of the Newborn 1998, p.1344)

Diphenhydramine (Benadryl)

Dose & Route: Children: 5 mg/kg/24 hr ÷ Q6 hr PO/IM/IV
Max dose: 300 mg/24 hr
For anaphylaxis or phenothiazine overdose: 1-2 mg/kg IV slowly.

Remarks: **Contraindicated** with concurrent MAO inhibitor use, acute attacks of asthma, GI or urinary obstruction. Use with **caution** in infants and young children, and do not use in neonates due to potential CNS effects. Side effects include sedation, nausea, vomiting, xerostomia, blurred vision and other reactions common to antihistamines. CNS side effects more common than GI disturbances. May cause paradoxical excitement in children. **Adjust dose in renal failure**.

(Siberry: The Harriet Lane Handbook 2000, pp.695-696)

DIPHTHERIA EQUINE ANTITOXIN

Available through CDC Drug Service, Division of Immunologic, Oncologic, and Hematologic Diseases, Center for Infectious Diseases, Centers for Diseases Control in Atlanta, Georgia.
Monday-Friday 8am to 4:30pm (404) 639-3356
After working hours (emergency requests only)
(404) 639-2888 (1).

Diphtheria antitoxin

Antitoxin. Because the condition of patients with diphtheria may deteriorate rapidly, a single dose of equine antitoxin should be administered on the basis of clinical diagnosis, even before culture results are available. to neutralize toxin as rapidly as possible, the preferred route of administration is intravenous. Before intravenous administration, however, tests for sensitivity to horse serum should be performed with a 1:1000 dilution of antitoxin in saline. If the patient is sensitive to equine antitoxin, desensitization is necessary. Although intravenous immunoglobulin preparations contain antibodies to diphtheria toxin, their use for therapy of cutaneous or respiratory tract diphtheria has not been approved, and optimal dosages have not been established. Antitoxin can be obtained from the National Immunization Program of the CDC. The site and size of the diphtheritic membrane, the degree of toxic effects, and the duration of illness are guides for estimating the dose of antitoxin; the presence of soft, diffuse, cervical lymphadenitis suggests moderate to severe toxin absorption. Suggested dose ranges are the following: pharyngeal or laryngeal disease of 48 hours' duration or less, 20 000 to 40 000 U; nasopharyngeal lesions, 40 000 to 60 000 U; extensive disease of 3 or more days' duration or diffuse swelling of the neck, 80 000 to 120 000 U. Antitoxin probably is of no value for cutaneous disease, but some experts recommend 20 000 to 40 000 U of antitoxin because toxic sequelae have been reported.

(American Academy of Pediatrics: Report of the Committee on Infectious Diseases. Red Book 2000, pp.231-232)

Diphtheria antitoxin

Route & Dose: IM, IV: 20,000-50,000 units/day for 2-3 successive days

Adverse Effects and Cautions: Hypersensitivity reaction
(Taeusch: Avery's Diseases of the Newborn 1998, p.1344)

DISOPYRAMIDE (Norpace)

Supplied: Capsules 100mg, 150 mg
Administration: PO

Disopyramide

Dosing: PO: 5-30 mg/kg/day (varies with age)
Warnings: Anticholinergic effects

Oral Administration, Kinetics, Metabolites:
The therapeutic plasma range of disopyramide is 2 to 5 μg/ml

Dosing and Interactions:
Dosing schedule has been as follows: younger than 2 years, 20 to 30 mg/kg/day; 2 to 10 years, 9 to 24 mg/kg/day. Older than 11 years, 5 to 13 mg/kg/day.

Coadministration of disopyramide with digoxin does not influence digoxin levels.

Side Effects: May patients receiving disopyramide have anticholinergic side effects, which limit the drug's use. Up to 50% of patients can have urinary retention, constipation, nausea, anorexia, vomiting, blurred vision, or dry mouth.

Exacerbation of AV block, sinus node disease, and new-onset VT are recognized clinical arrhythmic side effects.
(Gillette: Clinical Pediatric Arrhythmias 1999, pp.231-248)

Disopyramide

Class: IA

Uses: Similar to quinidine and procainamide

Dose (Level): PO: 1-3 mg/kg/dose q6hr (2-4 μg/mL)

Mode of Action: Similar to quinidine; some Ca^{++} channel blockade, potent anticholinergic

ECG/EP Changes: Similar to quinidine, more PR than QRS prolongation

Side Effects: Similar to quinidine; electromechanical dissociation; anticholinergic
(Garson: The science and practice of pediatric cardiology 1998, p.2952)

DOBUTAMINE (Dobutrex)

Supplied: Injection, concentrate for 250mg/20ml
Administration: IV, continuous infusion.
Must be DILUTED before administration to at least 50ml. The concentration of Dobutamine administered depends on the dosage and fluid requirements of the individual patient, but should not exceed 5000mcg/ml. Stable for 24 hours in D5W, D10W, NS. Pink discoloration of dobutamine solutions indicate slight oxidation of the drug; however there is no important loss of potency if the drug is administered within the recommended time period (3).

Dobutamine is physically and chemically stable with dopamine, tolazoline and theophylline (8).

Admixture incompatibility:
Incompatible with alkaline solutions (1). Also incompatible with hydrocortisone sodium succinate, cefazolin, cefamandole, penicillin, sodium ethacrynate, sodium heparin and aminophylline.

Dobutamine Hydrochloride (Dobutrex)

Indications and use:
To increase cardiac output during states of depressed contractility such as septic shock, organic heart disease, or cardiac surgical procedures.

Actions: A direct $ß_1$ agonist; actions on $ß_2$ and α-adrenergic receptors are much less marked than those of dopamine. Unlike dopamine, dobutamine does not cause release of endogenous norepinephrine, nor does it have any effect on dopaminergic receptors.

Route: IV
Dosage: 2-10 mcg/kg/min by continuous infusion. Maximum dosage is 40 mcg/kg/min.

Adverse effects: Generally dose-related. Chiefly ectopic heart beats, increased heart rate, and blood pressure elevations.

Comments: Contraindicated in idiopathic subaortic stenosis and atrial fibrillation.

(Gomella: Neonatology 1999, p.563)

Dobutamine

Dosage: 2-50 μg/kg/min

Comments: Titrate dose to target effect; in young infants increased heart rate may occur; tolerance may develop with prolonged use (>3 days)

(Fanaroff: Neonatal-Perinatal Medicine 1997, p.1743)

Dobutamine

Dose: 5-20 μg/kg/min

Mode of Action: β-Adrenergic agonist; low dose: α-agonist, high dose: peripheral vasodilator

Adverse Effects: Ventricular ectopy, may increase PCWP, cause pulmonary edema

Comment: Potent inotrope; useful in combination with dopamine

(Garson: The science and practice of pediatric cardiology 1998, p.2950)

Dobutamine

THERAPY FOR ACUTE CONGESTIVE CARDIAC FAILURE

A recommended starting infusion rate for dobutamine is 2 to 5 μg/kg/minute. This infusion rate may be titrated up based on clinical response, but adverse reactions including arrhythmias and significant hypotension increase in frequency at higher infusion rates. Like dopamine, dobutamine should not be mixed with alkaline solutions.

In an effort to minimize the untoward effects of each agent while taking advantage of their beneficial hemodynamic properties, we often combine "renal" dopamine at 3 to 5 μg/kg/minute with dobutamine at 5 to 10 μg/kg/minute, along with an afterload-reducing agent such as milrinone or nitroprusside in postoperative patients so that inotropic support and afterload reduction may be titrated separately.

(Garson: The science and practice of pediatric cardiology 1998, pp.2329-2341)

Dobutamine

Dose & Route: Continuous IV infusion:
2.5-15 mcg/kg/min.
Max. recommended dose: 40 mcg/kg/min

Remarks: **Contraindicated** in IHSS. Tachycardia, arrhythmias (PVC's) and hypertension may occasionally occur (especially at higher infusion rates).

Correct hypovolemic states before use. Increases AV condition, may precipitate ventricular ectopic activity.

Monitor BP and vital signs. $T_{1/2}$: 2 min. Peak effects in 10-20 min.

(Siberry: The Harriet Lane Handbook 2000, p.697)

DOMPERIDONE

Domperidone is investigational in the United States with Janssen as Motilium (R). Domperidone is available on a compassionate basis by contacting Cynthia Seymore, Janssen Research Foundation, PO Box 200, 1125 Trenton-Harbortown Road, Titusville, NJ 08560, (609) 730-3155.

Clinical trials with intravenous domperidone were discontinued in the US by Janssen. The company voluntarily withdrew the intravenous preparation from worldwide markets following reports of cardiovascular adverse effects. (12)

Domperidone

The dosage for domperidone is 0.3 mg/kg given orally three or four times a day.

(Walker: Pediatric Gastrointestinal Disease 2000, pp.1813-1814)

DOPAMINE (Intropin)

Supplied: Injection 40mg, 80mg, 160mg/ml in 5ml vials, syringes 80mg/100ml, 160mg/100ml, 320mg/100ml in 250ml and 500ml

Administration: IV, continuous infusion.

Concentrated product must be diluted before administration. The concentration of Dopamine administered depends on the dosage and fluid requirements of the individual patient. Concentrations as high as 3.2mg/ml have been used. Stable in D5W,NS (3).

Dopamine is physically and chemically stable with dobutamine, tolazoline, theophylline, Lidocaine, and Ranitidine (8).

Infuse into a large vein to prevent extravasation. For extravasation, use phentolamine. See phentolamine monograph (author). Extravasation may cause necrosis and sloughing of surrounding tissue (1).

Preparing Solution:

A formula commonly used follows:

$$6 \times \frac{\text{Desired dose (mcg/kg/min)}}{\text{Desired rate (ml/hr)}} \times \text{Wt (kg)} = \frac{\text{mg drug}}{\text{100mL fluid}}$$

Dopamine Hydrochloride (Dopastat, Intropin)

Indications and use:

To increase tissue perfusion after adequate fluid volume replacement in septic states, improve cardiac output and stroke volume with severe congestive heart failure refractory to digoxin and diuretics; and increase cardiac output, blood pressure, and urine flow in patients in shock.

Actions: Actions are dose-dependent. Low doses act directly on dopaminergic receptors to produce renal and mesenteric vasodilation; in moderate doses, β_1-adrenergic effects become prominent, resulting in a positive inotropic effect on the myocardium; high doses stimulate α-adrenergic receptors, producing increased peripheral resistance and renal vasoconstriction.

Route: IV by continuous infusion

Dosage: **Note**: Dose-effect relationship is speculative in neonates.

Low dose:
0.5-5 mcg/kg/min causes increased renal perfusion

Moderate dose:
5-10 mcg/kg/min causes increased cardiac output

High dose:
10-40 mcg/kg/min causes systemic vasoconstriction

Suggested drip administration:

mg dopamine per 100 mL of solution =

$$\frac{6 \times \text{Infant's weight [kg]} \times \text{Desired dose mcg/kg/min}}{\text{Rate in (mL/h)}}$$

Adverse effects:
Dopamine may cause ectopic heart beats, tachycardia, hypotension, hypertension, and excessive diuresis. Gangrene of the extremities has occurred with high doses over prolonged periods. Extravasation may cause tissue necrosis and sloughing of surrounding tissues; if this occurs, inject phentolamine, 0.1 to 0.2 mg/kg diluted to 1 mL saline throughout the affected area.

Comments: Administration of phenytoin IV to patients receiving dopamine may result in severe hypotension and bradycardia; therefore, use with extreme caution.

(Gomella: Neonatology 1999, pp.563-564)

<u>Dopamine</u>

Dosage: 0.5-3 μg/kg/min
Comments: "Renal dose" to promote splanchnic blood flow and cortical redistribution of renal blood flow

Dosage: 3-8 μg/kg/min
Comments: Cardiotonic dose; pharmacodynamic response similar to dobutamine

Dosage: >8 μg/kg/min
Comments: Pressor dose; vasoconstrictive action both direct and indirect

(Fanaroff: Neonatal-Perinatal Medicine 1997, p.1743)

Dopamine

Dose: 3-30 μg/kg/min

Mode of Action: Renal vasodilator at low concentrations, β-1 and β-2 stimulation, mild α-agonist, norepinephrine release

Adverse Effects: Tachyarrhythmia; may increase pulmonary resistance, nausea, vomiting

Comments: Drug effect may attenuate secondary to catecholamine depletion; useful in combination with nitroprusside; *do not* mix with bicarb or aminophylline

(Garson: The science and practice of pediatric cardiology 1998, p.2950)

Dopamine

THERAPY FOR ACUTE CONGESTIVE CARDIAC FAILURE

As an inotropic agent, low-dose dopamine offers the advantage of having less chronotropic effect than isoproterenol and is less arrhythmogenic than may other catecholamines. Low infusion rates of dopamine (5 μg/kg/minute or less) may be used to enhance renal blood flow and to produce natriuresis. Moderate rates of infusion (5 to 15 μg/kg/minute) are used for an inotropic effect, but a dose-dependent α-adrenergic effect should be anticipated and avoided. Infusion rates over 20 μg/kg/minute may compromise renal blood flow. Because of the immaturity of myocardial and vascular adrenergic receptors in the newborn, infusion rates of dopamine higher than those above have been used, but this therapeutic modality is not well studied.

Although efficacious in many situations, dopamine has several hemodynamic effects that must be considered before it is used as an inotropic agent. Dopamine increases pulmonary vascular resistance, particularly in the setting of hypoxemic pulmonary hypertension, and also may suppress the central respiratory drive. Dopamine increases ventricular afterload at higher doses, thereby increasing myocardial oxygen demand. Dopamine also should be infused through a central intravenous line, with frequent inspection of the infusion site, because local extravasation leads to tissue necrosis. Extravasated dopamine should be treated with local infiltration of phentolamine, as outlined for norepinephrine. Because strongly alkaline solutions inactivate dopamine, the agent should not be infused with sodium bicarbonate.

(Garson: The science and practice of pediatric cardiology 1998, pp.2329-2341)

Dopamine

Dose & Route: Low dose: 2-5 mcg/kg/min IV; increases renal blood flow; minimal effect on heart rate and cardiac output

Intermediate dose: 5-15 mcg/kg/min IV; increases heart rate, cardiac contractility, and cardiac output, and to a lesser extent, renal blood flow.

High dose: >20 mcg/kg/min IV; alpha adrenergic effects are prominent; decreases renal perfusion
Max dose recommended: 20-50 mcg/kg/min IV

Remarks: **Do not use** in pheochromocytoma, tachyarrhythimas, or hypovolemia. Monitor vital signs and blood pressure continuously. Correct hypovolemic states. Tachyarrythmias, ectopic beats, hypertension, vasoconstriction, vomiting may occur. Use cautiously with phenytoin since hypotension and bradycardia may be exacerbated.

Should be administered through a central-line or large vein. Extravasation may cause tissue necrosis; treat with phentolamine. Do not administer into an umbilical arterial catheter.

(Siberry: The Harriet Lane Handbook 2000, p.698)

DOXAPRAM (Dopram)

Supplied: Injection 20mg/ml in 20ml vials (contains benzyl alcohol)

Administration: IV
Stable in D5W, NS, D10W. Dilute to a concentration of 1 to 2mg/ml (1, 3).

Admixture incompatibility:
Admixture of doxapram with alkaline solution such as 2.5% thiopental sodium, bicarbonate or aminophylline will result in precipitation or gas formation(1).

Doxapram Hydrochloride (Dopram)

Indications and use:
Apnea of prematurity resistant to methylxanthine therapy.

Actions: Analeptic agent with potent respiratory and CNS stimulant properties.

Route: IV.

Dosage: 0.5-1.5 mg/kg/h (maximum: 2.5 mg/kg/h) by continuous IV infusion; decrease the infusion rate when control of apnea is achieved.

Therapeutic range: < 5 mcg/mL. At a dose of a 1.5 mg/kg/h, the mean serum concentration reported was 3.2 mcg/mL (assay not available in most centers).

Adverse effects: Increase in blood pressure, heart rate, cardiac output; and skeletal muscle hyperactivity may occur. Abdominal distention, increased gastric residuals, vomiting, jitteriness, hyperglycemia, glycosuria, and seizures have been reported in neonates.

Comments: Efficacy of doxapram in premature neonates with severe idiopathic apnea resistant to theophylline has been documented. Use cautiously because of its side effects. Should not be given during the first few days of life, when hypertensive episodes may be associated with an increased risk of intraventricular hemorrhage. Has a narrow therapeutic range, and its use warrants serum drug level monitoring. Contraindicated in cardiovascular and seizure disorders. Benzyl alcohol is contained in the formulation, which may accumulate to toxic levels after prolonged use.

(Gomella: Neonatology 1999, p.564)

Doxapram

Dosage: 2 mg/kg loading dose followed by 4 mg/kg/hr IV

Comments: Not recommended for long-term use because of insidious acidosis and CO_2 retention; not recommended for newborns because of benzyl alcohol preservative

(Fanaroff: Neonatal-Perinatal Medicine 1997, p.1749)

Doxapram

Dose/kg: Loading dose: 3 mg

Route & frequency: IV infusion over 1 h

Dose/kg: Maintenance dose: 1-2.5 mg/kg/h

Route & frequency:

Continuous IV infusion; start at 1 mg/kg/h and titrate up to minimum effective dose

maximum conc: 2 mg/mL

Comments: Maintain therapeutic caffeine or theophylline levels while on doxapram. Taper drug to avoid rebound apneic episodes. Increases oxygen consumption and may cause hypertension, tachycardia, and seizures

(Avery: Neonatology Pathophysiology and Management of the Newborn 1999, p.1555)

Doxapram

Generic Available: No

Use: Respiratory and CNS stimulant; idiopathic apnea of prematurity refractory to xanthines

Warnings: Should be used with caution in newborns as the U.S. product contains benzyl alcohol (0.9%); recommended doses of doxapram for neonates will deliver 5.4-27 mg/kg/day of benzyl alcohol; large amounts of benzyl alcohol (>100 mg/kg/day) have been associated with fatal toxicity (gasping syndrome); the use of doxapram in newborns should be reserved for neonates who are unresponsive to the treatment of apnea with therapeutic serum concentrations of theophylline or caffeine

Usual Dosage: I.V.:
Neonatal apnea (apnea of prematurity): Initial loading dose: 2.5-3 mg/kg followed by a continuous infusion of 1 mg/kg/hour titrated to the lowest rate at which apnea is controlled (maximum dose: 2.5 mg/kg/hour)

Administration: Parenteral: I.V. use only: Dilute loading dose to a maximum concentration of 2 mg/mL and infuse over 15-30 minutes; for infusion, dilute in NS or dextrose to 1 mg/mL (maximum concentration: 2 mg/mL); irritating to tissues; avoid extravasation

Reference Range: Initial studies suggest a therapeutic serum level of at least 1.5 mg/L; toxicity becomes frequent at serum levels >5 mg/L

(Taketomo: Pediatric Dosage Handbook 1999-2000, pp.321-322)

<u>Doxapram HCl</u>

Dose & Route: Methylxanthine-refractory neonatal apnea: Load with 2.5-3 mg/kg over 15 min, followed by a continuous infusion of 1 mg/kg/hr titrated to the lowest responsive dose;
Max dose: 2.5 mg/kg/hr

Remarks: Hypertension occurs with higher doses (greater than 1.5 mg/kg/hr. May also cause tachycardia, arrhythmias, seizure, hyperreflexia, hyperpyrexia, and sweating. Avoid extravasation into tissues.

(Siberry: Then Harriet Lane Handbook 2000, p.699)

EDROPHONIUM (Enlon, Reversol, Tensilon)

Supplied: Injection 10mg/ml in 1ml, 10ml, 15ml
Administration: IM, IV

Edrophonium

Dose/kg: Myasthenia gravis test:
Neonates: 0.1 mg (single dose, not per Kg)
Infants: 0.04 mg/kg/dose X 1 (max of 1 mg for body weight ≤34 kg)

Route & frequency: IV once. If no IV access available, may give IM or SC

Comments: Keep atropine and resuscitation equipment available
Antidote: Atropine 0.01-0.04 mg/kg/dose

(Avery: Neonatology Pathophysiology and Management of the Newborn 1999, p.1555)

Edrophonium

Route & Dose: Tensilon test for myasthenia gravis
SC, IM: 0.2-0.5 mg/kg, IV: preliminary test dose = 0.04 mg slow push, test dose = 0.16 mg/kg (1 min later)

Adverse Effects and Cautions:
Cardiac arrhythmia, diarrhea, tracheal secretions may require atropine antagonism

(Taeusch: Avery's Diseases of the Newborn 1998, p.1344)

Edrophonium

Uses: PSVT
Dosing: 0.04 mg/kg test for bronchospasm; then 0.16 mg/kg over 2 min
Acute Side Effects:
Sinus bradycardia; atrioventricular (AV) block; bronchospasm; abdominal pain
Other Considerations:
Atropine for excessive vagal response; less effective in infants

PSVT, paroxysmal supraventricular tachycardia.

(Gillette: Clinical Pediatric Arrhythmias 1999, p.153)

Edrophonium Chloride

Dose and Route: Test for Myasthenia Gravis (IV):
Neonate: 0.1 mg single dose

Infants and children:
Initial: 0.04 mg/kg/dose x 1
Max: 1 mg for <34 kg, 2 mg for ≥34 kg
If no response after 1 min, may give 0.16 mg/kg/dose for a total of 0.2 mg/kg
Total max dose: 5 mg for <34 kg, 10 mg for ≥34 kg

Remarks: May precipitate cholinergic crisis, arrhythmias, bronchospasm. Keep atropine available in syringe and have resuscitation equipment ready. Hypersensitivity to test dose (fasciculations or intestinal cramping) is indication to stop giving drug. **Contraindicated** in GI or GU obstruction, or arrhythmias. Dose may need to be reduced in chronic renal failure.

Short duration of action with IV route (5-10 minutes). Antidote: Atropine 0.01-0.04 mg/kg/dose.

(Siberry: The Harriet Lane Handbook 2000, p.701)

EMLA CREAM

Supplied: 2.5% lidocaine, 2.5% prilocaine
(in 5 g with tegaderm dressings and 30g)
Patches, in 2's 10's

Administration: Topical

EMLA (Lidocaine/prilocaine)

Before the scheduled time of the circumcision, the cream (0.5 mL), either EMLA or sterile petroleum jelly, was applied with a cotton-tipped swab on the outside of the prepuce and covered with an occlusive gauze dressing that was taped to itself. The newborn was then swaddled and left in a crib for the next 45 to 60 minutes.

Circumcision procedure produces pain responses that EMLA diminishes....

(Benini: Topical Anesthesia During Circumcision in Newborn Infants. JAMA 1993;270:850-853)

Lidocaine and Prilocaine (EMLA)

Use: Topical anesthetic for use on normal intact skin to provide local analgesia for minor procedures such as I.V. cannulation or venipuncture; has also been used for painful procedures such as lumbar puncture and skin graft harvesting

Usual Dosage: Topical:
Neonates: Safety and efficacy have not been established; preliminary results in a study of 30 preterm neonates (n=30) using a single 0.5 g dose of EMLA applied to the heal for 1 hour resulted in no measurable changes in methemoglobin levels

Administration: Topical: Do not use on mucous membranes or the eyes; apply a thick layer of cream to intact skin and cover with an occlusive dressing

Patient Information:
Not for ophthalmic use; for external use only. EMLA® may block sensation in the treated skin.

Nursing Implications:
In small infants and children, an occlusive bandage should be placed over the EMLA cream to prevent the child from placing the cream in his/her mouth or smearing the cream on the eyes

(Taketomo: Pediatric Dosage Handbook 1999-2000, pp.533-534)

EMLA (Lidocaine/prilocaine)

Each neonate was randomly assigned to receive 0.5 ml of EMLA on the right or left heel. The exact dose was measured with a 1 ml tuberculin syringe...We used 0.5 mg of EMLA because it covers a significant portion of the neonatal heel (surface area □ 5cm^2)...The heel was the site of application because it is the most common site of blood collection in neonates...These results are in agreement with those of other investigators who used similar or higher doses (up to 1.25 gm for 1 hour) and measured either Met-Hb or drug concentrations or both. None of the studies to date have indicated a significant risk of toxic effects.

(Taddio: Safety of Lidocaine-prilocaine cream in the treatment of preterm neonates. J Pediatr 1995:1002-1005)

Emla

Remarks: Use with **caution** in patients with G6PD deficiency and in patients with renal and hepatic impairment. Prilocaine has been associated with methemoglobinemia.

Must apply 60-90 minutes in advance under an occlusive dressing. Wipe cream off before procedure.

(Siberry: The Harriet Lane Handbook 2000, p.703)

ENALAPRIL MALEATE (Vasotec)
ENALAPRILAT (Vasotec IV)

Supplied: Injection: 1.25 mg/ml in 1ml, 2ml vials (contains benzyl alcohol)
Tablets: 2.5mg, 5mg, 10mg, 20mg

Administration: Give as a slow IV infusion, over at least 5 minutes. The appropriate dose may be diluted in D5W, NS. Stable for 24 hours (1).

Comment: Clinical response is usually seen within 15 minutes. Peak effects after the first dose may not occur for up to four hours. The peak effects of subsequent doses may exceed those of the first (1).

Extemporaneous Compounding (Recipe)

Dosage form: Oral suspension
Made from: Tablets
Concentration: 0.1 mg/mL
Stability: 91 d (4°C); 56 d (25°C)
Store: Room temperature
Label: Shake well

Ingredient	Strength	Quantity
Enalapril tablets	10 mg	1
Ora-Sweet or Ora-Sweet SF		
Ora-plus		aa qs 100 mL

Instructions: Crush the tablet in a mortar. Add a small amount of the vehicle and triturate to make a smooth paste. Add increasing amounts of the vehicle to make the suspension pourable. Transfer to a graduate and qs to final volume with the vehicle. If Ora-Sweet and Ora-Plus products are not available, water may be used. Reduce the stability to 6 wk in water at 25°C. (11)

Enalapril (PO)
Enalaprilat (IV) (Vasotec)

Indications and use:
Manage hypertension and heart failure.

Actions: Inhibits conversion of angiotensin I to angiotensin II and the breakdown of bradykinin, causing vasodilation.

Route: IV, PO

Dosage: IV: 5-10 mcg/kg/dose q8-24h
PO: 100 mcg/kg/dose as a single daily dose. May increase gradually over 2 weeks as needed to a maximum of 500 mcg/kg/day PO. Reduce the dose in renal dysfunction. Use a low initial dose to avoid a profound drop in blood pressure, especially in patients on diuretics who are hyponatremic or hypovolemic. Monitor blood pressure hourly for the first 12 h.

Adverse effects: Hypotension, hyperkalemia, decreased renal function, oliguria, cough, decreased hemoglobin and hematocrit, and, rarely, bone marrow depression, neutropenia, and thrombocytopenia.

Comments: Note that the IV dose is much smaller than the PO dose. Use caution to adjust the dose when changing routes of administration.

(Gomella: Neonatology 1999, pp.564-565)

Enalapril

Vasodilator Therapy in children with CHF

Dose/Route of Administration:
0.08 mg/kg/dose PO q 12-24 hr
0.3 mg/kg/day max

Disadvantages: Risk of renal failure

(Garson: The science and practice of pediatric cardiology 1998, p.2322)

Enalapril (Vasotec)

Dose: 0.08 mg/kg/dose q12-24hr in older children

Mode of Action: Same as captopril

Adverse Effects: Same as captopril, ? lower incidence of renal toxicity?

Comments: Same as captopril

(Garson: The science and practice of pediatric cardiology 1998, p.2951)

Enalaprilat (IV)

Dose/kg: 5-10 µg

Route & Frequency: IV q8h-q24h administer over 5 min

Comments: CrCl <10 mL/min: give 50% of dose
May cause hypoglycemia, hyperkalemia, neutropenia, anemia, and deterioration of renal function

(Avery: Neonatology Pathophysiology and Management of the Newbron 1999, p.1555)

Enalapril (PO)

Dose/kg: 0.05-0.1 mg

Route & frequency: PO qd titrate to maximum of 0.5 mg/kg

Comments: Adjust dose in renal impairment: CrCl 10-50 mL/min: give 75% of dose

(Avery: Neonatology Pathophysiology and Management of the Newborn 1999, p.1555)

Enalapril Maleate, Enalaprilat

Dose & Route: Infants & Children:
PO: 0.1 mg/kg/24 hr ÷ QD-Bid; increase PRN over 2 wk
Max dose: 0.5 mg/kg/24 hr
IV: 0.005-0.01 mg/kg/dose Q8-24 hr

Remarks: Use with **caution** in bilateral renal artery stenosis. Side effects: nausea, diarrhea, headache, dizziness, hyperkalemia, hypoglycemia, hypotension, and hypersensitivity. Cough is a reported side effect of ACE inhibitors.

Enalapril (PO) is converted to its active form (Enalapriat) by the liver. Administer IV over 5 min. Reduce dose in renal impairment. **Adjust dose in renal failure**.

(Siberry: Then Harriet Lane Handbook 2000, p.704)

ENOXAPARIN (Lovenox)

Supplied: Injection: 30mg/0.3ml (also available in amps) 40mg/0.4ml, 60mg/0.6ml, 80mg/0.8ml, 100mg/1ml
All strengths available as syringes with 27 gauge x ½ inch needle.

Administration: Administer as SC injection only; do not administer IM. Screen patients prior to prophylactic administration of enoxaparin to rule out a bleeding disorder. There is usually no need for daily monitoring of the effect of enoxaparin in patients with normal presurgical coagulation parameters (1).

Enoxaparin

Dose & Route: DVT treatment:
Infants (limited information):
1.5 mg/kg Q12 hr SC
Children: 1 mg/kg Q12 hr SC

Remarks: Inhibits thrombosis by inactivating factor Xa without significantly affecting bleeding time, platelet function, PT or APTT at recommended doses. Dosages of enoxaparin, heparin, or other low molecular weight heparins **cannot** be used interchangeably on a unit-for-unit (or mg-for-mg)

basis because of differences in pharmacokinetics and activity. Peak anti-factor Xa activity is achieved after 4 hours of dose.

Contraindicated in major bleeding and drug-induced thrombocytopenia. May cause fever, confusion, edema, nausea, hemorrhage, thrombocytopenia, hypochromic anemia, and pain/erythema at injection site.

Administer by deep SC injection by having the patient lie down. Rotate administration between the left and right anterolateral and left and right posterolateral abdominal wall. See package insert for detailed SC administration recommendations. To minimize bruising, do not rub the injection site.

(Siberry: The Harriet Lane Handbook 2000, p.704)

Low Molecular Weight Heparin

Children admitted to the Hospital for Sick Children, Toronto, Canada, between March 1994 and July 1997 were treated with the LMWH enoxaparin (Rhone Poulenc Rorer, Canada) if the treating physician estimated that the risk/benefit ratio of traditional therapy (UFH/oral anticoagulants) was potentially compromised (high risk of bleeding, required diet or medication alterations, no venous access). For therapy of an established thrombosis or high-risk prophylaxis (cardiomyopathy, prosthetic mitral valve, cardiovascular shunts, systemic lupus erythematosus, central venous line-related thrombosis with a previous thrombotic event), children ≤2 months of age received LMWH at a rate that was a 50% increase over the initial dosing regimen for children >2 months of age (1.5 mg/kg or 1.0 mg/kg, respectively), subcutaneously every 12 hours, as established in the previous pharmacokinetic study. Dosing alterations for therapy were made according to a published nomogram to maintain the antifactor Xa level between 0.5 and 1.0 U/mL. For low-risk prophylaxis (CVL-related thrombosis with no thrombotic history, trauma after surgery), children received 50% of the therapeutic dose with a target anti-factor Xa range of 0.1 to 0.4 U/mL. Anti-factor Xa levels were measured at 4 hours after the second or third dose, then weekly for the duration of therapy.

Age and Sex Distribution.

The age distribution of children who received therapeutic doses ranged from 1 day to 18 years (median 3.5 years, mean 6.1 years)...

In conclusion, LMWH appears to offer a safe and effective form of anticoagulation in children with or at risk of TEs. The use of subcutaneous catheters reduces the trauma from daily injections. The results of this study support the need for a randomized clinical trial comparing LMWH with

UFH and warfarin in the prevention of TEs and the treatment of children with or at risk for TEs.

(Dix: The use of low molecular weight heparin in pediatric patients: A prospective cohort study. J Pediatr 2000;136:439-45)

Enoxaparin

Low-Molecular-Weigh Heparin

Low-molecular-weight heparin (LMWH) is an alternative to heparin therapy. A starting dose of 1 to 1.5 mg/kg q 12 hours subcutaneously is begun, and adjusted to achieve an anti-factor Xa range of 0.5 to 1 units/mL. A nomogram for dose adjustment is reviewed in the article by Edstrom and Christensen earlier in this issue. LMWH is monitored by anti-factor Xa levels drawn 4 hours following each adjusted dose and at least weekly thereafter. change in renal function, protein status, circulatory status (e.g., shock), and addition of antibiotics can affect LMWH clearance. Check anti-factor Xa levels if these situations occur.

(Calhoun: Consistent approaches to procedures and practices in neonatal hematology. Clinics in Perinatology 2000, 27:733-753)

EPINEPHRINE (Adrenalin)

Supplied: Injection 1:10,000 (0.1mg/ml) in 10ml syringe
Injection 1:100,000 (0.01mg/ml) in 5ml syringe
Injection 1:1000 (1mg/ml) in 1ml amps, 30mL vials

Administration: IV, Endotracheal, Intraosseous, SQ

Administer by DIRECT IV INJECTION. Using 0.1mg/ml or 0.01mg/ml concentrations. Doses may be repeated every 3-5 minutes during a resuscitation effort.

For continuous IV infusion, a initial rate of 0.1 μg/kg per minute, the rate of infusion may be increased in increments of 0.1 μg/kg per minute, if necessary, to a maximum of 1 mcg/kg/min (3).

For ENDOTRACHEAL ADMINISTRATION, the dose is equivalent to the IV dose. To aid delivery of the drug via the endotracheal tube, the dose may be diluted with 0.9% NaCl (3).

Epinephrine

Administration of epinephrine is indicated when the heart rate remains <60 bpm after a minimum of 30 seconds of adequate ventilation and chest compressions (Class I). Epinephrine is particularly indicated in the presence of asystole.

Epinephrine has both α- and β-adrenergic-stimulating properties; however, in cardiac arrest, α-adrenergic-mediated vasoconstriction may be the more important action. Vasoconstriction elevates the perfusion pressure during chest compression, enhancing delivery of oxygen to the heart and brain. Epinephrine also enhances the contractile state of the heart, stimulates spontaneous contractions, and increases heart rate.

The recommended intravenous or endotracheal dose is 0.1 to 0.3 mL/kg of a 1:10 000 solution (0.01 to 0.03 mg/kg), repeated every 3 to 5 minutes as indicated. The data regarding effects of high-dose epinephrine for resuscitation of newly born infants is inadequate to support routine use of higher doses of epinephrine (Class Indeterminate, LOE 4). Higher doses have been associated with exaggerated hypertension but lower cardiac output in animals. The sequence of hypotension followed by hypertension likely increases the risk of intracranial hemorrhage, especially in preterm infants.

MedicationsDrugs are rarely indicated in resuscitation of the newly born infant. Bradycardia in the newly born infant is usually the result of inadequate lung inflation or profound hypoxia, and adequate ventilation is the most important step in correcting bradycardia. Administer medications if, despite adequate ventilation with 100% oxygen and chest compressions, the heart rate remains <60 bpm.

Routes of Medication Administration

The tracheal route is generally the most rapidly accessible route for drug administration during resuscitation. It maybe used for administration of epinephrine and naloxone, but it should not be used during resuscitation for administration of caustic agents such as sodium bicarbonate. The tracheal route of administration may result in a more variable response to epinephrine than the intravenous route; however, neonatal data is insufficient to recommend a higher dose of epinephrine for tracheal administration.

Attempt to establish intravenous access in neonates who fail to respond to tracheally administered epinephrine. The umbilical vein is the most rapidly accessible venous route; it may be used for epinephrine or naloxone administration as well as for administration of volume expanders and bicarbonate. Insert a 3.5F or 5F radiopaque catheter so that the tip is just below skin level and a free flow of blood returns on aspiration. Deep insertion poses the risk of infusion of hypertonic and vasoactive medications into the liver. Take care to avoid introduction of air emboli into the umbilical vein.

Peripheral sites for venous access (scalp or peripheral vein) may be adequate but are usually more difficult to cannulate. Naloxone may be given intramuscularly or subcutaneously but only after effective assisted ventilation has been established and only if the infant's peripheral circulation is adequate. We do not recommend administration of resuscitation drugs through the umbilical artery because the artery is often not rapidly accessible and complications may result if vasoactive or hypertonic drugs (eg, epinephrine or bicarbonate) are given by this route.

Intraosseous lines are not commonly used in newly born infants because the umbilical vein is more accessible, the small bones are fragile, and the intraosseous space is small in a premature infant. Intraosseous access has been shown to be useful in the neonate and older infant when vascular access is difficult to achieve. Intraosseous access can be used as an alternative route for medications/volume expansion if umbilical or other direct venous access is not readily attainable (Clas IIb. LOE 5).

(American Heart Association: Part 11: Neonatal Resuscitation 2000;102 (suppl I):I-343-I-357)

Epinephrine

Indications and use: Bradycardia, cardiac arrest, cardiogenic shock, anaphylactic reactions, bronchospasm.

Actions: Acts directly on both α- and β-adrenergic receptors, with β_2 effects predominating at lower doses. Exerts both positive chronotropic and inotropic effects on the heart and relaxes bronchial smooth muscle. α-adrenergic stimulation produces an increase in systolic blood pressure and constriction of renal blood vessels.

Route: IV, ET

Dosage: 1:10,000 used IV

IV bolus: 0.1-0.3 mL/kg/dose q5min prn.
IV infusion: Start with 0.1 mcg/kg/min. Maximum 1.5 mcg/kg/min (titrate).

Intratracheal: 0.1-0.3 mL/kg/dose diluted 1:1 with normal saline.

Adverse effects: Hypertension, tachycardia, nausea, pallor, tremor, cardiac arrhythmias, increased myocardial oxygen consumption, and decreased renal and splanchnic blood flow.

(Gomella: Neonatology 1999, p.565)

Epinephrine

Dose: 0.05-1.0 μg/kg/min

Mode of Action: Potent β-agonist, $B_1 > B_2$, mild α-agonist

Adverse Effects: Tachycardia, arrhythmias, hyperglycemia, headache, restlessness

Comments: Combined inotropic, chronotropic effects with BP maintenance

(Garson: The science and practice of pediatric cardiology 1998, p.2950)

Epinephrine

THERAPY FOR ACUTE CONGESTIVE CARDIAC FAILURE

As is the case with all inotropic agents, epinephrine infusion requires titration dependent on serial examinations focused on the adequacy of cardiac output. In general, the starting infusion rate is 0.05 to 0.1 μg/Kg/minute, and this may be increased slowly as needed. Infusion rates greater than 0.3 μg/kg/minute should be avoided because of adverse side effects of the drug. Ventricular arrhythmias may result from subendocardial ischemia secondary to increased myocardial oxygen demand relative to delivery. There also may be peripheral ischemia at high infusion rates of epinephrine secondary to extreme vasoconstriction. Because of this side effect, infusion should be accomplished through a central catheter, which should be inspected frequently to identify early signs of infiltration. Splanchnic and renal blood flow may be compromised with epinephrine infusion, even at low infusion rates. Epinephrine also may raise serum glucose and lactate levels, and may induce a leukocytosis by mobilizing marginated white cells. In light of the deleterious side effects of this agent, we generally reserve epinephrine infusions as a short-term treatment for patients who are unresponsive to all other available therapies. Nonetheless, epinephrine can be life-saving in these circumstances. Once the patient is stabilized, the epinephrine is titrated down, as indicated by frequent clinical examination, and withdrawn as soon as possible.

(Garson: The science and practice of pediatric cardiology 1998, pp.2329-2341)

Epinephrine HCl

Dose & Route: Cardiac Uses:

Neonate:

Asystole and bradycardia: 0.1-0.3 ml/kg of 1:10,000 solution (0.01-0.03 mg/kg) IV/ET Q3-5 min

Infants and Children:

Bradycardia, asystole, and pulseless arrest (first dose): 0.01 mg/kg of 1:10,000 solution (0.1 ml/kg) IO/IV; **max dose**: 1 mg (10 ml)

Asystole and pulseless arrest (subsequent doses) and all ET doses: 0.1 mg/kg of 1:1000 solution (0.1 ml/kg) IO/IV/ET Q3-5 min. If doses are not effective, increase dose to 0.2 mg/kg of 1:1000 solution (0.2 ml/kg).

Respiratory uses:

Bronchodilator:

1:1000 (Aqueous)

Infants and Children: 0.01 ml/kg/dose SC (**max single dose** 0.5 ml); repeat Q15 min x 3-4 doses or Q4 hr PRN

1:200 (Susphrine suspension)

Infants and Children: 0.005 ml/kg/dose SC (**max single dose** 0.15 ml); repeat Q8-12 hr PRN

Inhalation: 1-2 puffs Q4 hr PRN

Nebulization: (alternative to racemic epinephrine): 0.5 ml/kg of 1:1000 solution diluted in 3 ml NS; **max doses**: ≤4 yr: 2.5 ml/dose; >4 yr: 5 ml/dose

Remarks: Hypersensitivity reactions: For asthma and certain allergic manifestations (e.g., angioedema, urticaria, serum sickness, anaphylactic shock) use epinephrine SC. The adult IV dose for hypersensitivity reactions or to relieve bronchospasm usually ranges from 0.1 to 0.25 mg injected slowly. Neonates may be given a dose of 0.01 mg/kg body weight; for the infant, 0.05 mg is an adequate initial dose and this may be repeated at 20 to 30 minute intervals in the management of asthma attacks.

May produce arrhythmias, tachycardia, hypertension, headaches, nervousness, nausea, vomiting. Necrosis may occur at site of repeated local injection.

Concomitent use of non-cardiac selective beta-blockers or tricyclic antidepressants may enhance epinephrine's pressor response. Chlorpromazine may reverse the pressor response.

ETT doses should be diluted with NS to a volume of 3-5 ml before administration. Follow with several positive pressure ventilations.

(Siberry: The Harriet Lane Handbook 2000, pp.705-706)

<u>Epinephrine</u>

Indication: Protocol for inborn infants with Congenital Diaphragmatic Hernia

An epinephrine infusion initiated at 0.1 µg/kg/min

(Finer: Congenital diaphragmatic Hernia: Developing a Protocolized Approach. J Pediatr Surg 1998;33:1331-1337)

<u>Epinephrine</u>

For Treatment of Hypoglycemia:

If hypoglycemia does not respond to intravenous glucose plus hydrocortisone, then a trial dose of epinephrine 1:1,000 (0.01 mL/kg) is administered subcutaneously. If this trial dose is successful, then a maintenance dose of epinephrine 1:200 in 25% glycerine solution (Sus-Phrine; 0.005 to 0.01 mL/kg every 6 hours) is administered subcutaneously or ephedrine sulfate (0.05 mg/kg/3 hr) is given orally.

(Yeh: Neonatal Therapeutics 1991, p.247)

EPINEPHRINE, RACEMIC (AsthmaNefrin, Vaponefrin)

Supplied: AsthmaNefrin: Solution for inhalation 2.25% racepinephrine HCL (Equiv. to 1.125% epinephrine base)
Vaponefrin: Solution for inhalation 2% racepinephrine base (equiv. to 1% epinephrine base)

Administration: Inhalation

Epinephrine, racemic (Vaponefrin)

Dose: 0.1-0.3 mL. Dilute with NS to 3 mL.
Dose: every 30 min-2 h four times.

$_{L}$-Epinephrine 1:1000: 0.05-0.15 mL. Dilute with NS to 3 mL. Dose: 30 min-2 h four times.

Side Effects: Tachycardia
Tremor
Hypertension
Racemic epinephrine, 2 mg = $_{L}$-epinephrine, 1 mg

(Gomella: Neonatology: Management, Procedures, On-call Problems, Diseases and Drugs 1999, p.56)

Epinephrine (racemic)
2.25% solution

Dose/kg: 0.25 mL total dose

Route & frequency: Inhalation via nebulizer over 15 min q4hr prn
Dilute with NS to total volume of 2.5-3 mL

Comments: May cause tachycardia and arrhythmias

(Avery: Neonatology Pathophysiology and Management of the Newborn 1999, p.1555)

Epinephrine, Racemic

Dose & Route: Croup (using 2.25% solution): 0.05 ml/kg/dose diluted to 3 ml with NS. Given via nebulizer over 15 minutes PRN, but not more frequently than Q1-2 hr. **Max dose**: 0.5 ml

Remarks: Tachyarrhythmias, headache, nausea, palpitations reported. Rebound airway edema may occur. Cardio-respiratory monitoring should be considered if administered more frequently than Q1-2 hr.

(Siberry: The Harriet Lane Handbook 2000, p.706)

Epinephrine, Racemic

Route: Inhalant

Neonatal Dose: 0.25 mL/dose diluted to 2 mL with saline

Pediatric Dose: <10 kg: 2 mL of a 1:8 dilution
10-15 kg: 2 mL of a 1:6 dilution

Discussion: Make dilutions with normal saline (preferred) or sterile water and use in a nebulizer; monitor for rebound congestion and tachyarrhythmias.

(Rudolph: Rudolph's Pediatrics 1996, p.2183)

EPINEPHRINE SUSPENSION (Sus-Phrine)

Supplied: 1:200 (5 mg/ml) suspension, in 0.3ml amps, 5ml vials
Administration: For SC use only.
Storage: Refrigerate the suspension, do not freeze.
Do not expose to temperatures >30°(86°F)
Shake well before using.

<u>Epinephrine Hydrochloride</u> (Susphrine)

Indications and Use:
Relaxation of bronchial smooth muscles, cardiac stimulation, and dilation of skeletal muscle vasculature.

Actions: Direct action on both alpha-adrenergic and beta-adrenergic receptors. Alpha-adrenergic effects are thought to occur from production of cAMP, whereas beta-adrenergic effects result from inhibition of adenyl cyclase activity.

Route: SC
Dosage: Suspension (1:200) give 0.005 mL/kg/dose (0.025 mg/kg) to a maximum of 0.15 mL q8-12h.

Adverse effects: Tremor, tachycardia, hypertension, increased myocardial oxygen consumption, decreased renal and splanchnic blood flow, and cardiac arrhythmias.

Comments: Longer-acting form of epinephrine useful in patients who require chronic therapy such as those with bronchopulmonary dysplasia (BPD).
(Gomella: Neonatology 1994, p.482)

<u>Epinephrine</u>

Administration: An epinephrine suspension (Sus-Phrine) 5 mg/ml (1:200) is available for a more prolonged effect; however, its high concentration and low dose (0.004-0.005 ml/kg/dose SC given every 6 hours, prn) make it difficult to measure accurately and make delivery of an overdose in small infants more likely. Therefore, its use in small infants is discouraged.
(Zenk: Neonatal Medications & Nutrition. A Comprehensive Guide 2000; pp.176-179)

EPOETIN ALFA (Erythropoietin, EPO, Epogen, Procrit)

Supplied: Injection 2,000 units; 3,000 units; 4,000 units; or 10,000 units in 1ml, 2ml multi-dose vial [With 2.5mg albumin (human) per vial]

Administration: IV, SQ

Comment: Do not shake. Prolonged vigorous shaking may denature the glycoprotein, rendering it biologically inactive (1). Discard 2ml multi-dose vial 21 days after initial entry.

Erythropoietin

A Consistent Approach to Recombinant Erythropoietin Administration in the NICU - Drug Administration:

rEpo is given in a dose of 1200 to 1400 U/kg/wk, either as 200 U/kg/d intravenously or 400 U/kg subcutaneously three times per week. We generally limit the administration to a course not exceeding 2 weeks, and we evaluate the need for additional treatment days or weeks later. If given intravenously, the drug should be mixed with a protein-containing solution (either hyperalimentation or 5% albumin) in a volume sufficient to run over 4 hours (we use 1 to 2 mL total volume). Alternatively, Epo (200 U/kg/d) can be added to the hyperalimentation solution and run over 24 hours. If given subcutaneously, 400 U/kg three times per week is given in undiluted form. Using the 2000 U/mL concentration gives an injection volume of 0.2 mL/kg three times per week, and using the 4000 U/mL concentration gives an injection volume of 0.1 mL/kg. Care should be given to allow room for the drug to enter the subcutaneous space by holding the skin loosely between the thumb and finger. We generally use the lateral thigh as the injection site, and usually alternate thighs.

(Calhoun: Consistent approaches to procedures and practices in neonatal hematology. Clinics in Perinatology 2000, 27:733-753)

Erythropoietin

Dose/kg: Anemia of prematurity: 50-100 U
Route & frequency: SC three times weekly
Titrate dose up based on clinical response
or
Dose/kg: 200 U
Route & frequency: IV/SC qd-qod for 2-6 wk

Comments: Must give iron supplementation. Monitor hematocrit, retics, serum Fe, smear, and ferritin levels. Contraindicated in newborns with neutropenia.

(Avery: Neonatology Pathophysiology and Management of the Newborn 1999, p.1555)

Erythropoietin

Dose & Route: Renal Failure: SC/IV
Initial: 50-100 U/kg 3x/wk; may increase dose if hematocrit does not rise by 5-6 points after 8 wk; maintenance doses are individualized

AZT treated HIV patients: SC/IV
100 U/kg/dose 3x/wk x 8 wk; the dose may be increased by 50-100 U/kg/dose given 3x/wk;
max dose 300 U/kg/dose given 3x/wk

Anemia of prematurity:
25-100 U/kg/dose SC 3x/wk; alternatively, 200 U/kg/dose IV/SC QD to QOD for 2-6 wk may be used

Remarks: Evaluate serum iron, ferritin, TIBC before therapy. Iron supplementation recommended during therapy unless iron stores are already in excess. Monitor Hct, BP, clotting times, platelets, BUN, serum creatinine. Peak effect in 2-3 wk. Reduce dose when target Hct is reached, or when Hct increases >4 points in any 2-wk period. May cause hypertension, seizure, hypersensitivity reactions, headache, edema, dizziness. SC route provides sustained serum levels compared to IV route.

(Siberry: The Harriet Lane Handbook, 2000, p.710)

Erythropoietin

Infants were stratified for gestational age < or = 27 weeks and 28 to 30 weeks, and then randomized to two different dosage schedules of r-EPO, two times a week and five times a week, each totaling 500 U/kg a week. The reason for stratification was to allow all infants to be available at 4 weeks and the younger ones at 8 weeks. r-EPO was administered for 4 weeks and then continued to discharge or 8 weeks, which every occurred sooner. The primary end-point was absolute reticulocyte counts at 4 weeks in all infants. The effect of dose frequency on several secondary outcome variables was also evaluated. At 4 weeks, these variables were hematocrit, transfusion, iatrogenic blood loss, infection, serum ferritin, and, at 8 weeks, were absolute reticulocyte count, hematocrit, iatrogenic blood loss, and infection. Feedings were begun depending on the infant's clinical condition. When infants were receiving at least 60 kcal/kg/d of feedings, oral iron supplements were started at an initial dose of 3 mg/kg/d and increased to 6 to 10 mg/kg/d for the remainder of the study. Additional vitamin supplements included vitamin E (15 units/d), folate (50 mcg/d), and a preparation of vitamins A, C, and D.

Erythropoietin Administration

Commercially available r-EPO (Procrit) was provided by Ortho Biotech, Raritan, NJ. Doses were prepared by the on-site pharmacist and administered subcutaneously in the lateral thigh with a 30-gauge needle; volume of the dose was maintained between 0.3 and 0.6 mL.

Conclusions

More frequent dosing of the same weekly amount of r-EPO produced a significant and sustained increase instimulated erythropoiesis in VLBW infants. The importance of this finding on reducing transfusions was not able to be demonstrated because this study was not intended to differentiate transfusions. In this population of infants and at the dose level of r-EPO, iatrogenic blood loss contributed more to transfusions than an lower level of erythropoiesis, the former primarily associated with mechanical ventilation. Based on this and other studies, when VLBW infants are at risk for greater phlebotomy losses, it may be justifiable to use more vigorous r-EPO treatment, and when at lower risk to use less frequent dosing to enhance cost-effectiveness.

(Brown: Comparison Between Two and Five Doses a Week of Recombinant Human Erythropoietin for Anemia of Prematurity: A Randomized Trail. Pediatrics 1999;104:210-215)

Recombinant Erythropoietin

Infants were randomly assigned to receive 200 units/kg per day of Epo for 10 consecutive days, either subcutaneously or added to their TPN solution. All infants received standard TPN solution containing amino acids (Travasol, Baxter Healthcare Corporation), lipids (Intralipid, Kabi Vitrum), pediatric multivitamins (M.V.I. Pediatric, Astra), and trace elements (P.T.E.-5, Lyphomed). All infants received 1 mg/kg per day of elemental iron, in the form of iron dextran (InFeD, Schein Pharmaceutical) added to their TPN fluids....We conclude that, in this population, adding Epo to the TPN solution was as effective as subcutaneous dosing and resulted in similar Epo concentrations and clearance. We speculate that adding Epo to the TPN solution will avoid the problems inherent in treating very low birth weight infants by the subcutaneous route. Further studies (including more conclusive evaluation of iron requirements) are needed to determine the pharmacokinetics of long-term administration of Epo in preterm infants.

(Ohls: Pharmacokinetics and effectiveness of recombinant erythropoietin administered to preterm infants by continuous infusion in total parenteral nutrition solution. J Pediatr 1996;128:518-523)

Erythropoietin

We treated 157 preterm infants born at 26.9 +/-1.6 weeks of gestation who weighed 924 +/- g at birth with either subcutaneous r-HuEPO (100U/kg/d, 5 days per week) or placebo for 6 weeks in a randomized, double-blind, controlled clinical trial... Infants were eligible... postnatal age at the first dose of study medication of 7 to 28 days for infants born at 28 to 30 weeks of gestation, 7 to 35 days for infants born at 27 weeks gestation, and 7 to 42 days for infants born before 27 weeks of gestation; ...oral or orogastric feedings for 48 hours before enrollment at a minimum total daily caloric intake from intravenous and enteral sources of 60 kcal/kg/d, at least 50% of which was from enteral intake...Patients received oral iron supplements at study entry to achieve a total enteral intake of 3 mg/k/d of elemental iron. Total iron intake was increased to 6 mg/kg/d when the infants tolerated full caloric feedings enterally. Infants also received 15 units of supplemental vitamin E and an additional 1 mL/d of an enteral multivitamin preparation....We conclude that treatment with r-HuEPO at a weekly dose of 500 U/kg stimulates erythropoiesis, moderates the course of anemia, is associated with a reduction in erythrocyte transfusions , and appears safe in very low birth weight preterm infants who are receiving iron supplements.

(Shannon: Recombinant human erythropoietin stimulates erythropoiesis and reduces erythrocyte transfusions in very low birth weight preterm infants. Pediatrics 1995;95:1-8).

EPOPROSTENOL (PGI$_2$, PGX, Prostacyclin, Flolan)

Supplied: Powder for reconstitution: 0.5 mg, in 17 ml, 1.5 mg, in 17 ml

<u>Prostacyclin</u> (PGI$_2$)

Long-Term PGI$_2$ Plus Conventional Therapy

PGI$_2$ was administered intravenously in children who failed to improve clinically and hemodynamically on conventional therapy. Calcium channel blockers were included as long as there were no adverse effects. For the infusion of PGI$_2$, a catheter was introduced into a jugular or subclavian vein as described previously; PGI$_2$ was delivered continuously via a portable pump. The initial dose ranged from 2 to 10 $ng \cdot kg^{-1} \cdot min^{-1}$ (4±2 $ng \cdot kg^{-1} \cdot min^{-1}$ and was increased to maintain an optimal therapeutic dose: at 1 year, the dose averaged 78±38 $ng \cdot kg^{-1} \cdot min^{-1}$ (n=28); at 2 years, 116±48 $ng \cdot kg^{-1} \cdot min^{-1}$ (n=17); and at 3 years, 122±36 $ng \cdot kg^{-1} \cdot min^{-1}$ (n=8).

Cardiac catheterizations were performed yearly, and more frequently if the clinical state deteriorated. PGI$_2$ infusion was continued until either transplantation or death.

(Barst: Vasodilator Therapy for Primary Pulmonary Hypertension in Children. Circulation 1999;99:1197-1208)

ERYTHROMYCIN (EES, Pediamycin, Ilosone)

Injectable: Erythromycin lactobionate 500mg, 1gm vial

Supplied: E. estolate suspension 125mg/5ml, 250mg/5ml
E. ethylsuccinate suspension 200mg/5ml 400mg/5ml
Ophthalmic ointment 0.5% in 3.5gm

Administration: PO, Ophthalmic, IV

For prophylaxis of chlamydial or gonococcal ophthalmia neonatorum, a ribbon of erythromycin ophthalmic ointment approximately 1cm in length should be placed in the lower conjunctival sacs of neonates shortly after birth. The eyelids are then massaged gently to spread the ointment; after one minute, excess ointment can be wiped away with sterile cotton. The ointment should not be flushed from the eye following application. A new tube or single-use container of erythromycin ointment should be used for each neonate (3).

<u>Erythromycin</u>

Antibacterial Drugs for Newborn Infants:
Dose (mg/kg or Units [U]/kg) and Frequency of Administration
Route: PO

Dose: Infants 0-4 wk
BW <1200 g: 10 every 12 h

Infants <1 wk old
BW ≤1200-2000 g: 10 every 12 h
BW >2000 g: 10 every 12 h

Infants ≥1 wk old
BW ≤2000-2000 g: 10 every 8 h
BW >2000 g: 10 every 6 or 8 h

Antibacterial Drugs for Pediatric Patients Beyond the Newborn Period: Dosage per kg/d

Route: PO
Mild to Moderate Infections: 30-50 mg in 2-4 doses

Severe Infections: Inappropriate

Comments: Available in base, stearate, ethyl succinate, and estolate preparations

Route: IV
Mild to Moderate Infections: Inappropriate

Severe Infections: 15-50 mg in 4 doses

Comments: Administer in a continuous drip or by slow infusion over 60 min or longer; may cause cardiac arrhythmia

(American Academy of Pediatrics: Report of the Committee on Infectious Diseases. Red Book 2000, pp.651,657)

Erythromycin

Suggested Dosage Schedules for Antibiotics Used in Newborns
Route: PO

Dosage (mg/kg) and Interval of Administration:
Weight <1200 g
Age 0-4 WK: 10 q12h

Weight 1200-2000 g
Age 0-7 Days: 10 q12h
Age >7 Days: 10 q8h

Weight >2000 g
Age 0-7 Days: 10 q12h
Age >7 Days: 10 q8h

(Remington: Infectious Diseases of the Fetus and Newborn Infant 2001, p.1454)

Erythromycin

Routes: IV, PO

Dosages (mg/kg/day) and Intervals of Administration:
Body weight < 2000g
0-7 days old: 20 div q12h
8-28 days old: 30 div q8h

Body weight >2000g
0-7 days old: 20 div q12h
8-28 days old: 40 div q8h

>28 days old: 40 div q6h

(Nelson: Pocket Book of Pediatric Antimicrobial Therapy 2000-2001, p.16)

Erythromycin (Ilosone, others)

Classification: Macrolide antibiotic

Action and spectrum:

Acts by suppression of protein synthesis. Action may be bactericidal or bacteriostatic at normal therapeutic concentrations. Spectrum of activity is broad and includes the streptococci (except enterococci), *Staphylococcus aureus*, *Clostridia spp*, *Corynebacterium diphtheriae* *Listeria monocytogenes*, *Haemophilus influenzae*, *Bordetella pertussis*, *Brucella* spp, *Campylobacter fetus*, *Branhamella catarrhalis*, *Neisseria gonorrhoeae*, *Legionella micdadei*, *Legionella pneumophila*, *Rickettsia* spp, *Mycoplasma pneumoniae*, *Chlamydia trachomatis*, *Treponema pallidum*, and some *Bacteroides* spp. Ophthalmic form is routinely instilled into the eyes of newborn infants as prophylaxis against ophthalmia neonatorum.

Route: PO, IV over 60 min, ophthalmic.

Dosage: <1200 g: 20 mg/kg/day divided q12h
0-7 days old: 20 mg/kg/day divided q12h
>7 days old: 30 mg/kg/day divided q8h

Ophthalmic as prophylaxis: Instill 0.5-1 cm in each eye once.
Ophthalmic for acute infection: Instill 0.5-1 cm in each eye q6h.

Elimination and metabolism:

Hepatic metabolism, excreted via the bile and kidneys. Half-life is 1.5-3 h (prolonged in renal failure).

Adverse effects: Stomatitis, epigastric distress, oral or perianal candidiasis. Transient cholestatic hepatitis and allergic reactions occur rarely. May cause increased serum levels of theophylline, digoxin, and carbamazepine.

Comments: Parenteral forms are painful and irritative; dilute to 5mg/mL and infuse over 60 min.. Do not use IM. Lactobionate formulation contains 180 mg of benzyl alcohol per gram of erythromycin.

(Gomella: Neonatology 1999, p.565)

Erythromycin

The effective dose of erythromycin used to stimulate gastrointestinal motility is smaller than the dose usually used to treat infection. The adult dose used to treat gastroparesis is 250 mg orally before meals. Intravenous erythromycin is more effective than long-term oral dosing. Using kinetic data, one paper suggested suspension rather than tablet form may be more effective. Tolerance does seem to develop, and higher doses may be needed. Doses in children have been suggested at 3 mg/kg per dose, or 20 mg/kg per day divided in two to four doses.

(Walker: Pediatric Gastrointestinal Diseases 2000, p.1815)

Erythromycin

Prevention of Neonatal Ophthalmia

Ophthalmia neonatorum, defined as conjunctivitis occurring within the first 4 weeks of life, occurs in 1% to 12% of neonates. The prevalence of infection with *Chlamydia trachomatis* and *Neisseria gonorrhoeae* is related directly to the prevalence of infection among pregnant women and whether pregnant women are screened and treated or newborn infants are given ophthalmia prophylaxis.

Screening of all pregnant women for chlamydia and gonorrhea infection followed by appropriate treatment and follow-up of all infected women and their partner(s) can minimize the risk of perinatal transmission.

Gonococcal Ophthalmia

For newborn infants, topical 1% silver nitrate solution, 0.5% erythromycin ointment, and 1% tetracycline ointment are considered equally effective for prophylaxis of ocular gonorrheal infection. Each is available in single-dose tubes. Povidone-iodine in a 2.5% solution also might be useful for preventing gonococcal ophthalmia, but more studies are required, and a product for this purpose currently is not available in the United States. Silver nitrate causes more chemical conjunctivitis than other agents but is recommended in areas where the incidence of penicillinase-producing *Neisseria gonorrhoeae* (PPNG) is appreciable. The efficacy of erythromycin or povidone-iodine prophylaxis against PPNG is not known; 1 study has demonstrated tetracycline to be effective for prophylaxis of PPNG infections. Infants born to women with untreated gonococcal infection should receive 1 dose of ceftriaxone (25-50 mg/kg) or cefotaxime (100 mg/kg), as well as topical prophylaxis. Infants who have gonococcal ophthalmia should be hospitalized and evaluated for signs of disseminated infection.

Chlamydial Ophthalmia

Neonatal ophthalmia due to *Chlamydia trachomatis*, although not as severe as gonococcal conjunctivitis, is common in the United States. Results of studies on the clinical efficacy of erythromycin and of tetracycline ointment for prophylaxis of chlamydial conjunctivitis have been conflicting. Topical antibiotics and silver nitrate do not have proven efficacy in preventing conjunctivitis or nasopharyngeal colonization. One study has shown that 2.5% povidone-iodine is likely to be more effective than either topical erythromycin or silver nitrate for preventing chlamydial conjunctivitis but does not prevent nasopharyngeal colonization and subsequent risk of pneumonia. Infants with ophthalmia neonatorum caused by *C trachomatis* should be evaluated and treated.

(American Academy of Pediatrics: Report of the Committee on Infectious Diseases. Red Book 2000, pp.735,741)

<u>Erythromycin Lactobionate</u>

Case 1. A small for gestational age premature infant....On the 14th day of life...treatment was started with 30-minute infusions of erythromycin lactobionate (25 mg/kg every 12 hours).

On the 4th day of erythromycin treatment the patient developed a marked QT interval prolongation (480 milliseconds) preceding an atrioventricular block.... and the patient died.

Case 2. A small for gestational age preterm infants....At the end of the 8th erythromycin infusion, the neonate developed a lethal ventricular tachycardia, unresponsive to cardiopulmonary resuscitation.

In the present report the dosage of erythromycin lactobionate was 20 to 25 mg/kg every 12 hours intravenously infused over 30 minutes. This therapeutic regimen could lead to higher peak erythromycin serum concentrations than in patients treated with 40 mg/kg/day in four divided dose infused over 60 minutes.

Waites et al. provided important pharmacokinetic data but we feel that erythromycin lactobionate should be strongly limited in newborn infants meanwhile pending safe recommendations from further prospective studies.

(Gouyon: Cardiac Toxicity of Intravenous Erythromycin Lactobionate in Preterm Infants. Pediatric Infect Dis J 1994;13:840-841

ERYTHROMYCIN ETHYLSUCCINATE/SULFISOXAZOLE

(Pediazole)

Supplied: Oral suspension, granules Erythromycin ethyl-succinate 200 mg, sulfisoxazole 600 mg per 5 ml in 100, 150, 200, 250 ml.

Administration: PO

Do not administer to infants <2 months old; systemic sulfonamides are contraindicated in this age group.

<u>Erythromycin Ethylsuccinate and Acetyl Sulfisoxazole</u> (Pediazole)

Dose & Route: Otitis Media:

50 mg/kg/24hr (as erythromycin) and

150 mg/kg/24hr (as sulfa)÷Q6hr PO or

give 1.25 ml/kg/24hr÷Q6hr PO

Remarks: See adverse effects of erythromycin and sulfisoxazole. **Not** recommended in infants <2 month old. Do **not** use in renal impairment because dosage adjustments are inconsistent for sulfisoxazole and erythromycin.

(Siberry: The Harriet Lane Handbook 2000, p.708)

ESMOLOL (Brevibloc)

Supplied: Injection: 10mg/ml, 10ml vials; 250mg/ml, 10ml vials

Comment: The use of Esmolol infusions up to 24 hours has been well documented. Limited data indicate that Esmolol is well tolerated up to 48 hours.

The 250mg/ml strength is concentrated, and is not for direct IV injection; dilute prior to infusion. DO NOT mix with sodium bicarbonate. DO NOT mix with other drugs prior to dilution in a suitable IV fluids. The 10mg/ml vial is ready to use (1). Avoid concentrations >10mg/ml.

Esmolol

Uses: Same as propranolol

Dosing: 500 µg/kg bolus; then 50 µg/kg/min; repeat load every 4 min, and increase infusion by 50 µg/kg/min up to 400 µg/kg/min, as needed

Acute Side Effects:
Same as propranolol

Other Considerations:
May require very large doses in young children

(Gillette: Clinical Pediatric Arrhythmias 1999, p.152)

Esmolol

Esmolol is given for therapy of a wide spectrum of tachyarrhythmias, especially in the postoperative setting, and for control of blood pressure elevations, especially after cardiac transplantation.

Dosing: IV: 500 mcg/kg load, 50-200 mcg/kg/min infusion

Warnings: Hypotension

Dosing: A loading dose of 500 mcg/kg is used, given over 1 to 2 minutes, followed by a maintenance infusion starting at 50 mcg/kg/min. Additional bolus doses can be administered, with subsequent increases in the infusion rate up to 200 mcg/kg/min or higher.

Side Effects: The most frequent adverse effect is hypotension during bolus therapy. In small children and those with single-ventricle physiology, this effect can be profound, requiring volume and inotropic support.

(Gillette: Clinical Pediatric Arrhythmias 1999,pp.231-248)

Esmolol

Dosage: Pediatrics: Loading dose = 500-600 µg/kg i.v. over 2-4 min; initial maintenance = 100-200 µg/kg/min

Comments: May increase in 50-100 μg/kg/min increments up to maximum of 1,000 μg/kg/min. Mean effective dose = 500-600 μg/kg/min.

(Allen: Moss and Adam's Heart Disease in Infants, Children, and Adolescents 2001, pp.1460-1468)

ETHACRYNIC ACID (Edecrin)

Supplied: Tablets 25mg, 50mg
Injection, powder for 50mg/vial

Administration: IV, PO

Add 50ml D5W or NS to vial. D5W solutions may have a low pH (<5); the resulting solution may be hazy or opalescent. Use of such a solution is not recommended. Discard unused, reconstituted solution after 24 hours (1). For DIRECT IV INJECTION, administer over a period of several minutes (2).

For INTERMITTENT INFUSION, ethacrynic acid may be infused slowly over a period of 20 to 30 minutes (3).

DO NOT give SQ or IM because of local pain and irritation.

Extemporaneous Compounding (Recipe)

Dosage form: Oral suspension
Made from: Powder
Concentration: 1 mg/mL
Stability: 220 d, room temperature
Store: Room temperature

Ingredient	Strength	Quantity
Ethacrynic acid powder		120 mg
Alcohol USP		13 mL
Parabens[a]		
Sodium hydroxide	0.1N	qs to pH7
Sorbitol solution	50%	qs ad 120 mL

[a] Methylparaben 0.005% and propylparaben 0.002% final concentration.

Instructions: Mix ethacrynic acid powder, parabens, alcohol, and some of the sorbitol. Adjust pH to 7 with sodium hydroxide solution. Then qs with sorbitol solution, methylparaben 0.005%, and propylparaben 0.002% final concentration. (11)

Ethacrynic Acid (Edecrin)

Indications and use:
When prompt diuresis is needed inpatients refractory to other diuretics. Other diuretics should be tried first because ethacrynic acid is more toxic.

Actions: Loop diuretic. Inhibits reabsorption of sodium and chloride in the proximal and distal tubules and the loop of Henle. Inhibits sodium reabsorption to a greater degree than other diuretics. Does not appear to have a direct effect on the pulmonary vasculature, as furosemide does.

Route: PO, IV

Dosage: 0.5-1 mg/kg/dose qd in preterm infants; q12h in full-term neonates; or more frequently, if needed, in older infants. Maximum: 2 mg/kg IV or 6 mg/kg PO.

Adverse effects: Inject the IV dose slowly over several minutes. May cause dehydration, electrolyte depletion, diarrhea, GI upset, GI bleeding, hearing loss, rash, local irritation and pain, hematuria, and rarely, hypoglycemia and neutropenia.

(Gomella: Neonatology 1999, p.566)

Ethacrynic acid

Route & Dose: IV: 0.5-1.0 mg/kg/dose q 12-24 h

Adverse Effects and Cautions:
Ototoxicity with aminoglycosides; hypokalemia and hyponatremia

(Taeusch: Avery's Diseases of the Newborn 1998, p.1345)

Ethacrynic acid (Edecrin)

Dose: 0.5-2 mg/kg IV

Mode of Action: Loop diuretic; blocks Na^+ reabsorption

Adverse Effects: Hypokalemia, alkalosis

Comments: Possible ototoxicity

(Garson: The science and practice of pediatric cardiology 1998, p.2951)

Ethacrynic Acid

Dosage: 2-3 mg/kg/day divided every 12hr PO
0.5-2.0 mg/kg/dose every 6-8 hr PO

Comments: Ototoxicity may occur
Dosage for infants not well established

(Fanaroff: Neonatal-Perinatal Medicine 1997, p. 1749)

ETHAMBUTOL (Myambutol)

Supplied: Tablets 100 mg, 400 mg

Administration: PO

Warning: Not recommended for use in children <13 years (1).
May cause stomach upset; take with food.

Ethambutol

Antituberculosis Drugs in Children

Daily Dose (mg/kg)	Twice Weekly Dose (mg/kg/per dose)
15-25	50

Ethambutol (EMB) has been used for many years as a companion drug for INH in adults. The usual oral dose is 15 mg/kg per day. At this dose the drug primarily is bacteriostatic, its major role being to prevent emergence of resistance to other drugs. However, at doses of 25 mg/kg per day or 50 mg/kg given twice a week, EMB has some bactericidal action. Unfortunately, at these higher doses, optic neuritis or red-green color blindness has occurred in some adults. Although the incidence of ophthalmologic toxicity in children is extremely low, if it occurs at all, EMB is not recommended for routine use in young children in whom visual field and color discrimination tests are difficult and inaccurate. However, it is used frequently and safely in children with life-threatening forms of tuberculosis or with drug-resistant tuberculosis.

(Remington: Infectious Diseases of the Fetus an Newborn Infant 2001 pp.1188-1189)

ETHYL ALCOHOL (Dehydrated Ethanol Alcohol)

Supplied: 1ml amps

Administration: IV

Comment: Each ml of dehydrated alcohol, USP contains not less than 98% by volume of ethanol.

Ethyl Alcohol (Ethanol)

Central Occluded Catheters

Dose: Instill 0.3-0.6 ml of 70 percent ethyl alcohol solution into catheter.

Administration: Instill catheter-specific volume into the catheter and allow to dwell for 1-2 hours then aspirate.

Concentration: 70 percent.

Pharmacist Compounding Directions

70 Percent Ethyl Alcohol Solution

Draw up 3.5 ml of 98 percent ethyl alcohol (dehydrated alcohol injection. USP) using appropriate aseptic technique. Add 1.5 ml sterile water for injection to make 5 ml. Filter with a 0.22 micron filter.

Use: Re-establishment of central venous catheter patency for occlusions caused by IV fat emulsion. Successful in restoring patency in 80 percent of catheters occluded with lipids.

Adverse Effects: Systemic toxicity should not occur as long as the alcohol is instilled into the catheter and aspirated back out.

If alcohol is inadvertently injected systemically, however, the following may occur: sedation, alcohol intoxication, increased liver function tests, increased urine uric acid, alcohol odor to breath, vein irritation, extravasation injury, fever.

May cause hypoglycemia in diabetic patients.

Nursing Implications:

Procedure is usually performed by a physician.

Monitor patient closely for adverse effects.

(Zenk: Neonatal Medications & Nutrition. A Comprehensive Guide 2000; p.187)

ETIDRONATE DISODIUM (Didronel)

Supplied: Oral: 200mg, 400mg tablets
IV: 300 mg/amp, 6ml amps

Administration: Oral:
To maximize absorption avoid the following within 2 hours of dosing:

1. Food, especially items high in calcium, such as milk or milk products.
2. Vitamins with mineral supplements or antacids high in metals (eg. Calcium, iron, magnesium, aluminum).

Parenteral:
Administer the diluted dose IV over a period ≥ 2 hours. The daily dose must be diluted in ≥ 250 ml of sterile normal saline (1). Regardless of the volume of solution in which Etidronate IV infusion is diluted, slow infusion is important (1).

Etidronate

Indication: For hypercalcemia

The patient was treated with intravenous infusions of normal saline solution, oral NaCl (3 meq/kg/d), furosemide (4 mg/kg/d intravenous every 6 hours), and prednisone (up to 2 mg/kg/d). Initially, serum calcium levels decreased. Furosemide was changed from intravenous to oral administration, saline solution infusions were stopped, and a diet low in calcium and vitamin D was started. When the serum calcium level rose again furosemide was changed back to intravenous administration (6 mg/kg/d every 4 hours), normal saline solution infusions were restarted, the prednisone dose was increased (3 mg/kg/d), and the oral feedings were stopped. Because hypercalcemia and elevated urinary calcium to creatinine ratios persisted the patient was given etidronate (5 mg/kg/dose orally twice a day), which acts to decrease the release of skeletal calcium into the circulation.

The child was discharged on a low-calcium and vitamin D free formula (Calcilo XD; Ross, Columbus, Ohio), oral NaCl supplements (3 meq/kg/d), prednisone (2 mg/kg/d for 2 weeks followed by a 1-month taper), and etidronate (5 mg/kg/d).

(Rice: Etidronate therapy for hypercalcemia in subcutaneous fat necrosis of the newborn. J Pediatr 1999;134:349-51)

FAMOTIDINE (Pepcid)

Supplied: Tablets 10mg, 20mg, 40mg
Injection 10mg/ml in 2ml (preservative free)
Injection 10mg/ml in 4ml (with benzyl alcohol)
Powder for oral suspension; 40mg/5mL when reconstituted.

Administration: IV, PO

For direct IV injection, dilute to a concentration of 2-4mg/ml and inject over not less than 2 minutes.

For intermittent IV infusion, dilute to a concentration of 0.2mg/ml and infuse over 15 to 30 minutes.

Stable in D5W, D10W, NS for 48 hours at room temperature (1).

<u>Famotidine</u>
Therapy for Reflux

Common doses: 0.5 mg/kg/dose bid or tid; adult 40 mg HS
(Wyllie: Pediatric Gastrointestinal Disease 1999, p.180)

<u>Famotidine</u>

Dose & Route: Children:
IV: Initial: 0.6-0.8 mg/kg/24 hr ÷ Q8-12 hr up to a **max** of 40 mg/24 hr
PO: Initial: 1-1.2 mg/kg/24 hr ÷ Q8-12 hr up to a **max** of 40 mg/24 hr

Remarks: A 12 hr dosage interval is generally recommended; however, infants and young children may require an 8 hr interval because of enhanced elimination. Headaches, dizziness, constipation, diarrhea, and drowsiness have occurred. **Adjust dose in severe renal failure**
(Siberry: The Harriet Lane Handbook 2000, p.713)

<u>Famotidine</u>

Dose: An initial dose of 0.4 mg/kg was given and repeated only after the intragastric pH had dropped to <4.0 for 2 hours. Increased doses were given (0.8, 1.2 and 1.6 mg/kg) if the previous dose did not raise the intragastric pH to >4.0 for ≥6 hours.

We conclude that intravenous famotidine therapy raises gastric pH to >4.0 for approximately 9 hours in most children. Prolonged intravenous use of famotidine rapidly leads to a decreased duration of efficacy, necessitating intragastric pH monitoring to assess the effectiveness of treatment.
(Treem: Suppression of gastric acid secretion by intravenous administration of famotidine in children. J Pediatr 1991;118:812-816)

FAT EMULSION (Intralipid, Liposyn II and III)

Supplied: Injection 10%, 20% in multiple size units

Administration: IV, not greater than 0.15 gm/kg/hr over 18 to 24 hrs.

Intravenous lipid solutions may be given through a peripheral or central venous line via a Y or T connector, distal to the filter. It may also be admixed directly with the amino acid/glucose solution. Although an admixture of lipids and amino acid/glucose solutions is widely used in adults, experience in pediatric patients, particularly in the newborn, is limited.

Composition of Intravenous Fat Emulsions:

	INTRALIPID (CLINTEC)	LIPOSYN II (ABBOTT)	LIPOSYN III (ABBOTT)
Source	Soybean	Soybean/safflower	Soybean
Egg phospholipid	1.2%	1.2%	1.2%
Glycerin	2.25%	2.5%	2.5%
Fatty acids			
Linoleic	50%	65.8%	54.5%
Oleic	26%	17.7%	22.4%
Palmitic	10%	8.8%	10.5%
Linolenic	9%	4.2%	8.3%
Steric	3.5%	3.4%	4.2%
Calories (kcal/ml)			
10%	1.1	1.1	1.1
20%	2.0	2.0	2.0

(Drug, Facts and Comparisons, Facts and Comparisons 1999.)

Jandice in premature infants:
Use with caution because free fatty acids displace bilirubin bound to albumin.

Fat Emulsion is supplied in single dose containers; do not store partially used bottles or resterilized for later use. Do not use filters. Do not use any bottle in which there appears to be separation of the emulsion (1).

Fat Emulsion

Fats: Because of their high caloric density, intravenous fat solutions (eg, Intralipid, Lyposyn II, Nutralipid, and Soyacal) provide a significant portion of daily caloric needs. Most intravenous fat solutions are isotonic (270-300 mosm/L) and therefore are not likely to increase the risk of infiltration of peripheral lines. When administering fat solutions to neonates with unconjugated hyperbilirubinemia, caution may be needed because of the competitive binding of bilirubin and nonesterified fatty acids on albumin, which may increase significantly during infusion.

Concentrations: Lipid emulsions are supplied either as 10% or 20% solutions providing 10 or 20 g of triglyceride, respectively. A common regimen is 0.5 g/kg/day on the first day, 1 g/kg/day on the second day, and 2 g/kg/day (maintenance dose) on the third day. The infusion is given continuously over 20-24 h, and the rate should not exceed 0.12 g/kg/h. For example, in an infant weighing 2 kg who is to start at an amount of 0.5 g/kg/day:

2 kg x 0.5 g/kg/day = 1 g/day
1 mL of 10% Intralipid = 0.1 g
1 mL/0.1 g = x mL/g
0.1 x = 1
x = 10 mL

This infant should receive a total of 10 mL of 10% Intralipid in a 24-h period to equal 0.5 g/kg/day. The volume (eg, 10 mL) is divided by 24 h. It should run at 0.4 mL/h for 24 h. In the very low birth weight infant (<1000 g), the 20% emulsion is recommended because of the excessive phospholipid liposomes present in the 10% solution.

Complications: Fat intolerance (hyperlipidemia) may be seen. "Lipidcrits" (visual checks of the serum for cloudiness caused by excessive fats) are of value only when positive. Periodic determination of blood triglyceride levels is recommended. Such levels should be <150 mg/dL when the child is jaundiced and <200 mg/dL otherwise. The infusion of fats should be decreased or stopped when these levels are exceeded.

(Gomella: Neonatology: Management, Procedures, On-call Problems, Diseases and Drugs 1999, pp.90-91)

Fat Emulsion (Lipids, Intralipids, Intravenous Fat)

Fat. Intravenous fat (IVF) is an integral part of the PN regimen. It provides a concentrated isotonic source of calories (20% solution supplies 2.0 kcal/mL) and prevents or reverses essential fatty acid (EFA) deficiency.

The IVF should be infused over 24 hours, whenever possible. Continuous IVF infusions (24 hr/d) are better tolerated than intermittent infusions (8 to 18 hr/d), with less fluctuation and lower concentrations of plasma lipids especially at higher rates of infusion. Early studies argued against exceeding a rate of 0.15 g/kg/hr (3.6 g/kg/d). Slower infusion rates are required for small-for-gestational-age (SGA) infants. Infusion rates of 0.12 g/kg//hr or less resulted in less elevation of plasma lipid levels than rates of 0.17 g/kg/hr or more.

Interestingly, 15 mL twice a day of corn oil, sunflower oil, or safflower oil enterally provides as much linoleic acid as 150 mL of 10 percent IVF at less than 5 percent of the cost. Many PN patients not on complete bowel rest tolerate such a regimen. An EFA deficiency can be prevented by providing 2 to 4 percent of total calories as IVF (1 to 2% linoleic acid)-an IVF dose of 0.5 to 1.0 g/kg/d. Linoleic and linolenic acids are EFAs.

Fat may frequently contribute 30 to 40 percent of total non-nitrogen calories, but generally, it should not exceed 60 percent. Four grams per kilogram per day of 20 percent IVF caused less increase of plasma lipids than 2 g/kg/d of 10 percent IVF. Hyperlipidemia occurs when PN with 10 percent IVF but not 20 percent IVF and is caused by an increase in lipoprotein X. The phospholipid/triglyceride ratio is 0.12 in 10 percent IVF and 0.06 in 20 percent IVF (see Table). Phospholipid is believed to inhibit lipoprotein lipase, which is the main enzyme responsible for IVF clearance probably explaining why 20 percent IVF is cleared more rapidly than 10 percent IVF. Twenty percent IVF is currently used exclusively in our institution. The dose should not exceed 0.15 g/kg/hr. Thirty percent IVF has been shown to be safe and has similar metabolic effects to 20 percent IVF. It is administered as a three-in-one solution and cannot be given alone via a peripheral intravenous line. Suggested dosing for IVF is shown in Table.

TABLE DOSING* FOR INTRALIPID

AGE	STARTING DOSE	DAILY DOSE INCREASE	MAXIMUM DOSE
Preterm	0.5-1.0	1.0	3.5
Full-Term (0 to 6 mo)	1.0-1.5	1.0-1.5	3.5
Older infant (6 to 12 mo)	1.0-1.5	1.0-1.5	3.0

*In g/kg/d

(Walker: Pediatric Gastrointestinal Disease 2000, pp.1712-1721)

Lipid Metabolic Complications

Use of Intravenous Fat

The incidence of complications associated with the use of IVF is low. If the IVF infusion exceeds its maximal clearance rate, hyperlipidemia occurs, which may cause impairment of pulmonary function, displacement of albumin-bound bilirubin by plasma free fatty acids (which may lead to kernicterus), and a fat overload syndrome (hypertriglyceridemia, fever, lethargy, liver damage, and coagulopathy). Thus, careful monitoring of the use of IVF emulsions is essential by regularly checking serum triglyceride levels.

After boluses of IVF are infused into newborn infants, several investigators have demonstrated significant drops of arterial oxygen tension (PaO_2) without alteration in other pulmonary function tests. Two hypotheses exist to explain the fall in arterial oxygen saturation: (1) lipid microemboli block pulmonary capillaries and alter perfusion ventilation rations; and (2) fat metabolism leads to increased production of certain prostaglandins, which leads to pulmonary hypertension. The use of IVF in patients with pulmonary compromise has yielded conflicting results. While fat emboli were found on postmortem examination of pulmonary capillaries in neonates and infants who received Intralipid, other reports have found no consistent association.

We recommend that IVF be started at 0.5 to 1.0 g/kg/d (preterm) and 1.0 to 1.5 g/kg/d (full term) in the first week of life, and that the dose be increased depending on the triglyceride level and clinical status of the baby.

(Walker: Pediatric Gastrointestinal Disease 2000, pp.1712-1721)

Lipids

Absolute lipid requirements are limited to the requirements for essential fatty acids (EFAs), ie, form 1% to 4% of total energy intake as linoleic acid ([LA],18:2*w*6) and approximately 1% of total energy intake as α-linolenic acid 9[LNA], 18:3*w*3).

The concern for bilirubin toxicity attributable to increased plasma unesterified fatty acids is based on the potential for unesterified fatty acids to displace bound bilirubin from albumin, thereby increasing free bilirubin and the risk of bilirubin encephalopathy. However, displacement of bilirubin form albumin is minimal at fatty acid /albumin ratios < 4.1 and higher ratios are unlikely. Further, clinical studies have shown that infusion of lipid at rates up to 3g/d/kg does not increase plasma concentrations of free fatty acids or free bilirubin.

Available parenteral lipid emulsions contain large proportions of LA and LNA. Failure to provide LA results in biochemical signs of deficiency within 72 hours, but this can be prevented by administration of as little as .5 g/d/kg of available lipid emulsions. These emulsions do not contain arachidonic acid (AA, 20:4*w*6) and docosahexaenoic acid (DHA, 22:6*w*3); thus, concerns have been expressed about availability of sufficient amounts of these fatty acids for the developing central nervous system. In this regard, plasma, liver, lung, and kidney lipid levels of both AA and DHA fall during infusion of lipid emulsions, although the short-term effect on brain lipid levels is relatively small. The long-term effects of lower intakes of AA and DHA on brain development are unknown but should be determined given the large contribution of these EFAs to brain growth and development at this early state of development.

(Hay: Workshop Summary: Nutrition of the Extremely Low Birth Weight Infant. Pediatrics 1999;104:1360 -1368)

Fat Emulsions

There is much controversy over early introduction of intravenous lipid emulsions particularly in a sick VLBW infant. Theoretical concerns include increased free bilirubin concentrations, impairment of oxygenation, microembolization of lipid particles, reduced rates of fat oxidation, and the effect on immune function. Early studies found increases in the incidence and severity of chronic lung disease in VLBW infants started on intravenous lipids in the first week of life. However, more recent studies have demonstrated no increase in ventilator requirements or the incidence of bronchopulmonary dysplasia in VLBW infants started on 1 gm/kg/day of lipids on the first day of life. Sosenko and coworkers also found that VLBW infants given early intravenous lipids had no significant differences in mortality, including the incidence of chronic long disease. A study by Brans and colleagues confirmed that VLBW infants, particularly those weighing less than 1,000 gm, tend to clear lipids more slowly than their more mature peers, supporting the AAP's recommendation to limit the dosage of fat emulsions to 3 mg/kg/day, especially in VLBW infants. Routine monitoring of serum triglyceride is necessary as lipids are being advanced, with a triglyceride level obtained with each increase of 1 gm/kg/day. Once maximum lipid intake is achieved, weekly monitoring should be continued while intravenous lipids are being infused. Triglyceride levels should be kept below the empirical value of 150 mg/dl, although that number remains controversial.

(Fanaroff: Neonatal-Perinatal Medicine 1997, pp.595-596)

FENTANYL (Sublimaze)

Supplied: Injection 50mcg (0.05mg)/ml in 2ml, 5ml, 10ml, 20ml amps

Administration: IM, IV

Methemoglobinemia has occurred rarely in premature neonates undergoing emergency anesthesia and surgery including combined use of fentanyl, pancuronium, and atropine; a cause-and effect-relationship has not been established (1).

Fentanyl (Sublimaze)

Indications and use: Analgesia, anesthesia, sedation.

Actions: A synthetic opiate agonist. Acts similarly to morphine and meperidine but without cardiovascular effects of those drugs and with shorter respiratory depressant effects.

Route: IV

Dosage: Analgesia: 1-2 mcg/kg/dose q2-4h prn or by continuous infusion at 0.1-3 mcg/kg/h.

Anesthesia: Major surgery, 25-50 mcg/kg/dose; minor surgery, 2-10 mcg/kg/dose.

Sedation: 2 mcg/kg/dose q2-4h prn or by continuous infusion of 0.5-1 mcg/kg/h (titrate).

Adverse effects: Bradycardia, muscular rigidity with reduced pulmonary compliance or apnea, bronchoconstriction, laryngospasm.

Comments: Limited experience in neonates. 0.1 mg of fentanyl = 10 mg of morphine or 75 mg of meperidine. Concurrent

ventilatory assistance is suggested with its use.
Tachyphylaxis occurs after several days of therapy.
Adheres to extracorporeal membrane oxygenation (ECMO) filter membranes; may have to adjust dose.

(Gomella: Neonatology 1999, p.566)

Fentanyl

Indication: Protocol for inborn infants with Congenital Diaphragmatic Hernia

Continuous sedation was provided with fentanyl infusion of 5 to 10 µg/kg/hr

(Finer: Congenital diaphragmatic Hernia: Developing a Protocolized Approach. J Pediatr Surg 1998;33:1331-1337)

Fentanyl

The infants were randomized in 5 blocks with closed envelopes and stratified for birth weight of less and equal or more than 1500 g to receive a loading dose of 10.5 mcg/kg fentanyl or 140 mcg/kg morphine in 1 hour. Thereafter, the infusion was continued at a maintenance rate of 1.5 mcg/kg/hr fentanyl or 20 mcg/kg/hr morphine for at least 24 hours.

Conclusions: With at least as effective analgesia as with morphine, fentanyl had fewer side effects. Fentanyl may be superior to morphine for short-term postnatal analgesia in newborn infants.

(Saarenmaa: Advantages of fentanyl over morphine in analgesia for ventilated newborn infants after birth: a randomized trial. J Pediatr 1999;134:144-50)

Fentanyl

Use: Sedation; relief of pain; preoperative medication; adjunct to general or regional anesthesia; management of chronic pain (transdermal product)

Warnings: I.V. use: Rapid I.V infusion may result in skeletal muscle and chest wall rigidity → impaired ventilation → respiratory distress → apnea, bronchoconstriction, laryngospasm; inject slowly over 3-5 minutes; nondepolarizing skeletal muscle relaxant may be required; due to risk of hypoventilation, oral transmucosal product should only be used in a closely monitored setting that has immediate access to advanced life support equipment and medications; patients receiving oral transmucosal fentanyl must be directly observe and monitored carefully (eg, a patient-dedicated observer and pulse oximetry); fentanyl should be administered by qualified health care professionals trained in anesthetic drug use and advanced cardiac life support. (eg, anesthesiologists); doses should be titrated, use lowest effective dose

Adverse Reactions:

Cardiovascular: Hypotension, bradycardia, flushing

Central nervous system: CNS depression, drowsiness, dizziness, sedation, euphoria

Dermatologic: Erythema, pruritus, facial pruritus with oral transmucosal product

Endocrine & metabolic: ADH release

Gastrointestinal: Nausea, vomiting, constipation, biliary tract spasm

Genitourinary: Urinary tract spasm

Local: Transdermal system: Edema, erythema, pruritus

Neuromuscular & skeletal: Skeletal and thoracic muscle rigidity especially following rapid I.V. administration

Ocular: Miosis

Respiratory: Respiratory depression, apnea

Miscellaneous: Physical and psychological dependence with prolonged use. **Note**: Neonates who receive a total fentanyl dose >1.6 mg/kg or continuous infusion duration >5 days are more likely to develop narcotic withdrawal symptoms; children 1 week to 22 months who receive a total dose of 1.5 mg/kg or duration >5 days have a 50% chance of developing narcotic withdrawal and those receiving a total dose >2.5 mg/kg or duration of infusion >9 days have a 100% chance of developing withdrawal. Doses should be tapered to prevent withdrawal symptoms.

Stability: Protect from light

Usual Dosage: Doses should be titrated to appropriate effects; wide range of doses, dependent upon desired degree of analgesia/anesthesia, clinical environment, and patient's status

Neonates and younger Infants:
Sedation/analgesia: Slow I.V. push: 1-4 mcg/kg/dose; may repeat every 2-4 hours

Continuous sedation/analgesia: Initial I.V. bolus: 1-2 mcg/kg, then 0.5-1 mcg/kg/hour; titrate upward
Mean required dose: Neonates with gestational age <34 weeks: 0.64 mcg/kg/hour; Neonates with gestational age ≥34 weeks: 0.75 mcg/kg/hour

Continuous sedation/analgesia during ECMO: Initial I.V. bolus: 5-10 mcg/kg slow I.V. push over 10 minutes, then 1-5 mcg/kg/hour; titrate upward; tolerance may develop; higher doses (up to 20 mcg/kg/hour) may be needed by day 6 of ECMO

Administration: Parenteral: I.V: Administer b slow I.V. push over 3-5 minutes or by continuous infusion; larger bolus doses (>5 mcg/kg) should be given slow I.V. push over 5-10 minutes

Monitoring Parameters:
Respiratory rate, blood pressure, heart rate, oxygen saturation, bowel sounds, abdominal distention

Nursing Implications:
Patients with elevated temperature may have increased fentanyl absorption transdermally, observe for adverse effects, dosage adjustment may be needed; pharmacologic and adverse effects can be seen after discontinuation of transdermal system, observe patients for at least 12 hours after transdermal product removed; destroy unused portion of fentanyl Oralet according to hospital policy on controlled substances.

Additional Information:
An opioid antagonist, resuscitative and intubation equipment, and oxygen should be available; fentanyl is 50-100 times as potent as morphine; morphine 10 mg I.V. = fentanyl 0.1-0.2 mg I.M.; fentanyl has less hypotensive effects than morphine or meperidine due to minimal or no histamine release; keep transdermal product (both used and unused) out of the reach of children; do **not** use soap, alcohol, or other solvents to remove transdermal gel if it accidentally touches skin as they may increase transdermal absorption, use copious amounts of water; fentanyl Oralet 5 mcg/kg = fentanyl 0.75-1.25 mcg/kg I.M.

(Taketomo: Pediatric dosage Handbook 1999-2000, pp.378-381)

Fentanyl

We observed chest wall rigidity in 8 patients after low dosage of fentanyl (3-5 mcg/kg body weight). All patients presented with respiratory distress, hypercapnia, and hypoxemia leading to bradycardia. In two patients, laryngospasm was noted and associated with muscle rigidity, thus making intubation impossible. Naloxone (20-40 mcg/kg body weight) reversed the laryngospasm and muscle rigidity immediately, allowing restitution within 1 min. In our patient population, we found fentanyl-induced chest wall rigidity in 4% of neonates after fentanyl administration.

Conclusion: Even low doses of fentanyl can lead to thoracic rigidity in neonates. Additionally, we observed laryngospasm in two patients and speculate that it might be a variant of muscle rigidity.

(Fahnenstich: Fentanyl-induced chest wall rigidity and laryngospasm in preterm and term infants. Crit Care Med 2000;28:836-839)

Fentanyl

Route & Dose: IV, IM: 1-2 µg/kg/dose, q 4-6 h prn

Adverse Effects and Cautions:

50-100 times the potency of morphine. Muscle rigidity ("stiff man" syndrome) may occur

(Taeusch: Avery's Diseases of the Newborn 1998, p.1345)

Fentanyl

Dose & Route: **Titrate dose to effect.**

IV/IM: 1-2 mcg/kg/dose Q30-60 min PRN

Continuous IV infusion: 1 mcg/kg/hr; titrate to effect; usual infusion range 1-3 mcg/kg/hr

PO (Oralet): Sedation: 10-15 mcg/kg/dose up to max of 400 mcg/dose

Transdermal: Safety and efficacy have not been established in pediatrics.

Remarks: Highly lipophilic and may deposit into fat tissue. IV onset of action 1-2 minutes with peak effects in 10 minutes. IV duration of action 30-60 minutes. Give IV dose over 3-5 minutes. Rapid infusion may cause respiratory depression and chest wall rigidity. Respiratory depression may persist beyond the period of analgesia. Transdermal onset of action 6-8 hours with a 72 hour duration of action

(Siberry: The Harriet Lane Handbook 2000, pp.714-715

FERROUS SULFATE (Fer in sol, Fer Iron)

Supplied: Ferrous Sulfate Elixir 220mg/5ml (44mg elemental Iron/5ml), contains 5% alcohol.

Fer in sol Drops 75mg (15mg elemental iron) / 0.6ml

Administration: PO

When iron-containing drops are given to infants, some darkening of the membrane covering the teeth may occur. Iron-containing liquids may temporarily stain the teeth. Dilute the liquid to reduce this possibility (1).

Ferrous Sulfate

Iron Supplementation

In neonates who are receiving an enteral intake of at least 60 mL/kg/d, we provide an enteral additive of 3 mg/kg/d elemental iron. The amount of supplemental iron is increased as enteral feedings increase. Patients on full feedings receive 6 mg/kg/d elemental iron. In patients receiving hyperalimentation, we have the pharmacy add rEpo and iron dextran (1 mg/kg/d) to the hyperalimentation solution. Alternatively, iron dextran can be added to the hyperalimentation at a dose of 3 to 5 mg/kg/once a week. It is sometimes useful to check a serum ferritin for patients who do not appear to respond adequately to the course of rEpo, to determine adequacy of iron supplementation.

(Calhoun: Consistent approaches to procedures and practices in neonatal hematology. Clinics in Perinatology 2000, 27:733-753)

Ferrous Sulfate (20% Elemental Iron) (Various)

Indications and use: Treatment and prevention of iron deficiency anemia.

Actions: Iron is needed for the production of heme proteins. The use of iron-fortified formulas during the first year of life will usually prevent iron deficiency anemia in both the preterm and term infant. Iron-fortified formulas can be fed safely to preterm infants. Of the ferrous salts available (sulfate, fumarate, gluconate), sulfate is preferred.

Route: PO

Dosage: Recommendations of the American Academy of Pediatrics; dosages are for elemental iron.

Term infants: 1mg/kg/day starting no later than 2 months of age.

Preterm infants: 2 mg/kg/day starting no later than 2 months of age.

Iron deficiency anemia: 6 mg/kg/day in 4 divided doses.

Iron implementation with erythropoietin: 6 mg/kg/day

Adverse effects: GI irritation (vomiting, diarrhea, constipation, darkened stool color).

Comments: Caution parents to guard against iron poisoning from accidental ingestion. Antidote is chelation with deferoxamine; consult specialized references and regional poison control center for further information.

(Gomella: Neonatology 1999, p.566)

Ferrous sulfate

Iron deficiency anemia:

Dose/kg: 2-3 mg elemental Fe

Route and frequency: PO q12h

With Erythropoietin:

Dose/kg: 3-6 mg elemental Fe

Route and frequency: PO q12h-q8h. Max 12 mg/kg/d

Premature supplement:

Dose/kg: 1 mg

Route and frequency: PO q12h or give formula with Fe

Comments: Do not give concurrently with antacids, milk. or cereal

Cimetidine decreases absorption of iron

May cause GI irritation; colors stools black

(Avery: Neonatology Pathophysiology and Management of the Newborn 1999, p.1556)

Iron Preparations

Dose: Iron deficiency anemia:

Premature Infants:

2-4 mg elemental Fe/kg/24 hr ÷ QD-BID PO;

max dose: 15 mg elemental Fe/24 hr

Prophylaxis:

Premature: 2 mg elemental Fe/kg/24 hr

Full-term: 1-2 mg elemental Fe/kg/24 hr

(Siberry: The Harriet Lane Handbook 2000, p.744)

FLECAINIDE ACETATE (Tambocor)

Supplied: Tablets 50, 100, 150 mg.

Administered: PO

Safety and efficacy for use in children <18 years of age have not been established. The majority of patients treated successfully had trough plasma levels between 0.2 and 1 mcq/mL. The probability of adverse experiences, especially cardiac, may increase with higher trough plasma levels, especially levels >1mcg/mL (1).

Extemporaneous Compounding (Recipe)

Dosage form: Oral suspension
Made from: Tablets
Concentration: 20mg/mL
Stability: 60 days
Store: Refrigerate
Label: Shake well

Ingredient	Strength	Quantity
Flecainide acetate tablets	100 mg	24
Ora-Sweet or Ora-Sweet SF		
Ora-plus	1:1 mixture	qs 120 mL

Instructions: Crush the tablets in a mortar and reduce to a fine powder. Add 20 mL of vehicle and mix to a uniform paste. Add vehicle in geometric amounts to almost desired volume. Transfer to a graduate and qs with vehicle. Mix well. (11)

Flecainide

Dosing: PO: 80-200 mg/m^2/day (varies with age)
IV: 1-2 mg/kg

Warnings: Avoid in abnormal hearts.

Oral Administration:

After an oral dose, flecainide reaches its maximum concentration in 1 to 2 hours. Milk products can block the absorption of flecainide such that, when patients are put on clear liquid diets (e.g., infants with gastroenteritis), flecainide levels can rise substantially. Doses should be reduced, perhaps by 25 to 30%, in this setting.

Intravenous Parameters:

Intravenous flecainide is available for use outside the United States. Its bolus dose is 1 to 2 mg/kg given over 5 to 10 minutes.

Dosing: The starting dosage in infants is often 80 to 90 mg/m^2/day, on a schedule of every 12 hours because of the prolonged $t_{1/2}$ at that age. The dosage for older patients is closer to 100 to 110 mg/m^2/day. This stating dosage tends to give trough levels of 200 to 400 ng/ml. A trough level of from 200 to 1000 ng/ml is considered therapeutic. Trough levels should be drawn 1 hour before the sixth or seventh maintenance dose. There is no loading dose.

Flecainide suspensions must be shaken vigorously to prevent inadvertent administration of drug doses that are too low or too high.

A rise in digoxin levels has been reported for adults on flecainide, but his experience has not been corroborated in pediatric patients. Flecainide can be used in combination with amiodarone for resistant arrhythmias, and with mexiletine for some infant ventricular tachyarrhythmias resulting from tumors.

Side Effects: On the basis of published data, side effects of flecainide are related to high levels and administration of the drug to patients with abnormal hearts. This drug is generally safe for those with normal cardiac anatomy. At peak concentration or with overdose, some patients may experience blurry vision and oral paresthesia. In patients with paroxysmal SVT, flecainide can result in slow conduction in more than one limb of a re-entrant circuit and bring about slower but incessant SVT. This phenomenon is most often observed during the first 1 to 2 days of therapy and argues for in-hospital initiation of the drug. Proarrhythmic effects beyond this are rare, but they occur most commonly in the patient with an atrial tachyarrhythmia and abnormal anatomy (e.g., atrial flutter in a patient who has undergone a Mustard or Fontan procedure).

(Gillette: Clinical Pediatric Arrhythmias 1999,pp.231-248)

Flecainide

Class: IC

Uses: PJRT
AET/IAH
SVT
PVCs/VT

Dose (Level): 100-225 mg/m^2/day divided q8-12hr PO (0.2-1 µg/mL) no active metabolites

Mode of Action: Depress abnormal automaticity; slows conduction in AVN, accessory connection, ventricle

ECG/EP Changes: Mild increase in PR, mild increase in QRS at high doses; prolongs AH, HV, ERP-Kent

Side Effects: Blurred vision, nausea, use with caution in CHF, may decrease contractility; proarrhythmic; may change intermittent SVT-WPW to incessant at slower rate; may increase pacing threshold

(Garson: The science and practice of pediatric cardiology 1998, p.2953)

Flecainide

Guidelines for Dosage: Antidysrhythmics

Dosage: Pediatrics: 2-5 mg/kg/day p.o. (divide t.i.d. or b.i.d.)

Comments: Reserved for resistant dysrhythmias; may have proarrhythmic effect; monitor plasma concentrations.

(Allen: Moss and Adam's Heart Disease in Infants, Children, and Adolescents 2001, pp.1460-1468)

Flecainide Acetate

Dose & Route: Children: Initial: 1-3 mg/kg/24 hr ÷ Q8 hr PO; usual range: 3-6 mg/kg/24 hr ÷ Q8 hr PO, monitor serum levels to adjust dose if needed.

Remarks: May aggravate LV failure, sinus bradycardia, preexisting ventricular arrhythmias. May cause AV block, dizziness, blurred vision, dyspnea, nausea, headache, increased PR or QRS intervals. **Reserve for life-threatening cases**.

Therapeutic trough level: 0.2-1 mg/L. Recommended serum sampling time at steady-state: obtain trough level within 30 minutes prior to the next scheduled dose after 2-3 days of continuous dosing for children.

Adjust dose in renal failure.

(Siberry: The Harriet Lane Handbook 2000, p.716)

FLUCONAZOLE (Diflucan)

Supplied: Tablets 50mg, 100mg, 150mg, 200mg
Injection 200mg/100ml; 400mg/200ml
Powder for oral suspension 10mg/mL, 40mg/ml when reconstituted.

Administration: PO, IV
Shake oral suspension well before using. Store between 4° and 86°F. Discard unused portion after 2 weeks (1).

Fluconazole

Recommended Doses of Parenteral and Oral Antifungal Drugs
Route: IV
Dose: Children 3-6 mg/kg per day, single dose
Adverse Reactions:
Rash, gastrointestinal tract symptoms, hepatotoxicity, Steven-Johnson syndrome, anaphylaxis

Note: Limited or no information about use in newborn infants is available.

(American Academy of Pediatrics: Report of the Committee on Infectious Diseases. Red Book 2000, pp.670-671)

Fluconazole

Suggested Dosage of Antifungal Agents for Infants with systemic or Severe Local Fungal Infection:
Dosage (mg/kg per day): 6

Fluconazole is an azole antifungal agent and is available in an intravenous as well as oral preparation. This agent has been shown to achieve good penetration into CSF, acular fluid, and skin. It is effective against many fungi, including *Candida, Coccidioides,* and *dermatophytes*. Its use in neonates is limited. Wiest and associates used fluconazole in a premature infant with disseminated candidiasis unresponsive to amphotericin B and 5-fluorocytosine. The infant received 6 mg/kg per day intravenously, achieving peak and trough serum levels of 10.3 and 6.98 mg/ml, respectively. Gürses and Kalayci reported successful use of fluconazole alone in a premature infant with candidal meningitis. Dreissen and co-workers in two reports indicated fluconazole was effective and associated with fewer side effects than amphotericin B. Fluconazole has also been used in pregnancy without harmful effects on the fetus.

(Remington: Infectious Diseases of the Fetus and Newborn Infant 2001, p.838

<u>Fluconazole</u> (Diflucan)

Indications and use: Antifungal agent for systemic candidiasis and meningitis. Advantages over amphotericin B are once-a-day dosing, good distribution characteristics with similar CSF and serum levels, oral as well as IV administration, and fewer adverse effects. Check the sensitivity of the organism.

Actions: Inhibits fungal cytochrome P450 and sterol C-14 α-demethylation, resulting in a fungistatic effect.

Route: PO, IV.

Dosage: 6mg/kg/day as a single daily dose. Infuse IV over 1-2 h. Reduce the dose in renal dysfunction.

Adverse effects: Usually well tolerated. Vomiting, diarrhea, rash, and elevations in liver function tests.

Comments: Monitor liver function tests. Use caution in preexisting renal dysfunction. Cimetidine and rifampin decrease fluconazole levels. Hydrochlorothiazide increases fluconazole levels. Fluconazole increases phenytoin and zidovudine levels, and increases the prothrombin time for patients on warfarin.

(Gomella: Neonatology 1999, p.566)

<u>Fluconazole</u>

In Summary, Kicklighter et al have produced a thoughtful preliminary study that begins to answer the ultimate question whether invasive candidiasis can be safely prevented in VLBW infants with fluconazole prophylaxis. By applying criteria designed to assess the usefulness of a prophylactic regimen, it is clear that there are several issues left to address before this question can be answered. This preliminary study dose not measure a clinically relevant endpoint; it does not refine the definition of a truly high risk population; it does not define optimal duration of prophylaxis; it does not address the issue of organism resistance with the pressure of long-term prophylaxis in a sizable proportion of neonates in an average NICU; and it provides no information on cost-effectiveness. These data do suggest that fluconazole can be safely used in VLBW infants (with appropriate concerns for drug-drug interactions), and that it can reduce rectal colonization. The authors plainly acknowledge that this study is preliminary and more work must be done. Their final conclusion is important and should be adhered to: routine fluconazole prophylaxis is not presently justified in VLBW infants.

(Neely: Fluconazole Prophylaxis in the Very Low Birth Weight Infant: Not Ready for Prime Time Pediatrics 2001;107:404-406)

Fluconazole

Infants were randomized to either fluconazole (6 mg/kg) or placebo (normal saline) intravenously. The investigational drug center (IDC) at MUSC performed randomization by random number assignment with all others blinded to the assignment group. The drug was given every 72 hours until DOL 7 and then every 24 hours on DOL 8 to 28. The drug was given by feeding tube once the infant had tolerated gavage feeding for a 48-hour period.

Conclusion: Prophylactic administration of fluconazole to the VLBW infant for the first 28 days of life is safe and results in a decreased risk of rectal colonization by candidal species. Larger studies to determine the effect of prophylaxis on candidal septicemia and development of resistance in such a selective high-risk group are warranted before initiation of routine prophylaxis.

(Kicklighter: Fluconazole for Prophylaxis Against Candidal Rectal Colonization in the Very Low Birth Weight Infant. Pediatrics 2001;107:293-298)

Fluconazole

Indication	Day 1	Daily Therapy	Minimum Duration of Therapy
Neonates 0-14 days: Same dosage as older children but administered every 24-72 h			
Neonates > 14 days, infants and children			
Oropharyngeal candidiasis	6 mg/kg	3 mg/kg	14 d
Esophageal candidiasis	6 mg/kg	3 mg/kg up to 12 mg/kg/d	21 d
Systemic candidiasis	6-12 mg/kg/d		28 d
Cryptococcal meningitis Acute	12 mg/kg	6 mg/kg up to 12 mg/kg/d	10-12 wk after CSF culture becomes negative
Relapse	6 mg/kg		

Usual Dosage: Daily dose of fluconazole is the same for oral and I.V. administration:

Oral, I.V.:
Premature neonates:
≤29 weeks gestation:
Postnatal age 0-14 days: 5-6 mg/kg/dose every 72 hours

Postnatal age >14 days: 5-6 mg/kg/dose every 48 hours

30-36 weeks gestation:

Postnatal age 0-14 days: 3-6 mg/kg/dose every 48 hours

Neonates >14 days, Infants, Children: Once daily: See table

Safety profile of fluconazole has been studied in 577 children ages 1 day to 17 years. Doses as high as 12 mg/kg/day once daily (equivalent to adult doses of 400 mg/day) have been used to treat candidiasis in immunocompromised children; 10-12 mg/kg/day doses once daily have been used prophylactically against fungal infections in pediatric bone marrow transplantation patients. Do not exceed 600 mg/day.

Administration: Parenteral: Fluconazole must be administered by intravenous infusion over approximately 1-2 hours at a rate not to exceed 200 mg/hour and a final concentration for administration of 2 mg/mL; for pediatric patients receiving doses ≥6 mg/kg/day, administer I.V. infusion over 2 hours

Monitoring Parameters: Periodic liver function and renal function tests

Additional Information:

Oral suspension contains sucrose and sodium benzoate as inactive ingredients

(Taketomo: Pediatric Dosage Handbook 1999-2000, pp.386-388)

Fluconazole

Dose & Route: Loading dose: 6-12 mg/kg IV;PO, then maintenance (see table)

NEONATAL MAINTENANCE DOSING

Postconceptional Age (wk)	Postnatal age (days)	Dose (mg/kg/dose)	Dosing interval (hr) & time (hr) to start 1st maint. dose after load
≤ 29	0-14	5-6	72
	>14	5-6	48
30-36	0-14	3-6	48
	>14	3-6	24
37-44	0-7	3-6	48
	>7	3-6	24
≥ 45	>0	3-6	24

Children:
Loading dose: 10 mg/kg IV/PO, then
Maintenance: (begin 24 hr after loading dose) 3-6 mg/kg/24 hr IV / PO QD

Remarks: Cardiac arrhythmias may occur when used with cisapride, terfenadine, astemizole. Concomitant administration of fluconazole with any of these drugs is **contraindicated**. May cause nausea, headache, rash, vomiting, abdominal pain, hepatitis, cholestasis, and diarrhea.

PO and IV doses are equivalent. Loading doses (mg/kg or mg amounts) are twice the maintenance dose amount.

Inhibits CYP 450 2C9/10 and CYP 450 3A3/4 (weak inhibitor). May increase effects of levels of cyclosporin, phenytoin, theophylline, warfarin, oral hypoglycemics, and AZT. Rifampin increases fluconazole metabolism.
Adjust dose in renal failure.

(Siberry: The Harriet Lane Handbook 2000, p.717)

FLUCYTOSINE (Ancobon, 5-Fluorocytosine)

Supplied: Capsules 250mg, 500mg
Administration: PO
May cause GI upset.

Extemporaneous Compounding (Recipe)
Dosage form: Oral suspension
Made from: Capsules
Concentration: 10 mg/mL
Stability: 60 days
Store: Refrigerate
Label: Shake well

Ingredient	Strength	Quantity
Flucytosine capsules	250 mg	4
Ora-Sweet or Ora-Sweet SF		
Ora-plus		aa qs 100 mL

Instructions: Empty the capsules in a mortar and reduce to a fine powder. Add approximately 10 mL of vehicle and mix to a uniform paste. Add vehicle in geometric portions to almost desired volume while mixing. Transfer to a graduate and qs to volume with vehicle. Mix well. (11)

5-Fluorocytosine

Suggested Dosage of Antifungal Agents for Infants with systemic or Severe Local Fungal Infection

Dosage (mg/kg per day): 100-150

(Remington: Infectious Diseases of the Fetus and Newborn Infant 2001, p.838)

5-Fluorocytosine

5-Fluorocytosine, a fluoropyrimidine, has been shown to have in vitro activity against some fungi and has been effective in some patients with fungal infection. The drug is absorbed well form the gastrointestinal tract, and, with doses of 100 to 150 mg/kg daily, serum levels vary from 17 to 44 μg/ml. In CSF, levels of 5-fluorocytosine may be as high as 88% of the serum concentration. The drug is administered orally at a dose of 50 to 150 mg/kg per day in four divided doses for 2 to 6 weeks in adults. There is increasing experience with this agent in infants. Hill and co-workers treated a premature infant who had disseminated candidiasis with 5-fluorocytosine at a dose of

100 mg/kg per day. After an initial oral dose of 25 mg/kg, serum levels of 5-fluorocytosine were 40 μg/ml at 2 hours and 27 μg/ml at 4 and 6 hours. The level in CSF at 6 hours was 40 μg/ml. Of interest was the rapid emergence of resistance of the *Candida* isolated from synovial fluid in their patient 12 days after initiation of 5-flourocytosine therapy. This had previously been reported for *Candida* as well as for *C. neoformans*. 5-Fluorocytosine has been used extensively in infants and children, usually with amphotericin B. Few untoward side effects have been noted, even with prolonged use. Schönebeck and Segerbrand reported a woman with *Candida* septicemia during pregnancy who was treated with 5-fluorocytosine with no apparent ill effects to her infant.

Toxicity of 5-fluorocytosine includes transient neutropenia and hepatocellular damage. Because the drug is cleared by the kidneys, the dose should be reduced and serum levels determined in patients with impaired renal function. Accumulation of 5-fluorocytosine in the blood can result in serious toxicity to the bone marrow, and monitoring levels in body fluids is recommended.

There is experimental evidence that suggests that amphotericin B and 5-fluorocytosine act synergistically against some fungi, notably *Candida* and *Cryptococcus*.

(Remington: Infectious Diseases of the Fetus and Newborn Infant 2001, pp.836-837)

<u>Flucytosine</u>

Recommended Doses of Parenteral and Oral Antifungal Drugs

Route: PO

Dose: 50 to 150 mg/kg per day in 4 doses at 6-h intervals (adjust dose if renal dysfunction)

Adverse reactions:

Bone marrow suppression; renal dysfunction, gastrointestinal tract symptoms, rash, neuropathy, hepatotoxicity, confusion, hallucinations

Among pyrimidine antifungal agents, only flucytosine (5-fluorocytosine) is approved for use in children. This drug has a limited spectrum of activity against fungi, a potential for toxicity, and when used as a single agent resistance often emerges. Flucytosine is used in combination with amphotericin B for cryptococcal meningitis and some life-threatening *Candida* infections such as meningitis.

(American Academy of Pediatrics: Report of the Committee on Infectious Diseases. Red Book 2000, pp.669, 671)

<u>Flucytosine</u>

Candidiasis, Disseminated infection

Therapy: Amphotericin B (for dose see Amphotericin B, Nelson reference), but daily dosage 0.5-0.75 mg/kg <u>OR</u> amphotericin B <u>PLUS</u> flucytosine 100 mg/kg/day PO div q6h or Albelcet AmBisome or Amphotec (for dose see

Amphotericin B, Nelson reference); Fluconazole 6-12 mg/kg IV or PO daily for noncompromized host (some strains resistant to fluconazole).

Comments: Hematologic toxicity and diarrhea with flucytosine; Keep serum concentration <100 µg/ml; Replace IV catheter in catheter-associated candidemia.

Candidiasis, urinary infection.

Therapy: Fluconazole 3-6 mg/kg once daily <u>or</u> flucytosine 50 mg/kg/day div q6h; Amphotericin B (50 µg/ml) bladder irrigation if catheter in place.

Comments: Stopping antibiotic or removing Foley catheter sometimes leads to spontaneous cure in the normal host

Chromomycosis, systemic infection

Therapy: Flucytosine <u>OR</u> itraconazole (as above)

(Nelson: Pocket Book of Pediatric Antimicrobial Therapy 2000-2001, pp.56-57)

<u>Flucytosine</u> (Ancobon)

Classification: Antifungal agent.

Action and spectrum:

Penetrates fungal cells, where it acts as antimetabolite, ultimately interfering with protein synthesis. It is active in vivo against some strains of *Cryptococcus* and *Candida*. May be synergistic with amphotericin B.

Route: PO.

Dosage: 50-100 mg/kg/day divided q6h. Renal impairment: 12.5-25 mg/kg/day divided as follows:
q12h for creatinine clearance of 20-40 mL/min.
q24h for creatinine clearance of 10-20 mL/min.
q24-48h for creatinine clearance of <10 mL/min.

Serum concentrations: 24-120 mcg/mL.

Pharmacokinetics: Volume of distribution, 0.68 L/kg; half-life, 3-5 hours; renal elimination.

Adverse effects: Vomiting, diarrhea, rash, anemia, leukopenia, thrombocytopenia, elevated liver function tests, increased BUN and creatinine, CNS disturbances.

(Gomella: Neonatology 1999, p.567)

<u>Flucytosine</u>

Dose & Route: Neonates: 80-160 mg/kg/24 hr ÷ Q6 hr PO

Remarks: Monitor CBC, BUN, serum creatinine, alkaline phos, AST, ALT. Common side effects: nausea, vomiting, diarrhea, rash, CNS disturbance, anemia, leukopenia, and thrombocytopenia.

Therapeutic Levels: 25-100 mg/L. Recommended serum sampling time at steady-state: obtain peak level 2-4 hours after oral dose following 4 days of continuous dosing. Peak levels of 40-60 mg/L have been recommended for systemic candidiasis.

Prolonged levels above 100 mg/L can increase risk of bone marrow suppression.
Adjust dose in renal failure
(Siberry: The Harriet Lane Handbook 2000, p.718)

FLUDROCORTISONE (Florinef)

Supplied: Tablets 0.1mg
Administration: PO

Fludrocortisone is an adrenal cortical steroid with potent mineralocorticoid activity and higher glucocorticoid activity, (about 15 times as potent as hydrocortisone), but is used only for its mineralocorticoid affects (1).
Warning: supplemental measures: Use mineralocorticoid therapy preferably in conjunction with other supplemental measures (e.g. glucocorticoids, control of electrolytes, control of infections) (1).

Fludrocortisone Acetate

For Treatment of Congenital Adrenal Hyperplasia:

Treatment: Administration of glucocorticoids inhibits excessive production of androgens and prevents progressive virilization. A variety of glucocorticoids (hydrocortisone, prednisone, dexamethasone) and dosage schedules have been used for this purpose. Most often, hydrocortisone (10-20 mg/m^2 per 24 hours) is administered orally in 3 divided doses. There have been recent problems with consistent dosing with the liquid formulation of hydrocortisone. Tablets may give more reliable levels. Infants usually require 2.5 to 5 mg 3 times daily and children, 5 to 10 mg 3 times daily. The morning dose should be given as early as possible to blunt the early morning corticotropin increase that begins during the predawn hours. Doses must be individualized by monitoring growth, bone age, and hormonal levels. Patients with disturbances of electrolyte regulation (salt losers) and elevated plasma renin activity require a mineralocorticoid and sodium supplementation in addition to the glucocorticoid. Maintenance therapy with fludrocortisone acetate (Florinef) (0.05-0.3 mg daily) and sodium chloride (1-3 g) is usually sufficient to normalize plasma renin activity. Increased doses of glucocorticoid are indicated during periods of stress, such as infection or surgery, for salt-losing and non-salt-losing patients.

ABSTRACT. The Section on Endocrinology and the Committee on Genetics of the American Academy of Pediatrics, in collaboration with experts from the fields of pediatric endocrinology and genetics, developed this policy statement as a means of providing up-to-date information for the practicing pediatrician about current practice and controversial issues in congenital adrenal hyperplasia (CAH), including the current status of pre-natal diagnosis and treatment, the benefits and problem areas of neonatal screening programs, and the management of children with nonclassic CAH. The reference list is designed to allow physicians who wish more information to research the topic more thoroughly.

(American Academy Of Pediatrics: Section on Endocrinology and Committee on Genetics. Technical Report: Congenital Adrenal Hyperplasia. Pediatrics 2000;106:1511-1518)

Fludrocortisone Acetate

Dose & Route: Infants: 0.05-0.1 mg/24 hr QD PO
Children: 0.05-0.2 mg/24 hr QD PO

Remarks: **Contraindicated** in CHF and systemic fungal infections. Has primarily mineralocorticoid activity. May cause hypertension, hypokalemia, acne, rash, bruising, headaches, GI ulcers and growth suppression.

Monitor BP and serum electrolytes.

Drug Interaction: drug's hypokalemic effects may induce digoxin toxicity; phenytoin and rifampin may increase fludrocortisone metabolism.

(Siberry: The Harriet Lane Handbook 2000, p.718)

FLUMAZENIL (Romazicon)

Supplied: Injection 0.1mg/ml in 5, 10mL vials
Administration: IV
Admixture compatibility: D5W, NS, LR

Flumazenil

Dose and Route: Children, IV: reversal of benzodiazepine sedation:
Initial dose: 0.01 mg/kg (**max dose**: 0.2 mg), then 0.005-0.01 mg/kg (**max dose**: 0.2 mg), given Q 1 minute to a maximum total cumulative dose of 1 mg. Doses may be repeated in 20 minutes up to a **maximum** of 3 mg in 1 hour.

Remarks: **Does not reverse narcotics**. Onset of benzodiazepine reversal occurs in 1-3 minutes. Reversal effects of flumazenil ($T_{1/2}$ approx 1 hr) may wear off sooner than benzodiazepine effects. If patient does not respond after cumulative 1-3 mg dose, suspect agent other than benzodiazepines.

(Siberry: The Harriet Lane Handbook 2000, p. 719).

Flumazenil

Dosage: Children: 0.01 mg/kg (maximum = 0.2 mg) i.v.;
infuse 5-10 μg/kg/h to maximum cumulative dose of 1 mg

Comments: Benzodiazepine receptor antagonist; pediatric dosage not well established.

(Allen: Moss and Adam's Heart Disease in Infants, Children, and Adolescents 2001, pp.1460-1468)

FLUORIDE (Luride, Flura Drops, Pediaflor)

Supplied: 0.5mg per ml (from 1.1mg sodium fluoride) (Luride) in 50mL
0.25mg per drop (from 0.55mg sodium fluoride) (Flura Drops) in 30ml
0.5mg per ml(from 1.1mg sodium fluoride) (Pediaflor) in 50ml

Administration: PO
Milk and other dairy products may decrease absorption of sodium fluoride; avoid simultaneous ingestion (1).

Fluoride

Fluoride is of established value in the prevention of dental caries and may also have beneficial effect on the skeletal system. No specific recommendations for fluoride supplementation have been made for premature infants. However, prematurity is associated with an increased incidence of dental caries, and there appears to be particular reason for ensuring adequte fluoride supplementation in premature infants. It is not clear to what extent, if any, that fluoride will exert a beneficial effect on nonerrupted teeth, or what if any benefits can be conferred by systemic fluoride as opposed to the local effect in the oral cavity. However, it is prudent to provide 0.1mg fluoride/kg body weight/day up to a maximum of 0.25mg fluoride/day to premature infants, other than those who are fed with formula that has been made up with water in a fluoridated area. Infant formulas and packaged water marketed for making up powdered formula provide less than 0.3mg fluoride per liter.

(Hay: Neonatal Nutrition and Metabolism 1991, p.224)

Fluoride

Route: PO
Neonatal Dose: >2 wk: 0.25 mg daily if fluoride in water is <0.3 ppm
Pediatric Dose: 1-24 mo: 0.25 mg daily if fluoride in water is <0.3 ppm;
Discussion: Use if fluoride content of drinking water <0.7 ppm; mix with infant foods or formulas to reduce nausea.

(Rudolph: Rudolph's Pediatrics 1996, p.2184)

Fluoride (Luride, Fluoritab)

Dose & Route: All doses/24 hr:
Recommendations from American Academy of Pediatrics and American Dental Association.

Concentration of fluoride in drinking water (ppm):

Age	<0.3	0.3-0.6	>0.6
Birth-6mo	0	0	0
6mo-3yr	0.25 mg	0	0

Remarks: **Acute overdose**: GI distress, salivation, CNS irritability, tetany, seizures, hypocalcemia, hypoglycemia, cardiorespiratory failure. Chronic excess use may result in mottled teeth or bone changes.

Take with food, but **not** milk, to minimize GI upset. The doses have been decreased due to concerns over dental fluorosis.
(Siberry: The Harriet Lane Handbook 2000, p.720)

FOLIC ACID (Folvite)

Supplied: Tablets 0.4mg, 0.8mg, 1mg
Injection 5mg/ml, 10ml vial

Administration: PO, IV, IM, SC

Folic acid

Route & Dose: PO: 50 µg/day for preterm newborns after feeding is established for maintenance; 500 µg/day for therapy
(Taeusch: Avery's Diseases of the Newborn 1998, p. 1345)

Folic Acid

Dose & Route: Folic Acid Deficiency PO, IM, IV, SC
Infants:
Initial Dose: 15 mcg/kg/dose, max dose 50 mcg/24 hr
Maintenance: 30-45 mcg/24 hr QD

Children:
Initial Dose: 1 mg/dose
Maintenance: 0.1-0.4 mg/24 hr QD

Remarks: Normal levels: serum >3ng/ml. RBC 153-605 ng/ml. May mask hematologic effects of vitamin B_{12} deficiency, but will not prevent progression of neurologic abnormalities. Women of child-bearing age considering pregnancy should take at least 0.4 mg QD before and during pregnancy to reduce risk of neural tube defects in the fetus.
(Siberry: The Harriet Lane Handbook 2000, p.723)

Folic Acid

Requirements: Recommended dietary intake in term infants is 25 µg/day. Parenteral requirements are 140 µg/day for term infants and 56 µg/day for preterm infants.

Goat's milk is virtually free of folate with levels of 7 µg/L compared with 52 µg/L for cow's milk, necessitating routine folate supplementation for the infant exclusively fed goat's milk.

Inborn defects in folate metabolism have been described, including impairment of intestinal and blood-brain barrier transport of the vitamin, as well as defects of specific enzymes of folate metabolism.

Toxicity: Folate is remarkably free of toxicity even in the large doses (up to 60 mg/day) used to treat certain inborn errors of metabolism. Hypersensitivity reactions characterized by an erythematous rash with urticaria and pruritus have been described.
(Hay: Neonatal Nutrition and Metabolism 1991, pp.157-159)

FOSCARNET (Foscavir)

Supplied: 24 mg/ml in 250, 500 ml

Administration: IV infusion, carefully control rate of infusion with an infusion pump.
DO NOT administer by rapid or bolus IV injection. Toxicity may be increased as a result of excessive plasma levels (1).

The standard 24 mg/ml solution may be used without dilution when using a central venous catheter for infusion

When a peripheral vein catheter is used, dilute the 24 mg/ml solution to 12 mg/ml with Dextrose 5% or NS.

Administration rate:
Induction treatment - minimum 1 hour
Maintenance treatment - 2 hours

Foscarnet (Foscavir)
Antiviral Drugs for Non-Human Immunodeficiency Virus Infections

Indication: CVM retinitis in patients with AIDS
Route: IV
Dosage: 180 mg/kg per day in 3 divided doses for 14-21 d, then 90-120 mg/kg once a day as maintenance dose

Indication: HSV infection resistant to acyclovir in immunocompromised host
Route: IV
Dose: 80-120 mg/kg per day in 2-3 divided doses until infection resolves

Notes: Dose should be decreased in patients with impaired renal function
(American Academy of Pediatrics: Report of the Committee on Infectious Diseases. Red Book 2000, pp.676-677)

FOSPHENYTOIN (Phenytoin, Cerebyx)

Supplied: 150 mg (100 mg phenytoin sodium) in 2 ml vials
750 mg (500 mg phenytoin sodium) in 10 ml vials

Comments: The dose, concentration in dosing solutions and infusion rate of IV fosphenytoin is expressed as phenytoin sodium equivalents (PE) to avoid the need to perform molecular weight-based adjustments when converting between fosphenytoin and phenytoin sodium doses. Fosphenytoin has important differences in administration from those for parenteral phenytoin sodium. (1)

Dilute fosphenytoin in 5% Dextrose or 0.9% saline solution for injection to a concentration ranging from 1.5 to 25 mg PE/ml.

Storage/stability: Refrigerate at 2° to 8° C (36° to 46° F). Do not store at room temperature for more than 48 hours. (1)

Phenytoin-fosphenytoin

Indication: For Neonatal Seizures

In the unusual infant who continues to exhibit active seizures after as much as 40mg/kg of phenobarbital, or in the severely asphyxiated infant in whom only the initial 20 mg/kg dose of phenobarbital is deemed appropriate, phenytoin is administered intravenously in a loading dose of 20 mg/kg. when this approach is used in an infant who continues to exhibit seizures after 20 mg/kg of phenobarbital, approximately 20% to 40% respond with cessation of seizures, when it is used in an infant who continues to exhibit seizures after 40 mg/kg of phenobarbital, approximately 15% respond with cessation. The cumulative result with either sequence of phenobarbital and phenytoin is not markedly different. The dose should be administered at a rate of no more than 1 mg/kg/min to avoid disturbance of cardiac function, particularly cardiac rhythm. Cardiac rate and rhythm should be monitored during the infusion. The drug should be administered directly into the intravenous line, because it is relatively insoluble in aqueous solutions and precipitates in standard dextrose intravenous solutions. The pH of the parenteral solution is 12 and is irritating to the vein; thus the dose should be followed by a few milliliters of normal saline. The 20-mg/kg loading dose results in a therapeutic blood level of approximately 15 to 20 µg/kg. *Fosphenytoin*, a phosphate ester prodrug of phenytoin, has proved to be a major advance in therapy of status epilepticus in children and adults. The drug's advantages include high water solubility and a pH value closer to neutral, ease of preparation in standard intravenous solutions, safe intramuscular administration, no tissue injury with intravenous infiltration, and a faster allowable rate of intravenous administration. The drug is converted to phenytoin, primarily by plasma phosphatases, in approximately 8 minutes. The effective dose, in phenytoin, equivalents (i.e., 1.5 mg of fosphenytoin yields approximately 1.0 mg of phenytoin), is essentially identical to that just described for phenytoin. Initial data indicate that the rate of conversion of fosphenytoin to phenytoin is similar in newborns, infants, and older children. Although the safety of this agent has not been established unequivocally in the newborn, fosphenytoin appears to be clearly preferred.

(Volpe: Neurology of the Newborn 2001, pp.204-205)

SEE ALSO: THERAPY FOR NEONATAL SEIZURES p.657

FUROSEMIDE (Lasix)

Supplied: Oral solution 10mg/ml; 40mg/5mL
Injection 10mg/ml in 2ml, 4ml, 10ml

Administration: PO, IM, IV

Discard opened containers of oral solution according to the manufacturer's recommendations.

For DIRECT IV INJECTION, administer IVP slowly over a period of 1 to 2 minutes (1).

For a more accurate dose delivery, furosemide may be diluted in NS. (Authors).

For IV infusion, furosemide should be diluted with a infusion solution of NS, LR, or D5W, adjusting the pH to greater than 5.5 when necessary (3).

Furosemide (Lasix)

Indications and use:

Fluid overload, pulmonary edema, congestive heart failure, hypertension.

Actions: Inhibits active chloride transport in the ascending limb of the loop of Henle. Furosemide-induced diuresis results in enhanced excretion of NaCl, potassium, calcium, magnesium, bicarbonate, ammonium, hydrogen, and possibly phosphate. IV administration increases venous capacitance independently of its diuretic effect, resulting in rapid improvement of pulmonary edema.

Route: PO, IV, IM.

Dosage: PO: 1-2 mg/kg/dose q12h as initial dose and increase slowly if needed, since more may be required due to highly variable bioavailability.

IV or IM: 1 mg/kg/dose q12-24h slowly. If there is no increase in urine output, double the above doses and repeat.

Adverse effects: Hypokalemia, hypocalcemia, hyponatremia. With prolonged use, nephrocalcinosis, hypochloremic metabolic alkalosis.

(Gomella: Neonatology 1999, p.567)

Furosemide (Lasix)

Dose: 0.5-2 mg/kg dose IV
0.5-3 mg/kg dose PO generally BID

Mode of Action: Loop diuretic; blocks Na^+ reabsorption in ascending loop

Adverse Effects: Hypokalemia, hyponatremia, hypocalcemia, alkalosis, nephrocalcinosis, hyperuricemia

Comments: Possible ototoxicity; augmented response when used with captopril

(Garson: The science and practice of pediatric cardiology 1998, p.2951)

Furosemide

Dosage: Pediatrics: 1 mg/kg i.v. or p.o. once or twice daily; continuous infusion 0.05 mg/kg/h, titrate up as necessary.

Comments: Maximum pediatric dose = 4-5 mg/kg/24 h. Dose interval may be shortened to 8 h. May produce hypokalemia (Allen: Moss and Adam's Heart Disease in Infants, Children, and Adolescents 2001, pp.1460-1468)

Furosemide

Adverse Reactions:

Cardiovascular: Orthostatic hypotension

Central nervous system: Dizziness, vertigo, headache

Dermatologic: Urticaria, photosensitivity

Endocrine & metabolic: Hypokalemia, hyponatremia, hypochloremia, alkalosis, dehydration, hyperuricemia

Gastrointestinal: Pancreatitis, nausea; oral solutions may cause diarrhea due to sorbitol content; anorexia, vomiting, constipation, abdominal cramping

Hematologic: Agranulocytosis, anemia, thrombocytopenia

Hepatic: Ischemic hepatitis, jaundice

Otic: Potential ototoxicity

Renal: Nephrocalcinosis, prerenal azotemia, interstitial nephritis, hypercalciuria

Drug Interactions: Indomethacin decreases the effect of furosemide; decreased lithium excretion; decreased glucose tolerance with antidiabetic agents; increased ototoxicity with aminoglycosides and ethacrynic acid; drugs affected by potassium depletion (ie, digoxin); increased anticoagulant activity of warfarin; increased salicylate toxicity due to decreased excretion; decreased furosemide effects when administered at the same time as sucralfate

Stability: Protect from light

Usual Dosage: Neonates, premature: (see Additional Information)
Oral: Bioavailability is poor by this route; doses of 1-4 mg/kg/dose 1-2 times/day have been used
I.M., I.V.: 1-2 mg/kg/dose given every 12-24 hours

Infants and Children:
Oral: 1-6 mg/kg/day divided every 6-12 hours
I.M., I.V.: 1-2 mg/kg/dose every 6-12 hours

Administration: Oral: May administer with food or milk to decrease GI distress

Parenteral: May be administered undiluted direct I.V at a maximum rate of 0.5 mg/kg/minute for doses <120 mg and 4 mg/minute for doses >120 mg; may also be diluted for infusion 1-2 mg/mL (maximum concentration: 10 mg/mL) over 10-15 minutes (following maximum rate as above)

Monitoring Parameters:

Serum electrolytes, renal function, blood pressure, hearing (if high dosages used)

Additional Information:

Nebulized furosemide at 1 mg/kg/dose (diluted to a final volume of 2 mL with NS) has been shown to be effective in improving pulmonary function in eight preterm infants with bronchopulmonary dysplasia undergoing mechanical ventilation; no diuresis or systemic side effects were noted

(Taketomo: Pediatric Dosage Handbook 1999-2000, pp.416-417)

<u>Furosemide</u>

Indication: For hypercalcemia

The patient was treated with intravenous infusions of normal saline solution, oral NaCl (3 meq/kg/d), furosemide (4 mg/kg/d intravenous every 6 hours), and prednisone (up to 2 mg/kg/d). Initially, serum calcium levels decreased. Furosemide was changed from intravenous to oral administration, saline solution infusions were stopped, and a diet low in calcium and vitamin D was started. When the serum calcium level rose again furosemide was changed back to intravenous administration (6 mg/kg/d every 4 hours), normal saline solution infusions were restarted, the prednisone dose was increased (3 mg/kg/d), and the oral feedings were stopped. Because hypercalcemia and elevated urinary calcium to creatinine ratios persisted the patient was given etidronate (5 mg/kg/dose orally twice a day), which acts to decrease the release of skeletal calcium into the circulation.

The child was discharged on a low-calcium and vitamin D free formula (Calcilo XD; Ross, Columbus, Ohio), oral NaCl supplements (3 meq/kg/d), prednisone (2 mg/kg/d for 2 weeks followed by a 1-month taper), and etidronate (5 mg/kg/d).

(Rice: Etidronate therapy for hypercalcemia in subcutaneous fat necrosis of the newborn. J Pediatr 1999;134:349-51)

GALLAMINE TRIETHIODIDE (Flaxedil)

Supplied: Injection 20 mg/ml
Administration: IV

Gallamine

Route: IV
Neonatal Dose: Initial: 0.25-0.75 mg/kg
Maintenance: 0.1-0.5 mg/kg given q30-40 min as needed

Pediatric Dose: Initial: 1.0 mg/kg
Maintenance: 0.5-1 mg/kg given q30-40 min as needed
Max: 100 mg

Discussion: Do not use in patients in renal failure or those in shock.
(Rudolph: Rudolph's Pediatrics 1996, p.2185)

GAMMA BENZENE HEXACHLORIDE (Kwell, Lindane)

Supplied: Cream 1%; Lotion 1%; Shampoo 1%, in 30ml, 60ml
Administration: Topical
Contraindications:
Premature neonates, because their skin may be more permeable than that of full-term infants and their liver enzymes may not be sufficiently developed; patients with known seizure disorders; hypersensitivity to lindane or any component of the products (1).

Gamma benzene hexachloride

Route: Topical
Neonatal Dose: Avoid
Pediatric Dose: >2 y: apply and may repeat in 7 days if needed
Discussion: Apply to affected areas for lice, mites, and scabies, and remove as directed to avoid central nervous system toxicity
(Rudolph: Rudolph's Pediatrics 1996, p.2185)

GAMMA GLOBULIN INTRAMUSCULAR

(Gamastan, Gammar, Gamma Globulin, Immune Serum Globulin)

Supplied: Injection 2ml, 10ml vials
Administration: IM
Following IM administration serum concentrations of IgG peak within 2 days (3).

Gamma Globulin Intramuscular

Measles postexposure immunoprophylaxis
Immune globulin (IG)
Indications: Prevents or modifies disease if given within 6 days of exposure; indicated for the following group:
Infants <6 months old if mother is susceptible

Dosing Standard dose IG for children and pregnant women:
0.25 mL/kg (max. 15 mL) IM
(Siberry: The Harriet Lane Handbook 2000, pp.365-366)

GAMMA GLOBULIN INTRAVENOUS

(Sandoglobulin, Gamimune N, Gammagard, Venoglobulin-I)

Supplied: Gamimune N Injection 5%, 10% in 10, 50 and 100 ml
Gammagard S/D Solution in 2.5, 5 and 10 gm
Sandoglobulin Powder for Injection 1, 3, 6, 12 gm vials
Venoglobulin Powder for Injection 2.5, 5 gm vial
Venoglobulin S Solution for Injection 5% in 50, 100 and 200 mL
Polygram S/D 2.5 gm, 5gm, 10gm

Administration: IV
See specific product information for preparation and administration (author).
IGIV provides immediate antibody levels, whereas IM administration involves a 2-5 day delay before adequate serum levels are attained. Half-life is ≈ 3 weeks (1).
Discard partially used vials.

Immune Gamma Globulin

Immune Globulin Intravenous:

Immune Globulin Intravenous is derived from pooled plasma of adults by an alcohol-fractionation procedure, which is modified by individual manufactures so as to yield a product suitable for IV use. The donor pool is like that of IG. The FDA specifies that all preparations must have a minimum concentration of measles, diptheria, polio, and hepatitis B antibodies. Antibody concentrations against common pathogens, such as *Streptococcus pneumoniae*, very widely between products and even among lots of the same product. Immune Globulin Intravenous consists primarily of the immunoglobulin fraction (more than 95% IgG and trace amounts of IgA and IgM). The protein content varies, depending on the product; both liquid and dried products are available. Immune Globulin Intravenous does not contain thimerosal.

Indications for the use of IGIV

During the 1980s, IGIV was developed as an infusion product that allowed patients with primary immunodeficiencies to receive enough immune globulin at monthly intervals to protect them from infection until their next infusion. Since then, the FDA and the National Institutes of Health have expanded the recommended uses for IGIV (see Table 1.6). This product also may be useful for other conditions. Since November 1997, a shortage of IGIV has existed in the United States Because of production impediments related to compliance and withdrawals based on the theoretical risk for contamination with the Creutzfeldt-Jakob disease (CJD) agent. Other problems include increased administration for approved and unapproved uses, wastage, and export of IGIV. In August 1998, the US Surgeon General recommended that plasma derivatives including IGIV be withdrawn only if the blood donor developed variant CJD. The FDA is using several methods to improve IGIV distribution to patients. Clinicians should review their IGIV use to ensure consistency with current recommendations. The use of IGIV for other conditions needs to be supported by adequate scientific evidence of effectiveness.

Table 1.6. US Food and Drug Administration and National Institutes of Health (NIH) Recommendations for Use of Immune Globulin Intravenous
Primary immunodeficiencies Pediatric human immunodeficiency virus infection Immune-mediated thrombocytopenia

Approval by the FDA of specific indications for a manufacturer's IGIV product is based on availability of data from one or more clinical trials. Thus, not all licensed products are approved for each of the indications listed in Table 1.6 (see above); in some cases only a single product has the indication in its product label. Therapeutic differences among IGIV products of different manufacturers may exist but have not been demonstrated. Recommended indications in children and adolescents for the prevention or treatment of infectious diseases include the following:

Pediatric HIV infection.
The value of IGIV in children with HIV infection has been evaluated in several trials. The Working Group on Antiretroviral Therapy and Medical Management of Infants, Children, and Adolescents with HIV Infection* has recommended IGIV therapy for children with any of the following: (1) significant recurrent bacterial infections despite appropriate anti-microbial prophylaxis in infants and children who have humoral immune defects, (2) absence of detectable antibody to measles in children who have received 2 doses of measles vaccine and who live in regions with a high prevalence of measles, (3) HIV-associated thrombocytopenia despite antiretroviral therapy, and (4) chronic bronchiectasis that is suboptimally responsive to antimicrobial and pulmonary therapy.

Low-birth-weight infants.
Results of some clinical trials have indicated that IGIV decreases the incidence of late-onset infections in infants who weigh less than 1500 g at birth, but other studies have not confirmed these results. Trials have varied in IGIV dosage, time of administration, and other aspects of study design. A large multicenter placebo-controlled trial, however, concluded that IGIV was beneficial for very-low-birth-weight infants. At present, IGIV is not recommended for routine use in preterm infants to prevent late-onset infection.

May be useful.
Anemia because of parvovirus B19, patients with stable

multiple myeloma who are at high risk for recurrent infection, CMV-negative recipients of CMV-positive organs, hypogammaglobulinemic neonates with a risk factor for infection or morbidity, intractable epilepsy, systemic vasculitic syndromes, warm-type autoimmune hemolytic anemia, neonatal alloimmune thrombocytopenia when unresponsive to other treatments, immune-mediated neutropenia, decompensation in myasthenia gravis, dermatomyositis, polymyositis, and severe thrombocytopenia that is unresponsive to their treatments.

Adverse Reactions to IGIV

The reported incidence of adverse events associated with the administration of IGIV ranges from 1% to 15% but usually is less than 5%. Most of these reactions are mild and self-limited. Severe reactions occur infrequently and usually do not contraindicate further IGIV therapy. Adverse events include the following:

- Pyrogenic reactions marked by high fever, chills, and systemic symptoms
- Minor systemic reactions with headache, myalgia, anxiety, light-headedness, nausea, or vomiting
- Vasomotor or cardiovascular manifestations, marked by flushing, changes in blood pressure, and tachycardia
- Aseptic meningitis
- Hypersensitivity reactions
- Acute renal failure

Anaphylactic reactions induced by anti-IgA can occur in patients with primary antibody deficiency who have a total absence of circulation IgA and Have IgG antibodies to IgA. These reactions are rare in panhypogammaglobulinemic persons and potentially more common in patients with selective IgA deficiency and subclass IgG deficiencies. In the rare instances in which reactions related to anti-IgA antibodies have occurred, use of IgA-depleted IGIV preparations will reduce the likelihood of further reactions. Avoidance of anaphylactic reactions, however, may require the use of globulin preparations that are completely devoid of IgA. Because of the extreme rarity of these reactions, screening for IgA deficiency is not recommended routinely.

An outbreak of hepatitis C occurred in the United States in 1994 among recipients of IGIV lots from a single domestic manufacturer. Procedures and requirements in the preparation of IHIV subsequently have been instituted to prevent transmission of HCV by IGIV.

Precautions for the use of IGIV

- Caution should be used when giving IGIV to a patient with a history of adverse reactions to immune globulin.
- Because systemic reactions to IGIV may occur (see Adverse Reactions to IGIV), epinephrine and other

means for treating acute reactions should be immediately available.

- Adverse reactions often can be alleviated by reducing either the rate or the volume of infusion. For patients with repeated severe reactions unresponsive to these measures, hydrocortisone, 1 to 2 mg/kg, can be given intravenously 30 minutes before infusion. Using a different IGIV preparation or pretreatment with diphenhydramine, acetaminophen, or aspirin also may be helpful.
- Seriously ill patients with compromised cardiac function who are receiving large volumes of IGIV may be at increased risk of vasomotor or cardiac complications manifested by elevated blood pressure, cardiac failure, or both.
- Screening for IgA deficiency is not recommended routinely for potential recipients of IGIV (see Adverse Reactions to IGIV).

(American Academy of Pediatrics: Report of the Committee on Infectious Diseases. Red Book 2000, pp.44-47)

Immune Globulin, Intravenous (IVIG) (Gamimune N, Sandoglobulin, Gammagard)

Indications and use:

Immunodeficiency syndromes, suspected sepsis (controversial). Sandoglobulin is also indicated for treatment of idiopathic thrombocytopenic purpura.

Action: Establishes immediate (passive) IgG antibody serum levels.

Route: IV only.

Dosage: Suspected sepsis: IV IgG 400-500 mg/kg/dose for 1-2 dose; repeat weekly.

Immunodeficiency syndrome:
Sandoglobulin: 200 mg/kg (initial rate: 0.08 –0.1 mL/kg/min) once per month. If desired clinical response or level of IgG is insufficient, then increase the dose to 300 mg/kg or repeat the dose more frequently.

Gamimune N: 100 mg/kg or 2 mL/kg (at an initial flow rate of 0.01-0.02 mL/kg/min for 30 min, may dilute in D_5W) once per month. If no adverse effects are observed, then increase the rate to 0.02-0.04 mL/kg/min. If desired clinical response is not achieved or level of IgG insufficient, increase the dose to 200 mg/kg (4 mL/kg) or repeat the dose more frequently than once per month.

Gammagard: 100 mg/kg once per month (initial rate of 0.5 mL/kg/h). If desired clinical response is not achieved or the level of IgG is insufficient, increase the dose to 200-400 mg/kg to maintain a serum IgG level >500 mg/dL.
Idiopathic thrombocytopenia purpura: Sandoglobulin: 400mg/kg/day for 5 consecutive days. (See above administration rate for immunodeficiency syndrome.)

Adverse effects: Hypotension and anaphylaxis. If either occurs, the rate of infusion should be decreased or stopped until resolved, then resumed at a slower rate as tolerated. Preparations contain antibodies to group B streptococcus and *Escherichia Coli*. Substantial variation among lots and manufacturers.

(Gomella: Neonatology 1999, p.570)

Gamma Globulin Intravenous

Dose: Indications

Antibody deficiency disorders (replacement therapy)

1) Dosage: 300-400 mg/kg IV per month.
2) Determine optimal frequency and dose of IVIG by monitoring clinical response and IgG trough levels. (IgG trough levels ideally >300-400 mg/dL over initial pretreatment level.)

Idiopathic thrombocytic purpura (ITP)

1) Initial therapy for acute ITP: 0.8-1.0g/kg IV in one or two doses.
2) Alternatively for acute ITP: Prednisone (2 mg/kg per day) or Rh_0(D) immune globulin may be added or substituted.

General Guidelines for administration (see package insert of specific products): Begin infusion at 0.01 ml/kg/min, double rate every 15-30 min, up to max of 0.08 ml/kg/min. If adverse reactions occur, stop infusion until side effects subside and may restart at rate that was previously tolerated.

Comments: May cause flushing, chills, fever, headache, hypotension.

Hypersensitivity reaction may occur when IV form is administered rapidly. Gamimune-N contains maltose and may cause an osmotic diuresis. May cause **anaphylaxis** in IgA-deficient patients due to varied amounts of IgA. Some products are IgA depleted. Consult a pharmacist.

Delay immunizations after IVIG administration.

(Siberry: The Harriet Lane Handbook 2000, p.739)

Immunoglobulin Intravenous (IVIG)

Therapy with IVIG at 500 mg/kg per day was begun on day 1 of life and continued for 5 days. In addition, the dosage of neostigmine was increased from 0.05 to 0.2 mg/kg per dose every 3 to 4 hours, until a maximum effect was obtained. Severe weakness that affects some infants with NMG can be life threatening. It was disappointing to discover that therapies widely used in older children and adults was myasthenia gravis were ineffectual in this infant with severe NMG. Our case demonstrates that supportive care is the mainstay of patient management in NMG.

(Tagher: Failure of intravenously administered immunoglobulin in the treatment of neonatal myasthenia gravis. J Pediatr 1999;134:233-5)

Immunoglobulin intravenous, human

Route & Dose: IV: 400-750 mg/kg/dose infused over 2-6 h

Adverse Effects and Cautions:

Studies in newborns are preliminary. Necrotizing enterocolitis, volume overload

(Taeusch: Avery's Diseases of the Newborn 1998, p.1345)

Gamma Globulin Intravenous

A Consistent Approach to IVIG Administration in the NICU

Treatment of Sepsis, Neutropenia and Shock. In our opinion, neonates with severe neutropenia and early onset or late-onset sepsis-shock syndrome are reasonable candidates for IVIG treatment. such treatment does not dramatically influence survival, but we think that the rationale for it's use in these infants (to provide specific antibody toward the organism with which they are infected) is sound and consistent with extensive animal data. Neonates with neutropenia from early onset bacterial sepsis almost invariably lack antibody to their infecting organism, and this is likely also to be the case with late-onset infection. Although any given vial of IVIG might or might not contain significant titers of antibody directed against the relevant organism, a single dose of 750 mg/kg might provide opsonins and effectuate an elevation in the blood neutrophil concentration more rapidly than a placebo. For neonates with severe neutropenia and septic shock, we use a single dose of 750 mg/kg intravenously, over a period of 2 to 4 hours.

(Calhoun: Consistent approached to procedures and practices in neonatal hematology. Clin Perinatol 2000;27:733-753)

GANCICLOVIR (Cytovene, DHPG)

Supplied: Injection, powder for 500mg/vial
Capsules 250mg

Administration: IV infusion over 1 hour.
Reconstitute vial with 10ml SWFI. Concentration equal to 50mg/ml. Do not refrigerate. Stable for 12 hours.

Dilute to a concentration of less than 10mg/ml prior to administration. Refrigerate, use within 24 hours. Stable in NS, D5W, LR. Infusion concentrations >10mg/ml are not recommended (1).

Handling and disposal:

Exercise caution in the handling and preparation of ganciclovir. Solutions of IV ganciclovir are alkaline (pH 11). Avoid direct contact with the skin or mucus membranes. Because ganciclovir shares some of the properties of antitumor agents (e.g., carcinogenicity and mutagenicity); give consideration to handling and disposal according to guidelines issued for antineoplastic drugs (1).

Ganciclovir (Cytovene)

Antiviral Drugs for non-human Immunodeficiency Virus Infections

Indication: Acquired CMV retinitis in immunocompromised host
Route: IV
Usually Recommended Dosage:
10 mg/kg per day in 2 divided doses for 14-21 d; for long-term suppression, 5 mg/kg per day for 5-7 d/wk

Indication: Prophylaxis of CMV in high-risk host
Route: IV
Usually Recommended Dosage:
10 mg/kg per day in 2 divided doses for 1 wk, then 5 mg/kg per day in 1 dose for 100 d

Route: PO
Usually Recommended Dosage:
1 g orally 3 times per day

Note: Dose should be decreased in patients with impaired renal function.

(American Academy of Pediatrics: Report of the Committee on Infectious Diseases. Red Book 2000, pp.676-677)

Ganciclovir

Major Indications: Congenital CMV (investigational)
Dosage: IV treatment symptomatic CNS 5 mg/kg q 12 hr IV
(Feigin: Textbook of Pediatric Infectious Diseases 1998, p.2665)

Ganciclovir

Ganciclovir is beneficial for treatment of retinitis caused by acquired or recurrent CMV infection in HIV-infected patients. This drug is approved in the United States for treatment of severe retinitis in immunocompromised adults. Limited data in children suggest that safety and efficacy are similar to those in adults. The combination of oral ganciclovir and intraocular ganciclovir implant is efficacious in adults with CMV retinitis, but data in children are not available. Ganciclovir often is useful in other types of CMV organ involvement. Although ganciclovir has been used to treat some congenitally infected infants, it is not recommended routinely because of insufficient efficacy data. In bone marrow transplant recipients, the combination of CMV Immune Globulin Intravenous (CMV-IGIV) and ganciclovir, given intravenously, has been reported to be synergistic in treatment of CMV pneumonia. Foscarnet also has been approved for treatment of CMV retinitis and is an alternative drug. This drug is more toxic but may be advantageous for some patients with HIV infection, such as those with disease caused by ganciclovir-resistant virus or those unable to tolerate ganciclovir. Cidofovir is efficacious for treatment of CMV retinitis in adults, but it has not been studied in children. Ganciclovir sustained-release implant is available for adults and adolescents. Cidofovir is nephrotoxic. Formivirsen is an antisense drug recently licensed for intraocular administration.

Cytomegalovirus disease in HIV-infected patients is not

cured by currently available antiviral agents. However, treatment with highly active antiretroviral therapy has significantly decreased severity and the need for long-term suppression.

(American Academy of Pediatrics: Report of the Committee on Infectious Diseases. Red Book 2000, p.229)

Ganciclovir

Dose & Route: Cytomegalovirus (CMV) infections:
Children >3 mo and adults:
Induction therapy (duration 14-21 days):
10 mg/kg/24 hr ÷ Q12 hr IV

Maintenance therapy: 5 mg/kg/dose QD IV or
6 mg/kg/dose QD IV for 5 days/wk

Prevention of CMV in transplant recipients:
Children and adults:
Induction therapy (duration 7-14 days):
10 mg/kg/24 hr ÷ Q12 IV

Maintenance therapy: same as above

Prevention of CMV in HIV-infected individuals:
Infants and Children: 5 mg/kg/dose QD IV

Remarks: Limited experience with use in children <12 yr old. Use with extreme caution. **Reduce dose in renal failure**. Oral absorption is poor. Common side effects: neutropenia, thrombocytopenia, retinal detachment, confusion. Drug reactions alleviated with dose reduction or temporary interruption. Minimum dilution is 10 mg/ml and should be infused IV over ≥1 hr. IM and SC administration are **contraindicated** because of high pH (ph=11)

(Siberry: The Harriet Lane Handbook 2000, pp.726-727)

GENTAMICIN (Garamycin)

Supplied: Injection 10mg/ml; 40mg/ml in 2ml
Injection, intrathecal 2mg/ml in 2ml amps, preservative-free
Ophthalmic 3mg/mL solution, 5ml, 15ml; 3mg/g ointment, 3.5 gm

Administration: IV, IM, Intrathecal

Direct IV injection is not recommended. The volume of diluent used depends on the fluid needs of the patient, but should be sufficient to allow a gentamicin infusion period of 30 minutes to 2 hours. Stable in D5W, NS for 24 hours at room temperature (3).

The recommended final concentration for administration is 2 mg/ml (6,2).

Gentamicin

Antibacterial Drugs for Newborn Infants:

Dose (mg/kg or Units [U]/kg) and Frequency of Administration
Route: IV, IM

Dose: Infants 0-4 wk
BW <1200 g: 2.5 every 18-24 h

Infants <1 wk old
BW ≤1200-2000 g: 2.5 every 12 h
BW >2000 g: 2.5 every 12 h

Infants ≥ wk old
BW ≤2000-2000 g: 2.5 every 8 or 12 h
BW >2000 g: 2.5 every 8 h

Notes: Optimal dosage should be based on determination of serum concentrations, especially in low-birth-weight (<1500 g) infants. In very low-birth-weight infants (<1200 g) every 18 to 24 hour dosing may be appropriate in the first week of life

Dosages for the aminoglycosides may differ from those recommended by the manufacturer in the package insert.

Antibacterial Drugs for Pediatric Patients Beyond the Newborn Period
Dosage per kg/d
Route: IV, IM
Mild to Moderate Infections: Inappropriate

Severe Infections: 3-7.5 mg in 3 doses

Comments: Once daily dosing (5-6 mg/kg every 24 h) is investigational in children

Note: Dosages for the aminoglycosides may differ from those recommended by the manufacturers (see package insert)
(American Academy of Pediatrics: Report of the Committee on Infectious Diseases. Red Book 2000, pp.651-653,662)

Gentamicin

Suggested Dosage Schedules for Antibiotics Used in Newborns
Route: IV, IM

Dosage (mg/kg) and Interval of Administration:
Weight <1200 g
Age 0-4 wk: 2.5 q18h

Weight 1200-2000 g
Age 0-7 days: 2.5 q12h
Age >7 days: 2.5 q8h

Weight >2000 g
Age 0-7 days: 2.5 q12h
Age >7 days: 2.5 q8h

Note: Appropriate dosage schedule should be based on serum concentration measurements.
(Remington: Infectious Diseases of the Fetus and Newborn Infant 2001, p.1454)

Gentamicin

Route: IV, IM

Dosage (mg/kg/dose) by Gestational age plus weeks of life:

≤26 Wks: 2.5 q24h

27-34 Wks: 2.5 q18h

35-42 Wks: 2.5 q12h

Once daily dosing regimen (4 mg/kg) is used by some neonatologists.

≥43 Wks: 2.5 q8h

Once daily dosing regimen (4 mg/kg) is used by some neonatologists.

Comment: Desired serum concentrations: 5-10 mg/ml (peak), < 2.5 mg/ml (trough)

(Nelson: Pocket Book of Pediatric Antimicrobial Therapy 2000-2001, p.17)

Gentamicin

Indication: For meningitis

Initial treatment: The optimal initial treatment in a newborn with bacterial meningitis of unknown cause is a combination of ampicillin and an aminoglycoside. The choice of aminoglycoside among gentamicin, kanamycin, amikacin, and tobramycin depends particularly on the susceptibility of gram-negative bacteria likely to be found in a given nursery population, but gentamicin is used most commonly. Although more readily demonstrated in vitro than in vivo, the combination of ampicillin and an aminoglycoside has been shown to be synergistic versus several common gram-negative and gram-positive organisms. The *usual doses, prior to results of cultures*, are for ampicillin, 100 to 150 mg/kg/day in the first week of life and 200 mg/kg/day after the first week, and for gentamicin, 5 mg/kg/day in the first week and 7.5 mg/kg/day after the first week. The drugs can be administered intramuscularly, but intravenous administration is preferred.

(Volpe: Neurology of the Newborn 2001, p.796)

Gentamicin

Indication: Ventriculitis

Ventriculostomy: Ventriculostomy (with intermittent intraventricular instillation of an antibiotic, usually through a reservoir) is indicated when the ventricular tap demonstrates purulent fluid with persistent infection. Antibiotics should be instilled in concentrations that generally exceed those usually sought in serum. Table shows the commonly used intraventricular antibiotics and the concentrations sought. Serial measurements of the CSF concentrations of the antibiotics are important. The best approach is to administer the agent at a dose calculated to produce a concentration approximately 20-fold greater than the measured minimal bactericidal concentration.

Ventriculostomy, with external drainage, may be required in neonatal bacterial meningitis when ventriculitis has caused obstruction to CSF flow and acute hydrocephalus, manifested by increased intracranial pressure and dilated lateral ventriculus. This condition may develop despite eradication of the ventricular infection by the systemic antibiotics and therefore with a sterile ventricular CSF. In such a circumstance, intraventricular instillation of antibiotic is not needed, and the task is management of the intracranial hypertension by CSF drainage, as described in Chapter 11 in relation to rapidly progressive posthemorrhagic hydrocephalus.

TABLE
Intraventricular Antibiotics for Ventriculitis

Antibiotic	Dose (mg)	Desired Peak Cerebrospinal Fluid concentration (μg/ml)
Gentamicin	1-5	80-120*
Vancomycin	4-5	80-100
Polymyxin	1-2	Unknown

*Histological change in white matter observed with concentrations >150 μg/ml.

(Volpe: Neurology of the Newborn 2001, p.798)

Gentamicin Sulfate

Classification: Aminoglycoside.

Action and spectrum: Bactericidal activity by inhibition of bacterial protein synthesis. Active chiefly against Gram-negative aerobic bacteria, including most *Pseudomonas*, *Proteus*, and *Serratia* spp. Some activity against coagulase-positive staphylococci but ineffective against anaerobes and streptococci. Provides some synergistic effect against group D streptococci (enterococci) when used in combination with a penicillin.

Route: IM, IV (infuse over 30 min), Intrathecal (not recommended)

Dosage: Base initial dose on body weight, then monitor levels and adjust using pharmacokinetics.
IV (preferred). IM:
<7 days' postnatal age:
- <1 kg and <28 weeks' gestational age:
  - 2.5 mg/kg/dose q24h.
- <1.5 kg and <34 weeks' gestational age:
  - 2.5 mg/kg/dose q18h.
- >1.5 kg and >34 weeks' gestational age:
  - 2.5 mg/kg/dose q12h.

>7 days' postnatal age:
- <1.2 kg: 2.5 mg/kg/dose q18-24h.
- >1.2 kg: 2.5 mg/kg/dose q8h.

Note: Once a day dosing using 4mg/kg IV has been reported in a few studies in term infants and for infants > 34weeks' gestation with normal renal functions.

Intrathecal or intraventricular: 1-2 mg qd.

Ophthalmic solution: Instill one drop into each eye q4-12h.

Elimination and metabolism:
Renal excretion by glomerular filtration.
Half-life is 4-8 h initially.

Adverse effects: Irreversible vestibular injury, proteinuria, uremia, oliguria, macular rash.

Comments: Desired serum peak is 4-10 mcg/mL (sample obtained 30 min after infusion has been completed) and desired serum trough is <2 mcg/mL (sample obtained 30 min to just prior to next dose). In general, a set of peak and trough levels should be obtained at about the fourth maintenance dose. Monitor serum creatinine. Excessive serum peak levels are associated with ototoxicity; excessive trough levels with nephrotoxicity. The aminoglycosides should not be used alone against Gram-positive pathogens.

(Gomella: Neonatology 1999 pp.567-568)

Gentamicin

Dose & Route: Parenteral (IM or IV):

Postconceptional age (wk)	Postnatal Age (days	Dose (mg/kg/dose)	Interval (hr)
≤29*	0-28	2.5	24
	>28	3	24
30-36	0-14	3	24
	>14	2.5	12
≥37	0-7	2.5	12
	>7	2.5	8

*Or significant asphyxia

Children: 6-7.5 mg/kg/24 hr ÷ Q8 hr.
Cystic Fibrosis: 7.5-10.5 mg/kg/24 hr ÷ Q8 hr.
Intrathecal/intraventricular: >3 mo: 1-2 mg QD
Ophthalmic ointment: apply Q6-8 hr
Ophthalmic drops: 1-2 drops Q4 hr

Remarks: Use with **caution** in patients receiving anesthetics or neuromuscular blocking agents, and in patients with neuromuscular disorders. May cause nephrotoxicity and ototoxicity. Ototoxicity may be potentiated with the use of loop diuretics. Eliminated more quickly in patients with cystic fibrosis, neutropenia, and burns.
Adjust dose in renal failure.

Monitor peak and trough levels:
Therapeutic peak levels:
6-10 mg/L general
8-10 mg/L in pulmonary infections, neutropenia, and severe sepsis.
Therapeutic trough levels: <2 mg/L.
Recommended serum sampling time at steady-state:
trough within 30 minutes prior to the 3rd consecutive dose and peak 30-60 minutes after the

administration of the 3rd consecutive dose.
(Siberry: The Harriet Lane Handbook 2000, pp.727-728)

Gentamicin

The charts of neonates receiving gentamicin and having at least one gentamicin SDL measured during the 6-month period of January through June of 1995 were retrospectively reviewed as a control group. At that time it was our practice to administer gentamicin to neonates weighing < 2000 g at 2.5 mg/kg/dose intravenously every 24 hours, and to neonates > 2000 g at 2.5 mg/kg/dose intravenously every 12 hours. Loading doses were not administered. Gentamicin doses were infused during a 30-minute period via an infusion pump. Initial trough SDL were routinely drawn immediately before the third dose and peak SDL were drawn 30 minutes after the end of the third dose infusion. SDL were subsequently routinely drawn twice a week or as needed to achieve the desired range. This set of patients served as a control group. Mean initial peak and trough SDL and the frequency distribution of peak and trough SDL in the desired range were determined.

All NICU patients with postnatal age < or = 7 days starting on gentamicin therapy from October 1995 through August 1996 were prospectively tracked and comprised the protocol group. The new gentamicin dosing and monitoring protocol included a loading dose of 5.0 mg/kg for all neonates, followed in 24 hours by a maintenance regimen. All term neonates who weighed > or = 2500 g received a maintenance regimen of 4.0 mg/kg every 24 hours. All other neonates received a maintenance regimen of 2.5 mg/kg every 24 hours. Previous studies using a loading dose of 3.75 to 5 mg/kg demonstrated an initial peak SDL > or = 5 mcg/mL in 92% to 100% of neonates, but a 23% to 56% incidence of elevated initial trough SDL was noted in premature infants, depending on gestational age and whether trough SDL were measured 12, 18, or 24 hours after the loading dose.Gentamicin sulfate (SoloPak Laboratories Inc, Elk Grove Village, IL) doses were diluted to 1 to 2 mg/mL and infused during a 60-minute period with metered syringe pumps and microbore tubing. After completion, the infusion was flushed, and peak SDL were drawn 60 minutes after the end of the infusion. Peak SDL were, therefore, measured a total of 2 hours after the beginning of the gentamicin infusion in the protocol group, versus 1 hour after the beginning of the infusion in the control group. Trough DL were measured immediately before a dose in both groups.

Conclusion. A loading dose followed by once-daily dosing was shown to result in SDL in the safe and therapeutic range in all term neonates in this study. In low birth weight neonates, this regimen resulted in peak and trough SDL throughout therapy that were similar to those observed in the control group. Delaying the initiation of maintenance once-daily dosing until 36-48 hours after the loading doe would be expected to result in a higher incidence of initial trough SDL in target range for very low birth weight neonates.

(Lundergan: Once-daily Gentamicin Dosing in Newborn Infants. Pediatrics 1999;103:1228-1234)

Gentamicin

Dose/kg: Loading dose: 5 mg
Route & frequency: IV, IM once

Dose/kg: Maintenance dose: 4 mg
Route & frequency: 24 h after loading dose
≥37 wk ≥2500 g: q24h

Dose/kg: Maintenance dose: 2.5 mg
Route & frequency: <37 wk <2500 g: q24h

Dose/kg: Alternate regimen: 2.5 mg
Route & frequency:
<28 wk: q24h
28-34 wk: q18h
>34 wk: q12h
>14 postnatal d, adjust dosing interval up one level

Comments: Monitor renal function. Ototoxicity is related to length of therapy. Therapeutic levels: Pk = 5-12 μg/mL, Tr = <2 μg/mL

(Avery: Neonatology Pathophysiology and Management of the Newborn 1999, p.1556)

Gentamicin

Drug Interactions: Increased toxicity: concurrent use of amphotericin B, cephalosporins, penicillins, loop diuretics, vancomycin, cisplatin, indomethacin; potentiates effect of neuromuscular blocking agents and botulinum toxin

Elimination: Clearance is directly related to renal function; eliminated almost completely by glomerular filtration of unchanged drug with excretion into urine
Clearance:
Neonates: 0.045 ± 0.01 L/hour/kg
Infants: 0.1 ± 0.05 L/hour/kg

Usual Dosage: Dosage should be based on an estimate of ideal body weight, except in neonates (neonatal dosage should be based on actual weight unless the patient has hydrocephalus or hydrops fetalis):

Neonates: I.M., I.V.:
Premature neonates,
<1000 g: 3.5 mg/kg/dose every 24 hours
0-4 week <1200 g: 2.5 mg/kg/dose every 18-24 hours
Postnatal age ≤7 days: 2.5 mg/kg/dose every 12 hours

Postnatal age >7 days:
1200-2000 g: 2.5 mg/kg/dose every 8-12 hours
>2000 g: 2.5 mg/kg/dose every 8 hours

Initial dose for term neonates receiving ECMO: I.V.: 2.5 mg/kg/dose every 18 hours; subsequent doses should be individualized by monitoring serum drug concentrations; when ECMO is discontinued, dosage may require readjustment due to large shifts in body water

Infants and Children <5 years: I.M., I.V.: 2.5 mg/kg/dose every 8 hours

Intraventricular/intrathecal (**use a preservative free preparation**):
Newborns: 1 mg/day
Infants >3 months and Children: 1-2 mg/day

Ophthalmic: Ointment: Apply 2-3 times/day

Administration: Parenteral: Administer by I.M., I.V. slow intermittent infusion over 30-60 minutes or by direct injection over 15 minutes; final concentration for I.V. administration should not exceed 10 mg/mL; administer other antibiotics, such as penicillins and cephalosporins, at least 1 hour before or after gentamicin

Monitoring Parameters:
Urinalysis, urine output, BUN, serum creatinine, peak and trough serum gentamicin concentrations, hearing test

Not all infants and children who receive aminoglycosides require monitoring serum aminoglycoside concentrations. Indications for use of aminoglycoside serum concentration monitoring include:
Treatment course >5 days
Patients with decreased or changing renal function
Patients with poor therapeutic response
Infants <3 months of age
Atypical body constituency
(obesity, expanded extracellular fluid volume)
Clinical need for higher doses or shorter intervals
(eg, cystic fibrosis, burns, endocarditis, meningitis, critically ill patients, relatively resistant organism)
Patients on hemodialysis or chronic ambulatory peritoneal dialysis
Signs of nephrotoxicity or ototoxicity
Concomitant use of other nephrotoxic agents

Reference Range:
Peak: 4-12 μg/mL; peak values are 2-3 times greater with once daily dosing regimens
Trough: 0.5-2 μg/mL

Nursing Implications:
Obtain drug levels after the third or fourth dose except in

neonates and patients with rapidly changing renal function in whom levels need to be measured sooner; peak gentamicin serum concentrations are drawn 30 minutes after the end of a 30-minute I.V. infusion, immediately on completion of a 1-hour I.V. infusion, or 1 hour after an intramuscular injection; infusion: trough levels are drawn within 30 minutes before the next dose; provide adequate patient hydration and perfusion

(Taketomo: Pediatric Dosage Handbook 1999-2000, pp.421-424)

<u>Gentamicin</u>

Objectives. To compare performance and cost analysis of two gentamicin regimens in infants > or = 34 weeks' gestation requiring antibiotics for a 72-hour rule-out sepsis evaluation. A once-daily dosing (ODD) regimen of 4 mg/kg was compared with a standard twice-daily dosing (TDD) regimen of 2.5 mg/kg every 12 hours.

Conclusion. ODD of gentamicin at 4 mg/kg in neonates > or = 34 weeks' gestation is the preferable treatment strategy based on:

1) significantly improved SGC performance compared with TDD;
2) elimination of the need for routine SGC collection in infants on short courses of therapy; and
3) significant antibiotic-associated hospital cost savings when compared with conventional therapy of TDD and SGC analysis.

(Thureen: Once- Verses Twice-daily Gentamicin Dosing in Neonates > or = 34 Weeks' Gestation: Cost-effectiveness Analyses. Pediatrics 1999;03:594-598)

GENTIAN VIOLET

Supplied: Topical Solution 1%, 2% in 30ml

Administration: Topical

Using cotton, apply gentian violet solution to lesions 2 or 3 times daily for 3 days. A 0.25% or 0.5% solution has been reported to be as effective as, and less irritating, than a 1% to 2% solution (3). Gentian violet will stain clothing and skin. Do not apply it to an ulcerative lesion because it may result in "tattooing" of the skin (1).

<u>Gentian Violet</u>

Topical Drugs for Superficial Fungal Infections

Strength: 1%-2%

Formulation: Solution

Applications per day 2

Adverse Reactions/Notes: Staining

(American Academy of Pediatrics: Report of the Committee on Infectious Diseases. Red Book 2000, p.674)

<u>Gentian violet</u>

Dose/kg: 1% topical solution

Route & frequency: Dilute to 0.5% solution 3-4 drops under the tongue or apply to lesions after feedings bid-tid

Comments: Stains skin and clothing; apply with cotton tip applicator. Do not apply to face

(Avery: Neonatology Pathophysiology and Management of the Newborn 1999, p.1556)

Gentian violet

Route & Dose: Top (skin): as 1-2% aqueous solution, bid
Top (oral): as 1% aqueous solution, bid

Adverse Effects and Cautions: Stains skin

(Taeusch: Avery's Diseases of the Newborn 1998, p.1345)

Gentian Violet

Use: Treatment of cutaneous or mucocutaneous infections caused by Candida albicans and other superficial skin infections refractory to topical nystatin, clotrimazole, miconazole, or econazole

Usual Dosage: Topical:
Infants: Apply 3-4 drops of a 0.5% solution under the tongue or on lesion after feedings

Administration: Topical: Apply to lesions with cotton; do not apply to ulcerative lesions on the face

Patient Information: Drug stains skin and clothing purple; proper hygiene and skin care need to be used to prevent spread of infection and reinfection

Nursing Implications: Keep affected area dry and exposed to air

Additional Information: 0.25% or 0.5% solution is less irritating than a 1% to 2% solution and is reported to be as effective

(Taketomo: Pediatric Dosage Handbook 1999-2000, pp.424-425)

GLUCAGON

Supplied: 1mg/vial (1 unit) and 10mg/vial (10 units) with Diluent

Administration: SC, IV, IM

After reconstitution use immediately. May be refrigerated for 48 hours if necessary (41°F) (1).

For IV ADMINISTRATION, use special diluent provided by the manufacturer to yield a concentration of 1 mg/ml.

For DIRECT IV INJECTION: Administer IV push without further dilution.

If glucagon is to be administered in doses exceeding 2mg, SWFI should be used as the diluent rather than the diluent provided by the manufacturer (3).

Compatible with dextrose IV solutions only (2).

Glucagon

Indications and use: Hypoglycemia as seen in infants of diabetic mothers (IDMs); hypoglycemia due to other causes unresponsive to routine treatment. Bowel spasm during barium enema.

Actions: Glucagon, a hormone produced by the alpha cells of the pancreas, causes increased breakdown of glycogen to form glucose and inhibition of glycogen synthetase. Blood glucose elevation occurs. Produces relaxation of smooth muscle in the GI tract when the drug is administered parenterally.

Route: SC, IM, IV.

Dosage: 0.025-0.3 mg/kg/dose; may repeat in 20 min prn. In IDMs: 0.3 mg/kg/dose. Maximum: 1 mg

Adverse effects: Hypersensitivity, nausea, and vomiting.

Comments: Incompatible with electrolyte-containing solutions; compatible with dextrose solutions. **Caution**: Do not delay initiation of glucose infusion while observing for glucagon effect.

(Gomella: Neonatology 1999, p.568)

Glucagon

Indications: Treatment of hypoglycemia when parenteral dextrose is unavailable or in cases of documented glucagon deficiency.

Dosage/Dosage Interval:
25-300 mcg/kg/dose (0.025-0.3 mg/kg/dose) IV push IM, SC, q20 min PRN. Maximum dose: 1 mg. **Continuous IV**: Administer in D10W solution, starting at 0.5 mg/day. Add hydrocortisone if no response within 4 h. Further dosage increases >2 mg/day unlikely to be effective. After effect seen, slowly taper over at least 24 h. **Infant of diabetic mother: Initial dose**: 0.3 mg/kg/dose up to 1 mg total as standard dose. Compatible with dextrose solutions.

Contraindications: Should not be used in small-for-gestational-age infants.

Precautions: Do not delay starting glucose infusion while awaiting effect of glucagon. Use caution in infants with history of insulinoma or pheochromocytoma. Incompatible with electrolyte-containing solutions.

Monitoring: Serum glucose concentration

Adverse Reactions: Vomiting, tachycardia, and GI upset.

(Cloherty: Manual of Neonatal Care 1998, p.707)

Glucagon

Dose: Intermittent:
0.3 mg/kg/dose given every 4 hours as needed.
Maximum: 1 mg/dose.

Continuous Infusion:
Begin with 0.5 mg/kg/day; increase every 30 minutes to 1 hour as needed to maintain normoglycemia. Wean gradually over 24-36 hours after normoglycemia is achieved.

Administration: Supplied as: Injection: As a lyophilized powder 1 mg (1 unit)/vial with 1 ml diluent.
IV Continuous Infusion: Reconstitute powder with diluent provided, then dilute with $D_{10}W$ to a volume based on the dose and the infant's fluid requirements.

Nursing Implications:
Monitor blood glucose.
Infuse IV glucagon slowly, over at least 1 minute, to decrease risk of nausea and vomiting.

(Zenk: Neonatal Medications & Nutrition. A Comprehensive Guide 2000; pp:216-218)

Glucagon

We report on a 35-week gestation infant who developed severe hyponatremia and thrombocytopenia after continuous infusion of glucagon for the treatment of intractable hypoglycemia. Given these serious side effects, glucagon infusion should be avoided in the treatment of premature infants.

Dexamethasone was discontinued and glucagon was begun at a dose of 1 mg/day infused over 24 hours.

Conclusion: Significant and severe side effects of glucagon infusion for the treatment of neonatal hypoglycemia in a premature infant are described. Until its safety is evaluated further, glucagon infusion for the treatment of hypoglycemia should be avoided in premature infants.

(Belik: Continuous Infusion of Glucagon Induces Severe Hyponatremia and Thrombocytopenia in a Premature Neonate. Pediatrics 2001;107:595-597)

Glucagon HCl

Dose & Route: Hypoglycemia, IM, IV, SC:
Neonates/Infants: 0.025-0.3 mg/kg/dose Q30 min PRN;
max dose: 1 mg/dose
Children: 0.03-0.1 mg/kg/dose Q20 min PRN;
max dose: 1/mg/dose

Remarks: High doses have cardiac stimulatory effect and have had some success in beta-blocker overdose. May cause nausea, vomiting, urticaria, and respiratory distress. Do **not** delay glucose infusion; dose for hypoglycemia is 2-4 ml/kg of Dextrose 25%

(Siberry: The Harriet Lane Handbook 2000, pp.728-729)

GLUCOSE (Dextrose)

Supplied: D5%W in 25ml, 50ml, 100ml, 150ml, 250ml, 500ml and 1000ml vials:, 10ml syringes
D10%W in 3ml amps, 250, 500, and 1000ml vials
D20%W in 500ml
D25%W in 10ml syringes
D50%W in 500ml, 1000ml, 50ml amps, and 50ml syringes

Glucose

Indication: For hypoglycemia

Therapy of Neonatal Hypoglycemia*
SYMPTOMATIC INFANT Glucose: 200 mg/kg as 2 ml/kg of 10% glucose IV
FOLLOWING BOLUS INFUSION, OR AT START OF THERAPY IF INFANT IS ASYMPTOMATIC Glucose: 8 mg/kg/min IV
IF GLUCOSE RATES OF 12 MG/KG/MIN REQUIRED FOR NORMOGLYCEMIA Hydrocortisone: 5 mg/kg every 12 hours IV or IM
TAPER AND WEAN IV GLUCOSE SLOWLY

IM, Intramuscularly; IV, Intravenously
*See text for references.

When to treat: The major issues in therapy related to when and how to treat. Detection of hypoglycemia at the bedside, previously dependent entirely on Dextrostix determinations, has been facilitated by portable reflectance meters and electrochemical glucose meters. Most physicians treat hypoglycemia with glucose infusion even if the infant is asymptomatic. The difficult issue in this context, of course, is the definition of hypoglycemia. The most frequently utilized definition of hypoglycemia in the past has been that of Cornblath and Schwartz, i.e., blood glucose levels of less than 30 mg/dl in the full-size term infant and less than 20 mg/dl in the low-birth-weight infant. The findings described earlier (see "Definition") suggest that the threshold values should be higher. At the present time, i consider that several factors support a recommendation to treat both the full-term and premature infant with blood glucose levels of less than 45 to 50 mg/dl. (Thresholds for treatment may be lower in the first 3 hours of life.) These factors include (1) the neurophysiological, epidemiological, and clinical observations that levels less than 50 mg/dl can be associated with evidence for neurophysiological or neurodevelopmental dysfunction, (2) the PET observation that cerebral glucose utilization in the premature infant may be limited by glucose transport at levels of plasma glucose less than approximately 54 mg/dl (3) the likelihood that degrees of hypoglycemia not sufficient to cause brain injury alone may do so when combined with other factors deleterious to the central nervous system, (4) the lack of precise information regarding the level of blood glucose below which neuronal injury is likely to occur, and (5) the ample experimental evidence that blood glucose levels are not accurate predictors of brain glucose levels, particularly in states such as asphyxia or seizures. It is essential that the physician consider the status of both *cerebral glucose delivery*, i.e., Cerebral blood flow as well as blood glucose content, and *cerebral glucose utilization*.

How to treat: If a decision is made to treat an infant, the next issue is the manner of therapy. A small group of infants requires specific therapies for hormonal or enzymatic aberrations; these therapies are discussed in detail elsewhere. For the large group of infants in whom glucose alone is the mainstay of therapy, the most frequent recommendation in the past has been to institute intravenous treatment with a bolus infusion of 0.5 to 1.0 g/kg as 2 to 4 ml/kg of 25% glucose (at a rate of 1 ml/min), to be followed with a continuous infusion of 8 to 10 mg/kg/min. However, later data indicated that this bolus infusion of glucose followed by continuous infusion may lead to *hyperglycemia*, especially in small preterm infants who exhibit impaired glucose homeostasis. Hyperglycemia has been shown to cause osmotic diuresis and dehydration, has been associated with increased mortality and perhaps, intracranial hemorrhage in premature infants, and often is followed by "rebound" hypoglycemia in hyperinsulinemic infants. (indeed, hyperglycemia can be an important contributory determinant of neurological sequelae even in infants without hypoglycemia.) Therefore it is prudent to avoid the relatively large bolus infusion, particularly in the premature infants. Pildes and co-workers have demonstrated particular effectiveness and apparent safety of a *minibolus infusion* of 200 mg/kg (2 ml of 10% glucose injected over 1 minute), immediately followed by a continuous glucose infusion of 8 mg/kg/min. The minibolus infusion results in rapid correction of blood glucose level (within 1 minute), and a relative stability of values between approximately 70 and 80 mg/dl occurs thereafter with the continuous infusion of 8 mg/kg/min, approximately the maximum utilizable dose of glucose in the newborn. Thus for the *symptomatic infant* i prefer the minibolus infusion. *Careful assessment of the initial clinical response after the minibolus infusion is essential*, especially if the indication for the infusion was seizure, because of variability in the response to blood glucose level; a second minibolus infusion may be necessary. *Continued careful monitoring of clinical response and blood glucose level* also is important because certain infants, e.g., Those with hyperinsulinism, may require higher maintenance doses of glucose, and some infants require lower maintenance doses to avoid hyperglycemia.

In general, after blood glucose levels are stable at 70 to 100 mg/dl, the dextrose concentration in the infusion is decreased by 2 mg/kg/min every 6 to 12 hours. Glucose levels are monitored closely and should be maintained above 50 mg/dl. For infants whose glucose levels do not increase adequately despite infusion rates of 12 mg/kg/min, or if hypoglycemia recurs, or if glucose infusion rates of >12 mg/kg/min are required, hydrocortisone (5 mg/kg every 12 hours) should be administered. Other therapies, e.g., subcutaneous epinephrine, diazoxide, glucagon, are utilized in rare,

specific clinical circumstances, discussed elsewhere.
(Volpe: Neurology of the Newborn 2001, pp.516-517)

Glucose

Indication: For Neonatal Seizures

An intravenous line is established and a blood glucose (Dextrostix) determination is performed on the first drops of blood. If hypoglycemia is present and if the infant is convulsing, 10% dextrose is given intravenously in a dose of 2 ml/kg (0.2 g/kg) and the baby maintained on intravenous dextrose at a rate as high as 0.5 g/kg/hr (8 mg/kg/min) if necessary. (This is approximately the maximum usable dose of glucose in the newborn.) Although constant infusion of glucose at 8 mg/kg/min corrects hypoglycemia in less than 10 minutes in most patients and is appropriate if the infant is not convulsing, the more rapid approach of bolus infusion is indicated for the convulsing infant. The possibility of maintaining supranormal levels of blood glucose in newborns with frequent seizures should be considered, in view of the experimental demonstrations of a decline in brain glucose concentrations with seizures and the protective effect of pretreatment with glucose. The potential hazards of this approach, especially in the premature infants, however, must be recognized. This remains an important topic for future clinical research.
(Volpe: Neurology of the Newborn 2001, p.203)

Glucose

Although the absolute glucose requirement of term infants is limited to that necessary to prevent hypoglycemia, about 3 to 4 mg/min/kg (or less), ELBW infants often require more. However, the absolute requirement for glucose (or carbohydrate) is probably much less than the usual amounts given to ELBW infants (often in excess of 12 to 14 mg/min/kg) as part of enteral and intravenous nutrition regimens. Actual measurements of glucose utilization and production rates in ELBW infants, even shortly after birth, average from 6 to 10 mg/min/kg. These rates are slightly higher than in term infants, in part because the brain-to-body-weight ratio of the ELBW infant is higher and in part because total energy requirements are higher.
(Hay: Workshop Summary: Nutrition of the Extremely Low Birth Weight Infant. Pediatrics 1999; 1360-1368.)

Glucose

Acute Treatment of Neonatal Seizures

Dose: 10% solution: 2 mL/kg IV followed by continuous infusion at 5 to 7 mg/kg per minute

(Hill: Neonatal Seizures Pediatrics in Review 2000;21:117-121)

SEE ALSO: THERAPY FOR NEONATAL SEIZURES p. 657

GLYCERIN SUPPOSITORIES

Supplied: Suppositories: Infant, Pediatric, Adult

Administration: PR

Glycerin 80 Percent

Dose: 0.2 ml per rectum daily as needed if no stool output for more than 24 hours.

Administration: Rectal: Place surgical lubricant on the syringe tip; insert into the rectum.

> **Pharmacist Compounding Directions**
> Glycerin 80 Percent Microenema for Neonates
>
> Measure 80 ml glycerin USP in a conical graduate; then add sufficient sterile water for irrigation to bring the volume to 100 ml. Mix; then pour into an amber glass bottle and shake well. This volume is sufficient to prepare approximately 500 doses. Draw up 0.2 ml into 0.5 ml oral syringes and label: Lubricate syringe tip before use. for ractal use only refrigerate. Do not add overfill.
>
> Stability: 3 months
> Storage:
> Refrigerate syringes in labeled zippered plastic bag.

Use: Laxative to promote bilirubin excretion by reducing enterohepatic circulation, decreasing gastrointestinal transit time, and encouraging passage of meconium. In healthy preterm infants, full intestinal motile function may not occur until 29-31 weeks postconceptional age.

May improve feeding tolerance, particularly in infants who have gastric residuals, emesis, and abdominal distention from gastrointestinal hypomotility.

Glycerin enemas are as effective and safe as glycerin suppository chips in stimulating bowel movements in neonates. The enemas offer the advantages of dose consistency as well as cleanliness, convenience, and staff safety.

Adverse Effects: Usually very well tolerated.
Overdose could result in diarrhea and dehydration.

Nursing Implications:

Allow to warm to room temperature before administration.
Administer carefully to avoid injuring the rectal mucosa.
Monitor for stool result.

Comments: Advantages of Enema over Suppository-chip Administration:

- Reduces nursing time required for dose preparation and administration
- Standardized dose saves pharmacy preparation time.
- ***Warning***: To prepare suppository chip, a sharp blade is often used to cut small pieces from pediatric glycerin

suppositories. This results in nonstandardized sizes and possible contamination of the material. Use of a blade presents a risk of injury to nurses, is cumbersome, and is time-consuming.

(Zenk: Neonatal Medications & Nutrition. A Comprehensive Guide 2000; pp:221-222)

Glycerin

Dose & Route: Constipation:
Neonate: 0.5 ml/kg/dose rectal solution PR as an enema QD-BID PRN
Children <6 yr: 2-5 ml rectal solution PR as an enema or 1 Infant suppository PR QD-BID PRN

Remarks: Onset of action: 15-30 min. May cause rectal irritation, abdominal pain, bloating, and dizziness. Insert suppository high into rectum and retain for 15 minutes.

(Siberry: The Harriet Lane Handbook 2000, p.729)

Glycerin

Use: Constipation; reduction of intraocular pressure; reduction of corneal edema; glycerin has been administered orally to reduce intracranial pressure

Usual Dosage: Constipation: Rectal: Administered in single doses only at infrequent intervals

Neonates: 0.5 mL/kg/dose of rectal solution as an enema
Children <6 years: 1 infant suppository as needed or 2-5 mL of rectal solution as an enema

Administration: Rectal: Insert suppository high in the rectum and retain 15 minutes

Monitoring Parameters: Blood glucose, intraocular pressure

Nursing Implications:
Use caution during insertion of suppository to avoid intestinal perforation, especially in neonates; instruct patient to lie down after oral glycerin administration to prevent or relieve headaches

(Taketomo: Pediatric Dosage Handbook 1999-2000, pp.426-427)

GLYCOPYRROLATE (Robinul)

Supplied: Injection 0.2mg/ml in 1ml, 2ml, 5ml, with benzl alcohol
Administration: IV, IM

Glycopyrrolate (Robinul)

Dose: IV or IM: 4-10 mcg/kg/dose given every 4-8 hours
PO: 40-100 mcg/kg/dose given every 8-12 hours

In Reversal of Neuromuscular Blockade: 0.2 mg for each 1 mg neostigmine given

Administration: Supplied as: Injection: 0.2 mg/ml ((=200 mcg/ml);
Tablets: 1 mg, 2 mg
IV-Rate: Maximum: 20 mcg/minute.
IV-Concentration: May give undiluted.

IM: May give undiluted.
PO: An oral liquid is not commercially available. May use the injectable form of the drug and give PO, or an oral liquid can be prepared by the pharmacist.

Pharmacist Compounding Directions
Glycopyrrolate 100 mcg/ml[1]

Crush tablets in syrup at 100 mcg/ml.
Stability: 2 weeks refrigerated.

Incompatible with: Drugs having an alkaline pH such as phenobarbital and sodium bicarbonate.

Cautions/Contraindications:
Note that the **PO dose is 10 times the parenteral dose**; be sure to recalculate the dose when changing routes of administration.
Should not be used in patients with narrow-angle glaucoma, urinary tract obstruction, ileus.

Infants, patients with Down syndrome, and children with spastic paralysis or brain damage may be hypersensitive to the antimuscarinic effects (e.g., mydriasis, tachycardia).

Adverse Effects: May delay gastric emptying.
May cause drowsiness, nervousness, tachycardia, rash, dry mouth, constipation, urinary retention, impaired sweating, and blurred vision.

Nursing Implications:
Monitor heart rate.
Observe for constipation and urine retention.

(Zenk: Neonatal Medications & Nutrition. A Comprehensive Guide 2000; pp.221-222)

Glycopyrrolate

Dose & Route: Respiratory Antisecretory:
IM/IV:
Children: 0.004-0.01 mg/kg/dose Q4-8 hr
Max dose: 0.2 mg/dose or 0.8 mg/24 hr

Oral:
Children: 0.04-0.1 mg/kg/dose Q4-8 hr

Reverse neuromuscular blockade:
Children and adults: 0.2 mg IV for every 1 mg neostigmine or 5 mg pyridostigmine

Remarks: Use with caution in hepatic and renal disease, ulcerative colitis, asthma, glaucoma, ileus, or urinary retention. Atropine-like side effects: tachycardia, nausea, constipation, confusion, bronchospasm, blurred vision, and dry mouth. These may be potentiated if given with other drugs with anticholinergic properties. IV dosage form may be used orally.

(Siberry: The Harriet Lane Handbook 2000, pp.729-730)

GRANULOCYTE COLONY STIMULATING FACTOR: G-CSF

(Filgastrim, Neupogen)

Supplied: Injection 300mcg/mL, 1ml, 1.6ml vials

Administration: SC, bolus injection, by short IV infusion (15-30 minutes) or by continuous SC or IV infusion.

If required, filgastrim may be diluted in 5% dextrose. Filgastrim diluted to concentrations between 5 and 15mcg/mL should be protected from absorption to plastic materials by addition of albumin (human) to a final concentration of 2mg/mL. When diluted in 5% dextrose or 5% dextrose plus albumin, filgastrim is compatible with glass bottles, PVC and pololefin IV bags.
Dilution to a concentration of <5mcg/ml is not recommended at any time. Do not dilute with saline at any time; product may precipitate (1).

Recombinant Granulocyt Colony Stimulating Factor (EG-CSF)

All study patients received a single daily intravenous dose of 10 mcg/kg of rG-CSF (Amgen, Thousand Oaks, CA) for 3 to 5 days. If the blood neutrophil concentration was >2000/uL after 3 doses, the rG-CSF administration was stopped (a 3-day course.) However, if it was <2000uL, 2 additional doses of rG-CSF were given (a 5-day course).

Speculation.

The principal means of clearing G-CSF from the serum is by saturable binding to specific G-CSF receptors (G-CSF-Rs). Therefore, the very high G-CSF serum and urine concentrations of group 2 patients before the first rG-CSF dose implies that their G-CSF-Rs were saturated before the dose was given. We speculate that if G-CSF-Rs are saturated with endogenous G-CSF, treatment with rG-CSF will add little or nothing to the granulocytopoietic efforts. On this basis, we judge that neonates with septic shock and neutropenia are unlikely to derive benefit from rG-CSF administration.

(Calhoun: Granulocyte Colony-Stimulating Factor Serum and Urine Concetrations in Neutropenic Neonates Before and After Intravenous Administration of Recombinant Granulocyte Colony-Stimulating Factor. Pediatrics 2000;105:392-397.)

rhu GM-CSF

Recombinant human granulocyte-macrophage colony-stimulating factor (rhu GM-CSF) versus placebo in VLBWNs.

Neonates were randomly assigned to receive rhu GM-CSF (8 µg/kg) or placebo, both to be administered intravenously in equal volumes over 2 hours through a microinfusion pump once daily for 7 days, then every other day for an additional 21 days for a total of 17 doses. VLBWNs were initially dosed by birth weight; thereafter, doses were adjusted weekly based exclusively on current weight.

Recombinant human GM-CSF, Leukine (specific activity: 5.6 x 10^6 IU/mg protein) produced in yeast was supplied by Immunex Crop as a lyophilized powder in vials for reconstitution to 10 µg/mL. Inactive ingredients in each rhu GM-CSF vial contained 40 mg of mannitol, 10 mg of sucrose, and 1.2 mg of tromethamine *USP*. The inactive placebo control was a lyophilized preparation containing 40 mg of mannitol, 10 mg of sucrose, and 1.2 mg of tromethamine *USP*. The storage, reconstitution, labeling, and administration of placebo were identical to those of rhu GM-CSF. Administration of study medication began on day 0 and continued through day 27, unless modified because of leukocytosis (ANC >20,000 cells/mm^3) or thrombocytosis (platelet count >750,000/mm^3).

Conclusion: In a large randomized placebo-controlled trial, prophylactic administration of rhu GM-CSF in VLBWNs does not appear to decrease the incidence of nosocomial infections.

(Cairo: A randomized, double-blind, placebo-controlled trail of prophylactic recombinant human granulocyte-macrophage colony-stimulating factor to reduce nosocomial infections in very low birth weight neonates. J Pediatr 1999;134:64-70)

<u>Granulocyte-Macrophage Colony-Stimulating Factor</u>

Infants were eligible for entry if born <32 weeks gestation. Recruitment was within 72 hours of birth. Subjects were excluded if there was life-threatening congenital abnormality or clinical evidence of sepsis at recruitment. Infants were randomized (computer-generated, block randomization), stratified by growth status AGA or SGA), either to receive GM-CSF for 5 consecutive days (study days 1-5), or to a control group. A dose of 10 µg/kg/d was chosen for its proliferative effect, while remaining within accepted safety margins. SGA infants were defined as being below the 10th centile birth weight for gestational age. GM-CSF (Leucomax, Novartis, UK) was supplied as lyophilized powder and reconstituted at a concentration of 10 µg in 0.1 mL. Administration was by subcutaneous injection into the thigh, using a 27 French gauge (FG) needle.

Conclusion: Five-day prophylactic GM-CSF completely abolishes postnatal neutropenia and sepsis-induced neutropenia in preterm neonates at high risk of sepsis, and so removes an important risk factor for sepsis and sepsis-related mortality.

(Carr: A Randomized, controlled Trial of Prophylactic Granulocyte-Macrophage Colony-Stimulating Factor in Human Newborns Less Than 32 Weeks Gestation. Pediatrics 1999;103:796-802)

rG-CSF

A Consistent Approach to rG-CSF Administration in the NICU

Approved Usage in Pediatrics:

The FDA has approved rG-CSF for "Severe chronic neutropenia." The varieties categorized as severe chronic neutropenia are virtually all diagnosed as pediatric disorders. Almost all patients with severe chronic neutropenia respond to rG-CSF doses of 5 to 10 μg/kg, given subcutaneously at intervals ranging from every day to less than once per week, as needed to titrate the blood neutrophil concentration to levels at or above 1000/μL. Very rarely a patient requires higher doses, and a few patients have been reported not to respond at all. Essentially, all infants with severe chronic neutropenia who we are aware of have responded favorably to rG-CSF. The varieties of severe chronic neutropenia where rG-CSF administration has been best studied are Kostmann's syndrome, Shwachman-Diamond syndrome, Barth syndrome, and cyclic hematopoiesis. At this time it is not clear whether patients with chronic idiopathic neutropenia or neonatal alloimmune neutropenia fit under the FDA indication of severe chronic, because they can be very severe, but are self-limited, and the chronicity rarely exceeds 6 months. Moreover, rG-CSF administration to patients with these latter neutropenic disorders has not been tested in randomized, placebo-controlled trials.

Dosing: rG-CSF can be given subcutaneously or intravenously. We start with 10 μg/kg/d for 3 days, with subsequent titration of any additional doses to keep the blood neurophil count at or over 1000/μL. If contemplating the use of rG-CSF for a neutropenia NICU patient, it is useful to consider the cause of the neutropenia.

If the cause of the neutropenia is unknown, we use rG-CSF treatment only if (1) the absolute neutrophil count (ANC) is less than 500/μL for more than 2 to 3 days, or (2) the ANC is 500 to 999/μL for more than 5 to 7 days.

If the cause of the neutropenia is known and it si a form of severe chronic neutropenia, we use rG-CSF treatment. These cases are rare and require considerable evaluation to establish the diagnosis. Such neonates are in the unknown category initially, awaiting diagnostic information, unless a family history suggests the diagnosis.

If the cause of the neutropenia is known and it is not a form of severe chronic neutropenia, we do not use rG-CSF treatment. In sepsis, necrotizing enterocolitis (NEC), and PIH, severe neutropenia rarely persists for more than 2 to 3 days. If a patient with sepsis, NEC, or PIH has an ANC less than 500/μL for 3 days or more, rG-CSF treatment could be considered.

(Calhoun: consistent approaches to procedures and practices in neonatal hematology. Clinics in Perinatology 2000, 27:733-753)

GRISEOFULVIN MICROSIZE (Grifulvin V, Grisactin 250, Fulvicin U/F)

Supplied: Oral suspension 125 mg/5ml, in 120 ml
Capsule 250 mg
Tablets 250 mg, 500 mg

Administration: PO

Griseofulvin

Griseofulvin has significantly altered morbidity of dermatophyte infection. This drug is deposited in epidermal structures before keratinization. As keratinized areas are exfoliated, they are replaced by noninfected tissue. In patients with tinea capitis, it may be necessary to clip the hair frequently because, as growth occurs, the ends of hairs may continue to harbor viable fungus. The oral dose of griseofulvin is 10 mg/kg per day for 7 to 10 days. Occasionally, a dose of 20 to 40 mg/kg per day is necessary for cure. In some instances, therapy must be continued for 3 weeks. There are few data on the use of griseofulvin in newborns. Ross reported of griseofulvin in an infant 1 month of age at a dose of 10 mg/kg per day for 4 weeks without untoward effects.

Griseofulvin is derived from a species of *Penicillium*, and cross-sensitivity may exist between penicillin and griseofulvin. The incidence of hypersensitivity reactions to griseofulvin inpatients allergic to penicillin, however, has not been reported. The most common untoward reaction to griseofulvin is rash. Occasionally, urticaria and angioneurotic edema occur. In on report, griseofulvin was shown to cross the placenta in low concentrations, but fetal effects were not discussed.

(Remington: Infectious Diseases of the Fetus and Newborn Infant 2001, p.838)

HEMOPHILUS b CONJUGATE VACCINE (HibTITER, ActHIB, OmniHIB, Pedvax HIB, ProHIBiT, Comvax)

Supplied: HibTITER-Injection: 10mcg, capsular oligosaccharide ≈25mcg diptheria CRM $_{197}$ protein/0.5mL dose (1, 5, 10 mL vials)

ActHIB-Powder for injection: 10mcg purified capsular polysaccharide 24mcg tetanus toxoid/0.5ml (7.5mL vials)

OminHIB-as above (in vials with 0.6ML syringes)

Pedvax HIB-Powder for injection: 15mcg purified capsular polysaccharide 250mcg Neisseria meningitidis OPM C/dose

ProHIBiT-Injection: 25 mcg purified capsular polysaccharide 18mcg conjugated diphtheria toxoid protein/0.5ML (1, 5, 10mL vials).

Comvax: 7.5mcg purified capsular polysaccharide, 125mcg Neisseria Meningitidis OMPC and 5mg hepatitis B surface antigen per 0.5ml.

Administration: IM

Data are not available regarding interchangeability of hemophilus b Conjugate vaccines with regard to safety, immunogenicity or efficacy (1).

<u>Haemophilus influenzae</u>

Hib capsular polysaccharide (PS)-tetanus toxoid conjugate vaccine (PRP-T) was given to 120 neonates at 2 days of age, followed by PRP-T or the Hib PS vaccine at 4 months and a PRP-T booster at 14 months. Their anti-Hib PS concentrations were compared with those in children receiving PRP-T at 2 and 4 months or at 4 months.

At 14 months a higher percentage of the infants who had received PRP-T at 2 days and 4 months than of those who had received PRP-T at 4 months only had anti-Hib PS concentrations greater than 0.15 μg/mL. All infants responded well to the booster at 14 months.

(Kurikka: Neonatal Immunization: Response to Haemophilus influenzae Type b-Tetanus Toxoid Conjugate Vaccine. Pediatrics 1995;95:815-821)

HEPARIN

Supplied: 10 units/ml, 100 units/ml, 1000 units/ml, 5000 units/ml, 10,000 units ml, 20,000 units ml

Administered: IV, SQ

Preservative-free products are available (1).

Comment: Avoid IM use. Local irritation, erythema, mild pain, hematoma, or ulceration may follow deep SQ use, but are more common after IM use (1).

<u>Heparin</u>

Continuous heparin therapy requires a dedicated intravascular line. A loading dose of 75 U/kg is given, followed by a continuous infusion of 28 U/kg/h. Four hours after initiating therapy, obtain a partial thromboplastin time (PTT), then adjust the heparin dose to achieve a PTT that corresponds to an anti-factor Xa level 0.3 to 0.7. This usually corresponds to a PTT of 60 to 85 seconds. PTTs should be obtained at least every 4 to 6 hours during the initiation of therapy, and then daily once therapeutic PTT values are obtained. If PTT values are erratic, monitor anti-factor Xa levels.

(Calhoun: Consistent approaches to procedures and practices in neonatal hematology. Clinics in Perinatology 2000, 27:733-753)

<u>Heparin Sodium</u> (Various)

Indications and use: Primary role is as an anticoagulant. Used to diagnose and treat disseminated intravascular coagulation and to maintain patency of arterial or venous lines.

Actions: In combination with antithrombin III (heparin cofactor), heparin inactivates coagulation factors IX, X, XI, XII, and thrombin, inhibiting conversion of fibrinogen to fibrin.

Route: SC, IV

Dosage: Loading dose: 50 units/kg as IV bolus.

Maintenance dosage:10-20 units/kg/h as continuous infusion.

To maintain line patency: 0.5-1.0 unit/mL of fluid.

Antidote: Protamine sulfate, 1 mg for each 100 units of heparin given in the preceding 3-4 h up to a maximum dose of 50 mg.

(Gomella: Neonatology 1999, p.568)

<u>Heparin</u>

Dose/kg: For maintenance of central catheters: 0.5-2 U/mL of IV fluid
Route & Frequency: IV

Dose/kg: Anticoagulation: bolus 50 U/kg
Route & Frequency: IV, once

Dose/kg: Maintenance: 10-25 U/kg/h
Route & Frequency: IV continuous infusion titrate up based on APTT/PTT

Dose/kg: Intermittent dosing: 50-100 U/kg/dose
Route & Frequency: IV q4h

Comments: See protamine sulfate for treatment of overdosage. Monitor clotting time; titrate dose to achieve 1.5-2.5 times normal physiologic values.

(Avery: Neonatology Pathophysiology and Management of the Newborn 1999, p.1556)

<u>Heparin</u>

Eligibility included (1) age >1 month and <18 years and (2) venous thrombosis confirmed by ultrasonography, venography, or ventilation-perfusion scan.

The treatment guidelines for combination therapy are as follows. Urokinase is given as a bolus infusion of 4400 U/kg over a 20-minute period, followed by a maintenance infusion of 4400 U/kg/h for a 48-hour period. Heparin is given as an infusion of 10 U/kg/h during urokinase infusion without a bolus; at 48 hours a heparin bolus of 50 U/kg is given, and the rate of infusion is increased to achieve a plasma heparin level of 0.4 to 0.7 U/mL. Heparin is continued to maintain this therapeutic level for at least 5 days; heparin is discontinued when the international normalized ratio is >2. Warfarin is given to maintain the international normalized ration >2 for 3 months to indefinitely.

Plasma concentrations of plasminogen, fibrinogen, and platelets were monitored at least daily during thrombolytic therapy. Transfusion support was administered routinely on the following schedule: plasminogen <0.50 U/mL was replaced with fresh-frozen plasma, 10 mL/kg; fibrinogen <50 mg/dL was replaced with cryoprecipitate, 10 mL/kg; platelet count <50,000/μL was replaced with single donor platelet concentrates, 10 mL/kg.

Conclusions: Combination therapy in children (urokinase and unfractionated heparin) was safe and efficacious. A prospective, randomized, controlled study in children is needed.

(Manco-Johnson: Combined thrombolytic and anticoagulant therapy for venous thrombosis in children. J Pediatr 2000;136:446-53)

Heparin Sodium

Dose & Route: Anticoagulation:
Infants and Children:
Initial: 50 U/kg IV bolus
Maintenance: 10-25 U/kg/hr as IV infusion or 50-100 U/kg/dose Q4 hr IV

Heparin Flush:
Peripheral IV: 1-2 ml of 10 U/ml solution Q4 hr
Central lines: 2-3 ml of 100 U/ml solution Q24 hr

TPN (central line) and arterial line: add heparin to make final concentration of 0.5 - 1 U/ml. **Flush dose should be less than heparinizing dose!**

Remarks: Adjust dose to give PTT 1.5-2.5 times control value. PTT is best measured 6-8 hr after initiation or changes in infusion rate. For intermittent injection, PTT is measured 3.5-4 hrs after injection. Toxicities; bleeding, allergy, alopecia, thrombocytopenia.

Use preservative-free heparin in neonates. **Note**: heparin flush doses may alter PTT in small patients; consider using more dilute heparin in these cases.

Antidote: **Protamine sulfate** (1 mg per 100 U heparin in previous 4 hr). For low molecular weight heparin ,see enoxaparin.

(Siberry: The Harriet Lane Handbook 2000, pp.732-733)

HEPATITIS B IMMUNE GLOBULIN

(H-BIG, Hep-B-Gammagee, HyperHep)

Supplied: H-Big in 4 and 5ml
Hep-B-Gammagee in 5ml
HyperHep in 1ml and 5ml

Administration: IM only
First dose (perinatal use) can be given the same time as the Hepatitis B vaccine (but at a different site) without impairing the active immune response from Hepatitis B vaccination (1).

Hepatitis B Immune Globulin

Dosages recommended for postexposure prophylaxis are for products licensed in the United States. Because the concentration of anti-HBs in other products may vary, different dosages may be recommended in other countries.

Table 3.18. Recommended Dosages of Hepatitis B vaccines*

	Vaccine †	
	Recombivax HB ‡ Dose, μg (mL)	Engerix-B § Dose μg (mL)
Infants of HBsAg-negative mothers, children and adolescents younger than 20 y of age	5 (0.5)	10 (0.5)
Infants of HBsAg-positive mothers (HBIG [0.5 mL] also is recommended)	5 (0.5)	10 (0.5)

* HBsAg indicates hepatitis B surface antigen; HBIG, Hepatitis B Immune Globulin

† Vaccines should be stored at 2°C to 8°C (36°F-46°F). Freezing destroys effectiveness. Both vaccines are administered in a 3-dose schedule. A 2-dose schedule, administered at 0 and 4 to 6 mo later, is available for adolescents 11-15 years of age using the adult dose of Recombivax, HB (10 μg).

‡ Available from Merck and Co, Inc, West Point, Pa. A combination of hepatitis B (Recombivax, 5 μg) and *Haemophilus influenzae* b (PRP-OMP) vaccine is licensed for use at 2, 4, and 12 to 15 months of age (Comvax).

§ Available from SmithKline Beecham Pharmaceuticals, Philadelphia, Pa. The US Food and Drug Administration has approved this vaccine for use in an optional 4-dose schedule at 0, 1, 2, and 12 mo.

(American Academy of Pediatrics: Report of the Committee on Infectious Diseases. Red Book 2000, pp.298-300)

Hepatitis B Immune Globulin (H-BIG)

Indications and use: Prophylaxis of hepatitis B exposure.

Actions: Passive immunization agent. Immune serum provides protection against the hepatitis B virus by directly providing specific antibody to hepatitis B surface antigen (HBsAg). The immunity is transient, usually lasting ~30 days.

Route: IM only.

Dosage: 0.5 mL administered within 12 h after delivery. (Repeat at 3 months and 6 months if vaccine was not given)

Adverse reactions:
Swelling, warmth. erythema, and soreness at injection site. Rarely, rash, fever, and urticaria.

Comments: Do not use in IgA deficiency, thrombocytopenia, or coagulopathy. Do not administer IV.
(Gomella: Neonatology 1999, p.569)

SEE ALSO: HEPATITIS B IMMUNIZATION

HEPATITIS B VACCINE (Recombivax-HB, Engerix-B)

Supplied: As hepatitis B surface antigen
Recombivax HB:
Injection 2.5mcg/0.5mL (pediatric formulation),
Injection 5mcg/0.5mL (adolescent/high-risk infant formulation).
Injection: 10mcg/ml (adult formulation)
Injection: 40mcg/ml (dialysis formulation)
Engerix-B:
Injection 20mcg/mL (adult formulation)
Pediatric inj. 10mcg/0.5mL (pediatric formulation)

Administration: IM

Preparation: After thorough agitation, the vaccine is a slightly opaque, white suspension. Use as supplied; no dilution or reconstitution is necessary (1).

Hepatitis B Vaccine

Two highly effective and safe hepatitis B vaccines produced by recombinant DNA technology have been licensed in the United States. The original plasma-derived vaccine is no longer produced in the United States, but plasma-derived vaccines are used widely in other countries. The recombinant vaccines contain 10 to 40 μg of HBsAg protein per milliliter adsorbed to aluminum hydroxide, and some contain thimerosal as a preservative. While the concentration of HBsAg protein differs in the two recombinant vaccine products, equal rates of seroconversion are achieved with both vaccines when given to healthy infants, children, adolescents, or young adults in the doses recommended (see Table 3.18).

Routes of Administration.
Vaccine is administered intramuscularly in the anterolateral thigh or deltoid area depending on the age of the recipient.

Table 3.18. Recommended Dosages of Hepatitis B vaccines*

	Vaccine †	
	Recombivax HB ‡ Dose, µg (mL)	Engerix-B § Dose µg (mL)
Infants of HBsAg-negative mothers, children and adolescents younger than 20 y of age	5 (0.5)	10 (0.5)
Infants of HBsAg-positive mothers (HBIG [0.5 mL] also is recommended)	5 (0.5)	10 (0.5)

* HBsAg indicates hepatitis B surface antigen; HBIG, Hepatitis B Immune Globulin

† Vaccines should be stored at 2ºC to 8ºC (36ºF-46ºF). Freezing destroys effectiveness. Both vaccines are administered in a 3-dose schedule. A 2-dose schedule, administered at 0 and 4 to 6 mo later, is available for adolescents 11-15 years of age using the adult dose of Recombivax, HB (10 µg).

‡ Available from Merck and Co, Inc, West Point, Pa. A combination of hepatitis B (Recombivax, 5 µg) and *Haemophilus influenzae* b (PRP-OMP) vaccine is licensed for use at 2, 4, and 12 to 15 months of age (Comvax).

§ Available from SmithKline Beecham Pharmaceuticals, Philadelphia, Pa. The US Food and Drug Administration has approved this vaccine for use in an optional 4-dose schedule at 0, 1, 2, and 12 mo.

(American Academy of Pediatrics: Report of the Committee on Infectious Diseases. Red Book 2000, pp.298-300)

<u>Hepatitis B Vaccine</u> (Heptavax-B, Recombivax HB, Engerix B)

Indications and use: Prophylaxis for hepatitis B.

Actions: Induces protective antibody formation to hepatitis B virus (anti-HBs).

Route: IM only.

Dosage: 0.5 mL IM (= Recombivax HB, 5 mcg; Engerix B, 10 mcg).

Adverse effects: Swelling, warmth, erythema, and soreness at injection site and, rarely, vomiting, rash, and low-grade fever.

Comments: Do not give intravenously or intradermally. Administer in anterolateral thigh.

(Gomella: Neonatology 1999, p.569)

<u>Hepatitis B Vaccination</u>

Thimerosal, a derivative of mercury, is used as preservative in hepatitis B vaccines. We measured total mercury levels before and after the administration of this vaccine in 15 preterm and 5 term infants. Comparison of pre- and post-vaccination mercury levels showed a significant increase in both preterm and term infants after vaccination. Additionally, post-vaccination mercury levels were significantly higher in preterm infants as compared with term infants. Because mercury is known to be potential neurotoxin to infants, further study of its pharmacodynamics is warranted.

(Stajich: Iatrogenic exposure to mercury after hepatitis B vaccination in preterm infants. J Pediatr 2000;136:679-81)

HYALURONIDASE (Wyadase)

Supplied: Injection, lyophilized powder 150 unit, 1500 unit
Injection, stabilized solution 150 units per 1ml, 10ml vials

Administration: NOT RECOMMENDED FOR IV USE
Sterile reconstituted solution may be stored below 30°C (86°F) for 2 weeks without significant loss of potency. Hyaluronidase solution must be refrigerated (1).

Hyaluronidase (Wydase)

Dose: 15 units SC. Dose may be repeated in 30-60 minutes, if needed, for severe swelling.

Administration: Supplies as: Wydase Lyophilized, 150 units/vial/ml.
SC: Concentration: 15 units/ml.

Preparation:

- **Reconstitute**: 150-units vial with 1 ml of normal saline injection (=150 units/ml).
- **Prepare at 1:10 Dilution**: Using a tuberculin syringe, withdraw 0.1 ml of the 150 unit/ml solution and add to 0.9 ml of normal saline injection to equal a total of 1 ml (=15 units/ml).

Administration Procedure:

- **Stop** infusion
- **Elevate** the extremity (can use a skin traction stockinette dressing with a window). Do not apply heat or cool compresses.
- **Inject** hyaluronidase locally by the subcutaneous or intradermal route using a 25 gauge needle. The dose is 15 units given in four 0.2 ml aliquots into the periphery or leading edge of the site, changing the needle after each injection.
- The additional 0.2 ml may be injected into the needle through which the IV was running before removing it from the extravasation site. This delivers hyaluronidase directly into the tissue plane in which the extravasation occurred.
- **Wrap** the extremity loosely for approximately 2 hours. do not apply heat, especially moist heat, because heat can damage and macerate the tissue even further.
- **Observe** and document the appearance of the lesion (induration, swelling, discoloration, blanching, and blister formation) every 15 minutes for approximately 2 hours.
- **Care for open wounds**. Apply silver sulfadiazine cream. consult plastic surgery and the burn unit services, if available, early in the course of treatment.

Smaller lesions will slough and heal spontaneously, whereas large ulcers will require excision and grafting.

Storage: Reconstituted 150 units/vial is stable for 24 hours if refrigerated.

Use: Used to treat extravasation of dextrose 10 percent, calcium salts, potassium salts, sodium bicarbonate, aminophylline, radiocontrast media, hypertonic saline, nafcillin, blood, parenteral nutrition, and may other drugs such as higher concentrations of dextrose. These drugs and/or solutions can sometimes cause severe tissue necrosis and sloughing on infiltration. Hyaluronidase may markedly reduce the amount of local tissue damage and destruction caused by infiltration. Promoting rapid absorption decreases the degree and duration of pain associated with the extravasation. It can reduce pressure necrosis from mechanical compression of tissues by large amounts of IV fluids trapped in a limited tissue space.

Administer within 1 hour after the toxic insult, if possible. **There is little or no advantage if the drug is given 3 or more hours after extravasation**.

Adverse Effects: Usually very well tolerated. Rarely, has caused allergic reactions in adults (urticaria). Inadvertent IV injection during local administration is not dangerous because hyaluronidase is rapidly inactivated by inhibitors in the blood. Do not inject into infected or cancerous tissue; doing so might promote the spread of these conditions.

(Zenk: Neonatal Medications & Nutrition. A Comprehensive Guide 2000; pp:230-232)

Hyaluronidase (Wydase)

Indications and use: Treatment of extravasation injuries.

Actions: An enzyme that temporarily breaks down hyaluronic acid (tissue "cement") and thereby allows the infiltrated drug or solution to be absorbed over a larger surface area. This speeds absorption and reduces tissue contact time with irritant substance.

Route: SC

Dosage: Dilute to 15 units/mL in normal saline. Before it is removed, inject 0.2 mL into the needle that was used to infuse the IV, and four 0.2 mL injections into the leading edge of the extravasation. Elevate the extremity. Do not apply heat. May repeat if necessary.

Adverse effects: Usually well tolerated. Urticaria (rare). Administer hyaluronidase within 1 h of the extravasation, if possible.

(Gomella: Neonatology 1999, p.569)

Hyaluronidase

Dose & Route: Infants and Children: Dilute to 15 U/ml; give 1 ml (15U) by injecting 5 separate injections of 0.2 ml (3U) at borders of extravasation site SC or ID using a 25- or 26-gauge needle

Remarks: **Contraindicated** in dopamine and alpha-agonist extravasation. May cause urticaria. Administer as early as possible (minutes to 1 hour) after IV extravasation.

(Siberry: The Harriet Lane Handbook 2000, p.733)

Hyaluronidase

Use: Increase the dispersion and absorption of other drugs; increase rate of absorption of parenteral fluids given by hypodermoclysis; management of I.V. extravasations

Usual Dosage: Infants and Children: Management of I.V. extravasation: S.C., intradermal: Reconstitute the 150 unit vial of lyophilized powder with 1 mL NS; take 0.1 mL of this solution and dilute with 0.9 mL NS to yield 15 units/mL; using a 25- or 26-gauge needle, five 0.2 mL injections are made subcutaneously or intradermally into the extravasation site at the leading edge, changing the needle after each injection; **Note**: some sites prepare a 150 units/mL solution and, without further dilution, administer 0.2 mL injections subcutaneously or intradermally into the extravasation site at the leading edge

Hypodermoclysis: S.C.: 15 units is added to each 100 mL of I.V. fluid to be administered

Premature Infants and Neonates: Volume of a single clysis should not exceed 25 mL/kg and the rate of administration should not exceed 2 mL/minute

Administration: Do not administer I.V.

Nursing Implications:

Administer hyaluronidase within the first few minutes to 1 hour after the extravasation is recognized

(Taketomo: Pediatric Dosage Handbook 1999-2000, p.450)

HYDRALAZINE (Apresoline)

Supplied: Tablets 10mg, 25mg, 50mg, 100mg
Injection 20mg/ml in 1ml

Administration: IV, PO, IM
Administer diluted or undiluted over 1 to 2 minutes.
Compatible in D5W, NS, LR (5).
Dilution recommended for more accurate dose administration, (authors).
Use hydralazine injection as quickly as possible after drawing through a needle into a syringe. Hydralazine changes color after contact with a metal filter (1).

Extemporaneous Compounding (Recipe)

Dosage form:	Oral suspension
Made from:	Injection
Concentration:	20 mg/5 mL
Stability:	30 days
Store:	Refrigerate

Ingredient	Strength	Quantity
Hydralazine injection	20 mg/mL	20 mL
Propylene glycol		8 mL
Purified water USP		qs ad 100 mL

Instructions: Withdraw the hydralazine injection from ampuls. Mix with the propylene glycol. Transfer to a graduate and qs with water. (11)

Hydralazine Hydrochloride
(Apresoline Hydrochloride)

Indications and use: For hypertension and as an afterload reducing agent to treat congestive heart failure.

Actions: Direct-acting vasodilator that reduces peripheral resistance and blood pressure and relaxes venous capacitance vessels. Reflex increase in heart rate, cardiac output, and stroke volume is probably produced in response to the decrease in peripheral vascular resistance.

Route: IM, IV, PO.

Dosage: IV or IM: 0.1-0.5 mg/kg/dose q6h (maximum: 2 mg/kg/dose).

PO: 0.5-7.0 mg/kg/day divided q6-8h.

Adverse effects: Most frequent are headache, palpitations, and tachycardia; most serious is a reversible lupus-like syndrome. Tachyphylaxis often occurs on chronic therapy.

Comments: Contraindicated in mitral valve rheumatic heart disease.
(Gomella: Neonatology 1999, p.569)

Hydralazine (Apresoline)
THERAPY FOR ACUTE CONGESTIVE CARDIAC FAILURE

Dose and Route of Administration:
0.1 to 0.5 mg/kg/dose i.v. q6-8h

Hemodynamic Effects:
Arteriolar dilation.

Complications and Comments Regarding Use:
Positive ANA

Notes: Hydralazine may be administered intravenously at 0.15 to 0.3 mg/kg over several minutes, or orally at a dose of 0.4 to 8.0 mg/kg/day divided every 6 hours. The maximum daily dose given to adult patients is usually about 400 mg. Effects occur as early as 5 minutes after parenteral infusion and 30 minutes after oral administration, with the peak effects occurring in 30 minutes to 2 hours. The half-life is 2 to 4 hours. Serum concentrations are lower after oral administration than after intravenous administration because of biotransformation by the intestinal wall and hepatic first-pass metabolism. Hydralazine undergoes hepatic acetylation.

The most serious adverse effect of hydralazine is a lupus-like syndrome that has been identified in up to 15% of adults receiving the maximum dose. In a pediatric series, 14% of patients developed positive antinuclear antibody tests. The lupus-like syndrome is most likely to develop in patients who are teated with high doses over long durations, particularly if they are slow acetylators. Although the syndrome may persist for several months, it is reversible after the drug is discontinued. Additional side effects of hydralazine include headaches, gastrointestinal disturbances, rash, fever, reflex tachycardia, and fluid retention.

(Garson: The science and practice of pediatric cardiology 1998, pp.2329-2341)

Hydralazine hydrochloride

Vasodilator Therapy in Children with CHF

Dose/Route of Administration:

0.25-1.0 mg/kg/dose PO q 6-8 hr
7 mg/kg/day max

Disadvantages: May cause lupus-like syndrome, reflex tachycardia, GI symptoms, neutropenia

Clinical Use of Orally Available Vasodilators

Hydralazine hydrochloride is the most common agent to be used as a pure arteriolar vasodilator. It appears to act directly to relax arteriolar smooth muscle, and it is available in both oral and parenteral forms. A common side effect from its use is the development of a lupus-like syndrome with the presence of antinuclear antibodies in the serum. Antibodies and symptoms usually disappear with discontinuation of the drug.

(Garson: The science and practice of pediatric cardiology 1998, pp.2321-2322)

Hydralazine Hydrochloride

Dose & Route: Hypertensive crisis:
Children: 0.1-0.2 mg/kg/dose IM or IV Q4-6 hr PRN; **max dose**: 20 mg/dose

Chronic hypertension:
Infants and children: Start at 0.75-1 mg/kg/24 hr PO ÷ Q6-12 hr (**max dose**: 25 mg/dose). If necessary, increase dose over 3-4 weeks up to a **maximum** of: 5 mg/kg/24 hr for infants.

Remarks: Use with caution in severe renal and cardiac disease. Slow acetylators, patients receiving high dose chronic therapy and those with renal insufficiency are at highest risk of lupus-like syndrome (generally reversible). May cause reflex tachycardia, palpitations, dizziness, headaches, and GI discomfort. Drug undergoes first pass metabolism. Onset of action: PO 45-60 minutes; IV: 10-20 minutes; IM: 5-10 minutes.

Adjust dose for renal failure.

(Siberry: The Harriet Lane Handbook 2000, p.734)

Hydralazine (Apresoline)

Dose:	0.1-0.5 mg/kg IV or IM 0.25-1 mg/kg PO q6-8hr, max. 7 mg/kg/day
Mode of Action:	Direct vasodilator
Adverse Effects:	Hypotension, tachycardia, lupus syndrome, neutropenia, GI upset
Comments:	Used in ventricular dysfunction; aortic, mitral insufficiency

(Garson: The science and practice of pediatric cardiology 1998, p.2951)

HYDROCHLORIC ACID HCL

Supplied: From chemical supply houses: 0.1 normal solution, 1 liter

Comments: Filtration with a 0.22 micron filter has been considered adequate cold sterilization, but pyrogens are not removed.

Hydrochloric Acid (HCL) 0. 1 N

Antidote: Occluded Central Catheters

Dose: 0.2 ml/dose IV per procedure described under Administration

Administration: IV-Concentration: 0.1 Normal (N).

Procedure for Restoring Patency of Occluded Central Catheters Using 0.1 N HCl:

1. Draw up 0.2 ml 0.1 N HCl in a syringe.
2. Instill into a secure central venous cathete, including percutaneous lines, positioned in the superior vena cava.
3. If the catheter will not irrigate or aspirate, instill HCl with gentle repeated push-pull action. The pressure may cause the catheter to balloon. Care must be taken to permit only a *small amount* of ballooning, or the catheter may crack and/or rupture.
4. If the catheter does not clear, allow the HCl to dwell in the catheter for 60 minutes.
5. Attempt to aspirate. When patency is restored, as determined by the ability to aspirate blood freely, withdraw the HCl and 0.5-1 ml of blood to remove residual clot or precipitate and the HCl. It is preferable not to push the HCl into the blood steam; however, Shulman and colleagues state that if the occlusion resolves as the HCl is injected, the excess HCl can be either injected into the patient or withdrawn.
6. Irrigate with normal saline; then flush with 2 ml of heparin/saline; then resume infusion. ***Note***: Before resuming infusion, reassess solution or medications begin infused through the central line to determine cause of occlusion so that it may be corrected. If the

cause may have been a calcium/phosphorus precipitation, reduce the concentration in parenteral nutrition solution.

7. If first attempt is unsuccessful, repeat the procedure.
8. If second attempt is unsuccessful, allow HCl to dwell in catheter overnight.

Compounding: HCl 0.1 N can be compounded by the pharmacy as follows using appropriate sterile technique:

Pharmacist Compounding Directions HCl 0.1 Normal
Using a glass syringe for transfer, add 4.3 ml of 37 percent weight to volume (w/v) HCl to 500 ml sterile water; filter through a filter suitable for strong acids. Use caution in preparing this solution accurately. Concentrated HCl is highly corrosive and should be handled as such. Filtration with a 0.22 micron filter has been considered adequate cold sterilization, but pyrogens are not removed. Package in 3 ml aliquots in sterile 10 ml evacuated glass vials.
Storage: Store at 4°C. Stability: 6 months.

Use: Clearance of central venous catheter occlusions caused by insoluble precipitates, such as calcium and phosphorus, or drugs. Occlusions from drugs that are incompatible with the solution infusing or minerals usually occur rapidly (within 1 day), whereas thrombosis is gradual, over 2-4 days. HCl 0.1 N has been used to clear occlusions from sequential administration of amikacin, piperacillin, vancomycin, and heparin. Salvage of catheters is preferable to premature removal and replacement. (Other agents used to clear occluded catheters are urokinase, ethyl alcohol, and sodium bicarbonate.

Treatment of severe metabolic alkalosis in a neonate and in adults.

Adverse Effects: Administered by the route and in the concentration and volume recommended, HCl is unlikely to cause adverse effects.

Hyperchloremia or metabolic acidosis may occur, but they are unlikely using the 0.2 ml dose recommended. For example, 9 ml of 0.1 N HCl must be given to a 3 kg infant to change the serum bicarbonate level by 1 nmol/liter.

Possible effects include pain and irritation at injection site, thrombophlebitis if used in a peripheral line, and tissue necrosis at extravasation sites. Use only in well-placed central venous catheters. Infiltration into the mediastinum could result in potentially lethal complications. Not for use in umbilical or arterial lines.

Transient febrile reactions have occurred when large volumes (4-17 ml) were infused into the systemic circulation during attempts to clear a line. This has not been reported in other studies where the HCl was aspirated, rather than injected systemically.

Hemolysis is possible with rapid infusion of large amounts.

Nursing Implications:

Generally injected by a physician.
Monitor patient for side effects.

(Zenk: Neonatal Medications & Nutrition. A Comprehensive Guide 2000, pp.236-238)

HYDROCHLOROTHIAZIDE (Esidrix, Hydrodiuril)

Supplied: Tablets 25mg, 50mg, 100mg
Oral solution 50mg/5ml

Administration: PO

<u>Hydrochlorothiazide</u>

Indications and use: Hypertension, pulmonary edema.

Actions: See Chlorothiazide.

Route: PO

Dosage: 1-3 mg/kg/day divided q12h.

Adverse effects & comments: See Chlorothiazide.

(Gomella: Neonatology 1999, p.570)

<u>Hydrochlorothiazide</u>

Route & Dose: PO: 2.0-2.5 mg/kg/day q 12 h

Adverse Effects and Cautions:

Hypercalcemia, hypokalemia, hyperglycemia

(Taeusch: Avery's Diseases of the Newborn 1998, p.1345)

<u>Hydrochlorothiazide</u>

Dose & Route: Neonates and Infants <6 months:
2-4 mg/kg/24 hr ÷ BID PO
≥6 months and Children: 2 mg/kg/ 24 hr ÷ BID PO

Remarks: See chlorothiazide. May cause fluid and electrolyte imbalances, hyperuricemia. Drug may not be effective when creatinine clearance is less than 25-50 ml/min.

(Siberry: The Harriet Lane Handbook 2000, p.734)

<u>Hydrochlorothiazide</u> (Hydrodiuril)

Dose: 2-4 mg/kg/day PO divided BID (200 mg/day max)

Mode of Action: Distal renal tubular inhibition

Adverse Effects: Same as chlorothiazide

Comments: Same as chlorothiazide

(Garson: The science and practice of pediatric cardiology 1998, p.2951)

Hydrochlorothiazide

Usual Dosage: Oral: (daily dosages should be decreased if used with other antihypertensives):

Neonates and Infants <6 months: 2-4 mg/kg/day in 2 divided doses; maximum daily dosage: 37.5 mg

Infants >6 months and Children: 2 mg/kg/day in 2 divided doses; maximum daily dosage: 200 mg

Administration: Oral: Administer with food

Monitoring Parameters:
Serum electrolytes, BUN, creatinine, blood pressure, fluid balance, body weight

(Taketomo: Pediatric Dosage Handbook 1999-2000, pp.452-453)

HYDROCORTISONE

HYDROCORTISONE CYPIONATE (Cortef oral susp.)

Supplied: Oral suspension 10mg/5ml in 120ml
Administration: PO

HYDROCORTISONE SODIUM SUCCINATE (SoluCortef, A-Hydrocort)

Supplied: Injection, powder for 100mg vial, univial, 250mg, 500mg, 1000mg vials
(some products contain benzyl alcohol)

Administration: IV, IM

Direct IV injection: It should be administered over a period of at least 30 seconds to several minutes. For IV infusion, diluted in D5W, NS to a concentration of 0.1-1mg/mL (5).

Hydrocortisone

According to divisional guidelines, a trial of HC administration may be considered by the attending neonatologist if the mean blood pressure remains at or below the 10th percentile for gestational and postnatal age-dependent norms despite volume administration and high-dose pressor/inotrope support. High-dose pressor/inotrope support is arbitrarily defined in the guidelines as the administration of dopamine at doses >20 µg/kg/min or the combined use of dopamine (≥10-15 µg/kg/min) with dobutamine and/or epinephrine. Although the dose of HC may vary according to the underlying pathology and previous steroid administration, in patients with no evidence for severe capillary leak or previous steroid administration, the guidelines recommend 1 mg/kg/dose of HC twice daily for 1 to 3 days. Accordingly, 16 patients in the study received HC at 1 mg/kg/dose twice daily for 1 to 3 days for a total of 17 treatment courses, while the 5 preterm infants with severe capillary leak syndrome and / or previous steroid treatment received 3 to 6 mg/kg/d of

HC divided twice daily or four times daily for 2 to 3 days for a total of 6 treatment courses.

Conclusion: The findings of the present study strengthen the notion that brief HC administration may restore cardiovascular stability in preterm infants with volume- and pressor-resistant hypotension. In addition, this study has demonstrated a rapid increase in blood pressure within 2 hours of the first HC dose followed by a sustained improvement in the cardiovascular status and urine output in this patient population. Based on these findings, we speculate that the non-genomic actions of HC may be responsible for the observed rapid cardiovascular response whereas the genomic actions contribute to the sustained normalization of the blood pressure and the decrease in pressor and inotrope requirements.

Preterm infants with volume- and pressor-resistant hypotension respond to hydrocortisone with rapid normalization of the cardiovascular status and sustained decreases in volume and pressor requirement.

(Seri: Cardiovascular Effects of Hydrocortisone in Preterm Infants With Pressor-Resistant Hypotension. Pediatrics 2001;107:1070-1074)

Hydrocortisone

Indications and use:

Acute adrenal insufficiency, congenital adrenal hyperplasia, and shock.

Actions: A steroid possessing glucocorticoid activity with some mineralocorticoid effects; most effects probably result from modification of enzyme activity, thus affecting almost all body systems. It promotes protein catabolism, gluconeogenesis, renal excretion of calcium, capillary wall permeability and stability, and red cell production; suppresses immune and inflammatory responses.

Route: PO, IV, IM, topical.

Dosage: Acute adrenal insufficiency: 1-2 mg/kg dose IV bolus; then 25-150 mg q24h divided q6h.

Congenital adrenal hyperplasia: Initial dose, 0.5-0.7 mg/kg/q24h divided ¼ in the morning, ¼ at noon, and ½ at night; maintenance dose, 0.3-0.4 mg/kg/q24h divided as above.

Topical (0.5%): Apply to area 3 times daily.

Adverse effects & comments:

See Dexamethasone. Application to large body surface areas may produce absorption with systemic effects. Avoid facial application.

(Gomella: Neonatology 1999, p.570)

HYDROCORTISONE

Indication: For hypoglycemia

Therapy of Neonatal Hypoglycemia*
SYMPTOMATIC INFANT Glucose:200 mg/kg as 2 ml/kg of 10% glucose IV
Following Bolus Infusion, or at Start of Therapy IF INFANT IS ASYMPTOMATIC GLUCOSE: 8 MG/KG/MIN IV
IF GLUCOSE RATES OF 12 MG/KG/MIN REQUIRED FOR NORMOGLYCEMIA HYDROCORTISONE: 5 MG/KG EVERY 12 HOURS IV OR IM
TAPER AND WEAN IV GLUCOSE SLOWLY

IM, INTRAMUSCULARLY; IV, INTRAVENOUSLY
*SEE TEXT FOR REFERENCES.

(Volpe: Neurology of the Newborn 2001, p.517)

SEE GLUCOSE: VOLPE: THERAPY OF NEONATAL HYPOGLYCEMIA

Hydrocortisone

For Treatment of Congenital Adrenal Hyperplasia:

Treatment: Administration of glucocorticoids inhibits excessive production of androgens and prevents progressive virilization. A variety of glucocorticoids (hydrocortisone, prednisone, dexamethasone) and dosage schedules have been used for this purpose. Most often, hydrocortisone (10-20 mg/m^2 per 24 hours) is administered orally in 3 divided doses. There have been recent problems with consistent dosing with the liquid formulation of hydrocortisone. Tablets may give more reliable levels. Infants usually require 2.5 to 5 mg 3 times daily and children, 5 to 10 mg 3 times daily. The morning dose should be given as early as possible to blunt the early morning corticotropin increase that begins during the predawn hours. Doses must be individualized by monitoring growth, bone age, and hormonal levels. Patients with disturbances of electrolyte regulation (salt losers) and elevated plasma renin activity require a mineralocorticoid and sodium supplementation in addition to the glucocorticoid. Maintenance therapy with fludrocortisone acetate (Florinef) (0.05-0.3 mg daily) and sodium chloride (1-3 g) is usually sufficient to normalize plasma renin activity. Increased doses of glucocorticoid are indicated during periods of stress, such as infection or surgery, for salt-losing and non-salt-losing patients.

ABSTRACT. The Section on Endocrinology and the Committee on Genetics of the American Academy of Pediatrics, in collaboration with experts from the fields of pediatric endocrinology and genetics, developed this policy statement as a means of providing up-to-date information for the practicing pediatrician about current practice and controversial issues in congenital adrenal hyperplasia (CAH), including the current status of pre-natal diagnosis and treatment, the benefits and problem areas of neonatal screening programs, and the management of children with nonclassic CAH. The reference list is designed to allow physicians who wish more information to research the topic more thoroughly.

(American Academy Of Pediatrics: Section on Endocrinology and Committee on Genetics. Technical Report: Congenital Adrenal Hyperplasia. Pediatrics 2000;106:1511-1518)

Hydrocortisone

Hydrocortisone was given as hydrocortisone sodium succinate (Solu-Cortef 100 mg Plain, Upjohn, NDC 0009-0825-01), reconstituted with sterile water for injection and diluted with normal saline. The initial dose and dosing interval, 1.0 mg/kg/day (~8-10 mg/m^2/day) given every 12 hours, was chosen based on preliminary data, and estimated to be ~1 to 1 1/2 times the normal basal endogenous production rate. Therapy was given for a total of 12 days: 9 days at 1.0 mg/kg/day, and a 3-day taper at a reduced dose of 0.5 mg/kg/day. All other care was provided at the direction of the attending physician, including the administration of any open-label glucocorticoid therapy.

Conclusions: First, early treatment with low-dose hydrocortisone in this population of extremely low birth weight infants increased the likelihood of survival without CLD. Second, the benefit was particularly apparent in infants with chorioamnionitis. Third, a larger multicenter trial is needed to verify the primary outcome and to better evaluate risks and benefits.

(Watterberg: Prophylaxis Against Early Adrenal Insufficiency to Prevent Chronic Lung Disease in Premature Infants. Pediatrics 1999;104:1258 -1263)

Hydrocortisone

Dose/kg: Congenital adrenal hyperplasia:
Initial: 20-35 mg/m^2/d
Maintenance: 12.5-37.5mg/m^2/d

Route & frequency:
PO divided as follows: 1.4 dose in morning and at noon, ½ dose at night

Comments: Increases chance of infection. May cause hypertension, salt and water retention, adrenal suppression, and hyperglycemia

Hydrocortisone

Dose/kg: Shock: Initial: 35-50 mg/kg
Route & frequency: IV, once

Dose/kg: Maintenance: 12.5-37.5 mg/kg
Route & frequency: IV q6h x 48-72

Dose/kg: Stress dose: 50 mg/m^2/d
Route & frequency: IV, IM divided q12h=q6h

Comments: Approximate weight to body surface area conversion table:

Weight (kg)	M^2
0.5	0.05
1	0.1
2	0.15
3	0.2
4	0.25

(Avery: Neonatology Pathophysiology and Management of the Newborn 1999, p.1557)

Hydrocortisone

Route & Dose: PO, IM, IV: adrenal crisis, 3-10 mg/kg/day;
PO: physiologic replacement, 1 mg/kg/day or
15-25 mg/m^2/day

Adverse Effects and Cautions:
See Cortisone
(Taeusch: Avery's Diseases of the Newborn 1998, p.1345)
(Avery: Neonatology Pathophysiology and Management of the Newborn 1999, p.1556)

IBUPROFEN

Supplied: Orphan drug status
Contact Farmacon Inc. at (203) 431-9989
Administration: IV

Supplied: Suspension: 100 mg/5 ml; in 119 ml and 473 ml
Drops: 100 mg/2.5 ml; in 7.5 ml, 40 mg/ml; in 15 ml
Tabs: chewable: 50 mg; in 24's and 50's, 100 mg, in 24's
Tabs: 100 mg, 200 mg, 400 mg, 600 mg, 800 mg
Administration: PO

Ibuprofen (Advil, Motrin)

Dose: Analgesic: 4-10 mg/kg/dose every 6-8 hours.
Maximum: 40 mg/kg/day.

Antipyretic:

- Temperature <102.5°F (39.2°C): 5 mg/kg/dose.
- Temperature ≥102.5°F (39.2°C): 10 mg/kg/dose.
- Maximum: 40 mg/kg/day in divided doses given every 4-8 hours.

The manufacturers state that neither the safety nor the efficacy of ibuprofen has been established in infants younger than 6 months of age; however, some clinicians are giving this drug to younger infants-for example, to 2-month-old term infants with their first immunizations, to reduce fever and discomfort.

Administration: Supplied as: Suspension: 100 mg/5 ml (=20 mg/ml).
Drops: 40 mg/ml.
PO: Give with feedings to reduce GI upset and risk of GI bleeding. Shake well before use.

Cautions/Contraindications:

Cautions:

- Use caution when administering to infants receiving anticoagulants or to those with decreased hepatic or renal function.
- The antipyretic, analgesic, and anti-inflammatory actions of ibuprofen may mask symptoms of or worsening of infections.
- Use with caution postoperatively.

Contraindications:

- Hypersensitivity to ibuprofen or aspirin.
- Active GI bleeding.
- Do not use in patients with a ductal-dependent lesion because ibuprofen may close the ductus arteriosus. For example, an infant receiving alprostadil (PGE) to maintain ductal patency should not receive ibuprofen.

Nursing Implications:

Monitoring:

- Temperature, if treating fever.

- For signs of pain relief, if treating pain.
- BUN, creatinine, and serum potassium periodically, especially with hepatic or renal dysfunction; in patients being given diuretics concurrently; or with signs of renal toxicity, such as increased blood pressure, fluid retention, or rapid weight gain.
- Periodic hemoglobin/hematocrit; occult blood loss in the stool with prolonged therapy.
- Liver function tests (AST [SGOT]; ALT [SGPT]) if signs and symptoms of hepatotoxicity occur.
- Periodic ophthalmologic exam for patients on long-term treatment for juvenile rheumatoid arthritis (JRA).

If ibuprofen is prescribed for infants outside the hospital, advise parents of the correct dose for the infant's weight; which concentration to use; and to call a health care practitioner if there is no improvement or the condition worsens in 24 hours, if they must give ibuprofen for longer than 3 days, or if inadvertent overdose occurs.

Sponging with tepid water should be considered along with antipyretic medications.

(Zenk: Neonatal Medications & Nutrition. A Comprehensive Guide 2000; pp.245-249)

<u>Ibuprofen</u>

Infants were randomly assigned to receive either intravenous indomethacin (0.2 mg/kg) or intravenous ibuprofen (10 mg/kg). Both drugs were continuously infused over 15 minutes. Regardless of the ductus closure after the first dose, all patients received a second and third dose of indomethacin (0.1 mg/kg) or ibuprofen (5 mg/kg) at 24-hour intervals.

In comparison with indomethacin, ibuprofen did not reduce cerebral BFV in preterm human infants. Ibuprofen, in contrast to indomethacin, does not affect renal or intestinal hemodynamics, although these effects have not been evaluated by Doppler ultrasonography.

We conclude that ibuprofen administration, when used to treat PDA in preterm infants, does not significantly reduce mesenteric and renal BFV.

(Pezzati: Effects of indomethacin and ibuprofen on mesenteric and renal blood flow in preterm infants with patent ductus arteriosus. J Pediatr 1999;135:733-8)

<u>Ibuprofen</u>

The parenteral ibuprofen preparation was obtained as ibuprofen lysine from Merckle Laboratories (Ulm, Germany). Based on an earlier study of ibuprofen for PDA in preterm infants, a loading dose of 10 mg/kg of ibuprofen followed by 5 mg/kg per dose at 12-hours intervals was administered. The route of administration was intravenous or oral depending on tolerance of enteral feeds. Ibuprofen was continued until 28 days of life or until the infants were weaned from the ventilator and oxygen (whichever occurred earlier).

Conclusion: Although a trend toward less ventilator and hospital days in the ibuprofen group was observed in this pilot study, the differences were not statistically significant. The incidence of BPD was similar in both groups. In the study group, two infants developed gastrointestinal complications and a third infant experienced reversible renal failure. The plasma ibuprofen levels were low. Further studies are needed to assess the use of ibuprofen for the prevention and/or treatment of BPD in preterm infants.

(Raju: Ibuprofen Use to Reduce the Incidence and Severity of Bronchopulmonary dysplasia: A pilot Study. Journal of Perinatology 2000; 1:13-16)

<u>Ibuprofen</u>

Study Design: The infants at each unit were randomly assigned to a treatment group by means of cards in sealed opaque envelopes. Each infant received three doses of either indomethacin (Indocin I.V., Merck, West Point, Pa.; 0.2 mg per kilogram at 12 hour intervals) or ibuprofen (an intitial dose of 10 mg per kilogram, followed by two doses of 5 mg per kilogram each, after 24 and 48 hours). The medications were infused continuously over a period of 15 minutes. The doses and intervals for ibuprofen were the same as in our earlier trial and were in accordance with recommendations for use in infants and neonates that were based on preliminary pharmacodynamic data. Ibuprofen was prepared for intravenous use from a commercially available product intended for parenteral administration (Imbun I.M., Merckle, Blaubeuren, Germany).

Results. The rate of ductal closure was similar with the two treatments: ductal closure occurred in 49 of 74 infants given indomethacin (66 percent), and in 52 of 74 given ibuprofen (70 percent) (relative risk, 0.94; 95 percent confidence interval, 0.76 to 1.17; P=0.41). The numbers of infants who needed a second pharmacologic treatment or surgical ductal ligation did not differ significantly between the two groups. Oliguria occurred in 5 infants treated with ibuprofen and in 14 treated with indomethacin (P=0.03). There were no significant differences with respect to other side effects or complications.

Conclusions: Ibuprofen therapy on the third day of life is as efficacious as indomethacin for the treatment of patent ductus arteriosus in preterm infants with the respiratory distress syndrome and is significantly less likely to induce oliguria.

(Overmeire: A Comparison of Ibuprofen and Indomethacin for Closure of Patent Ductus Arteriosus. N Engl J Med 2000;343:674-81)

Ibuprofen

Infants were consecutively assigned within 3 hours of age to treatment with either one dose of ibuprofen lysine (10 mg/kg intravenously) followed by 5 mg/kg per dose intravenously at 24 and 48 hours of age (n=12), one dose of ibuprofen lysine (10 mg/kg intravenously; n=11), or saline (n=11).

Administration of three doses of ibuprofen within 3 hours after birth in preterm neonates reduced the incidence of PDA without causing notable early adverse drug reactions in this phase 1 trial. Early closure of the ductus arteriosus was also associated with better respiratory outcome and earlier discharge from the hospital.

(Varvarigou: Early Ibuprofen Administration to Prevent Patent Ductus Arteriosus in Premature Newborn Infants. JAMA 1996;275:539-544)

IBUTILIDE FUMARATE (Corvert)

Supplied: Injection Solution: 0.1 mg/ml, in 10 ml vials

Administration: Dilution: Ibutilide may be administered undiluted or diluted in 50 ml diluent. Ibutilide may be added to 0.9% sodium chloride or 5% Dextrose injection before infusion.

Ibutilide

Ibutilide is an intravenous class III agent. The drug has not been studied in pediatric patients to date, and the adult data are not extensive, focusing primarily on the drug in acute termination of atrial fibrillation and atrial flutters.

Dosing: IV: 10-25 mcg/kg

Warnings: Torsades de pointes

Dosing: Adult studies have used 10 to 25µg/kg as a bolus over 10 minutes. The bolus may be repeated in 10 minutes.

Side Effects: About 8% of patients experience torsades de pointes ventricular tachycardia. AV block can occur. The drug is teratogenic.

(Gillette: Clinical Pediatric Arrhythmias 1999, pp.231-248)

IMIPENEM/CILASTATIN (Primaxin)

Supplied: Primaxin I.M. Powder for Injection; vials.
500mg imipenem/500mg cilastatin
750mg imipenem/750mg cilastatin
Primaxin I.V. Powder for Injection; vials, IVPB.
250mg imipenem/250mg cilastatin
500mg imipenem/500mg cilastatin

Administration: IM, IV

IM: Use lidocaine 1% as diluent (without epinephrine). The IM formulation is NOT for IV use.

IV: Add 10ML D5W, D10W, NS other to vial. Shake well and dilute this suspension to a final conc. of 2.5 to 5 mg/ML with one of the above diluents. The final solution should be clear. Administration: (adult) 125mg, 250mg, 500mg generally infused over 20-30 minutes; each 1gm dose over 40-60 minutes.

If nausea develops, slow the infusion rate (1).

<u>Imipenem-Cilastatin</u>

Antibacterial Drugs for Newborn Infants
Dose (mg/kg or Units [U]/kg and Frequency of Administration
Route: IV

Dose:

<u>Infants 0-4 wk</u>
BW <1200 g: 25 every 12 h

<u>Infants <1 wk old</u>
BW ≤1200-2000 g: 25 every 12 h
BW >2000 g: 25 every 12 h

<u>Infants ≥1 wk old</u>
BW ≤2000-2000 g: 25 every 8 h
BW >2000 g: 25 every 8 h

Notes: Safety in infants and children has not been established (American Academy of Pediatrics: Report of the Committee on Infectious Diseases. Red Book 2000, pp.651-652)

<u>Imipenem</u> (Primaxin)

Antibacterial Drugs for Pediatric patients Beyond the Newborn Period dosage per kg/d
Route: IV, IM
Mild to Moderate Infections: 40-60 mg in 4 doses
Severe Infections: 60 mg in 4 doses
Comments: Caution in use for therapy of meningitis because of possible seizures

Notes: Inpatient with history of allergy to penicillin or one of its many congeners, alternative drugs are recommended. In some circumstances, a cephalosporin or other β-lactam class drug may be acceptable. However, these drugs should not be used in patients with an immediate hypersensitivity (anaphylaxis) to penicillin because approximately 5% to 15% of penicillin-allergic patients will also be allergic to the cephalosporins.

Not approved for use in patients younger than 12 years old (American Academy of Pediatrics: Report of the Committee on Infectious Diseases. Red Book 2000, pp.657,662)

<u>Imipenem</u>

Route: IV, IM
Dosage (mg/kg) and Interval of Administration

<u>Weight 1200-2000</u>
Age 0-7 Days: 20 q12h
Age >7 Days: 20 q12h

Weight >2000
Age0-7 Days: 20 q12h
Age >7 Days: 20 q8h

(Remington: Infectious Diseases of the Fetus and Newborn Infant 2001, p.1454)

Imipenem-Cilastatin

Dose & Route: Neonates: <1 wk: 40-50 mg/kg/24 hr ÷ Q12 hr IV
1-4 wks: 60-75 mg/kg/24 hr ÷ Q8 hr IV
Children: (4 wks-3 months): 100 mg/kg/24 hr ÷ Q6 hr IV
Children (>3 months): 60-100 mg/kg/24 hr ÷ IV; **max dose**: 4 g/24 hr

Remarks: For IV use, give slowly over 30-60 minutes. Adverse effects: pruritus, urticaria, GI symptoms, seizures, dizziness, hypotension, elevated LFTs, blood dyscrasias, and penicillin allergy. CSF penetration is variable but best with inflamed meninges. Higher doses of 90 mg/kg/24 hr have been used in older children with cystic fibrosis.
Adjust dose in renal insufficiency

(Siberry: The Harriet Lane Handbook 2000, p.737)

IMMUNIZATION

All neonatal intensive care nurseries should implement a policy for the immunization of preterm infants. Preterm infants, including those of low birth weight, should be immunized at the usual chronologic age of 2 months, in most cases. Vaccine doses should not be reduced for preterm infants. If an infant is still in the hospital at 2 months of age, the immunization schedule, including the administration of whole cell or acellular diphtheria-tetanus-pertussis vaccine, *Haemophilus influenzae* conjugate, and hepatitis B and poliovirus in the nursery, oral poliovirus vaccine should not be used.

The dose and schedule for hepatitis B virus vaccination is determined according to the gestational age of the infant and the hepatitis B surface antigen status of the mother. Preterm infants who develop chronic respiratory disease should be given influenza immunization annually in the fall, beginning at 6 months of age.

(AAP/ACOG: Guidelines for Perinatal Care 1997, p.199)

Immunization

Infants born to HBsAg-negative mothers:

Should receive the 1st dose of hepatitis B (Hep B) vaccine by age 2 months. The 2nd dose should be at least 1 month after the 1st dose. The 3rd dose should be administered at least 4 months after the 1st dose and at least 2 months after the 2nd dose, but not before 6 months of age for infants.

Infants born to HBsAg-positive mothers:

Should receive hepatitis B vaccine and 0.5 mL hepatitis B immune globulin (HBIG) within 12 hours of birth at separate sites. The 2nd dose is recommended at 1 to 2 months of age and the 3rd dose at 6 months of age.

Infants born to mothers whose HBsAg status is unknown:

Should receive hepatitis B vaccine within 12 hours of birth. Maternal blood should be drawn at the time of delivery to determine the mother's HBsAg status; if the HBsAg test is positive, the infant should receive HBIG as soon as possible (no later than 1 week of age).

(American Academy of Pediatrics: Report of the Committee on Infectious Diseases. Red Book 2000, p.23)

Immunization in Special Clinical Circumstances

Preterm Infants

Prematurely born infants, including infants of low birth weight, should be immunized at the usual chronologic age in most cases. Some studies suggest a reduced immune response in very-low-birth-weight infants (≤1500 g) immunized by the usual schedule. Additional data are required to better define the optimal immunization schedule for these infants. Vaccine dosages should not be reduced for preterm infants. If an infant is still in the hospital at 2 months of age, the immunizations routinely scheduled at that age should be given, including diphtheria and tetanus toxoids and acellular pertussis (DTaP), *Haemophilus influenzae* type B (Hib) conjugate, and inactivated poliovirus (IPV) vaccine.

The optimal time to initiate hepatitis B immunization in preterm infants with birth weights less than 2 kg whose mothers are hepatitis B surface antigen (HBsAg)-negative has not been determined. Seroconversion rates in low-birth-weight infants in whom immunization was initiated shortly after birth have been reported in some studies to be lower than rates in preterm infants immunized at a later age and in term infants immunized shortly after birth. Hence, initiation of immunization in preterm infants with a birth weight of less than 2 kg whose mother are HBsAg-negative should be delayed until just before hospital discharge if the infant weights 2 kg or more or until approximately 2 months of age when other immunizations are given.

Preterm infants with birth weights less than 2 kg whose mothers are HBsAg-positive should receive Hepatitis B Immune Globulin (HBIG) within 12 hours of birth and concurrent hepatitis B vaccine at different sites. If the maternal HBsAg status is not known, vaccine also should be given in accordance with recommendations for the infant of an HBsAg-positive mother. The maternal HBsAg status should be determined, and HBIG should be given to the infant if the mother is HBsAg-positive. If the birth weight is less than 2 kg and the maternal status cannot be determined within the initial 12 hours of life, HBIG should be given. This initial vaccine dose should not be counted in the required 3 doses to complete the immunizations series. The maternal HBsAg status will determine the subsequent schedule for completion of hepatitis B immunization.

Preterm infants in whom chronic respiratory tract disease develops should be given influenza immunization annually in the fall once they reach 6 months of age. To protect premature infants and infants with other chronic conditions before this age, the family and other caregivers, including hospital personnel, should be immunized against influenza. In addition, infants with a history of premature birth, chronic lung disease, or both may benefit from immunoprophylaxis with palivizumab or Respiratory Syncytial Virus Immune Globulin Intravenous.

(American Academy of Pediatrics: Report of the Committee on Infectious Diseases. Red Book 2000, p.54)

SEE ALSO: HEPATITIS B IMMUNIZATION

IMMUNOSUPPRESSION REGIMEN

Immunosuppression Agents

Heart Transplantation Among 233 Infants During the First Six Months of Life: The Loma Linda Experience

The recipients were given cyclosporine by continuous infusion (0.1 mg/kg/hr) prior to transplantation. Following surgery, cyclosporine was converted to oral dosing after feeding was established (target levels 250-300 ng/ml, using a whole blood assay measuring parent compound). Methylprednisolone (20-25 mg/kg) was given at the induction of anesthesia and every 12 hours following transplantation for a total of 4 postoperative doses. Steroids were not used for maintenance therapy. Azathioprine (3 mg/kg/day) was begun on the first postoperative day and adjusted to keep the leukocyte count greater than 4,000 cells per microliter. Most infants transplanted beyond 30 days of age were also given induction therapy with antithymocyte serum daily for 5 days, beginning immediately after surgery (7).

Recipients were typically discharged on azathioprine and cyclosporine. Target cyclosporine levels were decreased to 150-200 ng/ml after 6 months and again to 100-150 ng/ml after the first year. A small cohort of neonatal recipients has been maintained on cyclosporine monotherapy.

Strategies for treating acute and indolent rejection have included bolus steroids, methotrexate, tacrolimus, mycophenolate mofetil, rabbit antithymocyte serum, equine antithymocyte globulin and, rarely, total lymphoid irradiation.

(Fortuna: Heart transplantation among 233 infants during the first six months of life: the Loma Linda Experience. Loma Linda Pediatric Heart Transplant Group. Clin Transpl 1999;263-272)

Corticosteroids

Transplantation for Congenital Heart Disease

The immunosuppression regimen consists of triple-drug therapy with cyclosporine A, azathioprine, and corticosteroids in many centers. For the first 6 postoperative months, the therapeutic range of blood cyclosporine A levels is 250 to 300 ng/mL. This target level is reduced to 100 to 200 ng/mL thereafter.

More recently, tacrolimus (FK 506) has been used instead of cyclosporine A in some pediatric patients. We have witnessed improved outcomes in high-risk recipients, in particular, children with congenital heart disease. Our criteria for the use of tacrolimus immunotherapy include the presence of congenital heart defects, failure to respond to cyclosporine A, and a history of blood transfusions.

Corticosteroids may result in long-term morbidity in children after heart transplantation. These complications include obesity, hypertension, hyperlipidemia, osteoporosis, cataracts, peptic ulcer disease, and growth retardation. Thus, every attempt is made to wean corticosteroids after the initial 6 months posttransplantation. In many instances these patients will remain immunologically stable on double-drug therapy.

(Odim: Transplantation for congenital heart disease. Adv Card Surg 2000;12:59-76)

INDINAVIR (Crixivan)

Supplied: Capsules 200 mg, 400 mg

Comment: For optimal absorption, administer without food, but with water, 1 hour before or 2 hours after a meal. (1)

Storage/Stability: Store in a tightly closed container at room temperature, 15° - 30°C (59° to 86° F). Protect from moisture. Indinavir capsules are sensitive to moisture. Dispense and store in the original container. Keep the desiccant in the original bottle. (1)

Indinavir/Crixivan

Dosage: Pediatric: Under study in clinical trials: 350-500 mg/m^2 q 8 h

Neonatal: Unknown

(American Academy of Pediatrics: Report of the committee on Infectious Diseases. Red Book 2000, p.687)

Indinavir

Children between the ages of 3 months and 18 years were eligible for enrollment.

Medication was given in following doses: indinavir, 400 mg/m^2 every 8 hours; zidovudine, 120 mg/m^2 every 8 hours; and lamivudine, 4 mg/kg every 12 hours. Indinavir was administered as standard capsules of 200 mg and 400mg or as capsules of 150 mg and 300 mg, which were prepared at the pharmacy. When patients were too young to swallow capsules, indinavir capsules had to be opened by the caregivers and dissolved in 5 to 10 mL of water. In children in whom problems were encountered with the ingestion of indinavir, the drug was changed to nelfinavir (30 mg/kg every 8 hours). Zidovudine was administered either as syrup (10 mg/mL) or as capsules of 100 mg and 250 mg, depending on the child's age. Lamivudine was administered as syrup (10 mg/mL) or as tablets of 150 mg. The importance of taking the indinavir 1hour before or 2 hours after meals was repeatedly emphasized.

Conclusions: Highly active antiretroviral therapy consisting of indinavir, zidovudine, and lamivudine in children reduced HIV-1 RNA to less than 500 copies/mL in 70% of the children within 6 months. Improved CD4 cell counts were observed in most patients, as was a better clinical condition (no invasive or opportunistic infections, increased weight gain). Side effects of the triple therapy were mild. Highly active antiretroviral therapy can be used as successfully in children as in adults.

(van Rossum: clinical and virologic response to combination treatment with indinavir, zidovudine, and lamivudine in children with human immunodeficiency virus-1 infections: A multicenter study in The Netherlands. J. Pediatr 2000;136:780-8)

Indinavir

Usual Dosage: Neonates: Should not be administered to neonates until further studies are performed due to side effect of hyperbilirubinemia

Children: Under study in clinical trials: 500 mg/m^2/dose every 8 hours; maximum dose: 800 mg/dose every 8 hours

(Taketomo: Pediatric Dosage Handbook 2000-2001; pp.514-515)

INDOMETHACIN (Indocin)

Supplied: Injection, powder for 1mg vial

Administration: IV - Administer IV push over a period of 5 to 10 seconds. Add 1 to 2ml NS or SWFI (without benzyl alcohol) to vial for a concentration of approximately 0.1mg/0.1ml and 0.05mg/0.1ml respectively. Discard any unused portion of the solution. Prepare a fresh solution just prior to each administration (1).

Indomethacin (Indocin IV)

Indications and use: Pharmacologic closure of patent ductus arteriosus (PDA).

Actions: Nonsteroidal anti-inflammatory drug (NSAID) with analgesic and antipyretic properties. Action is principally by inhibition of prostaglandin synthesis, thus inhibiting cyclooxygenase, an enzyme that catalyzes the formation of prostaglandin precursors (endoperoxides) from arachidonic acid. Decreases cerebral blood flow.

Route: IV

Dosage: PDA closure: IV at 12- to 24-h intervals. Indocin should be given q12h unless the patient has decreased urinary output.

Initial dose: 0.2 mg/kg.

Second dose: <48 hours: 0.1 mg/kg
2-7 days: 0.2 mg/kg
>8 days: 0.25 mg/kg

Third dose: <48 hours: 0.1 mg/kg
2-7 days: 0.2 mg/kg
>8 days: 0.25 mg/kg

Prevention of intraventricular hemorrhage: 0.1 mg/kg IV at 6 and 12 h postnatal and q24h for 2 more doses.

Adverse effects: May cause decreased platelet aggregation, transient oliguria (decreased glomerular filtration rate), increased serum creatinine, increased serum concentrations of renally eliminated drugs such as gentamicin, hyponatremia, hyperkalemia, hypoglycemia. Displaces bilirubin from albumin binding sites but is not considered clinically significant.

Comments: Contraindicated in necrotizing enterocolitis (NEC) or when stool Hematest > 3 +, BUN >30 mg/dL, serum creatinine >1.8 mg/dL, urine output <0.6 mL/kg/h for the preceding 8 h, in thrombocytopenia (<60,000/mm^3), with active bleeding, or if there has been intraventricular bleeding within the preceding 7 days (controversial).

(Gomella: Neonatology 1999, p.571)

Indomethacin

Indication: Prophylactic

All premature infants delivered at ≤27 6/7 weeks' gestation and admitted within the first 15 hours after birth to the William H. Tooley Intensive Care Nursery between January 1, 1992, and December 31, 1997, were eligible for this study. During this time interval 2 separate approaches were used to treat the patent ductus arteriosus: a "symptomatic approach" (from January 1992 through December 1994; n = 170) and a "prophylactic approach" (January 1995 through December 1997; n = 130). All infants in the prophylactic approach era received indomethacin within 15 hours after birth; none of these infants had an echocardiographic examination before they received indomethacin because it was assumed that 90% would still have a patent ductus arteriosus at that time.[7] In contrast, infants in the symptomatic treatment era did not receive indomethacin unless there were clinical signs of a PDA (see following text) or a PDA was visualized on a screening echocardiographic examination at 4 days after birth. All infants in the symptomatic approach era had an echocardiographic examination within the first 5 days.

Indomethacin treatment consisted of 3 doses (0.2 mg/kg, 0.1 mg/kg, and 0.1 mg/kg). Infants in the prophylactic group received their 3 doses during a 48-hour period (at 0, 24, and 48 hours, respectively); in contrast, infants in the symptomatic group or those infants receiving indomethacin outside the prophylactic period received their 3 doses during a 36-hour period (0, 12, and 36 ours).

Conclusion: Prophylactic indomethacin improved the rate of permanent ductus closure by increasing the degree of initial constriction. Prophylactic indomethacin did not affect the remodeling process, nor did it alter the inverse relationship between infant maturity and subsequent reopening. Even when managed with prophylactic indomethacin, the rate of ductus reopening remained unacceptably high in the most immature infants.

(Narayanan: Prophylactic indomethacin: Factors determining permanent ductus arteriosus closure. J Pediatr 2000; 136:330-7)

Indomethacin

Dose/kg:

Doses (mg/kg) No. 1	No. 2	No. 3	Route and frequency IV q8h-q12h x 3 doses:
0.2	0.1	0.1	<48 h of life
0.2	0.2	0.2	2-7 d
0.2	0.25	0.25	>7 d

Dose/kg: Extended treatment: 0.2 mg

Route & frequency: IV qd x 5 days following standard three-dose regimen with extended 1 x may decrease recurrence of PDA

Prevention of IVH; 0.1 mg/kg q24h for three doses, beginning at 6-12 h of age

Comments: Decreases GFR. Decreases platelet aggregation

(Avery: Neonatology Pathophysiology and Management of the Newborn 1999, p.1557)

Indomethacin (Indocin)

Dose: 0.05-0.25 µg/kg/min IV

Mode of Action: Prostaglandin inhibition (cyclooxygenase)

Adverse Effect: Decreased urine output, platelet inhibition

Comments: Contraindicated in patients with decreased urine output, elevated BUN/creatine, decreased creatine clearance, active IVH, NEC, and thrombocytopenia

(Garson: The science and practice of pediatric cardiology 1998, p.2954)

Indomethacin

Indomethacin Overdose:

Therefore we cannot conclude that this magnitude of dosing error does not increase morbidity in these fragile infants. What we can say is that the occurrence of a 10-fold indomethacin overdose does not necessarily lead to catastrophic complications in the preterm infant. We are currently using drug dosing tables that already have the appropriate dose calculated for infant weights between 450 and 3000 g. By removing the need to perform calculations, we hope to reduce the number of future overdoses.

(Narayanan: Incidence and outcome of a 10-fold indomethacin overdose in premature infants. J Pediatr 1999;135:105-7)

Indomethacin

Contraindications:

Hypersensitivity to indomethacin, any component, aspirin, or other nonsteroidal anti-inflammatory drugs (NSAIDs); active GI bleeding, ulcer disease; premature neonates with necrotizing enterocolitis, impaired renal function (eg, neonates with urine output <6.6 mL/kg/hour or serum creatinine ≥mg/dL), IVH, active bleeding, thrombocytopenia

Adverse Reactions:

Cardiovascular: Hypertension, edema

Central nervous system: Somnolence, fatigue, depression, confusion, dizziness, headache

Dermatologic: Rash

Endocrine & metabolic: Hyperkalemia, dilutional hyponatremia (I.V.), hypoglycemia (I.V.)

Gastrointestinal: Nausea, vomiting, epigastric pain, abdominal pain, anorexia, GI bleeding, ulcers, perforation

Hematologic: Hemolytic anemia, bone marrow suppression, agranulocytosis, thrombocytopenia, inhibition of platelet aggregation

Hepatic: Hepatitis

Ocular: Corneal opacities

Otic: Tinnitus

Renal: Renal failure, oliguria

Miscellaneous: Hypersensitivity reactions

Drug Interactions:

Indomethacin may increase serum concentrations of digoxin, methotrexate, lithium, and aminoglycosides (reported with I.V. use in neonates); may increase nephrotoxicity of cyclosporin; may decrease antihypertensive and diuretic effects of furosemide and thiazides; may increase serum potassium with potassium-sparing diuretics; may decrease antihypertensive effects of beta-blockers, hydralazine, and captopril; aspirin may decrease and probenecid may increase indomethacin serum concentrations; other GI irritants (eg, potassium supplements, NSAIDs) may increase GI adverse effects

Stability: I.V. product: Protect from light; not stable in alkaline solution; reconstitute just prior to administration; discard any unused portion; do not use preservative-containing diluents for reconstitution; will precipitate if reconstituted with solutions at pH <6 (product is not buffered)

Usual Dosage: Patent ductus arteriosus:
Neonates: I.V.: Initial: 0.2 mg/kg, followed by 2 doses depending on postnatal age (PNA)
PNA **at time of first dose** <48 hours: 0.1 mg/kg at 12-24-hour intervals
PNA **at time of first dose** 2-7 days: 0.2 mg/kg at 12-24-hour intervals
PNA **at time of first dose** >7 days: 0.25 mg/kg at 12-24-hour intervals

In general, may use 12-hour dosing interval if urine output >1 mL/kg/hour after prior dose; use 24-hour dosing interval if urine output is <1 mL/kg/hour but >0.6 mL/kg/hour; doses should be withheld if patient has oliguria (urine output <0.6 mL/kg/hour) or anuria

Administration: Parenteral: I.V.: Administer over 20-30 minutes at a concentration of 0.5-1 mg/mL in preservative free sterile water for injection or preservative free NS
Note: Do **not** administer via I.V. bolus or I.V. infusion via an umbilical catheter into vessels near the superior mesenteric artery, as these may cause vasoconstriction and can compromise blood flow to the intestines. Do not administer intra-arterially

Monitoring Parameters:
BUN, serum creatinine, liver enzymes, CBC with differential; in addition, in neonates treated for PDA: heart rate, heart murmur, blood pressure, urine output, echocardiogram, serum sodium, platelet count, and serum concentrations of concomitantly administered drugs which are renally eliminated (eg, aminoglycosides, digoxin); periodic ophthalmic exams with chronic use

Additional Information:
Indomethacin may mask signs and symptoms of infections; fatalities in children have been reported, due to unrecognized overwhelming sepsis, drowsiness, lethargy, nausea, vomiting, seizures paresthesia, headache, dizziness, tinnitus, GI bleeding, cerebral edema, and cardiac arrest have been reported with overdoses

(Taketomo: Pediatric Dosage Handbook 1999-2000, pp.482-484)

Indomethacin

Group A-Intravenous (IV) indomethacin at 0.2 mg/kg by a 1-minute rapid injection for the first dose and then 0.1 mg/kg, again by rapid injection, every 12 hours for two additional doses (total indomethacin dose 400 mcg/kg);

OR

Group B-IV indomethacin infusion at 11 mcg/kg/hour to run for 36 hours [total dose 396 mcg/kg], providing essentially the same total dose of indomethacin as received by Group A.

Slow, continuous infusion eliminated the decrease in cerebral flow velocity and appears to be effective in closing the PDA.

(Hammerman: Continuous Versus Multiple Rapid Infusions of Indomethacin: Effects on Cerebral Blood Flow Velocity. Pediatrics 1995;95:244-248)

INOSITOL

Supplied: Tablets: 250, 500, 650mg
Powder: ¼ tsp equals 375mg, in 25, 60, 100, 120, 500 grams

Administration: PO, no IV formulation available.

Comment: Inositol, an isomer of glucose, is present in cell membrane phospholipids and plasma lipoproteins. No specific role in human nutrition has been established.(1)

Inositol

Inositol (myo-inositol) or placebo (glucose) was given as a 5 percent (wt/vol) intravenous infusion for 5 to 30 minutes. The infusion was first given from 4 to 12 hours after birth and subsequently at 12-hour intervals. The dosage was 80 mg per kilogram of body weight per day, given for five days. If the infant remained dependent on a respirator, required supplemental oxygen, and could not tolerate the amount of fluid given during enteral feeding (80 ml per kilogram per day), the five-day treatment regimen was repeated beginning on day 10 or day 20 or both. The administration of inositol or placebo was discontinued if anuria or oliguria developed (urine output, <1 ml per kilogram per hour or blood urea nitrogen, >23 mmol per liter [>33 mg per deciliter]), if hyperglycemia necessitated lowering the glucose infusion rate to less than 2 mg per kilogram per minute, or if the amount of enteral fluid exceeded 80 ml per kilogram per day.

Eighty-one infants given inositol and 51 given placebo survived without bronchopulmonary dysplasia (71 percent vs 55 percent; P = 0.005). In the 65 infants given surfactant, however, inositol had no effect on the degree of respiratory failure. Thirteen infants given inositol and 21 given placebo had retinopathy of prematurity (13 percent vs 26 percent; P = 0.0222); none of the infants given inositol had stage 4 disease, whereas 7 of those given placebo did (0 percent vs 9 percent; $P = 0.012$).

We propose that in premature infants in the first week of life, parenteral nutrition and enteral feeding should be supplemented with inositol so that the intake of inositol equals that from breast milk.

(Hallman: Inositol supplementation in infants with respiratory distress syndrome. N Engl J Med 1992;326:1233-1239)

INSULIN, REGULAR

Supplied: (100 Units/ml)
Regular Insulin (from pork)
Regular Purified Pork
HUMULIN R human insulin (rDNA)
NOVOLIN R human insulin (rDNA)

Administration: IV, SQ

Insulin, Regular

Indications and use:
Hyperglycemia, hyperkalemia, increase caloric intake in infants with glucose intolerance on parenteral nutrition.

Actions: Hormone derived from the beta cells of the pancreas and the principal hormone required for glucose utilization. In skeletal and cardiac muscle and adipose tissue, insulin facilitates transport of glucose into these cells. Stimulates lipogenesis and protein synthesis and inhibits lipolysis and release of free fatty acids from adipose cells. Promotes intracellular shift of potassium and magnesium.

Note: Should be diluted by the pharmacy to 1 unit/mL in diluent provided by the manufacturer to improve accuracy in measurement and avoid overdose.

Route: IV, SC.

Dosage: Hyperglycemia: Loading dose, 0.1 unit/kg/dose infused IV over 15-20 min; maintenance dose, 0.02-0.1 unit/kg/h by continuous IV infusion (titrate with hourly determinations of blood glucose until stable, then q4h) (dilute insulin as above).

Hyperkalemia: Give calcium gluconate, 50 mg/kg/dose IV, and sodium bicarbonate IV, 1 meq/kg/dose IV, first; then give dextrose, 600-800 mg/kg/dose, and insulin, 0.2 unit/kg/dose IV (3-4:1 glucose:insulin ratio).

Increase caloric intake for infants on parenteral nutrition: 0.02-0.1 units/kg/h IV as continuous infusion. Monitor serum glucose q hour until stable, the q4h.

Adverse effects: Hypoglycemia (may cause coma, severe CNS injury), hyperglycemic rebound (Somogyi effect), urticaria, anaphylaxis.

Comment: Human insulin (preferred) is less antigenic than pork-derived insulin, which is less antigenic than beef-derived insulin. Insulin adsorbs to plastic surfaces of IV systems. In concentrations of 10 units/L, ~ 50% of the insulin binds to the tubing. At greater concentrations ~ 5 units/L binds to the IV tubing. Adjust dose as needed.

(Gomella: Neonatology 1999, pp.571-572)

<u>Insulin</u>

Dose/kg: Hyperglycemia:
Initial: 0.1 U
Route & Frequency: IV once, over 15-20 min

Dose/kg: Maintenance: 0.02-0.1 U/h
Route & Frequency: IV, continuous infusion

Dose/kg: Intermittent: 0.1-0.2 U
Route & Frequency: SC q6-12h

Dose/kg: Hyperkalemia:
0.3 U/g of glucose
Route & Frequency: IV, with glucose: 500 mg/kg/dose

Comments: Monitor blood glucose and titrate dose accordingly; may cause rebound hyperglycemia if discontinued abruptly. Use only human regular insulin for IV infusions.

(Avery: Neonatology Pathophysiology and Management of the Newborn 1999, p.1557)

<u>Insulin, Regular</u>

Indications: Hyperglycemia

Dosage/route/frequency:
Load: 0.1 U/kg/dose regular insulin, IV x 15-20 min;
Maintenance: 0.02-0.1 U/kg/h, regular insulin;
Intermittent dose: 0.1-0.2 U/kg/ q6-12h, SC

Clinical considerations:
Dilute initial concentration to 0.1-1 U/ml in 0.9% normal saline

Indications: VLBW with hyperglycemia

Dosage/route/frequency:
0.02-0.4 U/kg/h, IV; adjust conc. to keep infusion rates ≤ 0.1 ml/h

Clinical considerations:
Titrate to keep blood glucose: 100-150

Indications: Hyperkalemia

Dosage/route/frequency:
First administer calcium gluconate 50 mg/kg/dose IV, + sodium bicarbonate: 1 mEq/kg/dose IV; follow with dextrose 300-600 mg/kg/dose + regular insulin 0.2 U/kg/dose Iv (3-4:1 glucose to insulin ratio)

Monitoring: Follow blood glucose concentration, q30 min after starting infusion and after changes in infusion rate. Follow these parameters of q2-4h after achieving a stable euglycemic state.

Clinical Considerations:

Reduce loss of insulin due to adsorption to the plastic tubing by flushing tubing with the insulin solution prior to beginning the infusion or by adding albumin 0.3 g/100 ml of solution.

Adverse Reactions:

Hyperglycemic rebound (Somogyi effect), urticaria, anaphylaxis; may rapidly induce hypoglycemia. Insulin resistance may develop with prolonged use and necessitate an increased dose.

(Cloherty: Manual of Neonatal Care 1998, p.713)

<u>Insulin, Regular</u>

Indication: For diabetes mellitus

Patient 1:

A male infant was born by cesarean section at 36 weeks' gestation to a 39-year-old woman (gravida 4, para 3, abortion 1) of mixed European Descent.

Glucose control was maintained with a total insulin dose of 1 to 1.2 U/kg/d for the first 2 months of life. By 3 months of age, the child was euglycemic on every preprandial glucose determination, and the insulin dose was reduced. Insulin therapy was discontinued at 4 months, and hemoglobin A_{1c} (5.2% was normal at 5 months and remains normal.

Patient 2:

A 2.26 kg male infant was born at 39 weeks' gestation to a 23-year-old woman (gravida 1, para 1) by normal spontaneous vaginal delivery. On the third hospital day an insulin drip (0.05 U/kg/h) was started, and the infant was transferred to The University of Chicago Hospitals.

Physical examination demonstrated a normal-appearing infant. Initially, insulin supplementation up to 2.5 U/kg/D was required to control glucose levels. After blood sugar control was achieved, the child was weaned from the continuous insulin infusion to subcutaneous insulin (1 to 1.6 U/kg/d). At home the insulin requirement fell progressively over the first month of therapy to ~0.6 U/kg/day; however, the child could not be completely weaned. Home monitoring continued to show variation in blood glucose levels; the child continuously required insulin of at least 0.3 U/kg/d. The child continues to receive insulin therapy after 5 years.

(Christian: Significance of genetic testing for paternal uniparental disomy of chromosome 6 in neonatal diabetes mellitus. J Pediatr 1999;134:42-6)

<u>Insulin</u>

For both concentrations of insulin (0.5 and 0.25 U/ml), the intravenous system was "flushed" to the 7 ml mark on the syringe before initiation of collection....loss of insulin was noted with both solutions (0.5 U/ml), under the nonflushed condition only 55.9% of the prescribed dose for the first 2 hours was delivered before the delivery rate of the flushed system, 71.4%, was approached....This study supports the practice of preflushing intravenous administration sets to deliver a more predictable amount of insulin with time.

(Simeon: Continuous insulin infusion in neonates: Pharmacologic availability of insulin in intravenous solutions. J Pediatr 1994;124:818-820)

INTERFERON ALFA-2A (Roferon-A)

Supplied: Injection Soln.: 3 million IU/vial. 6 million units/ml, 9 million units/0.9ml, 36 million units/ml
Powder for Injection: 6 million IU/1mL in 18 million IU/vial with diluent.

Administration: SC or IM

Interferon Alfa-2A

We evaluated the effects of daily subcutaneous injections of interferon alfa-2a (up to 3 million units per square meter of body-surface area) in 20 neonates and infants with life-threatening or vision threatening hemangiomas that failed to respond to corticosteroid therapy... Interferon alfa-2a appears to induce the early regression of life-threatening corticosteroid-resistant hemangiomas in infancy.

(Ezekowitz: Interferon alfa-2a therapy for life-threatening hemangiomas of infancy. N Engl J Med 1992;326:1456-1463)

INTRAOSSEOUS ACCESS

Intraosseous Cannulation (Cannulation of Intramedullary Sinuses)

Intravenous access is difficult to achieve in an emergency, and delay in obtaining this access can compromise the effectiveness of resuscitation. Intraosseous access, initially described in the 1940s, provides a safe and reliable method for rapidly achieving a route for administration of drugs, fluids, and blood products into a noncollapsible marrow venous plexus during resuscitation of children, particularly those 6 years old or younger. Intraosseous access can be reliably achieved in 30 to 60 seconds in most cases, even by healthcare providers with minimal experience.

In general, any intravenous drug or fluid required during the resuscitation of children can be safely administered by the intraosseous route. Reports of successful administration of catecholamines, calcium, antibiotics, digitalis, heparin, lidocaine, atropine, sodium bicarbonate, phenytoin, neuromuscular blocking agents, crystalloids, colloids, and blood can be found in the literature.

Continuous infusions of catecholamines can also be accomplished by the intraosseous route. Onset of action and drug levels following intraosseous infusion during CPR are comparable to those achieved following intravenous administration, and levels similar to those achieved after central venous administration have been documented in pediatric arrest models. Fluid required for rapid volume resuscitation and administration of viscous drugs and solutions should be administered under pressure to overcome resistance of emissary veins that lead from the intramedullary cavity to the general circulation via microscopic channels in the bony cortex.

Complications: Animal studies have shown that local effects of intraosseous infusion on the bone marrow and long-term effect on bone growth are minimal. Microscopic pulmonary fat and bone marrow emboli have been reported but do not appear to be clinically significant. Complications following intraosseous infusion have been reported in fewer than 1% of patients, but they are often more serious than those associated with peripheral vein infusion. Reported complications include tibial fracture, compartment syndrome, skin necrosis, and osteomyelitis. Although uncommon, these complications may be severe. Therefore, intraosseous infusion should be reserved for the treatment of critically ill infants and children and used as a temporary measure until other venous access sites become available.

Devices: Two types of intraosseous needles are available for use in infants and children: specially designed intraosseous infusion needles and Jamshidi-type bone marrow aspiration needles. Short, wide-gauge spinal needles with internal stylets are not recommended for intraosseous use because they are thin-walled and bend easily. They can be used in an emergency if no alternative is available. Standard hypodermic needles should *not* be used for intraosseous infusion, because they often become clogged with bone and bone marrow.

Drugs administered via the intraosseous route must be followed by a sterile saline flush of at least 5 mL to ensure that the drug is delivered to the central circulation. Fluids must be administered under pressure using an infusion pump or pressure bag or with manual injection using a syringe.

Site: The flat, anteromedial surface of the tibia, approximately 1 to 3 cm below the tibial tuberosity, is the preferred site for infants and children less than 6 years of age, since the marrow cavity in that location is very large and the potential for injury to adjacent tissues is minimal.

Note: Whenever possible, hand washing and sterile technique should be performed. During resuscitation, however, vascular access must be achieved as quickly as possible, so some of the following steps (indicated by *) may have to be omitted. Universal precautions should always be taken.

1. Locate the site of cannulation. The tibial tuberosity is identified by palpation, and the site of intraosseous cannulation is approximately 1 to 3 cm below this tuberosity on the medial surface of the tibia, approximately one finger's width below and just medial to the tibial tuberosity. At this site the tibia is just under the skin surface.

*2. Wash hands.

3. Put on gloves.

4. Cleanse the skin over the insertion site with an antiseptic solution.

5. Check the needle and ensure that the bevels of the outer needle and internal stylet are properly aligned.

6. Grasp the thigh and knee above the lateral to the insertion site with the palm of the nondominant hand. Wrap the fingers and thumb around the knee to stabilize the proximal tibia. Do not allow any portion of your hand to rest behind the insertion site. The leg should be supported on a firm surface.

7. Palpate the landmarks and again identify the flat surface of the tibia just below and medial to the tibial tuberosity.

8. Insert the needle through the skin over the flat anteromedial surface of the tibia already identified.

9. Advance the needle through the bony cortex of the proximal tibia, directing the needle perpendicular (90°) to the long axis of the bone or slightly caudad (toward the toes) to avoid the epiphysial plate, using a gentle but firm twisting or drilling motion.

10. Stop advancing the needle when a sudden decrease in resistance to forward motion of the needle is felt. This decrease in resistance usually indicates entrance into the bone marrow cavity. It is possible to aspirate bone marrow at this point. Any aspiration of bone marrow must be followed by irrigation to prevent obstruction of the needle with marrow.

11. Unscrew the cap and remove the stylet from the needle.

12. Stabilize the intraosseous needle and slowly inject 10 mL of normal saline through the needle. Check for any signs of increased resistance to injection, increased

circumference of the soft tissues of the calf, or increased firmness of the tissue.

13. If the test injection is successful, disconnect the syringe, evacuate any air remaining in the connection tubing, and join an infusion set to the needle. Secure the needle and tubing with tape and support it with a bulky dressing.

14. If the test injection is unsuccessful (ie, infiltration of the normal saline into the leg tissue is observed), remove the needle and attempt the procedure on the other leg.

Insertion is successful and the needle is clearly in the marrow cavity if the following conditions are present:

- A sudden decrease in resistance to insertion occurs as the needle passes through the bony cortex into the marrow.
- The needle can remain upright without support.
- Marrow can be aspirated into a syringe joined to the needle, although this is not consistently achieved.
- Fluid flows freely through the needle without evidence of subcutaneous infiltration.

If the needle becomes obstructed with bone or bone marrow, it can be replaced with a second needle passed through the same cannulation site, provided no evidence of infiltration is observed. If evidence of infiltration is observed or if the test injection fails, a second attempt at intraosseous cannulation should be performed on the contralateral tibia.

(American Academy of Pediatrics. American Heart Association. Pediatric Advance Life Support. 1997, pp.5-5,5-6)

IODINE (Lugol's Solution, Iodide, Strong Iodine Solutin)

Supplied: 5% Iodine and 10% Potassium Iodide in 120ml, 480ml
Tablets: 130mg potassium iodide, scored

Administration: PO

Iodine

Dosage: One drop 3 times per day PO

(Fanaroff: Neonatal-Perinatal Medicine 1997, p.1750)

Iodide

Dose: Carefully, 2 mg/kg/day is administered to counter sympathomimetic over-stimulation. It has an additive effect when added to thioamides (propylthiouracil and methimazole).

Complications: Include bradycardia, hypoglycemia, and congestive heart failure.

(Rapaport: Neonatal thyrotoxicosis. Pediatr Rev 1989;10:216)

IOPANOIC ACID (Telepaque)

Supplied: Tablet 500 mg
Administration: PO

<u>Iopanoic Acid</u> (Telepaque)

For neonatal Graves disease

Treatment was initiated with propranolol, 1.4 mg/kg per day initially and later increased to 2 mg/kg per day, and iopanoic acid (Telepaque), 500 mg orally once every third day. Treatment with propranolol and iopanoic acid was discontinued at age 60 days. Diarrhea developed at age 6 weeks and persisted after all medications were discontinued. This problem responded to a change in formula.

(Transue: Management of neonatal Graves disease with iopanoic acid. J Pediatr 1992;121:472-474)

IPRATROPIUM BROMIDE (Atrovent)

Supplied: Aerosol: Each actuation in 14 gm metered dose inhaler delivers 18 mcg.
Solution for inhalation 0.02% (500mcg/vial). Preservative free.
Nasal spray: 0.03% each. Spray delivers 21mcg, 30ml bottle (345 sprays), 0.06% each spray delivers 42mcg, 15ml bottle (165 sprays)

Administration: Inhalation.
It is an anticholinergic (parasympatholytic) which appears to inhibit vagal mediated reflexes by antagonizing the action of acetylcholine (1).

<u>Ipratropium Bromide</u> (Atrovent)

Indications and use: Bronchodilator.

Actions: Anticholinergic drug that acts by antagonizing acetylcholine at the parasympathetic sites, thereby inhibiting parasympathetic bronchoconstriction.

Route: Nebulization

Dosage: Nebulization: 250 mcg given q8h. dilute to 3 mL with normal saline or concurrent albuterol.

Adverse effects: Rebound airway hyperresponsiveness following discontinuation. Nervousness, dizziness, nausea, blurred vision, dry mouth, exacerbation of symptoms, airway irritation, cough, palpitations, rash, and urinary difficulty. Use with caution in narrow-angle glaucoma or bladder neck obstruction.

Comments: Compatible when admixed with albuterol if given within 1h.

(Gomella: Neonatology 1999, p. 572)

<u>Ipratropium</u>

Use: Anticholinergic bronchodilator used in bronchospasm associated with asthma, COPD, bronchitis, and emphysema; symptomatic relief of rhinorrhea associated with allergic and nonallergic rhinitis

Usual Dosage: Neonates: Nebulization: 25 mcg/kg/dose 3 times/day
Infants and Children: Nebulization: 125-250 mcg 3 times/day

Administration: Nasal spray: Pump must be primed before usage by 7 actuations into the air away form the face; if not used for >24 hours, pump must be reprimed with 2 actuations; if not used >7 days, reprime with 7 actuations

Nebulization: May be administered with or without dilution

(Taketomo: Pediatric Dosage Handbook 1999-2000, pp.492-493)

IRON DEXTRAN (InFeD)

Supplied: Injection 50mg iron per mL in 2mL

Administration: IM, IV

Warning: The parenteral use of complexes of iron and carbohydrates has resulted in anaphylactic-type reactions. Deaths associated with such administration have been reported; therefore, use iron dextran injection only in those patients in whom the indications have been clearly established and laboratory investigations confirm an iron-deficient state not amenable to oral iron therapy (1).

Administration: Staining of the skin can be minimized by using a separate needle to withdraw the drug from the container and by displacing the skin laterally prior to injection ("Z-Track Technique") (5). Iron dextran also has been administered by intravenous infusion over one to six hours after dilution in N.S. (5).

Iron Dextran

Dose & Route: Inject test dose (see comments) Iron deficiency anemia: Total replacement dose of iron dextran (ml) = 0.0476 x wt(kg) x (desired Hgb [g/dl] – measured Hgb [g/dl]) + 1 ml/5 kg body weight (up to max of 14 ml).

Acute blood loss: Total replacement dose of iron dextran (ml) = 0.02 x blood loss (ml) x hematocrit expressed as fraction. Assumes 1 ml of RBC = 1 mg elemental iron.

If no reaction to test dose, give remainder of replacement dose ÷ over 2-3 daily doses.

Max daily (IM) dose:
<5 kg: 0.5 ml (25 mg)
5-10 kg: 1 ml (50 mg)
>10 kg: 2 ml (100 mg)

Remarks: Oral therapy with iron salts is preferred. Numerous adverse effects including anaphylaxis, fever, hypotension, rash, myalgias, arthralgias. Use "Z-track" technique for IM administration. **Inject test dose**: 25 mg IM/IV (12.5 mg for infants).

May begin treatment dose after 1 hour. **Maximum** rate of IV infusion: 50 mg/min. for IV infusion, diluting in NS may lower the incidence of phlebitis. Direct IV push administration is **NOT** recommended. **Not** recommended in infants <4 months of age. Compatible with parenteral nutrition solutions.

(Siberry: The Harriet Lane Handbook 2000, p.743)

Iron Dextran (Sucrose)

Forty-two premature infants (<33 weeks' gestation, <1500 gm at birth) were randomly assigned to receive either parenterally administered iron sucrose (elemental iron, 6 mg/kg per week) or ferrous lactate (elemental iron, 12 mg/kg per day), given orally. Both groups were given rHuEpo (Eprex, from Janssen-Cilag), 600 U/kg per week in three divided doses subcutaneously....The parenteral preparation of iron used was iron sucrose (Venofer, Vifor International, St. Gallen, Switzerland), which was given by intravenous infusion within 72 hours of entry; supplements were given weekly thereafter. The medication was administered for 1 hour in 10 ml of normal saline solution with the use of a syringe pump....High doses of both orally administered iron and intravenously administered iron sucrose appear to supply sufficient iron for erythropoiesis in stable infants. Storage iron may become depleted after oral supplementation. The intravenous preparation appears to be safe and maintains serum ferritin concentrations, and it may be indicated for patients with low ferritin levels and for those not established on enteral feedings.

(Meyer: A comparison of oral and intravenous iron supplementation in preterm infants receiving recombinant erythropoietin. J Pediatr 1996;129:258-263)

Iron Dextran

Twenty-six very-low-birth-weight newborns were randomized to receive a TPN solution with or without IV iron.

The Iron group received 200 to 250 μg/kg/d as iron dextran in addition to the iron that is normally present as a contaminant.

A total iron intake of 400 μg/kg/d, half of which was provided by IV iron, is not sufficient to maintain iron balance or to meet fetal accretion rates (1000 μg/kg/d) in very-low-birth-weight newborns receiving total parenteral nutrition. Furthermore, endogenous iron from blood transfusions does not provide an adequate supply of iron.

(Friel: Intravenous Iron Administration to Very-Low-Birth-Weight Newborns Receiving Total and Partial Parenteral Nutrition. Journal of Parenteral and Enteral Nutrition 1995;19:114-118)

SEE ALSO: FERROUS SULFATE

ISOETHARINE (Bronkosol)

Supplied:	Solution for nebulization: 1% solution (many more)
Administration:	Inhalation
Comment:	Products contain sulfites.

	Isoetharine
Route:	Inhalation
Neonatal Dose:	0.25 mL/dose q4-6h
Pediatric Dose:	0.25-0.5 mL/dose q4-6h
Discussion:	Dilute these doses with 2 mL of normal saline and inhale through nebulizer as needed.

(Rudolph: Rudolph's Pediatrics 1996, p.2188)

Isoetharine (Bronkosol)

Lung mechanics and lower airway function were measured and compared before and after administration of aerosolized isoetharine early in the course of ECMO and again several days after ECMO. . . . During the second test approximately 2 wks later (post-ECMO), isoetharine increased MEF25 by 123 +/- 29% and increased the MEF25/FVC by 40 +/- 13% compared with baseline values. . . . Airway obstruction in infants recovering from severe meconium aspiration syndrome is partially reversible with aerosolized isoetharine.

(Koumbourlis: Contribution of airway hyperresponsiveness to lower airway obstruction after extracorporeal membrane oxygenation for meconium aspiration syndrome. Crit Care Med 1995;23:749-54)

ISONIAZID (Nydrazid, INH)

Supplied: Tablets: 50 mg, 100mg, 300 mg
Syrup 50mg/5ml
Injection 100mg/ml in 10ml

Administration: PO, IM
Oral and IM doses of isoniazid are identical (3).

Comments: Take on an empty stomach, at least 1 hour before or 2 hours after meals; it may be taken with food to decrease GI upset.

Although the parenteral product is manufactured for intramuscular use several reports of its use as a constant infusion and rapid intravenous injection are published. Unfortunately these reports are scanty in detail regarding specific administration protocols and most do not document the patient's reactions to the injection. Because most of the reports have used rapid infusion injection of the parenteral form of isoniazid, this may be the best way to administer the parenteral form of Isoniazid. Until further information concerning isoniazid's stability in various diluents and the patients response to such administration are documented, infusion of Isoniazid in a diluted form cannot be recommended. (10)

Isoniazid (INH)
Antituberculosis Drugs in Children

Daily Dose (mg/kg)	Twice Weekly Dose (mg/kg/per dose)
10-15	20-40

Although neonates usually tolerate INH well, some experts recommend routine biochemical monitoring in the first several months of therapy. the usual dosage of INH in children is 10 to 20 mg/kg per day, to a maximum of 300 mg per day. INH is available in tablets of 100 to 300 mg. A syrup on INH in sorbitol (10 mg/ml) appears to be satisfactory; however, it is unstable at room temperature and should be kept cool. Many children develop significant gastrointestinal intolerance (nausea, vomiting) while taking the INH suspension, but neonates and infants tolerate the lower required volume of suspension well. If tablets are used, they are easily crushed in a dessert spoon and given with some soft food such as applesauce, mashed banana, thawed undiluted frozen orange juice, or another palatable medium. The crushed tablets should not be added to the nursing bottle or offered in milk or water because they will be ingested only partially.

(Remington: Infectious Diseases of the Fetus and Newborn Infant 2001, p.1188)

Isoniazid

Route: PO, IM.

Dosage: 50 mg/5 ml syrup
10-20 mg/kg/day q 12-24h (MAX: 300 mg)
NON-NEWBORN SECTION

(Nelson: Pocket Book of Pediatric Antimicrobial Therapy. 2000-2001, p.78)

Isoniazid (INH, Laniazid, Nydrazid)

Classification: Antituberculous agent.

Action & spectrum:
Bactericidal effect on growing tubercle bacilli by interfering with lipid and protein synthesis. Spectrum includes *Mycobacterium* spp (eg, *M tuberculosis, M kansasii, M avium*).

Route: PO, IM.

Dosage: Primary tuberculosis: 10-15 mg/kg/day divided q12-24h with rifampin for 9-12 months.

Skin test conversion: 10-15 mg/kg/day PO q24h for 9 months.

Adverse effects: Peripheral neuropathy, seizures, encephalopathy, blood dyscrasias, allergy.

(Gomella: Neonatology 1999, p.572)

Isoniazid (INH, Nydrazid, Laniazid)

Dose & Route: Prophylaxis:
Infants and Children: 10-15 mg/kg (up to 300 mg) PO QD. After 1 month of daily therapy and in cases where daily compliance cannot be ensured, may change to 20-40 mg/kg (up to 900 mg) per dose PO, given twice weekly.

Treatment:
Infants and Children: 10-15 mg/kg (up to 300 mg) PO QD or 20-30 mg/kg (up to 900 mg) per dose twice weekly with Rifampin for uncomplicated pulmonary tuberculosis in compliant patients.

Remarks: Should **not** be used alone for treatment. Peripheral neuropathy, optic neuritis, seizures, encephalopathy, psychosis, hepatic side effects may occur with higher doses, especially in combination with Rifampin. Follow LFT's monthly. Supplemental pyridoxine (1-2 mg/kg/24hr) is recommended. May cause false positive urine glucose test. Inhibits hepatic microsomal enzymes; decrease dose of carbamazepine, diazepam, phenytoin and prednisone. May be given IM (same as oral doses) when oral therapy is not possible. **Adjust dose in renal failure**

(Siberry: The Harriet Lane Handbook 2000, p.745)

Isoniazid

Route: PO
Neonatal Dose: Prophylaxis: 10 mg/kg/24 h as single dose or divided q12h

Pediatric Dose: Prophylaxis: 10 mg/kg/24 h as single dose or divided q12h and continue for 1 y

Route: IM, PO
Neonatal Dose: Therapy: 10-20 mg/kg/24 h q8-12h
Pediatric Dose: Therapy: 10-30 mg/kg/24 h q8-12h

Discussion: Monitor hepatic function monthly even though incidence of hepatitis in <20-y olds is rare; adverse reactions more common with slow acetylators; supplement adolescents with vitamin B_6 10 mg for each 100 mg of isoniazid taken; use vitamin B_6 as antidote for INH toxicity.

(Rudolph: Rudolph's Pediatrics 1996, p.2188)

ISOPROTERENOL (Isuprel)

Supplied: Injection, solution 1:5000 (0.2mg/ml) in 1ml, 5ml, 10ml
Injection: (1:50,000), 10ml
Solution for inhalation: 0.5%, 1%,
Aerosol: 0.25%; 0.2% (80 mcg/dose)

Administration: IV, Inhalation
Dilution for IV injection: Dilute 1ml of 1:5000 solution (0.2mg) to 10ml with NS or D5W
IV infusion: Dilute 10ml of 1:5000 solution (2mg) in 500ml D5W or dilute 5ml of 1:5000ml (1mg) in 250ml D5W (1).

Isoproterenol (Isuprel, Others)

Indications and use: Shock, cardiac arrest, Adams-Stokes syndrome, ventricular arrhythmia due to AV block, bronchospasm.

Actions: Acts on both β_1-and β_2-adrenergic receptors with minimal or no effect on alpha receptors in therapeutic doses. Relaxes bronchial smooth muscle, cardiac stimulation (inotropic and chronotropic), and peripheral vasodilation (reduces cardiac afterload).

Route: IV, inhalation.

Dosage: IV: 0.05-0.5 mcg/kg/min (titrate).
Inhalation/nebulization: 0.1 mL to maximum of 0.5 mL/dose. Dilute to 2 mL with normal saline, given q4h prn.

Adverse effects: Tremor, vomiting, hypertension, tachycardia, cardiac arrhythmias.

Comments: Contraindicated in hypertension, degenerative heart disease, hyperthyroidism, tachycardia caused by digoxin toxicity, and preexisting cardiac arrhythmias. Increases cardiac oxygen consumption out of proportion to increase in cardiac oxygen output. Not considered an inotropic agent of choice.

(Gomella: Neonatology 1999, p.572)

Isoproterenol

Dose: 0.05-0.4 µg/kg/min

Mode of Action: Potent β-agonist, peripheral vasodilator, transient decrease in PAP

Adverse Effects: Ventricular ectopy, tachycardia, hypotension if hypovolemic, headache

Comments: Useful in symptomatic bradycardia, *do not* mix with any drugs

(Garson: The science and practice of pediatric cardiology 1998, p.2950)

Isoproterenol

THERAPY FOR ACUTE CONGESTIVE CARDIAC FAILURE

Slow infusion rates of isoproterenol, beginning at 0.01 to 0.05 µg/kg/minute, are useful as a temporary measure in patients with some forms of symptomatic bradycardia. A positive inotropic response from isoproterenol usually requires higher infusion rates, in the range of 0.05 to 0.1 µg/kg/minute. The dosage can be increased as long as tachycardia is minimal, because excessive tachycardia has been associated with myocardial ischemia. As indicated earlier, isoproterenol may be particularly beneficial for the management of elevated pulmonary vascular resistance in patients with a limited chronotropic response. The intravascular volume may require supplementation in patients placed on isoproterenol infusion to avoid significant hypotension with reduced cardiac output.

(Garson: The science and practice of pediatric cardiology 1998, pp.2329-2341)

<u>Isoproterenol</u>

Dose & Route: Aerosol: 1-2 puffs up to 6x/24 hr

Nebulized solution:
Children: 0.05 mg/kg/dose = 0.01 ml/kg/dose of 0.5% Sol (**min dose**: 0.5 mg; **max dose**: 1.25 mg) diluted with NS to 2 ml Q4 hr PRN

IV Infusion:
Children: 0.05-2 mcg/kg/min; start at minimum dose and increase every 5-10 min by 0.1 mcg/kg/min until desired effect or onset of toxicity; **max dose**: 2 mcg/kg/min

Sublingual:
Children: 5-10 mg/dose Q3-4 hr; **max dose**: 30 mg/24 hr

Remarks: Use with care in CHF, ischemia, or aortic stenosis. May cause flushing, ventricular arrhythmias, profound hypotension, anxiety, and myocardial ischemia. Patients with continuous IV infusion should have heart rate, respiratory rate, and blood pressure monitored. **Not** for treatment of asystole or for use in cardiac arrests, unless bradycardia is due to heartblock. Continuous infusion use for bronchodilatation must be gradually tapered over a 24-48 hr period to prevent rebound bronchospasm. Tolerance may occur with prolonged use.

(Siberry: The Harriet Lane Handbook 2000, pp.745-746)

<u>Isoproterenol</u>

Indication: Raises both heart rate and cardiac output, lowers pulmonary vascular resistance.

Intravenous Dose: 0.01-0.5 μg/kg/min.

Major Side Effects: Increase in myocardiac oxygen consumption, sinus tachycardia, tachyarrhythmias.

(Klitzner: Pharmacology and Therapeutics in Pediatric Cardiology 1994, pp.1099-1125)

ITRACONAZOLE (Sporanox)

Supplied: Capsules 100 mg
Oral Solution 10 mg/ml, in 150 ml bottle
Injection 10 mg/ml, in kit including 25 ml amp, 50 ml bag of 0.9% NaCl injection, USP, and 1 filtered infusion set.

Comment: Do not use capsules and oral solution interchangeably. Only the oral solution has been demonstrated effective for oral or esophageal candidiasis. (1)

Oral Solution: If possible, do not take with food.

Itraconazole

Suggested Dosage of Antifungal Agents for Infants with systemic or Severe Local Fungal Infection

Dosage (mg/kg per day): 10

Itraconazole, another azole antifungal agent, has not been used extensively in children. Bhandari and Narange reported its use in two premature infants with disseminated candidiasis. Both received 10 mg/kg per day in two divided doses for 3 and 4 weeks, respectively. Both infants did well without any evidence of toxicity.

(Remington: Infectious Diseases of the Fetus and Newborn Infant 2001, p.838)

KANAMYCIN (Kantrex)

Supplied: Injection, pediatric 75mg/2ml
Injection 500mg/2ml, 1gm/3ml

Administration: IV, IM
Stable in D5W or NS for 24 hours (3).
Concentration for central catheter 6mg/mL, peripheral vein 5mg/ml. Duration of infusion 30 minutes (6)

<u>Kanamycin</u> (Kantrex)

Antibacterial Drugs for Pediatric Patients Beyond the Newborn Period
Dosage per kg/d

Route: IV, IM
Mild to Moderate Infections: Inappropriate

Severe Infections: 15-22.5 mg in 3 doses

Comments: 30 mg in 3 doses is recommended by some consultants

Note: Dosages for the aminoglycosides may differ from those recommended by the manufacturers (see package insert).
(American Academy of Pediatrics: Report of the Committee on Infectious Diseases. Red Book 2000, pp.653, 662)

<u>Kanamycin Sulfate</u> (Kantrex)

Classification: Aminoglycoside.

Action and spectrum:
Mechanism of action is identical to that of gentamicin sulfate. Active primarily against Gram-negative aerobic bacteria, including *Escherichia coli*, *Klebsiella*, *Enterobacter*, *Serratia*, *Proteus* spp; and some *Pseudomonas* spp. Some activity against staphylococci and mycobacteria. Not active against other Gram-positive organisms or anaerobes.

Route: IV (infuse over 30 min), IM.

Dosage: Base the initial dose on body weight, then monitor levels and adjust using pharmacokinetics.

<1.2 kg, 0-4 weeks old:
- 7.5 mg/kg/dose q18-24h.

1.2-2 kg:
- 0-7 days old: 7.5 mg/kg/dose q12-18h.
- >7 days old: 7.5 mg/kg/dose q8-12h.

>2 kg:
- 0-7 days old: 10 mg/kg/dose q12h.
- >7 days old: 10 mg/kg/dose q8h.

Elimination and metabolism:
Primarily renally excreted by glomerular filtration. Half-life is 4-8 h

Adverse effects: See Gentamicin Sulfate.

Comments: See Gentamicin Sulfate. Desired serum peak is 25-35 mcg/mL (sample obtained 30 min after infusion is complete) and serum trough is <10 mcg/mL (sample obtained 30 min to just prior to next dose). In general, a set of serum peak and trough levels should be obtained at about the fourth maintenance dose. Monitor serum creatinine every 3-4 days. Excessive serum peak levels are associated with ototoxicity; excessive trough levels with nephrotoxicity.

(Gomella: Neonatology 1999, pp.572-573)

KAYEXALATE (Sodium polystyrene sulfonate, SPS suspension)

Supplied: Powder for 1-pound jars
Oral, rectal suspension 15 gms in 60ml, Na content=65mEq per 60 ml

Administration: PO, PR
IN VIVO exchange rate of 1 mEq of potassium per gram of resin. In VITRO exchange rate is 3.1 mEq of potassium per gram. The range is so large that electrolyte balance must be monitored. Onset of action after oral administration ranges from 2 to 12 hours, and is longer after rectal administration (1).

Sodium Polystyrene Sulfonate (Kayexalate)

Indications and use: Treatment of hyperkalemia.

Actions: Cation exchange resin that releases sodium in exchange for other cations such as potassium. Each gram of resin exchanges 1 meq sodium for each milliequivalent potassium removed. Other cations such as calcium, magnesium, and iron are also bound.

Route: PO, PR (prepare in ~25% sorbitol solution).

Dosage: 1 g of resin will exchange 1 meq of potassium. Usual dose is 1 g/kg/dose PO q6h or q2-6h PR.

Adverse effects: Large doses may cause fecal impaction. Hypokalemia, hypocalcemia, hypomagnesemia, and sodium retention may occur.

(Gomella: Neonatology 1999, p.590)

Kayexalate

Dose & Route: Children:
Usual dose: 1 g/kg/dose Q6 hr PO or Q2-6 hr PR

Remarks: Note: Suspension may be given PO or PR.
Practical exchange ratio is 1 mEq K per 1 g resin. May calculate dose according to desired exchange.

1 mEq Na delivered for each mEq K removed. Use **cautiously** in presence of renal failure. May cause hypokalemia, hypomagnesemia, and hypocalcemia. Do **not** administer with antacids or laxatives containing Mg or Al. Systemic alkalosis may result. Retain enema in colon for at least 30-60 minutes.

(Siberry: The Harriet Lane Handbook 2000, pp.849-850)

Sodium Polystyrene Sulfonate

Use: Treatment of hyperkalemia

Contraindications: Hypernatremia; intestinal obstruction or perforation (oral use)

Warnings: Avoid using the commercially available liquid product in neonates due to the preservative content. Enema may be prepared with powder and diluted with sorbitol 10% solution or oral solution may be made by dilution with 25 % sorbitol solution. Treatment with this drug alone may be insufficient to rapidly correct severe hyperkalemia; other more rapidly effective appropriate measures should be used; enema will reduce the serum potassium faster than oral administration, but the oral route will result in a greater reduction over several hours.

Precautions: Use with caution in patients with severe CHF, hypertension, or edema; small amounts of magnesium and calcium may also be lost in binding

Adverse Reactions:

Endocrine & metabolic: Hypokalemia, hypocalcemia, hypomagnesemia, hypernatremia

Gastrointestinal: Anorexia, nausea, vomiting, constipation, intestinal necrosis

Usual Dosage: Children:
Oral: 1 g/kg/dose every 6 hours
Rectal: 1 g/kg/dose every 2-6 hours
(Taketomo: Pediatric Dosage Handbook 1999-2000, p.829)

KETAMINE (Ketalar)

Supplied: Injection 10mg/ml in 20ml
Injection 50mg/ml in 10ml
Injection 100mg/ml in 5ml

Administration: IM, IV

Comment: DO NOT inject 100mg/ml concentration IV without proper dilution.

Administer slowly (over 60 seconds). More rapid administration may result in respiratory depression and enhance pressor response.

Dilute the 100mg/ml concentration with an equal volume of water, NS or D5W for IV administration (1).

Ketamine Hydrochloride (Ketalar)

Indications and use:

Ketamine is a rapid-acting general anesthetic agent for short diagnostic and minor surgical procedures that do not require skeletal muscle relaxation.

Actions: Dissociates the cortex from the limbic system. Induces coma, analgesia, and amnesia. The patient appears to be awake but is immobile and unresponsive to pain. Increases cerebral blood flow and cerebral oxygen consumption; improves pulmonary compliance and relieves bronchospasm.

Pharmacokinetics: Onset and duration: Unconsciousness:
IV: 30 s, lasts 5 - 10 min.
IM: 3-4 min, lasts 12-25 min.
Analgesia lasts 30-40 min.
Amnesia lasts for 1-2 h. Concurrent narcotics or barbiturates prolong recovery time.

Route: IV, IM, PO.

Dosage: IV: 0.5 -1 mg/kg/dose.
IM: 3 -7 mg/kg/dose.
PO: 6 mg/kg/dose.
Dilute before administration. Repeat doses are 1/2 of initial doses. Reduce the dose in hepatic dysfunction.

Adverse effects: Avoid use of ketamine in patients in whom increased intracranial pressure, cerebral blood flow, CSF pressure, cerebral metabolism, or significant elevation in blood pressure may present a risk.

Cardiovascular: Elevated blood pressure (frequent), tachycardia, arrhythmia, hypotension, bradycardia, increased cerebral blood flow, and decreased cardiac output may occur.

Respiratory: Respiratory stimulation, transient and minimal respiratory depression, and apnea after rapid IV administration of high doses; laryngospasm; and hypersalivation. Gag and cough reflexes are generally preserved.

Ophthalmic: Nystagmus, increased intraocular pressure.

CNS: Emergence reactions (psychic disturbances such as hallucinations and delirium lasting up to 24 h). Minimize by reducing verbal, tactile, and visual simulation in the recovery period. These occur less commonly in pediatric patients than in adults. Severe reactions can be treated with a benzodiazepine. Increased muscle tone that may resemble seizures and extensor spasm with opisthotonos may occur in infants receiving high, repeated doses.

Dermatologic: Rash as well as pain and redness at the IM injection site.

Comments: Pretreatment with a benzodiazepine 15 min prior to ketamine may reduce side effects such as psychic, circulatory, increased intracranial pressure and cerebral blood flow; tachycardia; and jerky movements. Monitor heart rate, respiratory rate, blood pressure, and pulse oximetry. Observe for CNS side effects during the recovery period. Have equipment for resuscitation available.

(Gomella: Neonatology 1999, pp.573-574)

Ketamine (Ketalar)

Dose & Route: Children:
Sedation:
PO/PR: 4-6 mg/kg x 1
IM: 2-3 mg/kg x 1
Induction of General Anesthesia:
IV: 0.5-3 mg/kg

Remarks: **Contraindicated** in elevated ICP, hypertension, aneurysms, thyrotoxicosis, CHF, angina, and psychotic disorders. May cause hypertension, hypotension, emergence reactions, tachycardia, laryngospasm, respiratory depression, and stimulation of salivary secretions. Benzodiazepine may be added to prevent emergence phenomenon. Anticholinergic agent may be added to decrease hypersalivation. Rate of IV infusion should **not** exceed 0.5 mg/kg/min or be administered in less than 60 seconds.

(Siberry: The Harriet Lane Handbook 2000, pp.749-750)

Ketamine

Dosage: 0.5-4 mg/kg i.v. initially, supplement every 30-60 min p.r.n. with 0.25-2 mg/kg i.v.

Comments: Not recommended for infants less than 3 mo

(Allen: Moss and Adam's Heart disease in Infants, Children, and Adolescents 2001, pp.1460-1468)

Ketamine (Ketalar)

Dose: IV: 0.5-1 mg/kg/dose. Average amount is 2 mg/kg/dose for 5-10 minutes of surgical anesthesia.
Maximum: 4.5 mg/kg/dose.

- Continuous Infusion: 10-15 mcg/kg/minute IV.
- Alternatively: A loading dose of 1-2 mg/kg IV, followed by a continuous infusion of 0.5-1 mg/kg/hour has been recommended.

IM: 3-7 mg/kg/dose. **Maximum**: 13 mg/kg/dose.

PO: 6 mg/kg/dose, diluted.

Repeat doses are half the initial dose as often as required. The larger the dose, the longer the time to recovery.

Reduce dose in hepatic dysfunction.

Administration: IV-Rate: 0.5 mg/kg/minute. Infuse over at least 1 minute

IV-Concentration: Dilute to 1-2 mg/ml. may dilute with D_5W, NS, or sterile water. Maximum: 2 mg/ml.

IM-concentration: 100 mg/ml.

Compatibility: May dilute with sterile water, normal saline, or dextrose.

Nursing Implications:

Initiate conscious sedation precautions and monitoring, including frequent continuous vital sign monitoring and pulse oximetry, when used in the nonintubated patient for procedure.

Monitor for respiratory depression, heart rate, respiratory rate, and blood pressure postanesthesia, especially in infants with cardiac decompensation and/or hypertension. Observe for CNS side effects during recovery period.

Have emergency equipment at bedside.

(Zenk: Neonatal Medications & Nutrition. A Comprehensive Guide 2000; pp:271-273)

KETOCONAZOLE (Nizoral)

Supplied: Tablet 200mg
Cream 2%, Shampoo 2%

Administration: PO, Topical

Ketoconazole

Recommended Doses of Parenteral and Oral Antifungal Drugs

Route: PO

Dose (per day): Children-: 3.3-6.6 mg/kg per day, single dose

Adverse Reactions:

Hepatotoxicity, gastrointestinal tract symptoms, rash, anaphylaxis, thrombocytopenia, hemolytic anemia, gynecomastia, adrenal insufficiency; cardiac toxicity is possible inpatients also taking terfenadine or astemizole

Notes: Interactions with other drugs are common. Consult the *Physicians' Desk Reference*, a drug interaction reference or database, or a pharmacist before prescribing these medications.

For children 2 years old and younger, the daily dose has not been established

(American Academy of Pediatrics: Report of the Committee on Infectious Diseases. Red Book 2000, p.671)

Ketoconazole

Suggested Dosage of Antifungal Agents for Infants with systemic or Severe Local Fungal Infection

Dosage (mg/kg per day): 9

(Remington: Infectious Diseases of the Fetus and Newborn Infant 2001, p.838)

Ketoconazole

Ketoconazole, an oral, water-soluble imidazole derivative, has been demonstrated to have activity against *Candida,*

Coccidioides, Histoplasma, Blastomyces, and dermatophytes as well as other fungi. This antifungal agent has been effective in patients with a variety of cutaneous and systemic fungal infections. Of particular interest is the use of ketoconazole in patients with dermatophyte infections, especially when griseofulvin has failed. In addition, it appears to be very effective in patients with chronic mucocutaneous candidiasis. Heel reviewed the use of ketoconazole in newborns and infants with candidiasis, and Hensey and Cooke successfully treated a premature infant who had systemic candidiasis with ketoconazole. Yinnon and colleagues reported the successful use of ketoconazole with 5-fluorocytosine in an infant infected with *C. lusitaniae* that was resistant to amphotericin B.

(Remington: Infectious Diseases of the Fetus and Newborn Infant 2001, p.837)

<u>Ketoconazole</u>

Route: PO
Dosage: 3.3-6.6 mg/kg/day Q24 hr (max 800 mg/day)
NON-NEWBORN SECTION

(Nelson: Pocket Book of Pediatric Antimicrobial Therapy 2000-2001, p.79)

<u>Ketoconazole</u>

Blastomycosis (North American), systemic infection
Therapy: Itraconazole 200-400 mg/day (adults), (?) 4 mg/kg/day (pediatric dosage not established) PO <u>OR</u> amphotericin B (as above) for severe disease; x 6 mos.
Comments: Alternative: ketoconazole 6 mg/kg/day PO div q12-24 hr

Coccidioidomycosis, systemic infection
Therapy: Amphotericin B (as above) for severe, non-CNS disease <u>OR</u> (for non-life threatening disease) itraconazole 200 mg PO bid (adult dose) <u>OR</u> fluconazole 6-12 mg/kg once daily for meningitis
Comments: Consider intrathecal amphotericin B for Fluconazole failures in meningitis

Histoplasmosis, systemic infection
Therapy: Amphotericin B 0.5 mg/kg IV daily <u>OR</u> (for non-life-threatening disease) itraconazole 200 mg bid PO (adults)
Comments: Ketoconazole (as above) as alternative

Paracoccidioidomycosis, systemic infection
Therapy: Itraconazole 100 mg/day PO (adult) <u>OR</u> amphotericin B 0.5 mg/kg IV daily or longer
Comments: Ketoconazole (as above) as alternative; Sulfa drugs less effective but inexpensive

(Nelson: Pocket Book of Pediatric Antimicrobial Therapy 2000-2001, pp.56-57)

Ketoconazole (Nizoral)

Classification: Antifungal agent.

Action and spectrum:

A broad-spectrum antifungal agent that acts by disrupting cell membranes. Fungicidal against *Blastomyces dermatitidis*, *Candida* spp, *Coccidioides immitis*, *Histoplasma capsulatum*, *Paracoccidioides brasiliensis*, and *Phialophora* spp. Development of resistance is rare.

Route: PO

Dosage: 2.5-5 mg/kg/day q24h.

Elimination and metabolism: Hepatic metabolism.

Adverse effects: Gastric distress is the most common side effect. Hepatic damage is rare.

Comments: Penetration into CSF is poor, so do not use in the treatment of fungal meningitis. Minimum period of treatment for candidiasis is 1-2 weeks, but duration should be based on clinical response. Monitor liver function tests. Limited experience in neonates.

(Gomella: Neonatology 1999, p.574)

LABETALOL (Normodyne, Trandate)

Supplied:	Tablets 100mg, 200mg, 300mg Injection 5mg/ml
Administration:	IV, PO Administer by DIRECT IV injection over 2 minutes. Stable in D5W and NS, at a concentration of 1.25 to 3.75 mg/ml for 24 hours (1). The maximum effect usually occurs within 5 minutes of each injection (1).

Extemporaneous Compounding (Recipe)

Dosage form:	Oral suspension
Made from:	Tablets
Concentration:	40 mg/mL
Stability:	60 days
Store:	Refrigerate
Label:	Shake well

Ingredient	Strength	Quantity
Labetalol hydrochloride tablets	300 mg	16
Ora-Sweet or Ora-Sweet SF		
Ora-plus		aa qs 120 mL

Instructions: Crush the tablets in a mortar and reduce to a fine powder. Add a small amount of vehicle and mix to a uniform paste. Add geometric amounts of vehicle to almost desired volume while mixing. Transfer to a graduate and qs to volume while mixing. (11)

Labetalol Hydrochloride (Normodyne)

Indications and use:
Treatment of hypertension. IV form is used to control severe hypertension.

Actions: Causes a dose-related decrease in blood pressure through α-, β_1-, and β_2-blocking actions without causing significant reflex tachycardia or a decrease in heart rate. Reduces elevated renins.

Pharmacokinetics:
Peak effect PO is 1-4 h after the dose; peak effect IV is 5-15 min. Metabolized in the liver by glucuronidation. Oral labetalol has a bioavailability of only 25% due to extensive first-pass effect. Oral absorption is improved by taking with food. Concomitant oral cimetidine may increase the bioavailability of oral labetalol.

Route: PO, IV, continuous IV infusion.

Dosage: Limited experience in neonates; carefully monitor blood pressure, heart rate, and electrocardiogram, and adjust the dose accordingly, Use the lowest effective dose.
PO: 3-4 mg/kg/day PO in 2 divided doses.
IV: 0.2 -0.5 mg/kg/dose over 2-3 min.
Continuous IV infusion: 0.2-1 mg/kg/h (1 mg/mL dilution).

Adverse effects: Orthostatic hypotension, bronchospasm, nasal congestion, edema, congestive heart failure, bradycardia, myopathy, and rash. Intensifies AV block. Reversible hepatic dysfunction (rare). Do not discontinue chronic labetalol abruptly; rather, discontinue gradually over 1-2 weeks. Do not use in patients with asthma, overt cardiac failure, heart block, cardiogenic shock, or severe bradycardia. May cause a paradoxic increase in blood pressure in patients with pheochromocytoma. Use with caution in hepatic dysfunction. Incompatible wit sodium bicarbonate.

Comments: Use caution in converting from the PO to IV route of administration because a much smaller dose is required IV than PO.

(Gomella: Neonatology 1999, p. 574)

Labetalol

Dose/kg: Bolus: 0.25 mg

Route & frequency: IV over 2 min

Dose can be doubled and repeated every 10 min until desired clinical response or total dose of 4 mg/kg is reached

Comments: Absolute contraindications: CHF, heart block, sinus tachycardia

Maintenance:

Dose/kg: 0.25-1 mg

Route & frequency: IV q4h

Dose/kg: 1.5-2mg

Route & frequency: PO q12h

Dose/kg: 0.25-1.5 mg/kg/h

Route & frequency: Continuous IV infusion, max conc 1 mg/mL

Comments: May cause bradycardia, edema, and bronchospasm

(Avery: Neonatology Pathophysiology and Management of the Newborn 1999, p.1557)

Labetolol

Dosage: 0.25-1.0 mg/kg i.v.

Comments: May administer by continuous infusion (0.4-3.0 mg/kg/h)

(Allen: Moss and Adam's Heart Disease in Infants, children and Adolescents 2001, pp.1460-1468)

Labetalol

Dose & Route: Children:

PO: Initial: 4 mg/kg/24 hr ÷ BID. May increase up to 40 mg/kg/24 hr

IV: Hypertensive emergency:

Intermittent dose: 0.2-1 mg/kg/dose Q10 min PRN; **max** 20 mg/dose

Infusion: 0.4-1 mg/kg/hr, to **max** of 3 mg/kg/hr; may initiate with a 0.2-1 mg/kg bolus; **max bolus**: 20 mg

Remarks: **Contraindicated** in asthma, pulmonary edema, cardiogenic shock, and heart block. May cause orthostatic hypotension, edema, CHF, bradycardia, AV conduction disturbances, bronchospasm, urinary retention, and skin tingling. Patient should remain supine for up to 3 hours after IV administration.

Onset of action: PO: 1-4 hours; IV: 5-15 minutes

(Siberry: The Harriet Lane Handbook 2000, pp.751-752)

LAMIVUDINE (3TC, Epivir, Epivir-HBV)

Supplied: Tablets:

100 mg (Epivir-HBV)

150 mg (Epivir)

Oral solution:

5 mg/ml, in 240 ml (Epivir-HBV)

10 mg/ml in 240 ml (Epivir)

Warning: Lactic acidosis and severe hepatomegaly with steatosis, including fatal cases, have been reported with use of antiretroviral nucleoside analogs alone or in combination, including lamivudine. (1)

Lamivudine

Children between the ages of 3 months and 18 years were eligible for enrollment. Children were included when the plasma HIV-1 RNA test result was positive on 2 subsequent occasions (children <18 months old)...

Medication was given in following doses: indinavir, 400 mg/m^2 every 8 hours; zidovudine, 120 mg/m^2 every 8 hours; and lamivudine, 4 mg/kg every 12 hours. Indinavir was administered as standard capsules of 200 mg and 400 mg or as capsules of 150 mg and 300 mg, which were prepared at the pharmacy. When patients were too young to swallow capsules, indinavir capsules had to be opened by the caregivers and dissolved in 5 to 10 mL of water. In children in whom problems were encountered with the ingestion of indinavir, the drug was changed to nelfinavir (30 mg/kg every 8 hours). Zidovudine was administered either as syrup (10 mg/mL) or as capsules of 100 mg and 250 mg, depending on the child's age. Lamivudine was administered as syrup (10 mg/mL) or as tablets of 150 mg. The importance of taking the indinavir 1hour before or 2 hours after meals was repeatedly emphasized.

Conclusions: Highly active antiretroviral therapy consisting of indinavir, zidovudine, and lamivudine in children reduced HIV-1 RNA to less than 500 copies/mL in 70% of the children within 6 months. Improved CD4 cell counts were observed in most patients, as was a better clinical condition (no invasive or opportunistic infections, increased weight gain). Side effects of the triple therapy were mild. Highly active antiretroviral therapy can be used as successfully in children as in adults.

(van Rossum: clinical and virologic response to combination treatment with indinavir, zidovudine, and lamivudine in children with human immunodeficiency virus-1 infections: A multicenter study in The Netherlands. J. Pediatr 2000;136:780-8)

Lamivudine (3TC)/Epivir

Characteristics of Antiretroviral Drugs
Nucleoside Analogue Reverse Transcriptase Inhibitors

Dosage: Pediatric: 4 mg/kg q 12 h

Neonatal (<30 d of age): Under study in clinical trials. 2 mg/kg q 12 h

Major Toxic Effects:

Most frequent: Headache, fatigue, nausea, diarrhea, skin rash, abdominal pain
Unusual (more severe): Pancreatitis (primarily seen in children with advanced HIV infection receiving multiple other medications)

Drug Interactions:

TMP-SMX increases 3TC blood levels (possibly competes for renal tubular secretions); unknown significance. When used with ZDV may prevent emergence of resistance, and for ZDV-resistant virus, revision to phenotypic ZDV sensitivity may be observed

Special Instructions:

Can be administered with food.
For oral solution: Store at room temperature.
Decrease dosage for patients with impaired renal function

(American Academy of Pediatrics: Report of the Committee on Infectious Diseases. Red Book 2000, pp.679-680)

LEUCOVORIN CALCIUM (Leucovorin, Wellcovorin, Folinic Acid, Citrovorum)

Supplied: Tablets: 5 mg, 15 mg, 25 mg.
Injection: 3 mg/ml
Powder for injection: 50mg/vial, 100mg/vial, 350mg/vial

Administration: IM, PO.
To counteract hematologic toxicity from folic acid antagonists (1).

Oral solution, once reconstituted is stable for 14 days when refrigerated, stable for 7 days at room temperature. Alcohol content of 21% to 23% (1).

Leukovorin (Folinic acid)

Concentration: 5mg tablets
Dispense: 30 tablets
Dosage: Sig: 10mg (2 tablets) on Monday, Wednesday and Friday. Crush and give with formula or apple juice in one dosage.

Suspended in 2% sugar solution. Suspension at usual concentration must be made up each week. Store refrigerated.

(Remington: Infectious diseases of the Fetus and Newborn Infant 2001, pp.292-293)

<u>Leucovorin</u> (Folinic acid)

Congenital *Toxoplasma* infection in the infant

Dosage: 10 mg three times weekly

Duration of Therapy: During and for 1 wk after pyrimethamine therapy

(Remington: Infectious Diseases of the Fetus and Newborn Infant 2001, pp.292-293)

SEE ALSO: CONGENITAL TOXOPLASMA INFECTION p.656

LEVAMISOLE (Ergamisol)

Supplied: Tablet 50mg

Administration: PO

<u>Levamisole</u>

Route: PO

Neonatal Dose: Disseminated herpes: Initial: 6mg every other day, then 7-15mg twice weekly has been used to treat some neonates.

Discussion: Drug has also been used in children to treat Wiskott-Aldrich syndrome

(Rudolph: Rudolph's Pediatrics 1996, p.2189)

LEVOTHYROXINE (Synthroid, Levothroid, T_4)

Supplied: Tablets 25mcg, 50mcg, 75mcg, 88mcg, 100mcg, others
Injection, powder for 200mcg and 500mcg vial

Administration: PO, IV

Dosage equivalence: 0.05 to 0.06mg equals approximately 60mg (1 grain) thyroid (it was previously considered that 0.1mg levothyroxine equaled 60mg thyroid) (1).

Reconstitute by adding 5ml NS, use immediately after reconstitution. Discard any unused portion.
IV or IM injection can be substituted for the oral dosage form when oral ingestion is precluded for long periods of time. The initial parenteral dosage should be approximately one-half of the previously established oral dosage (1).

Levothyroxine tablets may be given to infants and children who cannot swallow intact tablets. Crush the proper dose tablet and suspend in a small amount of formula or water. The suspension can be given by spoon or dropper. DO NOT store the suspension for any period of time. The crushed tablet may also be sprinkled over a small amount of food, such as cooked cereal or applesauce (1).

Levothyroxine Sodium (T_4) (Synthroid)

Indications and use: Treatment of congenital hypothyroidism.

Actions: Thyroid hormones increase metabolic rate of body tissues noted by increases in oxygen consumption, respiratory rate, body temperature, cardiac output, heart rate, blood volume, rate of fat, protein, and carbohydrate metabolism, enzyme system activity, growth, and maturation. Thyroid hormones are very important in CNS development. Deficiency in infants results in growth retardation, and failure of brain growth and development.

Route: IV, IM, PO.

Dosage: **Note**: The parenteral dose should be approximately 1/2 of the previously established oral dose.

0-6 months: 25 - 50 mcg/day PO (8-10 mcg/kg/day).
6-12 months: 50-75 mcg/day PO (6-8 mcg/kg/day).
Alternatively, 8-10 mcg/kg/day PO has been recommended for infants from birth to 1 year.

Adverse Affects: Adverse effects are usually due to excessive dose. If the following occur, discontinue and reinstitute at a lower dose: tachycardia, cardiac arrhythmias, tremors, diarrhea, weight loss, and fever.

(Gomella: Neonatology 1999, pp.574-575)

Levothyroxine

Dose & Route: Children PO dosing:
0-6 mo: 8-10 mcg/kg/dose QD
6-12 mo: 6-8 mcg/kg/dose QD
IM/IV dose: 50%-75% of oral dose QD

Remarks: **Contraindications** include acute MI, thyrotoxicosis uncomplicated by hypothyroidism, and uncorrected adrenal insufficiency. May cause hyperthyroidism, rash, growth disturbances, hypertension, arrythmias, diarrhea, and weight loss.

Total replacement dose may be used in children unless there is evidence of cardiac disease; in that case, begin with ¼ of maintenance and increase weekly. Titrate dosage with clinical status and serum T_4 and TSH. Increases the effects of warfarin. Phenytoin, carbamazepine may decrease levothyroxine levels.

100 mcg levothyroxine = 65 mg thyroid USP. Administer oral doses on an empty stomach. Excreted in low levels in breast milk; preponderance of evidence suggest no clinically significant effect in infants.

(Siberry: The Harriet Lane Handbook 2000, pp.754-755)

Levothyroxine

Treatment Schedules:
In 1986 the therapy recommended by the National Advisory Committee on CH consisted of an initial dose of

6 to 8 µg/k/g/d of levothyroxine, to be increased after 1 week, if euthyroidism was not achieved by then. In 1993 a higher initial dose, 10 µg/kg/d, was introduced. dosage was to be reduced by 1 µg/kg/d as soon as FT_4 concentration exceeded 30 pmol/L. It was up to the pediatrician to decide which schedule to follow. Therapy was controlled during the first year by 14.7 ± 4.4 (mean ± 1 SD) hormone measurements and a median number of 3 therapy adjustments (range, 0-15).

(Bongers-Schokking: Influence of timing and ose of thyroid hormone replacement on development in infants with congenital hypothyroidism. J Pediatr 2000; 136:292-7)

Levothyroxine (IV)

For <32 Weeks' gestation.

Infants received intravenous T_4 (10 µg/kg per day once daily) or placebo beginning within 48 hours of birth. Levothyroxine sodium was lyophilized with 10 mg of mannitol and 0.7 mg of anhydrous tribasic sodium phosphate, dissolved in 0.9% NaCl solution, and infused over 3 minutes immediately after preparation. The placebo solution was 0.9% NaCl. Oral T_4 (20 µg/kg per day once daily) was administered as soon as oral feedings were begun. The T_4 (n = 29) and placebo (n = 22) preparations were of similar color and consistency and were given in identical volumes per body weight for a total of 21 days. The initial 10 infants were observed every 15 minutes for 2 hours following administration for adverse reactions (e.g., hyperthermia, tachycardia); no untoward effects were noted. Throughout the study course, iodine-containing solutions were avoided.

Conclusion: Early T_4 supplementation in preterm newborns less than 32 weeks' gestation does not decrease the incidence of chronic lung disease or other complications of prematurity.

(Smith: Postnatal Thyroxine Supplementation in Infants Less Than 32 Weeks' Gestation: Effects on Pulmonary Morbidity. Journal of Perinatology 2000; 20:427-431)

Levothyroxine

Dose/kg: 5-8 µg
Route & Frequency: IV push over 30-60 sec; q24h

Dose/kg: 8-14 µg
Route & Frequency: PO; q24h

Dose/kg: Alternate dose: 25-50 µg total
Route & Frequency: PO q24h

Comments: Monitor serum T4 and TSH levels. Do not mix with any other IV fluids; mix immediately prior to administration. Increases effects of oral anticoagulants.

(Avery: Neonatology Pathophysiology and Management of the Newborn 1999, p.1557)

LIDOCAINE (XYLOCAINE)

Supplied: Injection 1% (10mg/ml) in 5ml and 10ml syringe
Injection 2% (20mg/ml) in 5ml vial, syringe
IV infusion 2mg/ml: 500ml D5W bag; 4mg/ml: 250, 500ml D5W bag

Administration: IV, IM
Specific product utilized for IM administration (1)

Administer IV push slowly, undiluted, as a bolus dose over a period of 2 to 4 minutes. For continuous infusion, dilute to a concentration of 2mg/ml to 4mg/ml (D5W) preferred (3).

When fluid restriction is desirable, a more concentrated solution of up to 8mg/ml may be used (3).

<u>Lidocaine</u> (Xylocaine)

Indications and use:
IV lidocaine is used almost exclusively for the short-term control of ventricular arrhythmias (premature beats, tachycardia, and fibrillation) or for prophylactic treatment of such arrhythmias. Skin infiltration as a local anesthetic.

Actions: Type 1 antiarrhythmic agent, with most activity related to blockade of the fast sodium channels in Purkinje fibers. Also a CNS depressant with sedative, analgesic, and anticonvulsant properties.

Route: IV, SC, or Intratracheal.

Dosage: 1 mg/kg/dose as IV bolus q5min to maximum total dose of 5 mg/kg, followed by IV infusion of 10-50 mcg/kg/min.

Therapeutic levels:
1-5 mcg/mL. Toxicity associated with levels >5 mcg/mL.

Adverse effects: Adverse effects generally involve the CNS: drowsiness, dizziness, tremulousness, and paresthesias. Muscle twitching, seizures, coma, respiratory depression, and respiratory arrest may also occur.

Comments: Primarily metabolized by the liver; dosage adjustment is necessary in liver failure. Contraindicated in sinoatrial or AV nodal block.

(Gomella: Neonatology 1999, p.575)

<u>Lidocaine</u>

Dosing: IV: 1-2 mg/kg, 20-50 mcg/kg/min infusion

Warnings: CNS side effects.

Intravenous Administration:
Lidocaine has a rapid distribution phase. In congestive heart failure, metabolism is diminished, and the dose of lidocaine should be reduced.

Therapeutic lidocaine levels are in the range of 2 to 5 μg/ml.

Dosing and Interactions:

Lidocaine is given as an intravenous bolus of 1 mg/kg and may be repeated in several minutes. Infusions of lidocaine are in the range of 20 to 50 μg/kg/min. Low cardiac output, common in critically ill patients requiring lidocaine infusions, often necessitates a reduction in the infusion rate because of decreased hepatic clearance and metabolism.

Side Effects: The major adverse drug reactions are related to the central nervous system: seizures, apnea, and altered mental status. Plasma concentrations are most often in excess of 6 to 7 μg/ml in this setting. Rarely, in patients with atrial tachyarrhythmias or with variable degrees of AV block (especially when resulting from prolongation of the QT interval), lidocaine may increase the ventricular response rate.

(Gillette: Clinical Pediatric Arrhythmias 1999,pp.231-248

Lidocaine

Uses: VT, VF

Dosing: 1 mg/kg q 5 min x 3 (load); 20-50 μg/kg/min (infusion)

Acute Side Effects:

Tinnitus; perioral paresthesias; altered sensorium; seizure; rarely decreases CO

Other Considerations:

Lower dose with heart or liver failure

VT, ventricular tachycardia; VF, ventricular fibrillation.

(Gillette: Clinical Pediatric Arrhythmias 1999, p.152)

Lidocaine

Class: IB
Inhibit Na^+ fast channel
Shorten repolarization
Moderate Na^+ inhibition with fast rate

Uses: Multiform PVC, couplets, VT; precardioversion if on digoxin;? predicts response to mexiletine, phenytoin

Dose (Level): 1 mg/kg IV q5min x 3, then infusion 20-50 μg/kg/min (1-5μg/mL)

Mode of Action: Little effect on normal tissues; decreases Purkinje ERP, automaticity; increases VF threshold

ECG/EP Changes: Slight ↓ HP-ERP, slight ↓ QTc

Side Effects: Paresthesia, seizure; ↑ AV conduction in AFL, ↓ vent and junctional escape rates; may ↓ cardiac output

(Garson: The science and practice of pediatric cardiology 1998, p.2952)

Lidocaine

Dose & Route: Anesthetic:

Injection:

Without epi: **max dose** of 4.5 mg/kg/dose (up to 300 mg)
With epi: **max dose** of 7 mg/kg/dose (up to 500 mg): do **not** repeat within 2 hours.

Topical: 3 mg/kg/dose no more frequently than Q2 hr.

Antiarrhythmic: Bolus with 1 mg/kg/dose slowly IO, IV; may repeat in 10-15 minutes x 2; **max total dose** 3-5 mg/kg within the first hour.

ETT dose = 2-2.5 x IV dose

Continuous Infusion: 20-50 mcg/kg/min IV

Remarks: **Contraindicated** in Stokes-Adams attacks, SA, AV, or intraventricular heart block without a pacemaker. Side effects include hypotension, asystole, seizures, and respiratory arrest.

Decrease dose in hepatic failure or decreased cardiac output. Do **not** use topically for teething. Prolonged infusion may result in toxic accumulation of lidocaine, especially in infants. Do **not** use epinephrine-containing solutions for treatment of arrhythmias.

Therapeutic levels 1.5-5 mg/L. Toxicity occurs at >7 mg/L. Toxicity in neonates may occur at >5 mg/L. Elimination $T_{1/2}$: premature infant: 3.2 hrs.

(Siberry: The Harriet Lane Handbook 2000, pp.755-756)

Lidocaine

Indication: For Neonatal Seizures

Several reports from Europe indicate value for lidocaine as an adjunctive agent in the treatment of neonatal seizures. Data on approximately 100 infants treated primarily because of failure of phenobarbital and diazepam indicate cessation of seizures, usually within 10 minutes of the start of intravenous infusion, in approximately 75%. Dosage schedules have varied, but most commonly a stating infusion of approximately 4 to 6 mg/kg/hr, with or without a bolus infusion at the onset, has been used. The drug has been tapered over several days. Doses required in premature infants are somewhat lower than in term infants. Of the side effects observed in older patients infused with lidocaine, e.g., arrhythmias, seizures, and hypotension, only recrudescence of seizures upon decrease of dosage has been observed (and observed only rarely). More data are needed on this promising therapy.

(Volpe: Neurology of the Newborn 2001, p.206)

LIOTHYRONINE (Cytomel, Triostat, T_3, Triiodothyronine)

Supplied: Tablets: 5 mcg, 25 mcg, 50 mcg.
Injection 10mcg/ml in 1mL

Administration: PO, IV
Dosage equivalents: 15 to 37.5 mcg equals approximately 60 mg desiccated thyroid (1).
If switching to oral levoyrovine, keep in mind that there is a delay of several days in the onset of action, discontinue IV therapy gradually (1).

Triiodothyronine

Dosage: Calculate dosage as for desiccated thyroid using the equivalent: 65 mg desiccated thyroid = 25 A9 T_3 [sic] (IV)

(Fanaroff: Neonatal-Perinatal Medicine 1997, p.1750)

Liothyronine

Usual Dosage: Congenital hypothyroidism (Cretinism): Neonates, Infants, and Children <3 years: Oral: 5 mcg/day; increase by 5 mcg every 3 days to a maximum dosage of 20 mcg/day for neonates and infants, 50 mcg/day for children 1-3 years of age

Administration: Oral: Administer on an empty stomach

(Taketomo: Pediatric dosage Handbook 2000-2001, pp.574-575)

LOPERAMIDE (Imodium A-D)

Supplied: Capsules: 2mg
Liquid 1mg/5ml, 1mg/ml (pepto diarrhea control)

Administration: PO

Loperamide Hydrochloride (Imodium)

Indication: Management of infants with short bowel syndrome.

Dose: A dose of 0.1 mg/kg given 2 or 3 times daily appears to be well tolerated.

Comments: Loperamide hydrochloride (Imodium) non-narcotic agonist, prolongs transit time, allowing for improved fluid and nutrient absorption with minimal central nervous system side effects.

(Hay: Neonatal Nutrition & Metabolism 1991, p.444)

Loperamide (Imodium)

Dose: Acute: 0.1 mg/kg/dose given bid to tid.

Usual: 0.4-0.8 mg/kg/day divided every 12 hours.
Maximum: 0.8 mg/kg/day

Chronic: 0.08-0.24 mg/kg/day divided bid to tid. Reduce to the lowest effective dose.
Maximum: 2 mg/dose.

Reduce dose in hepatic dysfunction.
If clinical improvement is not seen in 48 hours, discontinue use.

Administration: PO: For oral use **only**. Available in liquid form 1 mg/5ml (=0.2 mg/ml). Contains 5.25 percent alcohol.

Use: An antidiarrheal agent that is used as an adjunct to the management of diarrhea refractory to standard treatment, such as dietary adjustment and provision of fluids and electrolytes. Reduces daily stool output and duration of diarrhea. Decreases volume of stool and electrolyte output in short gut syndrome and in infants with ileostomies.

Antidiarrheals are not used to treat ordinary acute watery diarrhea; they ar useless against that type of diarrhea and can be dangerous for infants. Rehydration with appropriate fluids and electrolytes and prevention or correction of the cause of the diarrhea are the most important aspects of care.

Adverse Effects: May cause constipation, vomiting, abdominal distention, ileus, dry mouth, rash (rare), nervousness, somnolence. Habituation and tolerance have not occurred. Overdose is reversed with naloxone.

Motala and associates reported that of 30 infants with acute infectious diarrhea given loperamide 0.8 mg/kg/day for 48 hours after admission with rehydration with IV fluids, 2 infants had to be withdrawn from the trial because ileus developed in 1 and the other had persistent, severe vomiting. Transient drowsiness developed in 4 other infants. These researchers and others caution that the use of this drug in infants be limited to closely monitored inpatients.

Nursing Implications:

Monitor for abdominal distention, presence/absence of bowel sounds, and feeding intolerance.
Monitor fluid and electrolyte status carefully as in any infant with diarrhea.
Check CNS status for drowsiness.
Observe for ileus.

(Zenk: Neonatal Medications & Nutrition. A Comprehensive Guide 2000; pp.291-292)

<u>Loperamide</u>

Dose & Route: Active diarrhea:
Children (Initial doses within the first 24 hrs).
2-6 yr (13-20 kg): 1 mg PO TID

Follow initial day's dose with 0.1 mg/kg/dose after each loose stool (not to exceed the above initial doses).

Chronic diarrhea:
Children: 0.08-0.24 mg/kg/24 hr ÷ BID-TID
Max dose: 2 mg/dose

Remarks: May cause nausea, rash, vomiting, constipation, cramps, dry mouth, CNS depression. **Avoid** use in children <2 yr. **Discontinue** use if no clinical improvement is observed within 48 hr. Naloxone may be administered for CNS depression.

(Siberry: The Harriet Lane Handbook 2000, pp.757-758)

LORACARBEF (Lorabid)

Supplied: Suspension, powder for 100mg/5ml in 50mg, 75ml,100ml
Suspension, powder for 200ml/5ml in 50ml, 75ml, 100ml
(Strawberry bubble gum flavor)

Administration: PO
After mixing, the suspension may be kept at room T (59 - 86 F), for 14 days without significant loss of potency. Keep tightly closed. Discard unused portion after 14 days. (1)

Loracarbef (Lorabid)

Antibacterial Drugs for Pediatric Patients Beyond the Newborn Period
Dosage per kg/d

Route: PO

Mild to Moderate Infections: 30 mg for otitis media and 15 mg for other indications in 2 doses

Severe Infections: Inappropriate

Note: In patients with history of allergy to penicillin or one of its many congeners, alternative drugs are recommended. In some circumstances, a cephalosporin or other β-lactam class drug may be acceptable. However, these drugs should not be used in patients with an immediate hypersensitivity (anaphylaxis) to penicillin because approximately 5% to 15% of penicillin-allergic patients will also be allergic to the cephalosporins.

(American Academy of Pediatrics: Report of the Committee on Infectious Diseases. Red Book 2000, pp.655,662)

Loracarbef

Clinical Diagnosis:
Otitis media, acute. Infants and Children
(pneumococcus, Haemophilus, Moraxella most common)

Therapy: Usual therapy: amoxicillin 80-90 mg/kg/day PO div q8h
For failures or recurrences: amoxicillin-clavulanate 80-90 mg of amoxicillin component/kg/day PO div q8h OR cefuroxime axetil 30 mg/kg/day PO div q12h OR ceftriaxone 50 mg/kg/day IM q24h; x 1-3 doses
Other approved drugs: azithromycin, cefaclor, cefdinir, cefixime, cefpodoxime, cefprozil, ceftibuten, clarithromycin, erythromycin-sulfisoxazole, loracarbrf, trimethoprim-sulfamethoxazole

Comment: Recommendations based on CDC Working Group report (Pediatr Infect Dis J, January 1999;18:1-9); Gram's stain and cultures of pus, if available; If compromised host, suspect unusual infection (Tympanocentesis for culture may be necessary)

A Note on Acute Otitis Media with Effusion:

Several antibiotic regimens are effective for acute otitis media (AOM). Customarily, amoxicillin is used initially and other drugs are given for amoxicillin failures or relapses. The physician should consider advantages and disadvantages regarding antibacterial spectrum, palatability of suspensions, and cost. TMP/SMX is not effective for group A streptococcal infection. When prophylaxis is indicated, use amoxicillin or sulfa drug in one-half the therapeutic dose once or twice daily. How penicillin resistance in pneumococci affects empiric therapy is an unresolved issue.

(Nelson: Pocket Book of Pediatric Antimicrobial Therapy 2000-2001, pp.24-25)

LORAZEPAM (Ativan)

Supplied: Tablets 0.5mg, 1mg, 2mg
Injection 2mg/ml and 4mg/ml

Administration: IM, IV
Parenteral dosage form must be refrigerated.
IM injections : inject undiluted, deep into the muscle mass.

IV administration: Immediately prior to IV use, dilute with an equal volume of SWFI, NS, or D5W. Following dilution, the drug lorazepam may be injected into a vein or into the tubing of a freely flowing, compatible IV infusion of NS or D5W (3). DO NOT exceed 2mg/min. Have equipment to maintain a patent airway available (1).

Lorazepam

Indication: For Neonatal Seizures

Approximately 15% of newborns with seizures do not respond to the sequential administration of phenobarbital and phenytoin. In this situation, I have utilized lorazepam.

Lorazepam is a benzodiazepine anticonvulsant of proven efficacy in older infants and children. The drug is usually compared to the other major benzodiazepine used as an anticonvulsant, diazepam (see next section). Lorazepam, like diazepam, enters brain rapidly and produces a pronounced anticonvulsant effect in less than 5 minutes. Of importance, however, is that lorazepam is less lipophilic than diazepam and thus does not redistribute from brain as rapidly. Duration of action is generally 6 to 24 hours. Moreover, lorazepam appears less likely to produce respiratory depression or hypotension. This agent has been investigated in the newborn in three separate studies. The drug has been uniformly effective in treatment of neonatal seizures, whether as a second drug, after phenobarbital, or a third drug, after phenobarbital and phenytoin. Onset of effect has been in 2 to 3 minutes, and duration has extended to 24 hours. The effective dose is 0.05 to 0.10 mg/kg, administered intravenously in 0.05 mg/kg increments over several minutes. The half-life of lorazepam, studied in asphyxiated newborns only, is approximately 40 hours, i.e., twofold to threefold higher values than in the adult. This prolonged half-life could relate to decreased hepatic glucuronidation activity, a normal neonatal finding perhaps accentuated by asphyxial injury to liver.

Experimental data concerning the expected value of diazepines in the newborn are conflicting. Thus the mechanism of action of benzodiazepines is related to the binding to a specific receptor that augments a GABA-regulated chloride channel to produce inhibition. Although there is evidence that the developing nervous system has increased affinity for benzodiazepines, related data show that benzodiazepines do not potentiate GABA responses in cultured neonatal hippocampal neurons. Moreover, GABA maybe an *excitatory* neurotransmitter in early development, at least in some regions. Although more data are needed on these issues, the clinical data support a strong anticonvulsant action in the human newborn.

(Volpe: Neurology of the Newborn 2001, p.205)

Lorazepam (Ativan)

Indications and use:

Treatment of status epilepticus resistant to conventional anticonvulsant therapy (ie, phenobarbital, phenytoin).

Actions: A benzodiazepine. Facilitates γ-aminobutyric acid (GABA), which mediates transmission and mimics the actions of glycine at its receptor sites. Penetrates the blood-brain barrier more slowly than diazepam; however, the duration of action of lorazepam in the control of seizure activity in children studied was at least 3 h in 83% of cases and 24 h or longer in nearly 59% of cases. Median onset of seizure control is 10 min.

Route: PO, IM, IV.

Dosage: Status epilepticus:

Initial dosage: 0.05 mg/kg/dose IV. If no response after 15 min, repeat initial dose. May dilute with an equal volume of sterile water, normal saline, or D_5W. Infuse the dose over 2-3 minutes.

Sedation, anxiety: 0.05-0.1 mg/kg/dose IV q4-8h prn.

Adverse effects: May cause respiratory depression, apnea, hypotension, bradycardia, cardiac arrest, and seizure-like activity. Paradoxic CNS stimulation may occur, usually early in therapy; the drug should be discontinued if this effect occurs. Overdose may be reversed using flumazenil (Romazicon) 5-10 mcg/kg/dose IV.

(Gomella: Neonatology 1999, pp.575-576)

Lorazepam

Acute Treatment of Neonatal Seizures

Dose: 0.05 to 0.10 mg/kg IV

(Hill: Neonatal Seizures Pediatrics in Review 2000;21:117-121)

Lorazepam (Ativan)

Dose & Route: Status Epilepticus:
Neonates, Infants, Children, and Adolescents:
0.05-0.1 mg/kg/dose IV over 2-5 min. May repeat 0.05 mg/kg x 1 in 10-15 min.
Max dose: 4 mg/dose

Antiemetic adjunct therapy:
Children:
0.04-0.08 mg/kg/dose IV Q6 hr PRN.
Max single dose: 4 mg

Anxiolytic/Sedation:
Children:
0.05 mg/kg/dose Q4-8 hr PO/IV. **Max dose**: 2 mg/dose

May also give IM for preprocedure sedation

Remarks: **Contraindicated** in narrow-angle glaucoma and severe hypotension. May cause respiratory depression, especially in combination with other sedatives. May also cause sedation, dizziness, mild ataxia, mood changes, rash, and GI symptoms. Injectable product may be given rectally. Benzyl alcohol may be toxic to newborns in high doses.

Onset of action for sedation: PO, 20-30 minutes; IM, 30-60 minutes; IV, 1-5 minutes. Duration of action: 6-8 hrs. **Flumazenil is the antidote.**

(Siberry: The Harriet Lane Handbook 2000, pp.759-760)

Lorazepam

For Neonatal Seizures

The benzodiazepines, including lorazepam, diazepam, and clonazepam, have all been used in the treatment of neonatal seizures. Diazepam has been administered as a continuous intravenous infusion at a rate of 0.3 mg/kg/hr (Gramstrop, 1982), and lorazepam has been used at doses of 0.05 mg/kg given intravenously over 2 to 5 minutes (Deshmukh, 1986). In almost all circumstances, the benzodiazepines have been used as adjunctive agents rather than primary therapy. The benzodiazepines have not been compared with other anticonvulsants regarding efficacy.

(Swaipman: Pediatric Neurology 1999; p.188)

Lorazepam (Ativan)

Stability: Do not use if injection is discolored or contains precipitate; protect from light; refrigerate injectable form and oral solution; injection is stable at room temperature for 8 weeks

Usual Dosage: Adjunct to antiemetic therapy: Children: I.V.: 0.04-0.08 mg/kg/dose (maximum dose: 4 mg) every 6 hours as needed

Status epilepticus: I.V.:
Neonates: 0.05 mg/kg over 2-5 minutes; may repeat in 10-15 minutes

Infants and Children: 0.1 mg/kg/slow I.V. over 2-5 minutes, do not exceed 4 mg/single dose; may repeat second dose of 0.05 mg/kg slow I.V. in 10-15 minutes if needed

Monitoring Parameters:
Respiratory rate, blood pressure, heart rate; CBC with differential and liver function with long-term use

Additional Information:
Single oral doses >0.09 mg/kg produced increased ataxia without increasing sedative benefit vs lower doses; since both strengths of injection contain 2% benzyl alcohol, Neofax recommends using the 4 mg/mL strength for dilution with preservative free sterile water to make a 0.4 mg/mL dilution for I.V. use in neonates (in order to decrease the amount of benzyl alcohol delivered to the neonate); however, the stability of this dilution has not been studied. Diarrhea in a 9 month old infant receiving high-dose oral lorazepam was attributed to the lorazepam oral solution that contained polyethylene glycol and propylene glycol (both are osmotically active); diarrhea resolved when crushed tablets were substituted for the oral solution

(Taketomo: Pediatric Dosage Handbook 1999-2000, pp.546-547)

MAGNESIUM ACETATE

Supplied: Crystal, Reagent grade
Administration: PO

Magnesium Acetate

For children with short bowel syndrome:

Dose: 1 mEq/kg/day of aqueous magnesium acetate and magnesium gluconate solutions each for 1 week (PO). Because a better stool pattern can be obtained with magnesium acetate as compared with magnesium gluconate, magnesium acetate may be a useful source of magnesium in pediatric patients with short bowel syndrome.

(Kaufman: Magnesium acetate vs. magnesium gluconate supplementation in short bowel syndrome. J Pedatr Gastroenterol Nutr 1993;16:104-105)

MAGNESIUM GLUCONATE

Supplied: Powder
Administration: PO

Magnesium Gluconate

For children with short bowel syndrome:

Dose: 1 mEq/kg/day of aqueous magnesium acetate and magnesium gluconate solutions each for 1 week (PO).

(Kaufman: Magnesium acetate vs. magnesium gluconate supplementation in short bowel syndrome. J Pedatr Gastroenterol Nutr 1993;16:104-105)

SEE ALSO: MAGNESIUM ACETATE

MAGNESIUM SULFATE

Supplied: Injection 10% (0.8mEq/ml) in 10ml, 20ml, 50ml,
Injection 50% (4.0mEq/ml) in 2ml,10ml, 20ml, 50ml

Administration: IV
Dilute IV infusions to a concentration of ≤ 20% prior to IV administration. The most commonly used diluents are 5% Dextrose injection and 0.9% Sodium Chloride injection (1).

Admixture Compatibilities:
Magnesium sulfate in solution may result in a precipitate formation when mixed with solutions containing: alcohol (high concentrations); alkali carbonates and bicarbonates; alkali hydroxides, arsenates, barium, calcium, clindamycin phosphate; heavy metals; hydrocortisone sodium; succinate; phosphates; polymixin B sulfate, procaine HCL; salicylates; strontium; tartrates (1).

Magnesium Sulfate

Indications and use: Hypomagnesemia and refractory hypocalcemia.

Actions: May depress CNS and peripheral neuromuscular transmission by decreasing acetylcholine release. Acts on cardiac muscle to slow sinoatrial nodal impulse formation and prolongs conduction time.

Route: IM, IV, PO

Dosage: Hypomagnesemia or refractory hypocalcemia:
Initial dosage: 0.2 meq/kg/dose IV or IM q6h until serum magnesium level is normal or symptoms resolve or 0.8-1.6 meq/kg/dose PO 4 times daily.
Maintenance dosage: 0.25-0.5 meq/24h IV (add to infusion or give IV).

Adverse effects: Hypotension, flushing, depression of reflexes, depressed cardiac function, CNS and respiratory depression.

Comments: Contraindicated in renal failure. Monitor serum magnesium, calcium, and phosphate levels. Infuse IV magnesium sulfate over several hours.

(Gomella: Neonatology 1999, p.576)

<u>Magnesium</u>

Indication: For Neonatal Seizures.

I do not administered calcium routinely to all newborns during the initial seizure, except in the unusual instance of a classic presentation for later-onset hypocalcemia. If hypocalcemia is present, 5% calcium gluconate is given intravenously in a dose of 4 ml/kg (200 mg/kg). Electrocardiogram, or at least cardiac rhythm by auscultation, should be monitored during administration. It is important to recognize that phenobarbital can suppress the seizures of hypocalcemia, and, thus a decrease in seizures after phenobarbital administration does not rule out hypocalcemia as cause. If hypomagnesemia is present, magnesium sulfate is best given intramuscularly as a 50% solution in a dose of 0.2 mg/kg. In this regard it should be recalled that approximately one half of newborns with seizures secondary to later-onset hypocalcemia also have hypomagnesemia. The importance of treating these hypocalcemic infants with magnesium is emphasized by the following facts: (1) the administration of calcium to such infants may increase renal excretion of magnesium, aggravate the hypomagnesemia, and maintain the convulsive state; and (2) the administration of magnesium has been shown to correct *both* the hypocalcemia and the hypomagnesemia, perhaps by increasing movement of calcium from bone to plasma. However, magnesium cannot be administered with abandon because magnesium can produce a neuromuscular blockade. Transient weakness and hypotonia (without range) are often noted in infants given magnesium. Moreover, it should be recalled that the maintenance doses of magnesium and calcium shown in table should be administered only as long as needed to avoid hypomagnesemia or hypocalcemia.

(Volpe: Neurology of the Newborn 2001, p.208)

Magnesium Sulfate

Dose: Hypomagnesemia:

- IM/IV: 25-50 mg/kg/dose (=0.2-0.4 mEq/kg) every 6 hours for 3-4 doses until symptoms resolve and serum magnesium levels return to normal.
- PO: 100-200 mg/kg/day divided every 6 hours.

Seizures and Hypertension:

- IM/IV: 25-100 mg/kg/dose given every 4-6 hours (children). Monitor serum magnesium concentrations.

Maintenance Requirement for Patients on Parenteral Nutrition: 30-60 mg/kg/day (=0.25-0.5 mEq/kg/day).

Persistent Pulmonary Hypertension of the Newborn PPHN): Abu-Osba and associates treated infants with PPHN using a loading dose of 200 mg/kg (1.6 mEq/kg), then a maintenance infusion of 20-50 mg/kg/hour (0.16-0.4 mEq/kg/hour) for up to 8 hours with frequent serum magnesium determinations. This treatment, however, is experimental. Other methods (such as alkalinization, tolazoline, ECMO, and nitric oxide) are more frequently used to treat this disorder.

Reduce dose and monitor serum magnesium concentrations in renal impairment.

Administration: Supplied as: A 50 percent solution or 500 mg $MgSO_4$/ml (=4 mEq/ml).
IV-Rate: Infuse over 3-4 hours.
IV-Concentration: $\leq$30 mg/ml preferred; maximum: 200 mg/ml.

IM: Not the preferred route in neonates because of their poor muscle mass. If used, maximum concentration is 200 mg/ml.

PO: May use the parenteral form PO and dilute in feedings.

Use: Treatment of hypomagnesemia. Symptoms of hypomagnesemia are similar to tetany from hypocalcemia, usually with magnesium serum levels <1.5 mEq/liter and a normal serum calcium.

Adverse Effects: Hypotension with Rapid IV Administration: Monitor blood pressure. Monitor for cardiac arrhythmias and respiratory and CNS depression during infusion. Monitor serum magnesium levels.

Flushing, sweating, depressed reflexes, flaccid paralysis, hypothermia, cardiac and CNS depression, respiratory paralysis.

Diarrhea may occur with oral administration. Dilute and give in divided doses.

Treat overdose of magnesium with calcium gluconate IV, resuscitation and assisted ventilation. Peritoneal dialysis and hemodialysis are effective.

Nursing Implications:

Continuously monitor blood pressure, heart rate, and respiratory rate during infusion.
Monitor electrolyte values, especially for hypocalcemia.
Monitor for diarrhea with oral doses.

Comments: Conversion Factor: 1 mg magnesium sulfate = 8 mEq magnesium.

Interpretation of Magnesium Levels:
Low Levels:

- Hypomagnesemia: <1.5 mEq/liter.

Normal Levels:

- Normal level: 1.5-2.5 mEq/liter.
- Therapeutic level for preeclampsia, eclampsia, treatment of convulsive toxemia: 4-7 mEq/liter (anticonvulsant levels have also been expressed as 2.5-7.5 mEq/liter).

Toxic Levels (see **Adverse Effects**, above, for treatment):

- Loss of deep tendon reflexes, hypotension, narcosis: 7-10 mEq/liter.
- Respiratory paralysis: 12-15 mEq/liter.
- Effects on cardiac conduction, with lengthened PR interval, widened QRS. and dysrhythmias, which may lead to complete heart block: >15 mEq/liter.
- Likelihood of cardiac arrest: >25 mEq/liter.

(Zenk: Neonatal Medications & Nutrition. A Comprehensive Guide 2000; pp297-299)

Magnesium Sulfate

Acute Treatment of Neonatal Seizures
Dose: 50% solution: 0.2 mL/kg IM
(Hill: Neonatal Seizures Pediatrics in Review 2000;21:117-121)

Magnesium Sulfate

All doses expressed in $MgSO_4$ salt

Dose & Route: Cathartic: Child: 0.25 g/kg/dose PO Q4-6hr

Hypomagnesemia or Hypocalcemia:
IV/IM: 25-50 mg/kg/dose Q4-6hr x 3-4 doses; repeat PRN.
Max single dose: 2 g

PO: 100-200 mg/kg/dose QID PO
Daily Maintenance: 30-60 mg/kg/24 hr or 0.25-0.5 mEq/kg/24 hr IV. **Max dose**: 1 g/24 hr

Adjunctive therapy for moderate to severe reactive airway disease exacerbation (bronchodilation):
Children: 25 mg/kg/dose (**max dose**: 2 g) x 1 IV over 20 minutes

Remarks: When given IV **beware** of hypotension, respiratory depression, complete heat block, hypermagnesemia. Calcium gluconate (IV) should be available as **antidote**. Use with **caution** in patients with renal insufficiency and with patients on digoxin. **Serum level-dependent toxicity** include the following >3 mg/dl: CNS depression; >5 mg/dl: decreased deep tendon reflexes, flushing, somnolence; and >12 mg/dl: respiratory paralysis, heart block.

Maximum IV intermittent infusion rate: 1 mEq/kg/hr or 125 mg $MgSO_4$ salt/kg/hr.

(Siberry: The Harriet Lane Handbook 2000, p.762-763)

Magnesium sulphate

A loading dose of 200 mg/kg $MgSO_4$ diluted to 10% in sterile water was given intravenously over 20 minutes, followed by a continuous infusion of 20 to 150 mg/kg/hour, to obtain a magnesium blood concentration between 3.5 and 5.5 mmol/l.... Mean (SD) duration of treatment was 75.5(19.8) hours. No other vasodilatory drug was administered before or during the treatment and patients were not hyperventilated. Mean (SEM) PaO_2 values significantly increased from 42.6 (8.8) before treatment to 70.3 (24.1) mm Hg after 24 hours, with no change in pH or Pco2.

It is concluded that magnesium sulphate is a non-aggressive and low-cost treatment of short duration which is easy to apply. It may have a role in the various treatment of PPHN.

(Tolsa: Magnesium sulphate as an alternative and safe treatment for severe persistent pulmonary hypertension of the newborn. Arch Dis Child 1995;72:F184-F187)

MANNITOL

Supplied: Injection 5%, 10% in 500, 1000ml
Injection 15% in 500ml
Injection 20% in 250, 500ml
Injection 25% in 50ml

Administration: IV

Mannitol dosage requirements for patients 12 years of age and younger have not been established. However, some clinicians have suggested the following dosages for pediatric patients. In oliguria or anuria a test dose of 0.2 g/kg or 6 g/m^2 may be given as a single dose over 3-5 minutes. For therapeutic purposes 2 g/m^2 or 60 g/m^2 may be given. For the treatment of edema and ascites, this dose may be given as a 15 or 20% solution over 2-6 hours. To reduce cerebral or ocular edema the dose may be given as a 15 or 20% solution over 30-60 minutes (3).

Preparation: When exposed to low temperatures mannitol sodium may crystallize. Concentrations >15% have a greater tendency to crystallize. If crystals are observed, warm the bottle in a hot water bath, a dry heat over or autoclave, then cool to body temperature or less before administering. When infusing concentrated mannitol, the administration set should include a filter (1).

Mannitol

Dose/kg: 0.25-1 g (15%-20% solution)
Route and frequency: IV once over 2-6 h
Comments: Always use a 5-μm filter
May cause rebound edema and circulatory overload

Dose: Oliguria test dose: 0.2 g
Route and frequency: IV over 3-5 min
(Avery: Neonatology Pathophysiology and Management of the Newborn, 1999, p.1558)

Mannitol

Dosage: 0.5-1 g/kg i.v.
Comments: After urine flow is established, lower doses (0.25-0.5 g/kg) are recommended. Repeat every 6 h as clinically indicated.
(Allen: Moss and Adam's Heart Disease in Infants, Children, and Adolescents 2001, pp.1460-1468)

Mannitol

Dose & Route: Anuria/Oliguria:
Test Dose: to assess renal function: 0 .2 g/kg/dose IV; **max** 12.5 g over 3-5 min. If there is no diuresis within 2 hr. discontinue mannitol.
Initial: 0.5-1 g/kg/dose
Maintenance: 0.25-0.5 g/kg/dose Q4-6 hr IV

Cerebral Edema:
0.25 g/kg/dose IV over 20-30 min. May increase gradually to 1 g/kg/dose if needed. (May give furosemide 1 mg/kg concurrently or 5 min before mannitol.)

Remarks: **Contraindicated** in severe renal disease, active intracranial bleed, dehydration, and pulmonary edema. May cause circulatory overload and electrolyte disturbances. For hyperosmolar therapy, keep serum osmolality at 310-320 mOsm/kg.

Caution: May crystallize with concentration ≥20%; use in-line filter. May cause hypovolemia, headache, and polydipsia. Reduction in ICP occurs in 15 minutes and lasts 3-6 hours.
(Siberry: The Harriet Lane Handbook 2000, p.763)

MEDIUM CHAIN TRIGLYCERIDES (MCT Oil)

Supplied: Oil, in quarts, Lipid fraction of coconut oil consisting primarily of the triglycerides of C_8 (≈67%) and C_{10} (≈23%) saturated fatty acids

Administration: PO
Contains 115 calories per 15ml (1).

Medium-Chain Triglycerides

Dose: Initial: 0.5 ml every 6 hours (or every other feeding).

- If tolerated, may advance in 24 ours to 0.5 ml every 3 hours (every feeding).
- May increase dose volume with a corresponding reduction in dose frequency after 24 hours to 1 ml every 6 hours as tolerated to simplify administration. MCT oil is a caloric supplement, providing 7.6 kcal/ml. **Maximum dose**: 55 percent of calories from fat.

Administration: PO: Mix with formula. In older infants on a more varied diet, may mix with fruit juice, vegetables, and other foods.

A significant portion of the MCT oil (about 33 percent) may adhere to the feeding tube during gavage feedings, so the infant may receive fewer than the intended calories administered.

Adverse Effects: Diarrhea may be an indication that the dose has exceeded the infant's tolerance for the oil. Reduce the dose.

Lipid pneumonia. Undiluted MCT oil may be aspirated; mix with formula before administration.

Large amounts of MCT's may cause elevated blood and spinal fluid levels of medium-chain fatty acids in patients with advanced hepatic cirrhosis because of their impaired hepatic clearance. May lend to coma.

May exacerbate ketosis in patients with acidosis.

Nursing Implications:

Mix well into feeding.
Monitor growth parameters (head circumference, weight, length) weekly.
Monitor for diarrhea.

(Zenk: Neonatal Medications & Nutrition. A Comprehensive Guide 2000; pp:300-301)

Medium Chain Triglycerides

Usual Dosage: Infants: Nutritional supplement; Initial: 0.5 mL every other feeding, then advance to every feeding, then increase in increments of 0.25-0.5 mL/feeding at intervals of 2-3 days as tolerated

(Taketomo: Pediatric Dosage Handbook 1999-2000, pp.560-561)

Medium-chain triglyceride (MCT)

Route & Dose: PO: 1-8 ml/24 h divided in feedings (7.7 cal/ml)

(Taeusch: Avery's Diseases of the Newborn 1998, p. 1346)

MEFLOQUINE

SEE CHLOROQUINE (Nelson: Pocket Book of Pediatric Antimicrobial Therapy 1998-1999, pp.64-65)

MEPERIDINE (Demerol)

Supplied: Injection 25mg, 50mg, 75mg, 100mg per ml
Oral syrup 50mg/5ml in 500ml

Administration: IV, IM, PO
Dilute oral syrup with water. If taken undiluted, it may exert a slight topical anesthetic effect on mucous membranes (3).

For DIRECT IV INJECTION, dilute to a concentration of 10mg/ml and infuse slowly. Compatible in D5W, NS (3).

When repeat doses are necessary, the IM route is preferred over subcutaneous administration because of occurrence of local tissue irritation and induration following subcutaneous injection (3).

Meperidine Hydrochloride (Demerol)

Indications and use: Preoperative medication and for relief of moderate to severe pain.

Actions: Stimulates opiate receptors in CNS. Meperidine produces respiratory depression proportionate to drug dose. Duration of respiratory depression can extend several hours beyond the plasma half-life.

Route: PO, IM, IV, SC

Dosage: 0.5-1.5 mg/kg/dose. Maximum: 2 mg/kg/dose IV, IM, and SC, and 4 mg/kg/dose PO.

Adverse effects: Normeperidine (active metabolite) has excitant effects that may precipitate tremors, myoclonus, or seizures. Other side effects include respiratory and circulatory depression, nausea, vomiting, constipation, and sedation.

Comments: Effects can be reversed by naloxone 0.1 mg/kg IV.
(Gomella: Neonatology 1999, p.576)

Meperidine (Demerol)

Dose: IV, IM, SC: 0.5-1 mg/kg/dose given every 4 hours, as needed.
PO: 1-2 mg/kg/dose given every 4 hours, as needed.

Premedication with Lytic Cocktail (DPT)
(**Caution**: Use of DPT is discouraged by the American Academy of Pediatrics, and its use has been decreasing with the availability of safer and more effective agents.):

- Demerol (meperidine) 0.5 mg/kg/dose
- Phenergan (promethazine) 0.25 mg/kg/dose
- Thorazine (chlorpromazine) 0.25 mg/kg/dose

May mix all 3 components in the same syringe so that DPT may be given as a single IM injection.

Administration: IV-Rate: Infuse over at least 1-2 minutes. Rapid IV administration increases the incidence of adverse effects.

IV-Concentration: May give undiluted; however, dilution with at least an equal volume of dextrose or saline is preferred.

IM, SC-Concentration: May give undiluted. the IV route is preferred to IM or SC in neonates because of poor absorption.

PO: Dilute oral dose in feedings or water to prevent the slight topical anesthetic effect on the mucous membranes.

Adverse Effects: Increasing the dose increases the adverse effects, such as respiratory and CNS depression.
Antidote: Naloxone 0.1 mg/kg/dose IV.

Cardiovascular: Bradycardia, hypotension (due to histamine release), especially in patients with inadequate blood volume. Meperidine is more likely than most other opioids to cause side effects associated with histamine release.

CNS: CNS depression and arrest requiring mechanical ventilation, increased intracranial pressure, sedation. May cause twitches, tremors, and/or seizures with prolonged, repeated use because of accumulation of normeperidine metabolite.

Endocrine: Antidiuretic hormone release.

GI: Nausea, vomiting (take with food to reduce GI upset). Delayed gastric emptying, cramping, and biliary tract spasm. Meperidine is more likely to cause constipation than most other narcotic analgesics.

GU: Urinary tract spasm.

Local: Repeated SC administration causes local tissue irritation and induration.

Ophthalmic: Pupillary contraction (miosis).

Respiratory: Respiratory depression. In general, neonates are more susceptible to the depressant effects of opioids than are older children or adults. Lower doses at more frequent intervals are less likely to cause respiratory depression than are higher doses at longer intervals.

Patients unable to tolerate meperidine may be able to tolerate another narcotic agent, particularly if it is in a different pharmacologic class (codeine and morphine: phenanthrenes; meperidine and fentanyl: phenylpiperidines; methadone: a diphenylheptane).

Causes addiction; do not discontinue abruptly after prolonged use. Tolerance develops to the drug.

Nursing Implications:
Observe for excessive sedation.

Monitor blood pressure and heart rate.
Observe the infant to see that pain is relieved adequately.
Watch for withdrawal after long-term administration.

(Zenk: Neonatal Medications & Nutrition. A Comprehensive Guide 2000; pp:302-304)

Meperidine HCl (Demerol)

Dose & Route: PO, IM, IV and SC:
Children: 1-1.5 mg/kg/dose Q3-4h PRN.
Max dose: 100mg.

Remarks: **Contraindicated** in cardiac arrhythmias, asthma, increased ICP. Potentiated by MAO inhibitors, tricyclic antidepressants, phenothiazines, other CNS-acting agents. Meperidine may increase the adverse effects of isoniazid. May cause nausea, vomiting, respiratory depression, smooth muscle spasm, pruritis, palpatations, hypotension, constipation, and lethargy.

Drug is metabolized by the liver and its metabolite (normeperidine) is renally eliminated. **Caution**: in renal failure, sickle cell disease, and seizure disorders, accumulation of normeperidine metabolite may precipitate seizures. **Adjust dose in renal failure**.

Onset of action: PO/IM/SC, 10-15 minutes; IV, 5 minutes

1983 MP statement lists as compatible with breast feeding; no reevaluations in subsequent statement.

(Siberry: The Harriet Lane Handbook 2000, p.765)

Meperidine (Demerol)

Dose: 0.5-2 mg/kg IV, IM, PO (40 mg max)

Mode of Action: Narcotic analgesia

Adverse Effects: Tachycardia, respiratory depression

(Garson: The science and practice of pediatric cardiology 1998, p.2955)

MEROPENEM (Merrem IV)

Supplied: Powder for injection: 500 mg, 1 gm

Administration: Give over ≈15 to 30 minutes or as an IV bolus injection (5 to 20 ml) over ≈ 3 to 5 minutes. (1)

Comment: Do not mix with solutions containing other drugs. (1)

Meropenem

Route: IV, IM

Dosage (mg/kg) and Interval of Administration:

Weight 1200-2000 g
Age 0-7 Days: 20 q12h
Age >7 Days: 20 q12h

Weight >2000 g
Age 0-7 Days: 20 q12h
Age >7 Days: 20 q8h

Note: Dosages of meropenem suggested are the same as those of imipenem.

(Remington: Infectious Diseases of the Fetus and Newborn Infant 2001, p.1454)

Meropenem (Merrem)

Dose: For Infants >3 Months of Age:

- Intra-abdominal infections: 20 mg/kg/dose given every 8 hours.
- Meningitis: 40 mg/kg/dose given every 8 hours.

Reduce dose in renal impairment.

Administration: IV—Rate: may give over 3-5 minutes, but infusion over 30 minutes is preferred.

IV—Concentration: 50 mg/ml. Table 1-28 shows how many hours meropenem is stable when reconstituted in various solutions in concentrations of 2.5-50 mg/ml.

Cautions/Contraindications:

Efficacy and tolerability have not yet been evaluated in infants less than 3 months of age, although kinetic studies have been done.

Adverse Effects: CNS: Well tolerated. Meropenem does not appear to cause seizures in infants with bacterial meningitis, as imipenem dose.

Dermatologic: Rash (1.9 percent). The rash is mostly diaper-area moniliasis.

GI: Diarrhea (4.3 percent), vomiting (1 percent), oral moniliasis, glossitis.

Hematologic: Hematologic problems such as increased or decreased platelets, increased eosinophils, prolonged prothrombin time, decreased WBC, decreased hemoglobin and hematocrit, and others occur in less than 1 percent of patients.

Hepatic: Increased liver enzymes and bilirubin (<1 percent).

Hypersensitivity: Allergic reaction may occur.
Local: Inflammation at injection site; phlebitis.

Nursing Implications: Observe for rash and diarrhea.

(Zenk: Neonatal Medications & Nutrition. A Comprehensive Guide 2000; pp:305-307)

METAPROTERENOL (Alupent, Metaprel)

Supplied: Aerosol: 75mg (100 inhalations) 150mg (200 inhalations)
Each dose delivers 0.65mg
Inhalation solution: 0.4%, 0.6% in 2.5ml
Solution for inhalation: 5.0% in 10ml, 30ml
Syrup:10mg/5ml in 480ml

Administration: Inhalation, PO

Metaproterenol

0.1-0.25 mL (5-12.5 mg) of 5% solution. Dilute with NS to 3 mL. Dose: every 6 h

Side Effects: Same as isoproterenol
Cardiac arrhythmias potentiated by hypoxia

(Gomella: Neonatology: Management, Procedures, On-call Problems, Diseases and Drugs 1999, p.56)

Metaproterenol (Alupent)

Dose: Nebulization: 0.01 ml (0.5 mg)/kg/dose of 5 percent (=0.13 ml/kg of 0.4 percent) given every 3-6 hours. **Maximum**: 0.3 ml (15 mg) of 5 percent. Dilute to a final total volume of 3 ml with normal saline or other concurrent medications.

Some clinicians recommend a dose of 0.1-0.25 ml (5-12.5 mg) of a 5 percent solution diluted to 1.5-2 ml with half-normal or normal saline every 6 hours.

Administration: Supplied as:

- Concentrate (usually for outpatient use): 5 percent (50 mg/ml).
- Unit Dose (usually for inpatient use): 0.4 percent (4 mg/ml).

Dose titration:

- Reduce the dose to the next smaller dose and/or increase the interval to the next longer interval when the heart rate exceeds 180 bpm (if baseline HR was <150 bpm) or 200 bpm (if baseline HR was >150 bpm). A moderate increase in heart rate is expected and may indicate absorption and therapeutic response. Lengthening the interval between doses should be tired when respiratory status has improved. Taper to the lowest effective dose.
- Increase the dose to the next larger dose and/or decrease the interval to the next shorter interval if the infant is still in respiratory distress after a trial of 1 to 3 doses. However, do not increase the dose if the infant is experiencing adverse effects from the current dose.

Discontinuation of Treatment: If adverse effects occur or if the drug is no longer needed, discontinue the drug. If there has been no improvement in respiratory status as measured by pulmonary mechanics, change in respiratory support, or clinical status after 3 doses, discontinue the drug.

TABLE 1-29 Metaproterenol Volume conversions: ml to mg

5% (50 mg/ml) Concentrate	0.4% (4 mg/ml) Unit Dos	mg
0.1 ml	1.3 ml	5 mg
0.15 ml	1.9 ml	7.5 mg
0.2 ml	2.5 ml (adult dose)	10 mg
0.3 ml	3.8 ml	15 mg

Adverse Effects: Tachycardia, arrhythmias, increased blood pressure, and hyperglycemia.

May cause, more cardiac stimulation than albuterol, especially in patients with hypoxia, because it is less β_2 selective.

Lower frequency of adverse effects than for isoproterenol.

Tolerance may develop after prolonged use.

Nursing Implications:

Monitor heart rate, blood pressure, and respiratory status.

(Zenk: Neonatal Medications & Nutrition. A Comprehensive Guide 2000; pp:308-309)

Metaproterenol

Dose & Route: Inhalation:
Aerosol: 2-3 puffs Q3-4 hr to max dose of 12 puffs/24 hr

Nebulized Solution:
Dilute 0.1-0.3 ml of 5% solution 2.5 ml NS; administer Q4-6 hr PRN

Single-dose solutions:
Infants: 2.5 ml of 0.4%
Oral: Children <2 yr: 0.4 mg/kg/dose Q6-8 hr

Remarks: **Contraindicated** in cardiac arrhythmias, or narrow angle glaucoma. Adverse reactions as with other beta-adrenergic agents. Excessive use may result in cardiac arrhythmias and death. Also causes tachycardia, increased myocardial O_2 consumption, hypertension, nervousness, headaches, nausea, palpitations, and tremor. The use of tube spacers may enhance efficacy of administering doses via metered dose inhaler. Nebulizers may be given more frequently in the acute setting.

(Siberry: The Harriet Lane Handbook 2000, p.766)

METHADONE HCL (Dolophine)

Supplied: Injection 10mg/ml in 1ml, 20ml
Oral solution 5mg/5ml, 10mg/5mL
Oral concentrate 10mg/ml in 30, 120ml

Administration: IM, PO, SC
Injection IM is preferred for repeated doses. SC use may cause local irritation (1).

Methadone Hydrochloride

Indications and use:

Long-acting narcotic analgesic used for severe pain and neonatal abstinence syndrome.

Actions: CNS opiate receptor agonist resulting in analgesia and sedation.

Route: IV, IM, PO, SC.

Dosage: 0.05 - 0.2 mg/kg/dose given q 12-24h. The daily dose can be divided q 8h.

Adverse effects: Respiratory depression, bronchospasm, constipation, hypotension, bradycardia, CNS depression, sedation, increased intracranial pressure, urinary tract spasm, urine retention, biliary tract spasm, and dependence with prolonged use. **Caution**: Methadone may accumulate; reassess for the need to adjust the dose downward after 3-5 days to avoid overdose. Smaller doses or less frequent administration may be required in renal and hepatic dysfunction.

Comments: Taper by 10 -20% weekly, based on the infant's symptoms of withdrawal. Tapering is difficult with methadone because of its long duration of action; consider morphine instead. Treat overdose with naloxone.

(Gomella: Neonatology 1999, p. 576)

Methadone

Indication: Drug therapy for withdrawal syndrome in infants

Methadone has been used in treatment of addicted infants; the initial dose is 0.05 to 0.10 mg/kg given every 6 to 12 hours, with increases of 0.05 mg/kg until symptoms are controlled. Methadone can be administered every 12 to 24 hours because of its relatively long half-life. Of these agents I have had most experience with tincture of opium.

(Volpe: Neurology of the Newborn 2001, p.882)

Methadone HCl

Dose & Route: Children: 0.7 mg/kg/24 hr ÷ Q4-6 hr PO, SC, IM or IV PRN pain. **Max dose** 10 mg/dose

Remarks: May cause respiratory depression, sedation, increased intracranial pressure, hypotension, and bradycardia. Average $T_{1/2}$: children 19 hr. Oral duration of action is 6-8 hours initially and 22-48 hours after repeated doses. Respiratory effects last longer than analgesia. Accumulation may occur with continuous use, making it necessary to adjust dose.

(Siberry: The Harriet Lane Handbook 2000, pp.766-767)

METHICILLIN (Staphcillin)

Discontinued by manfacturer

Supplied: Injection, powder for 1gm, 4gm vials
(Contains 3 mEq Na/gm)

Administration: IV, IM
For IM administration, add 1.5ml SWFI to the 1 gm vial for a concentration of approximately 500mg/ml. Stable for 24 hours at room temperature, or 4 days when refrigerated (3).

For DIRECT INTERMITTENT IV injection, further dilute to a concentration of 20mg/ml with 0.45% NaCl or NS. The appropriate dose should then be injected at a rate of 200mg per minute into the tubing of a free-flowing compatible IV solution (3).

For INTERMITTENT INFUSION, Dilute to a concentration of 2-20mg/mL. INjuse over 20-30 minutes (3).

<u>Methicillin</u>

Antibacterial Drugs for Newborn Infants
Dose (mg/kg or Units [U]/kg) and Frequency of Administration

Route: IV, IM

Dose: <u>Infants 0-4 wk</u>
BW <1200 g: 25 every 12 h

<u>Infants <1 wk old</u>
BW ≤1200-2000 g: 25-50 every 12 h
BW >2000 g: 25-50 every 8 h

<u>Infants ≥1 wk old</u>
BW ≤2000-2000 g: 25-50 every 8 h
BW >2000 g: 25-50 every 6 h

Note: For meningitis, the larger dose is recommended.

Antibacterial Drugs for Pediatric Patients Beyond the Newborn Period
Dosage per kg/d

Route: IV, IM
Mild to Moderate Infections: 100-150 mg in 4 doses

Severe Infections: 150-200 mg in 4-6 doses

Comments: Methicillin (oxacillin)-resistant staphylococci are usually resistant to all other semisynthetic antistaphylococcal cephalosporins
Interstitial nephritis (ie, hematuria) occurs in 0%-4% of patients

Note: In patients with history of allergy to penicillin or one of its many congeners, alternative drugs are recommended. In some circumstances, a cephalosporin or other β-lactam class drug may be acceptable. However, these drugs should not be used in patients with an immediate hypersensitivity (anaphylaxis) to penicillin because approximately 5% to 15% of penicillin-allergic patients will also be allergic to the cephalosporins.

(American Academy of Pediatrics: Report of the Committee on Infectious Diseases. Red Book 2000, pp. 651,660,662)

Methicillin

Route: IV, IM

Dosage (mg/kg) and Interval of Administration:

Meningitis:

Weight <1200 g
Age 0-4 WK: 50 q12h

Weight 1200-2000 g
Age 0-7 Days: 50 q12h
Age >7 Days: 50 q8h

Weight >2000 g
Age 0-7 Days: 50 q8h
Age >7 Days: 50 q6h

Other Infections:

Weight <1200 g
Age 0-4 Wk: 25 q12h

Weight 1200-2000 g
Age 0-7 Days: 25 q12h
Age >7 Days: 25 q8h

Weight >2000 g
Age 0-7 Days: 25 q8h
Age >7 Days: 25 q6h

(Remington: Infectious Diseases of the Fetus and Newborn Infant 2001, p.1454)

Methicillin Sodium (Staphcillin)

Classification: Penicillinase-resistant penicillin.

Action and spectrum: Mechanism of action identical to that of other ß-lactam antibiotics. Active chiefly against penicillinase-positive and penicillinase-negative staphylococci. Less effective than penicillin G against other Gram-positive cocci. No activity against enterococci.

Route: IM or IV (infuse over 20 minutes).

Dosage: Meningitis:
< 2000 g and 0-7 days old: 100 mg/kg/day divided q12h.
< 2000 g and > 7 days old: 150 mg/kg/day divided q8h.
> 2000 g and 0-7 days old: 150 mg/kg/day divided q8h.
> 2000 g and > 7 days old: 200 mg/kg/day divided q6h.

Other indications:
< 2000 g and 0-7 days old: 50 mg/kg/day divided q12h.
< 2000 g and > 7 days old: 75 mg/kg/day divided q8h.
> 2000 g and 0-7 days old: 75 mg/kg/day divided q8h.
> 2000 g and > 7 days old: 100 mg/kg/day divided q6h.

Elimination and metabolism: Renal. Half-life variable (60-120 minutes or longer).

Adverse effects: Nephrotoxicity (interstitial nephritis) occurs more often with methicillin than with other penicillins. May cause hypersensitivity reactions, anemia, leukopenia, thrombocytopenia, phlebitis at infusion site, and hemorrhagic cystitis (in poorly hydrated patients).

Comments: In cases of methicillin resistance, vancomycin becomes the antistaphylococcal drug of choice. Dosage adjustment necessary in renal impairment. Monitor serum urea nitrogen and creatinine. Contains 2.9 meq sodium per gram.

(Gomella: Neonatology 1999, pp.576-577)

METHIMAZOLE (Tapazole)

Supplied: Tablets 5mg, 10mg

Administration: PO

Methimazole

Dosage: Initial: 0.4 mg/kg/day divided every 8 hr PO
Maintenance: 0.2 mg/kg/day divided every 8 hr

(Fanaroff: Neonatal-Perinatal Medicine 1997, p.1750)

Methimazole (Tapazole)

Dose & Route: Children:
Initial: 0.4-0.7 mg/kg/24 hr or 15-20 mg/m^2/24 hr PO ÷ Q8 hr
Maintenance: 1/3-2/3 of initial dose PO ÷ Q8 hr.
Max dose: 30 mg/24 hr PO.

Remarks: Readily crosses placental membranes and distributes into breast milk. Blood dyscrasias, dermatitis, hepatitis, arthralgia. CNS reactions, pruritus, nephritis, hypoprothrombonemia, agranulocytosis, headache, fever, hypothyroidism may occur. Switch to maintenance dose when patient is euthyroid. Administer doses with food.

(Siberry: The Harriet Lane Handbook 2000, p.768)

METHYLDOPA (Aldomet)

Supplied: Oral suspension 250mg/5ml in 473ml
Injection 250mg/5ml; 5ml, 10ml vials

Administration: IV, PO

For IV administration, the appropriate dose should be added to D5W in a concentration of 10mg/ml (3).

Administer the dose over 30 to 60 minutes (3).

Methyldopa (Aldomet)

Indications and use: Hypertension

Actions: Mechanism of action is not fully understood. Metabolized to α-methylnorepinephrine in the CNS, where it lowers arterial pressure by stimulation of central α-adrenergic receptors. Reduction of plasma renin may also play a role in its antihypertensive effect.

Route: IV, PO.
Dosage: 5-40 mg/kg/day divided q6-8h.

Adverse effects: Most common adverse effect is drowsiness, which occurs within the first 48-72 hours and may cause marked depression, orthostatic hypotension, sodium retention, edema, a positive direct Coombs' test reaction in 10-20% of patients (reversible), and drug fever. Causes fluid and sodium retention and should be given with a diuretic.

Comments: Preferred route of administration is oral, but absorption from the GI tract is unpredictable (10-15%). Contraindicated with active hepatic disease.

(Gomella: Neonatology 1999, p.577)

<u>Methyldopa</u>

Route & Dose: IV, PO: 2-3 mg/kg q 6-8 h; increased as needed at 2-day intervals; maximum dosage 12-15 mg/kg/dose

Adverse Effects and Cautions:
Sedation, fever, false-positive Coombs' test, hemolysis, sudden withdrawal of methyldopa may cause rebound hypertension

(Taeusch: Avery's Disease of the Newborn 1998, p.1346)

<u>Methyldopa</u>

Dose & Route: Hypertension:
Children: 10 mg/kg/24 hr ÷ Q6-12 hr PO; increase PRN Q2 days. **Max dose**: 65 mg/kg or 3 g/24 hr, whichever is less.

Hypertensive Crisis:
Children: 2-4 mg/kg/dose IV to **max** of 5-10 mg/kg/dose IV Q6-8 hr. Max dose (whichever is less): 65 mg/kg/24 hr or 3 g/24 hr.

Remarks: **Contraindicated** in pheochromocytoma and active liver disease. Use with **caution** if patient is receiving haloperidol, propranolol, lithium, sympathomimetics. Positive Coombs' test rarely associated with hemolytic anemia, fever, leukopenia, sedation, memory impairment, hepatitis, GI disturbances, orthostatic hypotension, black tongue, and gynecomastia may occur. May interfere with lab tests for creatinine, urinary catecholamines, uric acid, ASST.

Adjust dose in renal failure

(Siberry: The Harriet Lane Handbook 2000, p.769)

<u>Methyldopa</u>

Dosage: Pediatrics: 10 mg/kg/24 h p.o. (divide b.i.d. or t.i.d.)

Comments: Pediatric dose may be increased to 60 mg/kg/24 h

(Allen: Moss and Adam's Heart Disease in Infants, children and Adolescents 2001, pp.1460-1468)

METHYLENE BLUE

Supplied: Tablet: 65mg
Injection 10mg/ml in 1 ml

Administration: IV, PO

Inject the appropriate dose over a period of several minutes. It must be injected slowly to prevent local high concentrations of the drug and production of additional methemoglobinemia. One authority reports that if the total methylene blue IV dosage exceeds 7mg/kg dyspnea, precordial pain, restlessness, apprehension, and fibrillar tremors may result (3). Methylene Blue has caused hemolysis, especially in young infants and in patients with G-6-PD deficiency.
Because Methylene Blue is a dye, preparations of the drug stain skin; stains on skin may be removed by use of a hypochlorite solution. Methylene Blue imparts a blue-green color to urine and sometimes feces (3).

Methylene Blue (Urolene Blue)

Dose: Methemoglobinemia in Infants:
IV: 1-1.5 mg/kg/dose (= 0.1-0.15 ml/kg/dose of a 1 percent solution) IV. May repeat after 1hours if methemoglobin persists. If two doses are unsuccessful, exchange transfusion may be required.

Methemoglobin Reductase Deficiency:
Oral: 1.5-5 mg/kg/day PO. Given as a single daily dose. (May give with ascorbic acid 5-8 mg/kg/day PO given in three to four divided doses.) This usually is sufficient to maintain the methemoglobin concentration below that which causes cyanosis. These patients usually require treatment only for cosmetic purposes.

Refractory Hypotension in Septic Shock:
1 mg/kg/dose IV infused over 1 hours. May repeat one time.

Diagnostic Indicator Dye: (such as to disclose aspirated dye in the tracheal material during suctioning in an infant with a tracheostomy): **Maximum**: 5 mg/kg/day (= 0.5 ml/kg/day of the 1 percent solution) PO divided in feedings. Mix well. Give for several feedings; then discontinue. **Caution**: Excessive amounts of methylene blue (MB) can be toxic (see **CAUTIONS / CONTRAINDICATIONS** and **ADVERSE EFFECTS** below); use the smallest volume that will adequately color the feeding. MB is visible at very low concentrations.

- Blue food coloring has been used in the place of MB to color feedings for diagnostic purposes because of the lower cost of the food coloring. However, it too could have adverse effects if given in excessive amounts, such as transiently blue colored diarrhea and skin. Use only the minimum volume that will adequately color the feeding and discontinue when no longer needed.

Reduce Dose in Renal Dysfunction:
Consider use of the low dose in the range in very low birth weight infants because of their immature renal function.

Administration: Supplied as: Injection: 10 mg/ml (= 1 percent).
IV—Rate:

- Infuse over 1 hours (preferred) or over 5-15 minutes.
- Do not give by rapid IV push because the high local concentration of MB may cause the formation of additional methemoglobinemia.

IV—Concentration: May give undiluted or diluted with normal saline.

PO: Administer after meals with water, per fluid tolerance of the infant.

Intraosseous (IO) Administration:
There is one report of successful use of MB by the IO route in a 6-week-old (3 kg) infant for acquired methemoglobinemia. This route was used on an emergency basis because IV access could not be established. The rate of infusion and concentration recommended for IV administration are suggested for IO use.

Contraindications:

- Glucose-6-phosphate Dehydrogenase (G6PD) Deficiency: Do not use in infants with G6PD deficiency who have methemoglobinemia because MB may aggravate the methemoglobinemia and precipitate acute hemolysis.
- Cyanide Poisoning: Do not give MB to treat excess methemoglobinemia induced by sodium nitrate during treatment of cyanide poisoning because MB will release cyanide from the cyanomethemoglobin complex, causing an increase in the blood cyanide concentration and increased toxicity. MB has been used as an antidote for cyanide poisoning; however, sodium nitrite with sodium thiosulfate is safer and more effective.
- Intraspinal/Intrathecal Injection: Not for intraspinal or intrathecal injection because neural damage, including paraplegia, has occurred.
- Subcutaneous Injection: do not give by subcutaneous (SC) injection because necrotic abscess may occur.
- Hypersensitivity to MB.

Nursing Implications:
Staining of skin of health car providers may be removed with a topical application of diluted sodium hypochlorite (NaClO) solution (= modified Dakin's solution, available in 0.25 percent and 0.5 percent concentrations). Avoid

contact with eyes; may cause skin irritation. Avoid using diluted sodium hypochlorite to remove blue staining on neonates' skin because of the risk of skin irritation and chemical burns of their delicate skin and because there are no data on safety of this solution in this age group.

Full-strength (5 percent) sodium hypochlorite solution (= laundry bleach) is too concentrated for application to tissues.

Blue staining of skin by MB hinders assessment of hypoxia, including use of pulse oximetry.

- Monitoring: Measure blood methemoglobin concentration before MB administration if patient is symptomatic (because MB itself can produce methemoglobinemia) and then 1 to 2 hours after administration of MB to assess effectiveness of therapy. Monitor CBC and reticulocyte count to assure that hemolysis has not occurred.

Comments: Interactions:

- Urine pH: MB may interfere with analysis of urine pH.
- Pulse Oximetry: MB will temporarily cause inaccurate, artificially low (perhaps as low as 0) pulse oximetry saturation readings within 30 seconds of MB infusion. These usually return to baseline values within 4 to 5 minutes after administration. The probable mechanism of the interference is with light wave emission of the pulse oximeter; the light emission of the pulse oximeter is mostly absorbed by the light emission of methylene blue. The oximeter interprets this as an indication of the presence of reduced hemoglobin, which leads to erroneously low values for oxygen saturation.

(Zenk: Neonatal Medications & Nutrition. A Comprehensive Guide 2000; pp:310-318)

<u>Methylene blue</u>

Dose/kg: 1-2 mg

Route & frequency: IV slow push over 5 min (1% soln) May repeat in 1 h

Comments: Methylene blue is a reducing agent; it may decrease hemoglobin O_2 capacity

(Avery: Neonatology Pathophysiology and Management of the Newborn 1999, p.1558)

<u>Methylene blue</u>

Route & Dose: IV: 0.1-0.2 mg/kg of 1% solution for methemoglobinemia, infused slowly

(Taeusch: Avery's Diseases of the Newborn 1998, p. 1346)

METHYLPREDNISOLONE (Solu-Medrol, Medrol)

Supplied: Tablets 2 mg, 4 mg, 8 mg, (other)
Injection, powder for 40mg/ml, 125mg/2ml
(benzyl alcohol contained in some products)

Administration: IV, IM, PO

For DIRECT IV INJECTION: It should be administered over a period of at least 1 to several minutes (3).

Methylprednisolone (Solu-Medrol)

Dose: As an Anti-inflammatory and Immunosuppressive: 0.16-0.8 mg/kg/day divided every 6-12 hours.

For Status Asthmaticus: 1-2 mg/kg IV as a single dose, then 0.5-1 mg/kg/dose IV every 6 hours for up to 5 days, then change to oral prednisone. Base dose on severity of disease and response of patient. Reduce dose gradually to the lowest effective level.

Administration: Supplied as:

- Oral: 2 mg tablets (scored) (Medrol), but not as an oral liquid. (Prednisone, hydrocortisone, and dexamethasone are available as oral liquids.)
- Injection: 40 mg/ml vial.

IV—Rate: Infuse over at least 1 to several minutes.

IV—Concentration: May give undiluted (40 mg/ml) or may dilute with dextrose or saline. The diluent provided in "Act-O-Vial" and "Univial" contains benzyl alcohol. Insert needle through center of plunger-stopper and withdraw this diluent; replace with non-preserved saline.

IV—Compatibility: See Appendix E: Y-Site Compatibility of Common NICU Drugs.

IM: May give undiluted.

Adverse Effects: Acute Adverse Effects:
Usually do not occur, except with too-rapid withdrawal after long-term use.

Acute Pituitary-Adrenal Insufficiency:
Results from too-rapid withdrawal of corticosteroids after prolonged use (receipt of corticosteroids for longer than 7-10 days). Taper dose gradually if infant has received steroids for longer than 7-10 days.

Adverse Effects with Prolonged Use:
Adrenal suppression, including severe growth retardation; hypokalemic alkalosis; sodium retention; hypertension; hyperglycemia; increased susceptibility to infections; cataracts; myopathy; hypocalcemia; osteoporosis with bone fractures; nephrocalcinosis; and nephrolithiasis. Use alternate-day treatment to minimize adverse effects in patients on chronic corticosteroid therapy.

Nursing Implications:

Monitor for hypertension, hyperglycemia after dose.

Monitor for signs and symptoms of infection.

Monitor growth parameters, such as head circumference, length, and weight, weekly, and plot on growth curve.

Monitor for serum electrolytes, glucose and fluid status, and glucose spillage in urine.

Comments: Sodium Content: Methylprednisolone sodium succinate contains 2 mEq sodium/gm.

(Zenk: Neonatal Medications & Nutrition. A Comprehensive Guide 2000; pp:319-321)

<u>Methylprednisolone</u>

Dosage: 1-5 mg/kg/dose every 6 hours IV for bronchodilation; 30 mg/kg/dose every 6 hours IV for life-threatening disease.

Comments: See Dexamethasone

(Fanaroff: Neonatal-Perinatal Medicine 1997, p.1750)

<u>Methylprednisolone</u>

Dose & Route: Antiinflammatory/immunosuppressive:
PO/IM/IV: 0.5-1.7 mg/kg/24 hr ÷ Q6-12 hr

Acute spinal cord injury: 30 mg/kg IV over 15 minutes followed in 45 minutes by a continuous infusion of 5.4 mg/kg/hr x 23 hr

Remarks: Steroid potencies and doses based on body surface area. Not all practitioners use loading dose for status asthmaticus. Acetate form may be used for intramuscular, intra-articular, and intralesional injection; it should **not** be given IV. Like all steroids, may cause hypertension, pseudotumor cerebri, ance, Cushing's syndrome, adrenal axis suppression, GI bleeding, hyperglycemia, and osteoporosis.

(Siberry: The Harriet Lane Handbook 2000, pp.770-771)

METOCLOPRAMIDE (Reglan)

Supplied: Oral syrup 5mg/5mL
Concentrated oral solution 10mg/mL in 30mL (intensol)
Injection 5mg/mL in 2mL

Administration: PO, IV

For IV administration in adults, doses greater than 10mg are administered over a minimum of 15 minutes in an IV infusion (1).

For direct IV injection, administer over 1 to 2 minutes, since a transient but intense feeling of anxiety and restlessness, followed by drowsiness, may occur with rapid administration (1).

<u>Metoclopramide Hydrochloride</u> (Reglan)

Indications and use: Used in a variety of GI disorders. In neonates and infants, the drug has been used investigationally for feeding intolerance and gastroesophageal reflux.

Action: Dopamine antagonist acting on the CNS and on other organs. GI smooth muscle stimulant. Increases the resting tone of the esophageal sphincter. In neonates, metoclopramide resulted in a significant decrease in gastric aspirate, increased weight gain, shortened GI transit time, and increased food intake.

Route: IM, IV, PO

Dosage: 0.1-0.2 mg/kg/dose given q6hr 20 min before feedings.

Adverse effects: CNS effects include restlessness, drowsiness, and fatigue. Extrapyramidal reactions may occur but usually subside 24 h after discontinuance of the drug, and most patients will respond rapidly to diphenhydramine.

Comments: Contraindicated with bowel obstruction and seizure disorders.

(Gomella: Neonatology 1999, p.577)

<u>Metoclopramide</u>

Therapy for Reflux

Common doses: 0.1 mg/kg/dose qid: AC, HS

Partial list of side effects:

Restlessness, drowsiness, dystonic reactions –antidote: diphenhydramine

Partial list of contraindications:

Gastrointestinal obstruction, perforation, hemorrhage; pheochromocytoma; extrapyramidal risk

(Wyllie: Pediatric Gastrointestinal Disease 1999, p.180)

<u>Metoclopramide</u>

The major drawback to the use of metoclopramide in patients of any age is its side effects. The incidence of side effects is reported to vary from 10 to 30 percent. Children seem to be particularly susceptible to the toxic effects of metoclopramide. Most side effects result from the drug's effect on the central nervous system. Commonly reported side effects are mild anxiety, fatigue, drowsiness, headache, and insomnia. Occasionally, depression has been reported which seemed to improve with lowering the dosage of the drug.

Cholinergic side effects, such as diarrhea and abdominal cramps may occur, but rarely necessitate stopping the drug. Methemoglobinemia has been reported with an overdose (10-fold increase in dose) in a 3-week-old infant.

The dose of metoclopramide in infants and children for both gastroesophageal reflux and delayed gastric emptying is 0.1 mg/kg per dose given up to 4 times a day, with a maximum dose of 0.5 mg/kg per day. Metoclopramide is available in both an oral and parenteral preparation.

(Walker: Gastrointestinal Disease 2000, pp.1810-1811)

<u>Metoclopramide</u> (Reglan)

Dose & Route: Gastroesophageal reflux (GER) or GI dysmotility: Infants and Children: 0.1-0.2 mg/kg/dose up to QID IV/IM/PO; **max dose**: 0.8 mg/kg/24 hr

Antiemetic:
1-2 mg/kg/dose Q2-6 hr IV/IM/PO. Premedicate with diphenydramine to reduce EPS.

Remarks: **Contraindicated** in GI obstruction, seizure disorder, pheochromocytoma, or in patients receiving drugs likely to cause extrapyramidal symptoms (EPS). May cause EPS, especially at higher doses.. Sedation, headache, anxiety, leukopenia, and diarrhea may occur.

For GER, give 30 min before meals and at bedtime.
Adjust dose in renal impairment,
(Siberry: The Harriet Lane Handbook 2000, p.771)

<u>Metoclopramide</u>

Usual Dosage: Gastroesophageal reflux: Oral, I.<M., I.V.:
Neonates, Infants and Children: 0.4-0.8 mg/kg/day in 4 divided doses.

Administration: Oral: Administer 30 minutes before meals and at bedtime

Parenteral: Dilute to 0.2 mg/mL (maximum concentration: 5 mg/mL) and infuse over 15-30 minutes (maximum rate of infusion; 5 mg/minute); rapid I.V. administration is associated with a transient but intense feeling of anxiety and restlessness followed by drowsiness
(Taketomo: Pediatric Dosage Handbook 1999-2000, pp.592-593)

METOCURINE IODIDE (Metubine Iodide)

Supplied: Injection 2mg/ml in 20ml
Administration: IV
Administer IV as a sustained injection over 30 to 60 seconds. DO NOT GIVE IM (1).

<u>Metocurine</u>

0.2 mg/kg in premature infants. (Does not alter arterial blood pressure).

A bolus dose of pancuronium can produce tachycardia and hypertension in children through its sympathomimetic effect, which is sometimes desirable to support the cardiac output of infants with relatively fixed stroke volumes. If tachycardia is undesirable, metocurine (Metubine), which causes minimal change in heart rate, blood pressure, and cardiac rhythm in small children (even at doses of 0.5 mg/kg), is often appropriate. For patients in whom a short-acting, nondepolarizing muscle relaxant is desirable, atracurium and vecuronium have few cardiovascular side effects in children when given in low doses.
(Gregory: Pediatric Anesthesia 1994, pp.365-490)

<u>Metocurine</u>

Dose: 0.2 to 0.3 mg/kg
Metocurine is dimethyl d-tubocurarine; it is approximately twice as potent as d-tubocurarine and has a similar

duration of action. There is, however, marked variation in the response of infants to the neuromuscular blocking effects of metocurine.

The drug causes very little change in blood pressure, though a slight increase in heart rate may occur. Metocurine is reported to cause less histamine release than d-tubocurarine.

(Steward: Manual of Pediatric Anesthesia 1995, pp.512,62)

Metocurine

Dosage: 0.2-0.4 mg/kg IV

Comments: Administered as an iodide salt; continuous use has not been performed in children.

(Fanaroff: Neonatal-Perinatal Medicine 1997, p.1752)

METOLAZONE (Zaroxolyn, Mykrox)

Supplied: Tablets 2.5mg, 5mg, 10mg (Zaroxolyn)
Tablets 0.5mg (Mykrox)
The metolazone formulations are not bioequivalent or therapeutically equivalent at the same doses. Mykrox is more rapidly and completely bioavailable. DO NOT interchange brands (1).

Administration: PO

Extemporaneous Compounding (Recipe)

Dosage form: Oral suspension
Made from: Tablets
Concentration: 1 mg/mL
Stability: 90 days
Store: Refrigerate
Label: Shake well

Ingredient	Strength	Quantity
Metolazone tablet	10 mg	1
Syrup		qs ad 10 mL

Instructions: Crush the tablet in mortar. Add small amounts of syrup while mixing. Transfer to a graduate and qs with syrup. (11)

Metolazone

Dose/kg 0.2 mg

Route & frequency: PO q12h-q24h

Comments: May cause metabolic alkalosis and hyperuricemia; monitor serum electrolytes

(Avery: Neonatology Pathophysiology and Management of the Newborn 1999, p.1558)

Metolazone

Dose & Route: Dosage based on Zaroxolyn (for Mykrox or oral suspension, see remarks):
Children: 0.2-0.4 mg/kg/24 hr ÷ QD-BID PO

Remarks: **Contraindicated** in patients with anuria, hepatic coma. Electrolyte imbalance, GI disturbance, hyperglycemia, marrow suppression, chills, hyperuricemia, chest pain, hepatitis, and rash may occur. Mykrox and oral suspension have increased bioavailability;; therefore lower doses may be necessary when using these dosage forms.

(Siberry: The Harriet Lane Handbook 2000, pp.771-772)

METOPROLOL (Lopressor)

Supplied: Tablets 50mg, 100mg
Injection 1mg/mL in 5mL

Metoprolol

Dosage: 1-2 mg/kg/day p.o. (divided b.i.d.)

(Allen: Moss and Adam's Heart Disease in Infants, children and Adolescents 2001, pp.1460-1468)

Metoprolol

Metoprolol is a beta blocker with a limited experience of use in pediatrics.

Dosing: PO: 50-200 mg bid (adult)

Warnings: Similar to atenolol

Dosing: There are no studies of dosing guidelines for metoprolol in children. In adults, a starting dosage of 50 mg twice daily may be used and increased to 150 to 200 mg twice daily.

Side Effects: Insufficient data exist for the side effect profile of metoprolol in children.

(Gillette: Clinical Pediatric Arrhythmias 1999, pp.231-248)

Metoprolol

Antihypertensive drug

In several young infants, we have used the selective beta 1-adrenoseceptor blocking agent, metoprolol, successfully. The suggested dose for children is 1 to 5 mg/kg/day in single or divided doses.

Route: PO*

(* Route added after personal communication with the author)

(Rasoulpour: Systemic hypertension. Clin Perinatol 1992;19:121-137)

METRONIDAZOLE (Flagyl)

Supplied: Tablets 250mg and 500mg
Injection, ready to use 500mg/100ml
(Flagyl RTU contains Na 14mEq/500mg)
Injection, powder for 500mg

Administration: IV, PO

To avoid the reconstitution and preparation requirements of injectable powder, use the appropriate dose from RTU products unless fluid requirements prohibit its use (Author). Administer IV by intermittent IV infusion. Both loading and maintenance doses are infused over 1 hour. The recommended final concentration for infusion is 5 to 8mg/ml (6), 7.5mg/ml (7). The duration of infusion is 60 minutes (6,7).

Newborns demonstrate a diminished capacity to eliminate metronidazole. The elimination half-life inversely relates to gestational age. In infants whose gestational age was between 28 and 40 weeks, the corresponding elimination half-lives ranged from 109 to 22.5 hours (1). The plasma half-life is reported to be 6 to 8 hours in adults with normal renal and hepatic function (3).

Extemporaneous Compounding (Recipe)

Dosage form: Oral suspension
Made from: Tablets
Concentration: 1 mg/mL
Stability: 60 days
Store: Refrigerate
Label: Shake well

Ingredient	Strength	Quantity
Metronidazole tablets	10 mg	12
Ora-Sweet or Ora-Sweet SF		
Ora-plus		aa qs 120 mL

Instructions: Crush the tablets in a mortar. Add small amounts of vehicle and mix to a uniform paste. Add vehicle in geometric amounts to almost desired volume while mixing. Transfer to a graduate and add vehicle to final volume. (11)

Metronidazole

Antibacterial Drugs for Newborn Infants
Dose (mg/kg or Units [U]/kg and Frequency of Administration

Route: IV, PO

Dose: Infants 0-4 wk
BW <1200 g: 7.5 every 48 h

Infants <1 wk old
BW ≤1200-2000 g: 7.5 every 24 h
BW >2000 g: 7.5 every 12 h

Infants ≥ 1 wk old
BW ≤2000-2000 g: 7.5 every 12 h
BW >2000 g: 15 every 12 h

Note: Safety in infants and children has not been established

Antibacterial Drugs for Pediatric patients Beyond the Newborn Period
Dosage per kg/d

Route: PO
Mild to Moderate Infections: 15-35 mg in 3 doses

Severe Infections: Inappropriate

Comments: Safety in infants and children has not been established (American Academy of Pediatrics: Report of the Committee on Infectious Diseases. Red Book 2000, pp.651,657)

Metronidazole

Tetanus Treatment:

Oral (or intravenous) metronidazole (30 mg/kg per day, given at 6-hour intervals) is effective in reducing the number of vegetative forms of *C tetani* and is the antibiotic of choice. Parenteral penicillin G (100 000 U/kg per day, given at 4- to 6-hour intervals) is an alternative treatment. Therapy for 10 to 14 days is recommended.

(American Academy of Pediatrics: Report of the Committee on Infectious Diseases. Red Book 2000, p.565)

Metronidazole

Route: IV, PO

Dosage (mg/kg) and Interval of Administration:

Weight <1200 g
Age 0-4 WK: 7.5 q48h

Weight 1200-2000 g
Age 0-7 Days: 7.5 q24h
Age >7 Days: 7.5 q12h

Weight >2000 g
Age 0-7 Days: 7.5 q12h
Age >7 Days: 15 q12h

Note: A loading intravenous dose of 15 mg/kg followed 24 hr later (term infants) and 48 hr later (preterm infants) by 7.5 mg/kg every 12 hr has been suggested by other investigators.

(Remington: Infectious Diseases of the Fetus and Newborn Infant 2001, p.1454)

Metronidazole

Route: IV, PO

Dosages (mg/kg/day) and Intervals of Administration:

Body weight < 2000g
0-7 days old: 7.5 div q24hr
8-28 days old: 15 div q12h

Body weight >2000g
0-7 days old: 15 div q12h
8-28 days old: 30 div q12h

> 28 days old: 30 div q6h

(Nelson: Pocket Book of Pediatric Antimicrobial Therapy 2000-2001, p.16)

Metronidazole (Flagyl)

Classification: Bactericidal antibiotic.

Action and spectrum: The mechanism of action is not established. Good activity against anaerobic protozoa, including *Trichomonas vaginalis*, *Entamoeba histolytica*, *Giardia lamblia*, and

Balantidium coli. Good activity also against Gram-positive bacteria (*Clostridium*, *Peptococcus*, *Peptostreptococcus*, and *Veillonella* spp) and anaerobic Gram-negative bacteria (*Bacteroides* and *Fusobacterium* spp). Nonsporulating Gram-positive bacilli are often resistant (eg, *Propionibacterium*, *Actinomyces* spp), and the drug has minimal activity against aerobic and facultative anaerobic bacteria.

Route: PO or IV (infuse commercial dilution over 1 h)

Dosage: <2000 g: 15 mg/kg/day divided q12h
>2000 g and 0-7 days old: 15 mg/kg/day divided q12h
>2000 g and > 7 days old: 30 mg/kg/day divided q12h

Elimination and metabolism:
Hepatic metabolism with final excretion via the urine and feces. Large volume of distribution (penetrates into all body tissues and fluids).

Adverse effects: Occasional vomiting, diarrhea, insomnia, weakness, rash, phlebitis at injection site. Rarely, leukopenia. Mutagenicity and carcinogenicity may occur, but not established in humans.

Comments: Some texts recommend an initial loading dose of 15 mg/kg, with the first maintenance dose either 48 h later (for premature infants <2000 g) or 24 hours later (for the infant >2000 g at birth). Effectively penetrates into the CSF and therefore indicated for meningitis due to susceptible anaerobic pathogens.

Note: Some centers use empiric coverage with ampicillin and gentamicin for NEC. Use of metronidazole in NEC remains controversial.

(Gomella: Neonatology 1999, pp.577-578)

<u>Metronidazole</u> (Flagyl)

Dose/kg: 7.5 mg
Route & Frequency: IV, PO
0-4 wk <1.2 kg: q24h
≤ 7 d >1.2 kg: q12h
> 7 d 1.2-2 kg: q12h

Dose/kg 15 mg
Route & Frequency: >7 d >2 kg: q12h

Comments: Penetrates effectively into the CSF; may cause leukopenia, rash, phlebitis, and seizures.
Low cost is an advantage over other agents with similar antimicrobial range.

(Avery: Neonatology Pathophysiology and Management of the Newborn 1999, p.1558)

MEXILETINE (Mexitil)

Supplied: Capsules 150mg, 200mg, 250mg

Administration: PO

Extemporaneous Compounding (Recipe)

Dosage form: Oral suspension
Made from: Capsules
Concentration: 10 mg/mL
Stability: 6 days
Store: Refrigerate
Label: Shake well

Ingredient	Strength	Quantity
Mexiletine capsules	150 mg	8
Purified water USP		qs add 120 mL

Instructions: Empty the powder from the capsules into a mortar and add water while mixing. Use no sugar. (11)

Mexiletine

Although mexiletine's use is not widespread in pediatrics at this time, it may become the first-line drug used in the form of the congenital long QT syndrome resulting from a sodium channel defect.

Dosing: PO: 2-8 mg/kg/dose (varies with age)

Warnings: Skin rash, nausea

Oral Administration, Kinetics, Metabolites:

Effective concentrations tend to be in the range of 0.8 to 2.0 µg/ml.

Mexiletine crosses the placenta, but its use in fetal arrhythmias is rare. We have treated one fetus with apparent torsades de pointes VT successfully by maternal mexiletine administration. The fetus proved to have a congenital prolonged QT and intractable VT soon after birth.

Dosing and Interactions:

The stating dosage of mexiletine is 2 mg/kg every 8 hours. The dose may be increased up to approximately 5 mg/kg and up to 7 to 8 mg/kg for infants. No loading dose is given. Antacids or cimetidine can slow mexiletine absorption. There are no reported interactions with digoxin.

Side Effects: Adverse side effects are fairly common during mexiletine administration. The most common ones are related to gastrointestinal upset and skin rash. Many of the gastrointestinal complaints can be avoided by giving the drug with food. The skin rash is a fine, sandpaper like rash, mostly on the dorsum of the hands. Neurologic side effects are less common.

(Gillette: Clinical Pediatric Arrhythmias 1999,pp.231-248)

Mexiletine

Class: IB

Uses: Chronic ventricular ectopy, useful in patients responsive to phenytoin but with side effects, useful in patients with decreased function and VA, especially post-op

Dose (Level): 2.9-5 mg/kg/dose q8hr PO (0.5-2 µg/mL)
Serum concentration may not predict effect

Mode of Action: Structural analog of lidocaine; depresses conduction, especially at higher rates

ECG/EP Changes: None

Side Effects: Nausea (take food with drug), headache, paresthesia, rash, hepatitis (rare)

(Garson: The science and practice of pediatric cardiology 1998, p.2952)

Mexiletine

Mexiletine is similar in structure and function to lidocaine. Although most antiarrhythmic agents are also negative inotropes, mexiletine has no negative inotropic activity; therefore, it is well tolerated in patients with decreased cardiac output. Mexiletine is an excellent drug for ventricular tachycardia responsive or resistant to lidocaine. Mexiletine is available only for oral administration, at a dose of 2.2 to 5.5 mg/kg every 8 hours. The liver metabolizes 80% of the drug; the remainder is excreted in the urine.

(Yeh: Neonatal Therapeutics 1991, p.178)

MEZLOCILLIN (Mezlin)

Supplied: Injection, powder for 1g, 2gm, 3gm, and 4gm vials (contains 1.85mEq Na/gm)

Administration: IV, IM

For DIRECT IV INJECTION, each gram of mezlocillin should be reconstituted with at least 9 to 10ml SWFI, NS, or D5W. The appropriate dose should then be injected over a period of 3 to 5 minutes directly into a vein or into IV tubing. To minimize venous irritation, the concentration of drug should not exceed 10% (1).

For INTERMITTENT INFUSIONS, reconstituted solutions of mezlocillin should be diluted to a concentration of 20 to 40mg/ml and administered over 30 minutes (1).

Stable for 24 hours at room temperature or refrigerated in D10W at a concentration of 10mg/ml and 100mg/ml. Stable in D5W or NS for 48 hours at room temperature or for 7 days refrigerated at concentrations of 10mg/ml and 100mg/ml (1).

Mezlocillin (Mezlin)

Antibacterial Drugs for Pediatric Patients Beyond the Newborn Period
Dosage per kg/d

Route: IV, IM

Mild to Moderate Infections: 100-150 mg in 4 doses

Severe Infections: 200-300 mg in 4-6 doses

Note: In patients with history of allergy to penicillin or one of its many congeners, alternative drugs are recommended. In some circumstances, a cephalosporin or other β-lactam class drug may be acceptable. However, these drugs should not be used in patients with an immediate hypersensitivity (anaphylaxis) to penicillin because approximately 5% to 15% of penicillin-allergic patients will also be allergic to the cephalosporins.

(American Academy of Pediatrics: Report of the Committee on Infectious Diseases. Red Book 2000, pp.658,662)

Mezlocillin

Route: IV, IM

Dosage (mg/kg) and Interval of Administration:

Weight <1200 g
Age 0-4 WK: 75 q12h

Weight 1200-2000 g
Age 0-7 Days: 75 q12h
Age >7 Days: 75 q8h

Weight >2000 g
Age 0-7 Days: 75 q12h
Age >7 Days: 75 q8h

(Remington: Infectious Diseases of the Fetus and Newborn Infant 2001, p.1454)

Mezlocillin Sodium (Mezlin)

Classification: Semisynthetic extended-spectrum penicillin.

Action and spectrum: Mechanism of action identical to that of other ß-lactam antibiotics. Effective principally against Gram-negative organisms, including *Haemophilus influenzae*, *Klebsiella pneumoniae*, *Proteus mirabilis*, *Escherichia coli*, *Pseudomonas aeruginosa*, and some *Serratia* spp. Active also against many anaerobes, including *Peptococcus*, *Peptostreptococcus*, and *Bacteroides* spp (eg, *Bacteroides fragilis*).

Route: IM, IV (infuse over 30 minutes)

Dosage: 0-7 days: 150 mg/kg/day divided q12h
> 7 days: 225 mg/kg/day divided q8h

Elimination and metabolism:
Excreted primarily unchanged with urine; <10% hepatically metabolized.

Adverse effects: See Penicillin G (Aqueous), Parenteral.

Comments: Does not cause platelet dysfunction. Avoid IM use if possible. Adjust dosage in renal impairment. Contains 1.85 meq sodium per gram.

Note: Limited experience in neonates.
(Gomella: Neonatology 1999, p.578)

Mezlocillin

Route: IV, IM

Dosages (mg/kg/day) and Intervals of Administration:

Body weight < 2000g
0-7 days old: 150 div q12h
8-28 days old: 225 div q8h

Body weight >2000g
0-7 days old: 150 div q12h
8-28 days old: 225 div q8h

> 28 days old: 300 div q6h
(Nelson: Pocket Book of Pediatric Antimicrobial Therapy 2000-2001, p.16)

Mezlocillin

Condition: Urinary tract infection, Pseudomonas aeruginosa
Therapy: Mezlocillin or ticarcillin IV, IM AND aminoglycoside IV, IM x 10 days
Comment: Ceftazidime is a suitable alternative
(Nelson: Pocket Book of Pediatric Antimicrobial Therapy 2000-2001, p.13)

MICONAZOLE (Monistat)

Supplied: 2% cream, solution, powder, spray, ointment
Administration: Topical

Miconazole

Topical Drugs for Superficial Fungal Infections

Strength: 2%
Applications per day 2

Adverse Reactions/Notes: Irritant dermatitis

Skin infections are treated with topical nystatin, miconazole, clotrimazole, amphotericin B, ketoconazole, econazole, or ciclopirox. Nystatin usually is effective and is the least expensive of these drugs.
(American Academy of Pediatrics: Report of the Committee on Infectious Diseases. Red Book 2000, pp.673,200)

Miconazole

Miconazole is an imidazole derivative with activity against many species of fungi, including *Candida, Coccidioides* and *Cryptococcus*. Sung and associates treated two infants with systemic candidiasis with miconazole, and both recovered. One infant received 11.4 mg/kg per day, which was later increased to 15 mg/kg per day, also for

14 days. Serum levels in both were well above the minimal inhibitory concentration of the organism. Clarke and colleagues also reported a case of disseminated candidiasis in an infant treated with miconazole. The drug was given initially intravenously at a dose of 10 mg/kg per day in two divided doses and then orally. This infant developed ventricular tachycardia while receiving the drug. It was discontinued, and the tachycardia did not recur when the drug was given for a second course. There is an additional report of cardiac toxicity in an infant who received an overdose of miconazole. Casneuf and associates found miconazole to be effective for oral candidiasis and recommended a dosage schedule of 50 mg three times a day for infants weighing less than 10 kg and of 100 mg three times a day for children weighing more than 10 kg. In a recent randomized trail, miconazole gel in a dose of 25 mg four times a day was far more effective than nystatin suspension in neonates with oral candidiasis. There is a single report of resistance of *Candida* developing during therapy with miconazole.

Although there are additional reports of successful results with miconazole alone or in combination with other antifungal agents, there are increasing reports of failure of miconazole therapy. Data are insufficient and concerns are increasing regarding the routine use of miconazole in infants with infection caused by susceptible fungi.

(Remington: Infectious Diseases of the Fetus and Newborn Infant 2001, p.837)

Miconazole

Route: IV

Dosage: 20-40 mg/kg/day 8 hours
NON-NEWBORN SECTION

(Nelson: Pocket Book of Pediatric Antimicrobial Therapy 2000-2001, p.80)

Miconazole

Usual Dosage: Neonates: I.V.: 5-15 mg/kg/day divided every 8-24 hours
Infants and Children:
Topical: Apply twice daily

Administration: Parenteral:
I.V.: Administer by slow I.V. intermittent infusion over 1-2 hours at a final concentration not to exceed 6 mg/mL

Intrathecal or intraventricular: When necessary the undiluted I.V. formulation may be used

Topical: Apply sparingly to the cleansed, dry affected area; if intertriginous areas are involved, rub cream gently into the skin

(Taketomo: Pediatric Dosage Handbook 1999-2000, pp.600-602)

MIDAZOLAM (Versed)

Supplied: Syrup: 2mg/ml, 118ml
Injection: 1 mg/ml in 2 ml, 5 mg/ml in 1 ml (others) (contains benzyl alcohol).

Administration: IV, IM, PO

Infusion: Midazolam injection that has been diluted to a final concentration of 0.5 mg/ml or less in D5W or 0.9% NaCl is stable for 24 hours (3).

For IV injection midazolam is injected in incremental doses (3).

Pharmacology: Clinical experience with the drug suggests that Midazolam is 3 to 4 times as potent per mg as diazepam (1).

DO NOT use IV loading doses in neonates, rather the infusion may be run more rapidly for the first several hours to establish therapeutic plasma levels. Frequently reassess the rate of infusion, particularly after the first 24 hours, so as to administer the lowest possible effective dose and reduce potential for drug accumulation. This is particularly important because of the potential for adverse effects related to metabolism of the benzyl alcohol (1).

Midazolam Hydrochloride (Versed)

Indications and use:
Antianxiety agent. May be used for infants on assisted ventilation who are agitated and need sedation, or as a sedative prior to procedures.

Actions: Short-acting benzodiazepine.

Route: IV, IM, IV continuous infusion

Dosage: Intermittent: 0.05-0.2 mg/kg/dose IV q2-4h prn.

Continuous infusion:
- Loading dose: 0.2 mg/kg IV.
- Infusion: 0.4-0.6 mcg/kg/min.
- Maximum: 6 mcg/kg/min.

Adverse effects: Respiratory depression and arrest with excessive doses or rapid IV infusions. May cause hypotension. Infuse IV slowly. Use caution, particularly if fentanyl is being used concurrently.

(Gomella: Neonatology 1999, p.578)

Midazolam

Dose/kg: 0.03-0.1 mg
Route & frequency: IV, IM q2h-q4h prn

Dose/kg: 0.05 mg/h
Route & frequency: Continuous IV infusion; titrate up based on clinical response

Comments: May cause respiratory depression, hypotension, and dependence

(Avery: Neonatology Pathophysiology and Management of the Newborn 1999, p.1558)

Midazolam

Route & Dose: IV, IM: 0.07-0.20 mg/kg/dose q 2-4 h prn for sedation

Adverse Effects and Cautions:

Limited experience in newborns. Respiratory depression, apnea

(Taeusch: Avery's Diseases of the Newborn 1998, p.1346)

Midazolam

Use: Sedation, anxiolysis, amnesia prior to procedure or before induction of anesthesia; conscious sedation prior to diagnostic or radiographic procedures; continuous I.V. sedation of intubated and mechanically ventilated patients, status epilepticus

Usual Dosage: Neonates: Conscious sedation during mechanical ventilation: I.V. continuous infusion:
<32 weeks: Initial: 0.03 mg/kg/hour (0.5 mcg/kg/minute)
>32 weeks: Initial: 0.06 mg/kg/hour (1 mcg/kg/minute)
Note: Do not use I.V. Loading doses in neonates; for faster achievement of sedation, infuse the continuous infusion at a faster rate for the first several hours; use the smallest dose possible

Infants >2 months and Children: Status epilepticus refractory to standard therapy: I.V.: Loading dose: 0.15 mg/kg followed by a continuous infusion of 1 mcg/kg/minute; titrate dose upward every 5 minutes until clinical seizure activity is controlled; mean infusion rate required in 24 children was 2.3 mcg/kg/minute with a range of 1-18 mcg/kg/minute

Infants ≥6 months and Children: Sedation, anxiolysis, and amnesia prior to procedure or before induction of anesthesia: Oral: Single dose: 0.25-0.5 mg/kg, depending on patient status and desired effect, usual: 0.5 mg/kg; maximum dose: 20 mg:

Preoperative sedation or conscious sedation for procedures:
I.M.: Usual: 0.1-0.15 mg/kg 30-60 minutes before surgery or procedure; range: 0.05-0.15 mg/kg; doses up to 0.5 mg/kg have been used in more anxious patients; maximum total dose: 10 mg

I.V.: Infants <6 months: Limited information is available in nonintubated infants; dosing recommendations are unclear; infants <6 months are at higher risk for airway obstruction and hypoventilation; titrate dose with small increments to desired clinical effect; monitor carefully

Infants 6 months to Children 5 years: Initial: 0.05-0.1 mg/kg; titrate dose carefully; total dose of 0.6 mg/kg may be required; usual total dose maximum dose; 6 mg

Intranasal: Usual: 0.2 mg/kg; may repeat in 5-15 minutes; range: 0.2-0.3 mg/kg/dose

Conscious sedation during mechanical ventilation: I.V.; Continuous infusion: Loading dose: 0.05-0.2 mg/kg given slow I.V. over 2-3 minutes, then follow with initial continuous infusion: 0.06-0.12 mg/kg/hour (1-2 mcg/kg/minute); titrate to the desired effect; range: 0.4-6 mcg/kg/minute

Administration: Intranasal: Administer using a 1 mL needleless syringe into the nares over 15 seconds; use the 5 mg/mL injection; ½ of the dose may be administered to each nare

Parenteral: I.V.; Administer by slow I.V. injection over at least 2-5 minutes at a concentration of 1-5 mg/mL or by I.V. infusion; avoid extravasation; do not administer intra-arterially

Monitoring Parameters:
Level of sedation, respiratory rate, heart rate, blood pressure, oxygen saturation (ie. pulse, oximetry)

Nursing Implications:
Abrupt discontinuation after prolonged use may result in withdrawal symptoms

(Taketomo: Pediatric dosage Handbook 1999-2000, pp.602-605)

<u>Midazolam</u> (Versed)

Titrate to effect under controlled conditions.

Dose & Route: Sedation for procedures:
Children: IV:
6 months-5 yrs:0.05-0.1 mg/kg/dose over 2-3 min. May repeat dose PRN in 2-3 min intervals up to **max total dose** of 6 mg. A total dose up to 0.6 mg/kg may be necessary for desired effect.

Sedation with mechanical ventilation:
Intermittent:
Infants and Children: 0.05-0.15 mg/kg/dose Q1-2 hr PRN

Continuous IV infusion: (initial doses, titrate to effect):
Neonates:
<32 weeks gestation: 0.5 mcg/kg/min
≥32 weeks gestation: 1 mcg/kg/min
Infants and Children: 1-2 mcg/kg/min

Remarks: **Contraindicated** in patients with narrow angle glaucoma and shock. Causes respiratory depression, hypotension and bradycardia. Cardiovascular monitoring is recommended. Use lower doses or reduce dose when given in combination with narcotics or in patients with respiratory compromise.

Drug is a substrate for CYP 450 3A4. Serum concentrations may be increased by cimetidine, erythromycin, itraconazole, ketoconazole, and protease inhibitors. Sedative effects may be antagonized by theophylline. **Adjust dose in renal failure**

(Siberry: The Harriet Lane Handbook 2000 p.775)

Midazolam (Versed)

Dose:
0.07-0.08 mg/kg IM
0.035 mg/kg IV
Max total 0.2 mg/kg or 2.5 mg IV
0.3 mg/kg PR

Adverse Effects: Respiratory depression
Hypotension
Bradycardia

(Garson: The science and practice of pediatric cardiology 1998, p.2955)

MILRINONE (Primacor)

Supplied: Injection 1 mg/ml, in 10 and 20 ml vials and 5 ml carpuject sterile cartridge needle units.

Injection pre-mix 200 in mcg/ml in 5% Dextrose injection, in 100 ml

Dilution: Dilute with 0.45% or 0.9% sodium chloride injection or 5% Dextrose injection only . (1)

Milrinone

THERAPY FOR ACUTE CONGESTIVE CARDIAC FAILURE

Dose and Route of Administration:

Load with 50 µg/kg over 10-15 minutes. Maintain on 0.35-0.75 µg/kg/minute.

Hemodynamic Effects:

Increases cardiac output if preload is normal or increased.

Complications and Comments Regarding Use:

Hypotension: hemodynamic monitoring required.

Notes: Milrinone is considered 10 to 30 times more potent than its parent drug, amrinone. After intravenous injection, the serum half-lives of amrinone and milrinone are 2.6 to 3.6 and 0.8 hours, respectively, in patients with congestive heart failure. Amrinone is primarily metabolized by the liver, but also is partially excreted unchanged in the urine to a variable degree. Milrinone is largely excreted by the kidneys.

When used acutely, amrinone and milrinone improve cardiac output, decrease right and left ventricular filling pressures, and decrease systemic vascular resistance. There typically are minimal effects on heart rate or blood pressure in patients with congestive heart failure and following cardiac surgery. Early concern was raised that amrinone achieved its effects solely as a function of its vasodilating action, but recent studies show that amrinone also increases left ventricular contractility.

Loading the patient with amrinone appears to be more difficult than loading with milrinone. Although the package insert calls for a loading dose of 0.75 mg/kg intravenously given over several minutes, we have found that two or sometimes three of these loading doses is preferable. The maintenance infusion rate is 5 to 10 µg/kg/minute. However, we generally prefer milrinone, which we have found to have fewer hemodynamic side effects than amrinone. We load patients with 50 µg/kg of intravenous milrinone over several minutes. The maintenance dose is 0.35 to 0.75 µg/kg/minute. Serous adverse side effects from intravenous amrinone and milrinone are not common, and consist of significant hypotension, reversible thrombocytopenia, and ventricular ectopy. Because of the vasodilating effect of the drug, blood pressure and cardiac output should be monitored carefully and intravascular volume must be adequate before intravenous loading. Amrinone may increase hepatic enzyme levels in the serum and may cause gastrointestinal symptoms.

(Garson: The science and practice of pediatric cardiology 1998, pp.2329-2341)

<u>Milrinone</u>

Dosage: Loading dose = 0.1 mg/kg i.v. over 15-30 min; continuous infusion = 0.5-0.75 µg/kg/min

(Allen: Moss and Adam's Heart Disease in Infants, children and Adolescents 2001, pp.1460-1468)

<u>Milrinone</u>

Use: Short-term treatment of refractory CHF

Usual Dosage: I.V.:

Neonates, Infants, and Children: A limited number of studies have used different dosing schemes (see Additional Information). Two recent pharmacokinetic studies propose per kg doses for pediatric patients with septic shock that are greater than those recommended for adults (Lindsay, 1998) and in infants and children after cardiac surgery (Ramamoorthy 1998). Further pharmacodynamic studies are needed to define pediatric milrinone guidelines. Several centers are using the following guidelines:

Loading dose: 50 mcg/kg administered over 15 minutes followed by a continuous infusion of 0.5 mcg/kg/minute; range: 0.25-0.75 mcg/kg/minute; titrate dose to effect

Administration: Loading dose: Administer slow I.V. push over 15 minutes for pediatric patients and over 10 minutes in adults; loading dose may be given as undiluted solution, but my dilute to 10-20 mL (in adults) for ease of administration

I.V. continuous infusion: Dilute with ½Ns, NS, or D_5W and administer via infusion pump or syringe pump; usual concentration: ≤200 mcg/mL; 250 mcg/mL in NS has been used (see Barton, 1996)

Monitoring Parameters:

Blood pressure, heart rate, cardiac output, CI, SVR, PVR, CVP, EKG, platelet count, serum potassium, renal function; clinical signs and symptoms of CHF

Nursing Implications:

Do not administer furosemide I.V. push via "Y" site into milrinone solutions as precipitate will occur; decrease the infusion rate if significant hypotension occurs

Additional Information:

Dosing schemes and proposed dosing based on pharmacokinetic data:

Neonates: A loading dose of 50 mcg/kg administered over 15 minutes, followed by a continuous infusion of 0.5 mcg/kg/minute for 30 minutes in 10 neonates (3-27 days old, median age 5 days) improved hemodynamic parameters and was well tolerated (see Chang, 1995). Further neonatal studies of longer duration are needed.

Infants and children with septic shock: Twelve patients (9 months to 15 years of age) were administered a loading dose of 50 mcg/kg, followed by a continuous infusion of 0.5 mcg/kg/minute. At 1 hours after the loading doe, if patients did not respond (defined as a ≥20% increase in CI or an improvement in peripheral perfusion), an additional loading dose of 25 mcg/kg was given and the infusion rate was increased to 0.75 mcg/kg/minute. Nine of 12 patients required the additional loading dose and increased rate of infusion (see Barton 1996). A subsequent pharmacokinetic analysis of these patients recommended larger loading doses of 75 mcg/kg and infusion rates of 0.75-1 mcg/kg/minute. However, these doses were based on a one-compartment pharmacokinetic model and are higher than the mean infusion rate of 0.69 mcg/kg/minute used in the study (see Lindsay 1998). Further studies are needed.

Infants and Children after open heart surgery: Group A: Eleven patients received a loading dose of 25 mcg/kg given over 5 minutes followed by an infusion of 0.25 mcg/kg/minute; 30 minutes later, a second 25 mcg/kg loading dose was given and the infusion was increased to 0.5 mcg/kg/minute. Group B: 8 patients received a loading dose of 50 mcg/kg given over 10 minutes followed by an infusion of 0.5 mcg/kg/minute; 30 minutes later, a second loading dose of 25 mcg/kg was given and the infusion was increased to 0.75 mcg/kg/minute. Patients in both groups received a third loading dose of 25 mcg/kg if needed. A two-compartment model and NONMEM pharmacokinetic analyses were performed. Based on the NONMEM analysis, the authors propose the following doses: Infants: Loading dose: 104 mcg/kg and continuous infusion of 0.49 mcg/kg/minute; children: loading dose: 67 mcg/kg and continuous infusion of 0.61 mcg/kg/minute. Further studies ar needed before these proposed doses can routinely be used in the pediatric population.

(Taketomo: Pediatric Dosage Handbook 1999-2000, pp.606-608)

Milrinone

Dose: 0.25-1 µg/kg/min

Mode of Action: Phosphodiesterase inhibitor

Adverse Effects: Like amrinone, but no thrombocytopenia

Comments: 50 µg/kg load over 15 minutes

(Garson: The science and practice of pediatric cardiology 1998, p.2950)

MIVACURIUM CHLORIDE (Mivacron)

Supplied: 0.5 mg/ml (in 5% Dextrose 50 ml)
2 mg/ml in 5 ml, 10 ml vials in water for injection

Administration: IV injection, continuous infusion

Mivacurium is a short acting, nondepolarizing skeletal muscle relaxant for IV administration. The clinically effective duration of action of the stereoisomers in mivacurium is one-third to one-half that of intermediate-acting agents and 2 to 2.5 times that of succinylcholine (1).

Mivacurium has not been studied on children < 2 years of age (1).

Mivacurium

Usual Dosage: Children require higher doses mg/kg than adults and more frequent maintenance doses; I.V.: Children 2-12 years: 0.2 mg/kg; continuous infusion: 10-14 mcg/kg/minute; doses as high as 31 mcg/kg/minute have been used

Administration: Parenteral: Administer undiluted by rapid I.V. injection; infusions diluted in D_5W to a maximum concentration of 0.5 mg/mL

Monitoring Parameters: Assisted ventilation status, heart rate, blood pressure, peripheral nerve stimulator measuring twitch response

Nursing Implications: Does not alter the patient's state of consciousness; addition of sedation is recommended

(Taketomo: Pediatric dosage Handbook 1998-1999, pp.746-747)

Mivacurium

Neuromuscular Blocking Drug:
0.2 mg/kg; incremental dose 0.1 µg/kg, infusion rate 10 µg/kg/min.

Mivacurium is a synthetic nondepolarizing neuromuscular blocking agent with a short duration of action; it is hydrolyzed by plasma cholinesterase. A dose of 0.1-0.2 mg/kg produces a profound degree of block in under 2 minutes, but the onset of block is not as rapid as that which follows succinylcholine. The duration of action is approximately 50% of that of vecuronium. The cardiovascular effects of the drug are minimal. Its short duration of action suggests that it may prove useful for intubation for minor procedures and possibly for use as an infusion, especially when the extent of neuromuscular block must be adjusted rapidly (e.g. when muscle power must be assessed or motor evoked potentials monitored). As the recovery time has been shown to relate to plasma cholinesterase activity, prolonged effects may be expected in those with abnormality of the plasma cholinesterases.

(Steward: Manual of Pediatric Anesthesia 1995, pp.512,63)

<u>Mivacurium</u>

Indication: Induction of neuromuscular blockade to facilitate intubation

Dose and Route of Administration: 0.3 mg/kg IV

Side Effects (partial list): Apnea, paralysis

(Gregory: Pediatric Anesthesia 1994, p.902)

MORICIZINE (Ethmozine)

Supplied: Tablets 200mg, 250mg, 300mg
Administration: PO

<u>Moricizine</u>

Dosing: PO: 200-600 mg/m²/day
Warnings: Neurologic effects

Dosing and Interactions:

The dose of moricizine has not been well established in children. Available data are based on body surface area with a starting dose of 200 mg/m²/day divided every 8 hours. The maximum is 600 mg/m²/day. There are no known significant interactions of moricizine with digoxin. As with other drugs with extensive hepatic transformation, cimetidine may reduce clearance and prolong the elimination $t_{1/2}$

Side Effects: At higher dose ranges, neurologic side effects include blurry vision, headache, paresthesia, and tingling. Gastrointestinal symptoms are also common and are often alleviated by coadministration with food.

(Gillette: Clinical Pediatric Arrhythmias 1999, pp.231-248)

<u>Ethmozine</u>

Class: IB
Uses: AET, Ventricular ectopy, AVN reentry?

Dose (Level): 200-600 mg/m²/day divided q8hr

Mode of Action: Phenothiazine derivative, suppresses abnormal automaticity, shortens repolarization

ECG/EP Changes: Slight ↑ Pr, ↑ QRS; increases AH, HV

Side Effects: Headache, vertigo, paresthesia, tinnitus, nystagmus

(Garson: The science and practice of pediatric cardiology 1998, p.2952)

MORPHINE SULFATE

Supplied: Injection 1mg, 2mg, 4mg, 5mg, 8mg, 10mg, 15mg, 25mg, 50 mg/ml

Administration: IV, IM, SC

For IV administration: May give by direct IV injection over 3 to 5 minutes. For intermittent infusion or continuous infusion, dilute as desired in D5W or NS. Titrate to response or side effects (2).

For appropriate dose to be administered, dilution of product may be needed (Author).

Rapid IV use increases the incidence of adverse reactions. DO NOT administer IV unless a narcotic antagonist is immediately available (1).

Morphine Sulfate (Various)

Indications and use: Analgesia, preoperative sedation, supplement to anesthesia, acute pulmonary edema.

Actions: CNS opiate receptor agonist resulting in analgesia, drowsiness, and alterations in mood and pain perception. Vasodilatory (especially coronary vessels).

Route: IM, IV, SC.

Dosage: 0.05-0.2 mg/kg/dose q2-4h or continuous administration of 0.01-0.04 mg/kg/h.

Adverse effects: Dose-dependent side effects include miosis, respiratory depression, drowsiness, bradycardia, and hypotension. Constipation, sedation, GI upset, urine retention, histamine release, and sweating may occur. Causes physiological dependence; taper the dose gradually after long-term use to avoid withdrawal.

(Gomella: Neonatology 1999, pp.578-579)

Morphine

Indication: Protocol for inborn infants with Congenital Diaphragmatic Hernia

Continuous sedation was provided with morphine infusion, initially 20 μg/kg/hr

(Finer: Congenital diaphragmatic Hernia: Developing a Protocolized Approach. J Pediatr Surg 1998;33:1331-1337)

Morphine

The infants were randomized in 5 blocks with closed envelopes and stratified for birth weight of less and equal or more than 1500 g to receive a loading dose of 10.5 mcg/kg fentanyl or 140 mcg/kg morphine in 1 hour. Thereafter, the infusion was continued at a maintenance rate of 1.5 mcg/kg/hr fentanyl or 20 mcg/kg/hr morphine for at least 24 hours.

Conclusions: With at least as effective analgesia as with morphine, fentanyl had fewer side effects. Fentanyl may be superior to morphine for short-term postnatal analgesia in newborn infants.

(Saarenmaa: Advantages of fentanyl over morphine in analgesia for ventilated newborn infants after birth: a randomized trial. J Pediatr 1999;134:144-50)

Morphine Sulfate

Titrate to effect

Dose & Route: Analgesia/tetralogy (cyanotic) spells:
Neonates: 0.05-0.2 mg/kg/dose IM, slow IV, SC Q4 hr.

Neonatal opiate withdrawal: 0.08-0.2 mg/dose Q3-4 hr PRN

Infants and Children:
PO: 0.2-0.5 mg/kg/dose Q4-6 hr PRN (immediate release) or 0.3-0.6 mg/kg/dose Q12 hr PRN (controlled release)

IM/IV/SC: 0.1-0.2 mg/kg/dose Q2-4 hr PRN;
max dose: 15 mg/dose.

Continuous IV infusion: (Dosing ranges, titrate to effect)
Neonates: 0.01-0.02 mg/kg/hr
Infants and Children: 0.025-2.6 mg/kg/hr

Remarks: Dependence, CNS and respiratory depression, nausea, vomiting, urinary retention, constipation, hypotension, bradycardia, increased ICP, miosis, biliary spasm, allergy may occur. **Naloxone may be used to reverse effects**, especially respiratory depression. Causes histamine release resulting in itching and possible bronchospasm. Neonates may require higher doses due to decreased amounts of active metabolites. Rectal dosing is same as oral dosing but is not recommended due to poor absorption.

Adjust dose in renal failure

(Siberry: The Harriet Lane Handbook 2000, pp.779-780)

Morphine Sulfate

Warnings: Some preparations contain sulfites which may cause allergic reactions; neonates and infants <3 months of age are more susceptible to respiratory depression, use with caution and in reduced doses in this age group; use only preservative free injections for epidural or intrathecal administration and in neonates.

Usual Dosage: **Doses should be titrated to appropriate effect**: when changing routes of administration in chronically treated patients, please note that oral doses are approximately one-half as effective as parenteral dose

Neonates: (see Warnings; use preservative free formulation):

I.M., I.V., S.C.: Initial: 0.05 mg/kg every 4-8 hours; titrate carefully to effect; maximum dose: 0.1 mg/kg/dose

I.V. continuous infusion: Initial: 0.01 mg/kg/hour (10 mcg/kg/hour); do **not** exceed infusion rates of 0.015-0.02 mg/kg/hour due to decreased elimination, increased CNS sensitivity, and adverse effects

Infants and Children:
Oral: Tablet and solution (prompt release): 0.2-0.5 mg/kg/dose every 4-6 hours as needed; tablet (controlled release): 0.3-0.6 mg/kg/dose every 12 hours

I.M., I.V., S.C.: 0.1-0.2 mg/kg/doe every 2-4 hours as needed; may initiate at 0.05 mg/kg/dose; usual maximum dose: 15 mg/dose

I.V., S.C. Continuous infusion:
Sickle cell or cancer pain: Range: 0.025-2.6 mg/kg/hour (median dose, cancer pain: 0.04-0.07 mg/kg/hour)
Postoperative pain: 0.01-0.04 mg/kg/hour

Sedation/analgesia for procedures: I.V.: 0.05-0.1 mg/kg 5 minutes before the procedure

Epidural (use preservative free): 0.03-0.05 mg/kg (30-50 mcg/kg): maximum dose; 0.1 mg/kg (100 mcg/kg) or 5 mg/24 hours

Administration: Oral: Administer with food; swallow controlled or sustained release products whole, do not chew or crush

Parenteral:
I.V. push: Administer over at least 5 minutes at a final concentration of 0.5-5 mg/mL (rapid I.V. administration may increase adverse effects)

Intermittent infusion: Administer over 15-30 minutes
Continuous I.V. infusion: 0.1-1 mg/mL in D_5W
Epidural and intrathecal: Use only preservative free injections.

Monitoring Parameters:
Respiratory and cardiovascular status, oxygen saturation, pain relief (if used for analgesia), level of sedation

Nursing Implications:
Do not administer rapidly I.V.

Additional Information:
Less adverse effects are associated with epidural compared to intrathecal route of administration;

equianalgesic doses: Codeine: 120 mg I.M. = morphine 10 mg I.M. = single dose oral morphine 60 mg or chronic dosing oral morphine 15-25 mg

(Taketomo: Pediatric Dosage Handbook 1999-2000, pp.616-619)

MULTIVITAMINS

Supplied: Multivitamins, Parenteral (MVI Pediatric, MVC 9+4 Pediatric)
Vitamin A, D, C Drops (Tri vi sol, Vi Daylin ADC)
Multivitamin Drops (Poly vi Sol, Vi Daylin)

Administration: PO, IV

Multivitamins

Dose: 1 ml PO as a single daily dose or divided every 12 hours mixed in a small amount of the infant's feeding.

Begin with 0.5 ml PO bid in infants receiving less than 20 ml of formula per feeding, then advance to 1 ml PO as a single daily dose when feeding tolerance has improved and feeding volumes are larger.

Begin vitamin supplementation only when infant has advanced to full-strength formula to avoid GI upset.

Continue vitamin supplement in formula-fed preterm infants until the infant's intake exceeds 300 kcal/day or a body weight of 2.5 kg is achieved.

Nursing Implications:

Monitor for feeding intolerance.

(Zenk: Neonatal Medications & Nutrition. A Comprehensive Guide 2000; pp.341-343)

MUPIROCIN (Bactroban, Pseudomonic Acid A)

Supplied: Cream, nasal ointment 1gm tube
Ointment 2%, 15 gms, 30 gms

Administration: Topical

Indications: For the topical treatment of impetigo due to *Staphylococcus aureus*, beta hemolytic *Streptococcus* and *S pyogenes*. (1)

Mupirocin (Bactroban)

Indications and use:

Topical treatment of impetigo due to *Staphyococcus aureus* (including methicillin-resistant and β-lactamase-producing strains), β-hemolytic *Streptococcus* spp, and *Streptococcus pyogenes*. Used for minor bacterial skin infections due to susceptible organisms.

Actions: A topical antibacterial ointment. Inhibits protein and RNA synthesis by binding to bacterial isoleucyl-tRNA synthetase.

Route: Topical.

Dosage: Apply sparingly 3 times a day. Reevaluate in 3-5 days if no response.

Adverse effects: Burning, rash, erythema, and pruritus.

Comments: Use with caution in burn patients and patients with impaired renal function. Avoid contact with eyes; not for ophthalmic use. When applied to extensive open wounds or burns, the possibility of absorption of the polyethylene glycol vehicle, resulting in serious renal toxicity, should be considered.

(Gomella: Neonatology 1999, p.579)

Mupirocin

Route: Topical
Dosage: Apply to infected skin or nasal mucosa
Interval: q8h
NON-NEWBORN SECTION

(Nelson: Pocket Book of Pediatric Antimicrobial Therapy 2000-2001, p.80)

Mupirocin

Condition: Skin and Soft Tissues, Impetigo neonatorum

Therapy: Cleansing alone OR oxacillin IV, IM OR cephalexin 50 mg/kg/day PO div q6-8h, OR mupirocin topically; x 5 days

Comment: No antibiotic for superficial impetigo; Chlorhexidine baths; Break lesions with alcohol swab.

(Nelson: Pocket Book of Pediatric Antimicrobial Therapy 2000-2001, p.12)

Mupirocin (Bactroban)

Dose: Apply a small amount to the affected area three times a day.

Duration of Therapy: Continue therapy for 5-14 days. Re-evaluate if there is no improvement within 3-5 days.

Use with caution in patients with impaired renal function.

Administration: Affected area may be covered with a gauze dressing if desired.

Nursing Implications: Monitor for improvement in infection.

Check for signs of intolerance to mupirocin, such as erythema, increased exudate, or rash.

(Zenk: Neonatal Medications & Nutrition. A Comprehensive Guide 2000; pp:344-346)

NADOLOL (Corgard)

Supplied: Tablets 20mg, 40mg, others
Administration: PO

Nadolol

Nadolol is an oral sustained-release preparation. It has been administered to pediatric patients for SVT and for autonomic dysfunction syndromes.

Dosing: PO: 1 mg/kg/day

Warnings: Similar to atenolol

Oral Administration:

Nadolol is poorly absorbed. And peak plasma levels occur 3 to 4 hours after administration.

Dosing and Interactions:

Nadolol is approximately 50% as effective a beta blocker as propranolol. Initial therapy is often recommended at 1 mg/kg/day.

Side Effects: Effects on sinus rate and AV node conduction are similar to those of other nonselective beta-blocking agent.

(Gillette: Clinical Pediatric Arrhythmias 1999,pp.231-248)

Nadolol

Dosage: 1-5 mg/kg p.o. daily (maximum daily dose = 640 mg)

(Allen: Moss and Adam's Heart Disease in Infants, children and Adolescents 2001, pp.1460-1468)

NAFCILLIN (Nafcil, Unipen)

Supplied: Injection, powder for 500mg, 1gm, 2gm vials (contains 2.9mEq Na/gm)

Administration: IV, IM

For INTERMITTENT INFUSION, administer slowly over 30 to 60 minutes. Concentration of the antibiotic should be 2-40mg/mL (3).

FOR TREATMENT OF EXTRAVASATION see Hyaluronidase.

Additives that may result in a final pH of above 8 or below 5 should not be mixed with nafcillin.

The osmolality of nafcillin sodium (Wyeth) 40 mg/ml was determined to be 403 mOsm/kg in D5W and 402 mOsm/kg in N.S.

The osmolality of nafcillin sodium (Wyeth) 250 mg/ml in sterile water for injection was determined to be 709 mOsm/kg. (3)

Nafcillin

Antibacterial Drugs for Newborn Infants
Dose (mg/kg or Units [U]/kg) and Frequency of Administration
Route: IV, IM

Dose: Infants 0-4 wk
BW <1200 g: 25 every 12 h

Infants <1 wk old
BW ≤1200-2000 g: 25 every 12 h
BW >2000 g: 25 every 8 h

Infants ≥1 wk old
BW ≤2000-2000 g: 25 every 8 h
BW >2000 g: 25-35 every 6 h

Note: For meningitis, the larger dosage is recommended

Antibacterial Drugs for Pediatric Patients Beyond the Newborn Period
Dosage per kg/d

Route: IV, IM
Mild to Moderate Infections: 50-100 mg in 4 doses

Severe Infections: 100-150 mg in 4 doses

Comments: Serum concentrations after oral administration are low compared with those after other orally administered antistaphylococcal drugs

Note: In patients with history of allergy to penicillin or one of its many congeners, alternative drugs are recommended. In some circumstances, a cephalosporin or other β-lactam class drug may be acceptable. However, these drugs should not be used in patients with an immediate hypersensitivity (anaphylaxis) to penicillin because approximately 5% to 15% of penicillin-allergic patients will also be allergic to the cephalosporins.

(American Academy of Pediatrics: Report of the Committee on Infectious Diseases. Red Book 2000, pp.651-652,660,662)

Nafcillin

Route: IV
Dosage (mg/kg) and Interval of Administration:

Weight <1200 g
Age 0-4 wk: 25 q12h

Weight 1200-2000 g
Age 0-7 days: 25 q12h
Age >7 days: 25 q8h

Weight >2000 g
Age 0-7 days: 25 q8h
Age >7 days: 37.5 q6h

(Remington: Infectious Diseases of the Fetus and Newborn Infant 2001, p.1454)

Nafcillin

Route: IV

Dosages (mg/kg/day) and Intervals of Administration:

Body weight < 2000 gm
0-7 days old: 50 div q12h
8-28 days old: 75 div q8h

Body weight > 2000 gm
0-7 days old: 75 div q8h
8-28 days old: 150 div q6h

> 28 days old: 150 div q6h

(Nelson: Pocket Book of Pediatric Antimicrobial Therapy 2000-2001, p.16)

Nafcillin Sodium (Unipen)

Classification: Semisynthetic penicillinase-resistant penicillin.

Action and spectrum:
Mechanism of action identical to that of other ß-lactam antibiotics. Spectrum identical to that of methicillin (ie, primarily antistaphylococcal).

Route: IV (infuse over 30 min), IM (avoid - very irritating)

Dosage: <2000 g and 0-7 days old: 50 mg/kg/day divided q12h.
<2000 g and >7 days old: 75 mg/kg/day divided q8h.
>2000 g and 0-7 days old: 50 mg/kg/day divided q8h.
>2000 g and >7 days old: 75 mg/kg/day divided q6h.

Elimination and metabolism: Hepatic metabolism; concentrated in bile.

Adverse effects: Thrombophlebitis, hypersensitivity, and leukopenia. Severe tissue injury after IV extravasation.

Comments: Avoid IM use. Contains 2.9 meq sodium per gram.
(Gomella: Neonatology 1999, p.579)

NALOXONE (Narcan)

Supplied: Injection 0.4mg/ml in 1ml, 2ml and 10ml
Injection 1.0mg/ml in 2ml and 10ml
Injection, Neonatal* 0.02mg/ml in 2ml

Administration: IV, IM, SC, ET
*See Committee citation for dosage form to be used with newborns (author).

Administer by DIRECT IV INJECTION. Use rapid IV push over a period of 30 seconds (4).

Duration of action of some narcotics may exceed that of naloxone. Keep patients under surveillance and give repeat doses as necessary. (1)

Naloxone

Naloxone hydrochloride is a narcotic antagonist without respiratory-depressant activity. It is specifically indicated for reversal of respiratory depression in a newly born infant whose mother received narcotics within 4 hours of delivery. Always establish and maintain adequate ventilation before administration of naloxone. Do not administer naloxone to newly born infants whose mothers are suspected of having recently abused narcotic drugs because it may precipitate abrupt withdrawal signs in such infants.

The recommended dose of naloxone is 0.1 mg/kg of a 0.4 mg/mL or 1.0 mg/mL solution given intravenously, endotrachealy, or-if perfusion is adequate-intramuscularly or subcutaneously. Because the duration of action of narcotics may exceed that of naloxone, continued monitoring of respiratory function is essential, and repeated naloxone doses may be necessary to prevent recurrent apnea.

Medications: Drugs are rarely indicated in resuscitation of the newly born infant. Bradycardia in the newly born infant is usually the result of inadequate lung inflation or profound hypoxia, and adequate ventilation is the most important step in correcting bradycardia. Administer medications if, despite adequate ventilation with 100% oxygen and chest compressions, the heart rate remains <60 bpm.

Routes of Medication Administration.

The tracheal route is generally the most rapidly accessible route for drug administration during resuscitation. It maybe used for administration of epinephrine and naloxone, but it should not be used during resuscitation for administration of caustic agents such as sodium bicarbonate. The tracheal route of administration may result in a more variable response to epinephrine than the intravenous route; however, neonatal data is insufficient to recommend a higher dose of epinephrine for tracheal administration.

Attempt to establish intravenous access in neonates who fail to respond to tracheally administered epinephrine. The umbilical vein is the most rapidly accessible venous route; it may be used for epinephrine or naloxone administration as well as for administration of volume expanders and bicarbonate. Insert a 3.5F or 5F radiopaque catheter so that the tip is just below skin level and a free flow of blood returns on aspiration. Deep insertion poses the risk of infusion of hypertonic and vasoactive medications into the liver. Take care to avoid introduction of air emboli into the umbilical vein.

Peripheral sites for venous access (scalp or peripheral vein) may be adequate but are usually more difficult to cannulate. Naloxone may be given intramuscularly or subcutaneously but only after effective assisted ventilation has been established and only if the infant's peripheral circulation is adequate. We do not recommend administration of resuscitation drugs through the umbilical artery because the artery is often not rapidly accessible and complications may result if vasoactive or hypertonic drugs (eg, epinephrine or bicarbonate) are given by this route.

Intraosseous lines are not commonly used in newly born infants because the umbilical vein is more accessible, the small bones are fragile, and the intraosseous space is small in a premature infant. Intraosseous access has been shown to be useful in the neonate and older infant when vascular access is difficult to achieve. Intraosseous access can be used as an alternative route for medications/volume expansion if umbilical or other direct venous access is not readily attainable (Clas IIb. LOE 5).

(American Heart Association: Part 11: Neonatal Resuscitation 2000;102 (suppl I):I-343-I-357)

<u>Naloxone Hydrochloride</u> (Narcan)

Indications and use:
Narcotic reversal and investigationally for the treatment of septic shock.

Actions: A pure opiate antagonist with little or no agonistic activity. It has minimal or no pharmacologic effect, even in high doses, in patients who have not received opiates. Onset of action is within 1-2 min after IV injection and 2-5 min following SC or IM injection. Duration of action is generally 45 min to 4 h.

Route: IV, IM, SC, Intratracheal

Dosage: 0.1 mg/kg. May repeat in 5 min.

Comments: Avoid in infants of narcotic-addicted mothers because naloxone may precipitate acute withdrawal syndrome. Infant must be monitored for reappearance of respiratory depression and need for repeated doses.

(Gomella: Neonatology 1999, p.579)

<u>Naloxone</u> (Narcan)

Dose: Reversal of Narcotic-induced Respiratory Depression:
0.1 mg/kg/dose. May repeat every 3-5 minutes as required.

- Consider the duration of action and elimination rate for the opiate being reversed.
- Reassess the infant every 1-2 hours because repeated doses may be needed.
- Continuous Infusion: 0.04-0.16 mg/kg/hour. Base continuous infusion dose on dose required with intermittent therapy.

Reversal of Respiratory Depression Induced by Narcotics Given to the Mother Within 4 Hours of Delivery: 0.1 mg/kg IV, ET, or if perfusion is adequate, SC or IM> Maintain adequate ventilation before administration of naloxone. Repeat every 2-3 minutes as needed. Avoid administration if mother is narcotic dependent because naloxone may precipitate withdrawal reaction in the newborn.

Septic Shock: 0.02-0.05 mg/kg IV push initially. followed by a continuous infusion of 2-8 mcg/kg/minute (0.13-0.5 mg/kg/hour).

Administration: IV Push--Rate: Infuse over at least 1 minute.

IV Push--Concentration: May give undiluted.

Continuous IV Infusion: Use naloxone 1 mg/ml; then dilute up to 25 ml with dextrose. Discard 24 ours after diluting. To calculate continuous drip, refer to Appendix A: Simplified Neonatal Calculations.

IM and SC: May give undiluted.

ET: Dilute in 1-2 ml NS.

Incompatible with: Alkaline drugs such as sodium bicarbonate.

Nursing Implications:

Monitor for response to therapy, including improved respiratory effect. Do not use if there is a history of intrauterine narcotic exposure.

(Zenk: Neonatal Medications & Nutrition. A Comprehensive Guide 2000; pp:349-351)

Naloxone

Indication: For seizures induced by opiates:
A single trial dose of naloxone, 0.1 mg/kg, was given intravenously because the baby had intermittent seizure-like muscle activity despite phenobarbital therapy.

Conclusion: Our observations indicate a potential for neurologic abnormalities, including induction of seizure activity and electroencephalogram abnormalities, suggesting caution when opiates are used for sedation and/or pain control in the newborn period.

(da Silva: Seizure and Electroencephalographic changes in the Newborn Period Induced by Opiates and Corrected By Naloxone Infusion. J Perinatol 1999;19(2):120-123)

NEOMYCIN (Mycifradin)

Supplied: Oral solution 125mg/5ml in 480ml
Administration: PO

Neomycin

Antibacterial Drugs for Newborn Infants
Dose (mg/kg or Units [U]/kg) and Frequency of Administration
Route: PO only

Dose: Infants <1 wk old
BW ≤1200-2000 g: 25 every 6 h
BW >2000 g: 25 every 6 h

Infants ≥1 wk old
BW ≤2000-2000 g: 25 every 6 h
BW >2000 g: 25 every 6 h

Note: Optimal dosage should be based on determination of serum concentrations, especially in low-birth-weight (<1500 g) infants. In very low-birth-weight infants (<1200 g) every 18 to 24 hour dosing may be appropriate in the first week of life.

Dosages for the aminoglycosides may differ from those recommended by the manufacturer in the package insert

Antibacterial Drugs for Pediatric Patients Beyond the Newborn Period
Dosage per kg/d
Route: PO only

Mild to Moderate Infections: 100 mg in 4 doses

Severe Infections: 100 mg in 4 doses

Comments: For some enteric infections

Note: Dosages for the aminoglycosides may differ from those recommended by the manufacturers (see package insert)

(American Academy of Pediatrics: Report of the Committee on Infectious Diseases. Red Book 2000, pp.651-653,662)

Neomycin Sulfate

For Newborn with EPEC gastroenteritis

On the basis of these data, there appears to be sufficient evidence to recommend oral administration of nonabsorbable antibiotics in the treatment of severely or moderately ill newborns with EPEC gastroenteritis. The drug most frequently used for initial therapy is neomycin sulfate in a dosage of 100 mg/kg per day administered PO every 8 hours in three divided doses. In communities in which neomycin-resistant EPEC has been prevalent, treatment should be started with colistin sulfate or polymyxin B in a dosage of 15 to 20 mg/kg PO daily, divided into three equal doses. However, it is rarely necessary to use the approach.

(Remington: Infectious Diseases of the Fetus and Newborn Infant 2001, p.1264)

Neomycin

Clinical Diagnosis: Gastrointestinal Infections, Escherichia coli-Enteropathogenic

Therapy: Neomycin 100 mg/kg/day PO div q6-8h

Comment: Most traditional "enteropathogenic" strains are not toxigenic nor invasive.

(Nelson: Pocketbook of Pediatric Antimicrobial Therapy 2000-2001, p.34)

Neomycin Sulfate (Mycifradin)

Classification: Aminoglycoside.

Action & spectrum:

Mechanism of action identical to that of gentamicin sulfate. Indicated in the treatment of diarrhea due to enteropathogenic *Escherichia coli* and as preoperative prophylaxis before intestinal surgery.

Route: PO
Dosage: 50-100 mg/kg/day divided q4-6h.

Elimination and metabolism:
Renal excretion if systemic absorption occurs; otherwise fecally excreted.

Adverse effects: Sensitization with allergic reaction.

Comments: Poorly absorbed from GI tract, but significant levels can occur, especially in impaired renal function. Inactive against anaerobic organisms.
(Gomella: Neonatology 1999, pp. 579-580)

NEOSTIGMINE METHYLSULFATE (Prostigmin)

Supplied: Injection 1:4000 (0.25mg/ml) in 1ml
Injection 1:2000 (0.50mg/ml) in 1ml and 10ml
Injection 1:1000 (1.00mg/ml) in 10ml
Tablets 15 mg

Administration: IV, IM, SC

Indications and use:
Improvement of muscle strength in the treatment of myasthenia gravis. Reversal of nondepolarizing neuromuscular blocking agents (eg, tubocurarine, pancuronium) and occasionally for postoperative distention and urinary retention.

Actions: Neostigmine inhibits hydrolysis of acetylcholine and thus produces generalized cholinergic responses.

Route: IM, IV, SC, PO.

Dosage: Myasthenia gravis:
Diagnosis: 0.04 mg/kg/dose IM once or 0.02 mg/kg/dose IV once.

Treatment: 0.01-0.04 mg/kg/dose IM, IV, or SC q2-3h prn.

Reversal of nondepolarizing neuromuscular blocking agents:
Infants: 0.025-0.1 mg/kg/dose. (Use with atropine: Dose 0.01-0.04 mg/kg; or 0.4 mg atropine for each 1 mg of neostigmine.)

Adverse effects: Cholinergic crisis, which may include bronchospasm, increased bronchial secretions, vomiting, diarrhea, bradycardia, respiratory depression, seizures, and coma.

Comments: Antidote is atropine 0.01-0.04 mg/kg/dose. Reversal of blocking agent should not be attempted for at least 30 min after a dose of pancuronium or tubocurarine.
(Gomella: Neonatology 1999, p.580)

<u>Neostigmine</u>

Dose: Reversal of Nondepolarizing Neuromuscular Blockade After Surgery: 0.025-0.1 mg/kg/dose. Give with atropine.

Commonly Used Regimen:

- Neostigmine 0.04-0.06 mg/kg/dose IV
- Atropine 0.02 mg/kg/dose IV
- Atropine may be given several minutes before or concomitantly with neostigmine to prevent bradycardia.

Diagnosis of Myasthenia Gravis (MG) and Neonatal Myasthenia Gravis:

- 0.04 mg/kg/dose IM x 1 **or** 0.02 mg/kg/dose IV x 1
- Give atropine IV immediately before or IM 30 minutes before neostigmine.
- Significant improvement in muscle weakness within several minutes to 1 hour after the dose usually indicates myasthenia gravis. Observe the patient for 1-2 hours after the dose.

Symptomatic Control of Myasthenia Gravis and Neonatal Myasthenia Gravis: Therapy is often required day and night. Give larger portions of the total daily dose at times of greater fatigue, such as in the afternoons, evenings, or at mealtimes.

- Oral: 2 mg/kg/day divided every 3-4 hours. Individualize interval between doses.
- IM, SC: 0.01-0.04 mg/kg/dose given every 2-3 hours. (Atropine 0.01 mg/kg/dose IM, SC may be given with each dose or with alternate doses to counteract the muscarinic side effects of neostigmine.)

Administration: IV--Rate: Infuse over several minutes.
IV--Concentration: May give undiluted.
IM, SC: May give undiluted.
PO: Administer with feedings to decrease possibility of side effects.

- Oral Liquid: Neostigmine is not commercially available as an oral liquid, and no stability information on an oral liquid compounded by the pharmacist was located. The following is suggested for preparation of an oral liquid if there is no alternative:

  Immediately prior to each dose the nurse can mix the crushed 15 mg tablet with 15 ml of water or simple syrup (= 1 mg/ml), shake well, and administer a volume equal to the mg dose using a calibrated oral syringe. Discard unused portion. Preparation just prior to each dose obviates concern about inactivation.

- Capsules or powder papers may be prepared by the pharmacist in the appropriate milligram dose from the crushed tablets.

Cautions/Contraindications:

Be sure to reduce the dose when converting from the oral to the parenteral route.

Overdose may cause cholinergic crisis which can be fatal.

Do not use neostigmine in patients with GI or GU obstruction. Use with caution in patients with bradycardia, cardiac arrhythmias, epilepsy, hyperthyroidism, and asthma.

Management of Overdose: Maintain adequate respiration. Discontinue neostigmine. Administer atropine 0.01-0.04 mg/kg/dose IV to counteract the muscarinic effects of neostigmine. Atropine does not alleviate the skeletal muscle effects and respiratory paralysis of neostigmine overdose. In myasthenic patients, weakness beginning about 1 hour after the dose is probably overdosage, whereas weakness occurring 3 or more hours after the dose is probably underdosage or resistance.

Nursing Implications:

For neonatal myasthenia gravis, keep a daily record of dosing and effects on condition during initial therapy to facilitate arranging an optimal therapeutic regimen.

Monitor heart rate, respiratory rate, and muscle strength.

(Zenk: Neonatal Medications & Nutrition. A Comprehensive Guide 2000; pp:352-354)

Neostigmine

Dose & Route: Myasthenia gravis-Diagnosis: **Use with atropine (see comments).**
Children: 0.025-0.04 mg/kg IM x 1

Myasthenia gravis-Treatment:
Children:
IM, IV, SC: 0.01-0.04 mg/kg/dose Q2-3 hr PRN
PO: 2 mg/kg/24 hr ÷ Q3-4 hr

Reversal of nondepolarizing neuromuscular blocking agents:
Administer with atropine or glycopyrrolate.
Infants: 0.025-0.1 mg/kg/dose IV
Children: 0.025-0.08 mg/kg/dose IV

Remarks: **Contraindicated** in GI and urinary obstruction. **Caution** in asthmatic. May cause cholinergic crisis, bronchospasm, salivation, nausea, vomiting, diarrhea, miosis, diaphoresis, lacrimation, bradycardia, hypotension, fatigue, confusion, respiratory depression, seizures. Titrate for each patient, but **avoid** excessive cholinergic effects.

For diagnosis of myasthenia gravis (MG), administer atropine 0.011 mg/kg/dose IV immediately before or IM (0.011 mg/kg/dose) 30 minutes before neostigmine. For treatment of MG, patients may need higher doses of neostigmine at times of greatest fatigue.

Antidote: Atropine 0.01-0.04 mg/kg/dose. Atropine and epinephrine should be available in the event of a hypersensitivity reaction

Adjust dose in renal failure.

(Siberry: The Harriet Lane Handbook 2000, p.786)

NETILMICIN SULFATE (Netromycin)

Supplied: Injection 100mg/ml in 1.5ml

Administration: IV, IM

For IV administration, the volume of infusion fluid depends on the patient's fluid requirements, but should be sufficient to allow an infusion period of from 30 minutes to 2 hours (1).

Netilmicin (Netromycin)

Antibacterial Drugs for Pediatric Patients Beyond the Newborn Period

Dosage per kg/d

Route: IV, IM

Mild to Moderate Infections: Inappropriate

Severe Infections: 3-7.5 mg in 3 doses

Note: Dosages for the aminoglycosides may differ from those recommended by the manufacturers (see package insert)

(American Academy of Pediatrics: Report of the committee on Infectious Diseases. Red Book 2000, pp.653,662)

Netilmicin

Route: IV, IM

Dosage (mg/kg) and Interval of Administration:

Weight <1200 g
Age 0-4 wk: 2.5 q18h

Weight 1200-2000 g
Age 0-7 days: 2.5 q12h
Age >7 days: 2.5 q8h

Weight >2000 g
Age 0-7 days: 2.5 q12h
Age >7 days: 2.5 q8h

(Remington: Infectious Diseases of the Fetus and Newborn Infant 2001, p.1454)

Netilmicin Sulfate (Netromycin)

Classification: Aminoglycoside.

Action and spectrum: See Gentamicin Sulfate.

Route: IM, IV (infuse over 30 min).

Dosage: Monitor and adjust by pharmacokinetics. Initial empiric dosing is based on body weight:

<1.2 kg: 2.5 mg/kg/dose q18-24h.
< 2kg and 0-7 days: 2.5 mg/kg/dose q12-18h.
< 2kg and > 7 days: 2.5 mg/kg/dose q8-12h.
>2kg and 0-7 days: 2.5 mg/kg/dose q12h.
>2kg and >7 days: 2.5 mg/kg/dose q8h.

Elimination and metabolism: Renal excretion. Half-life is 4-8h.

Adverse effects: Ototoxicity associated with serum peak concentrations >12 mcg/mL; nephrotoxicity associated with serum trough concentrations >4 mcg/mL.

Comments: Therapeutic ranges is 6-10 mcg/mL (sample obtained 30 min after the infusion completed); serum trough concentrations are <3 mcg/mL (sample obtained 30 min to just before next dose). Obtain initial set of serum peak and trough levels at about the fourth maintenance dose. Monitor serum creatinine every 3-4 days. Other comments: see Gentamicin Sulfate. Gomella reference. Limited experience in neonates.

(Gomella: Neonatology 1999, p.580)

NIFEDIPINE (Procardia)

Supplied: Capsules 10mg and 20mg
Administration: PO
Calcium channel blocker (1)

Nifedipine

Vasodilator therapy in Children with CHF
Dose/Route of Administration:
Infants: 0.1-0.3 mg/kg/dose
Children: 0.2-0.5 mg/kg/dose
sublingual q 6 hr or oral q 8 hr

Disadvantages: Depresses myocardial contractility; not to be used with β blocker

Clinical Use of Orally Available Vasodilators

Nifedipine is a calcium channel blocker and is a relatively pure arteriolar vasodilator. As there are calcium channels in the myocardium, however, it also can cause depressed contractility as well as delayed conduction through the atrioventricular node. Nifedipine has been used primarily in hypertensive patients, but it has also proven efficacious in patients with hypertrophic cardiomyopathy, due to its effect on diastolic filling properties of the left ventricle. Nifedipine is available in oral and sublingual forms only. Although it has few serious side effects, ti should not be used in conjunction with β-blockers or in patients in whom contractile function is severely impaired.

(Garson: The science and practice of pediatric cardiology 1998, pp.2322)

Nifedipine

Class: IV Ca^{++} Blocker

Uses: Pulmonary hypertension? CHF?

Dose (Level): Adults: 0.5-1.5 mg/kg SL divided q6-8hr

Mode of Action: Negative inotropism; peripheral vasodilation

Side Effects: CHF; peripheral edema, flushing, gingival hyperplasia (rare)

(Garson: The science and practice of pediatric cardiology 1998, p.2954)

Nifedipine

Dosage: 0.1-0.5 mg/kg p.o. every 8 h

Comments: Maximum = 20 mg/dose

(Allen: Moss and Adam's Heart Disease in Infants, children and Adolescents 2001, pp.1460-1468)

Nifedipine (Adalat, Procardia, Procardia XL)

Dose & Route: Children:

Hypertension/Hypertenisve: 0.25-0.5 mg/kg/dose Q4-6 hr PRN PO/SL. **Max dose**: 10 mg/dose or 3 mg/kg/24 hr

Hypertrophic Cardiomyopathy: 0.5-0.9 mg/kg/24 hr ÷ Q6-8 hr PO/SL

Remarks: Use with **caution** in patients with CHF and aortic stenosis. May cause severe hypotension, peripheral edema, flushing, tachycardia, headaches, dizziness, nausea, palpitations, syncope. Nifedipine is a substrate for CYP 450 3A/4. Do **not** administer with grapefruit juice; may increase bioavailability and effects. Nifedipine may increase phenytoin, cyclosporine, and digoxin levels.

(Siberry: The Harriet Lane Handbook 2000 pp.788-789)

NITRIC OXIDE (INO max)

Supplied: Size D: Portable aluminum cylinders containing 353 liters at STP of nitric oxide gas in 800 ppm concentration in nitrogen (delivered volume 344 liters) (NDC) 64693-002-01)

Size D: Portable aluminum cylinders containing 353 liters at STP of nitric oxide gas in 100 ppm concentration in nitrogen (delivered volume 344 liters) (NDC 64693-001-01)

Size 88: Aluminum cylinders containing 1963 liters at STP of nitric oxide gas in 800 ppm concentration in nitrogen (delivered volume 1918 liters) (NDC 64693-002-02)

Size 88: Aluminum cylinders containing 1963 liters at STP of nitric oxide gas in 100 ppm concentration in nitrogen (delivered volume 1918 liters) (NDC 64693-001-02)

Nitric Oxide

Abstract: Approval of inhaled nitric oxide by the US Food and Drug Administration for hypoxic respiratory failure of the term and near-term newborn provides an important new therapy for this serious condition. This statement addresses the conditions under which inhaled nitric oxide should be administered to the neonate with hypoxic respiratory failure.

iNO should be administered using FDA-approved devices that are capable of administering iNO in constant concentration ranges in parts per million or less throughout the respiratory cycle. Infants who receive iNO therapy should be monitored according to institutionally derived protocols designed to avoid the potential toxic effects associated with iNO administration. These effects include methemoglobinemia (secondary to excess nitric oxide concentrations), direct pulmonary injury (attributable toe excess levels of nitrogen dioxide), and ambient air contamination.

(American Academy of Pediatrics Committee on Fetus and Newborn: Use of Inhaled Nitric Oxide. Pediatrics 2000; 106:344-345)

Nitric Oxide

Summary: Inhaled NO improves oxygenation and decreases ECMO use in term newborns with PPHN. From the available information, a reasonable recommendation for a starting dose of iNO in the tern infant is 20 ppm, with reductions in dose over time. Toxicity is apparent at 80 ppm, causing increases in methemoglobinemia and inspired nitrogen dioxide. High dose (>20 ppm) of iNO may also prolong bleeding time, but clinically significant increases in bleeding complications have not been reported in term newborns. The use of iNO in non-ECMO centers must be done cautiously, with arrangements in place for transport to an ECMO center without interruption of iNO delivery in patients with suboptimal immediate responses. Finally, there is increasing evidence for the potential role of low-dose iNO (5 ppm) in premature newborns with hypoxemic respiratory failure. Low-dose iNO causes immediate improvement in oxygenation and may prove to be useful as a lung-specific anti-inflammatory therapy. However, clinical application should currently be limited to controlled trials that target outcomes of both safety and efficacy.

(Kinsella: Clinical approach to inhaled nitric oxide therapy in the newborn with hypoxemia. J Pediatr 2000;136:717-26)

Nitric Oxide

We studied 248 neonates who were born after 34 weeks' gestation, were 4 days old or younger, required assisted ventilation, and had an oxygenation index of 25 or higher. The oxygenation index was calculated as the mean airway pressure times the fraction of inspired oxygen times 100, divided by the partial pressure of arterial oxygen. The neonates had clinical or echocardiographic evidence of pulmonary hypertension without structural heart disease. Clinical evidence of pulmonary hypertension was defined as a difference of 5 percent between preductal and postductal oxygen saturation or recurrent (more than two) decreases in arterial oxygen saturation (to less than 85 percent) in a period of 12 hours despite optimal treatment of lung disease. Echocardiographic evidence of pulmonary hypertension was defined as an estimated peak systolic pulmonary-artery pressure that was higher than 35 mm Hg or more than two thirds of the systemic systolic pressure as indicated by a tricuspid regurgitant jet, a right-to-left ductus arteriosus shunt, or a right-to-left atrial-level shunt. In addition, we considered as study candidates neonates in whom extreme alkalosis (a pH higher than 7.55) was required to maintain a partial pressure of arterial oxygen of more than 60 mm Hg.

Pre-enrollment treatment with high-frequency ventilation (model 3100A, SensorMedics, Yorba Linda, Calif.) or surfactant was encouraged. Neonates were not eligible for the study if extracorporeal membrane oxygenation was urgently needed for refractory hypotension (a mean blood pressure lower than 35 mm Hg) or profound hypoxemia (a partial pressure of arterial oxygen lower than 30 mm Hg) or if they had a lethal congenital anomaly, a substantial bleeding diathesis, active seizures, or a history of severe asphyxia

The administration of the study gas (nitrogen or nitric oxide) was started at 20 ppm, and this amount was continued for four hours. At four hours, arterial-blood gases and methemoglobin were measured. The dose was decreased to 5 ppm if the neonate's condition was stable, the partial pressure of arterial oxygen was at least 60 mm Hg, and the pH was 7.55 or lower. If these criteria were not met, the administration of study gas was maintained at 20 ppm, and the neonate was evaluated every 4 hours until the criteria were met or the neonate had been treated for 24 hours. During the first 24 hours, the dose of study gas could be returned to 20 ppm if the neonate's partial pressure of arterial oxygen fell below 60 mm Hg when the fraction of inspired oxygen was 1.0. After 24 hours of treatment, the dose was decreased to 5 ppm. Treatment was continued at 5 ppm until the fraction of inspired oxygen was less than 0.7, the neonate had been treated for 96 hours, or the neonate was seven days old, whichever came first.

If the neonate did not tolerate the decreased dose at 24 hours or if at 96 hours the study gas could not be discontinued, the treatment was considered a failure. If a clinical decision was made to proceed with extracorporeal membrane oxygenation, the study gas was continued until it was started.

(Clark: Low-dose nitric oxide therapy for persistent pulmonary hypertension of the newborn. N Engl J Med. 2000;342:469-74)

iNO

Conclusion. In infants with PPHN, iNO 1): at 2 ppm does not acutely improve oxygenation or prevent clinical deterioration, but does attenuate the rate of clinical deterioration; and 2) at 20 ppm acutely improves oxygenation in infants initially treated with 0 ppm, but not in infants previously treated with iNO at 2 ppm. Initial treatment with subtherapeutic dose of iNO may diminish the clinical response to 20 ppm of iNO and have adverse clinical sequelae.

(Cornfield: Randomized Controlled Trial of Low-dose Inhaled Nitric Oxide in the Treatment of Term and Near-term Infants With Respiratory Failure and Pulmonary Hypertension. Pediatrics 1999;104:1089-1094.)

Inhaled Nitric Oxide

Conclusion. For infants classified as treatment successes, a dose response between the I-NO dose and decrease in PaO2 after discontinuing I-NO was found. A reduction in I-NO to 1 ppm before discontinuation of the drug seems to minimize the decrease in PaO2 seen. For infants failing treatment, discontinuation of I-NO could pose a life-threatening reduction in oxygenation should extracorporeal membrane oxygenation not be readily available or I-NO cannot be continued on transport.

(Davidson: Safety of Withdrawing Inhaled Nitric Oxide Therapy in Persistent Pulmonary Hypertension of the Newborn. Pediatrics 1999;104:231-236)

Nitric Oxide

Conclusions: Low-dose inhaled NO improved oxygenation but did not improve survival in premature neonates with severe hypoxemia. Low-dose NO in the most critically ill premature neonates does not increase the risk of intracranial hemorrhage and may decrease the risk of chronic lung injury.

(Kinsella: Inhaled nitric oxide for preterm infants-still an experimental therapy. J Pediatr 2000;136:416-417)

Inhaled Nitric Oxide

In conclusion, in this randomized trial of inhaled nitric oxide treatment for infants with persistent pulmonary hypertension of the newborn ventilated by HFOV, inhaled NO led to a significant improvement in oxygenation, reduced the need for ECMO rescue treatment, and was well tolerated. However, inhaled NO therapy did not improve survival among infants with persistent pulmonary hypertension of the newborn. We speculate ventilator strategies aimed at lung recruitment might increase the efficacy of inhaled NO in infants with persistent pulmonary hypertension of the newborn associated with parenchymal disease and should be considered before initiation of inhaled NO treatment.

(Christou: Inhaled nitric oxide reduces the need for extracorporeal membrane oxygenation in infants with persistent pulmonary hypertension of the newborn. Crit Care Med 2000; 28:3722-3727)

Inhaled Nitric Oxide

We conclude that the use of low-dose iNO may imporveoxygenation in some infants with severe PD, allowing decreased FIO2 and ventilator support without evidence of adverse effects. Randomized cllinical trials of low-dose iNO for BPD are warranted.

(Banks: Changes in Oxygenation With Inhaled Nitric Oxide in Severe Bronchopulmonary Dysplasia. Pediatrics 1999;103:610-618)

Nitric Oxide

We conclude that INO, when used according to the protocol of the NINOS study, is not associated with an increase in neurodevelopmental, behavioral, or medical abnormalities at 18 to 24 months of age. INO is a beneficial therapy for the hypoxic term and near-term neonate that will reduce the need for ECMO without an increase in neurodevelopmental abnormality.

(The Neonatal Inhaled Nitric Oxide Study Group: Inhaled nitric oxide in term and near-term infants: Neurodevelopmental follow-up of The Neonatal Inhaled Nitric Oxide Study Group (NINOS). J Pediatr 2000;136:611-7)

Nitric Oxide

Study design: A total of 108 children (median age 2.5 years) with severe acute hypoxemic respiratory failure from 7 centers were enrolled. After consent was obtained, patients were randomized to treatment with iNO (10 ppm) or mechanical ventilation alone for at least 72 hours. Patients with an oxygenation index ≥40 for 3 hours or ≥25 for 6 hours were considered treatment failures and exited the study.

Conclusions: We conclude that iNO causes an acute improvement in oxygenation in children with severe AHRF. Two subgroups (immunocompromised and an entry oxygen index ≥25) appear to have a more sustained improvement in oxygenation, and we speculate that these subgroups may benefit from prolonged therapy.

(Dobyns: Multicenter randomized controlled trial of the effects of inhaled nitric oxide therapy on gas exchange in children with acute hypoxemic respiratory failure. J Pediatr 1999;134:406-12)

NITROFURANTOIN (Furadantin)

Supplied: Oral suspension: 25 mg/5 ml in 60 and 470 ml

Administration: Give with food or milk to improve drug absorption and, in some patients, tolerance. (1)

<u>Nitrofurantoin</u> (Furadantin)

Antibacterial Drugs for Pediatric Patients Beyond the Newborn Period
Dosage per kg/d

Route: PO
Mild to Moderate Infections: 5-7 mg in 4 doses

Severe Infections: Inappropriate

Comments: Should not be used for young infants; prophylactic dose is 1-2 mg/kg per day in 1 dose
(American Academy of Pediatrics: Report of the Committee on Infectious Diseases. Red Book 2000, p.657)

NITROGLYCERIN (Tridil, Nitrostat, Nitro-Bid IV)

Supplied: Injection 0.5mg/mL (10ml); 5mg/mL 5, 10 mL NOT FOR DIRECT IV INJECTION (1,3).
Ointment 2% 30gm
Nitroglycerin in D5W injection solution
25mg in 250 ml
50mg in 250 ml and 500ml
100mg in 250ml
200mg in 500ml

Administration: IV infusion, dilute in D5W, NS prior to infusion.

Use only with glass IV bottles and administration set provided. Total amount of nitroglycerin (40-80%) in the final diluted solution for infusion could be absorbed by PVC tubing or IV administration sets in general use. Manufactures have developed non-PVC infusion tubing in which nitroglycerin loss is <5%. Use IV sets provided by manufacturers or use similar infusion sets. (1)

<u>Nitroglycerin</u>

THERAPY FOR ACUTE CONGESTIVE CARDIAC FALURE

Dose and Route of Administration: 1 to 5 μg/kg/minute i.v.

Hemodynamic Effects: Predominantly venodilation. Lowers preload.

Complications and Comments Regarding Use:
Hypotension: hemodynamic monitoring required
May develop methemoglobinemia

Notes: Nitroglycerin has been used in pediatric patients by intravenous infusions in doses from 0.5 to 20.0 μg/kg/minute. Sublingual nitroglycerin usually is administered to adults in doses of 0.4 mg, repeated as needed. Isosorbide dinitrate is given to adults in sublingual doses of 2.5 to 10 mg every 2 hours or oral doses 20 to 60 mg every 4 hours. Oral and sublingual use of these medications is not common in children. Nitroglycerin is metabolized rapidly and has not been associated with significant toxicity in infants and children. Methemoglobinemia is an extremely rare complication associated with long-term use in adults. Headache is a common adverse effect. These drugs cause a rapid significant reduction in cardiac preload and therefore may decrease cardiac output if ventricular filling pressures are not adequate. Severe hypotension and reflex tachycardia may develop.

(Garson: The science and practice of pediatric cardiology 1998, pp.2329-2341)

<u>Nitroglycerin</u>

Dose: 1-5 µg/kg/min IV max. 10 µg/kg/min

Mode of Action: Predominant venodilator, mediated by changes in intracellular cGMP

Adverse Effects: Do no use if low preload, hypotension, tachycardia, nausea, vomiting, headache

Comments: Postop low CO with high filling pressures, pulmonary HTN, systemic venous congestion

(Garson: The science and practice of pediatric cardiology 1998, p.2951)

<u>Nitroglycerin</u>

Dose and Route: Children:

Continuous IV infusion: Begin with 0.25-0.5 mcg/kg/min; may increase by 0.5-1 mcg/kg/min Q3-5 min PRN. **Max dose**: 20 mcg/kg/min

Sublingual: 0.2-0.6 mg Q5 min **Max** of 3 doses in 15 min

Remarks: **Contraindicated** in glaucoma and severe anemia. In small doses (1-2 mcg/kg/min) acts mainly on systemic veins and decreases preload. At 3-5 mcg/kg/min acts on systemic arterioles to decrease resistance. May cause headache, flushing, GI upset, blurred vision, methemoglobinemia. Use with **caution** in severe renal impairment, increased ICP, hepatic failure. IV nitroglycerin may antagonize anticoagulant effect of heparin.

Decrease dose gradually in patients receiving drug for prolonged periods to avoid withdrawal reaction. Must use polypropylene infusion sets to avoid adsorption of drug to plastic tubing.

(Siberry: The Harriet Lane Handbook 2000, p.790)

<u>Nitroglycerin Ointment 2%</u>

For complications of arterial catheters or vasopressor use. A dose of 4 mm/kg (or 2 mg measured as 0.1 ml in a syringe) would be equivalent to no more than 0.2 to 0.5 mcg/kg per minute given intravenously. Nitroglycerin is well absorbed topically through intact skin; hemodynamic effects are usually seen in 30 to 60 minutes and last from 6 to 8 hours. Continuous monitoring of vital signs is required because of nitroglycerin's potential hypotensive effect. Authors limited experience suggests that topically applied 2% nitroglycerin ointment may be a safe and convenient method of improving capillary blood flow to ischemic tissues in neonates with complications of arterial catheter or vasopressor use, and may be safer than injection of phentolamine or hyaluronidase for extravasation of vasoconstrictor drugs.

(Wong: Treatment of peripheral tissue ischemia with topical nitroglycerin ointment in neonates. J Pediatr 1992;121:980-983)

Nitroglycerin

Dosage: 0.5-3 μg/kg/min i.v.

Comments: Maximum = 10 μg/kg/min

(Allen: Moss and Adam's Heart Disease in Infants, children and Adolescents 2001, pp.1460-1468)

Nitroglycerin

Dose: IV:

- Initial: Try 0.1-1 mcg/kg/minute initially. If needed, increase at 1 mc/kg/minute increments every 30-60 minutes.
- Usual: 1-5 mcg/kg/minute. Maximum: 10 mcg/kg/minute.
- Higher doses may be required if proper administration precautions are not followed.
- Titrate cautiously to desired hemodynamic effect.
- Dose has not been well established in neonates.

Topical:

- Ribbon of 2 percent ointment, up to 2.4 mg/kg (4 mm/kg).

Administration: IV--Rate: Continuous IV infusion

IV—Concentration: Dilute before use.

Maximum: 400 mcg/ml

IV—Compatibility: See Appendix E: Y-Site Compatibility of Common NICU Drugs.

Nursing Implications:

Continuously monitor vital signs, especially blood pressure and heart rate.

Monitor for hypotension and tachycardia.

(Zenk: Neonatal Medications & Nutrition. A Comprehensive Guide 2000; pp:355-357)

NITROPRUSSIDE (Nipride, Nitropress)

Supplied: Injection, powder for 50mg vial

Administration: IV infusion

Administered by continuous IV infusion in D5W. Dissolve the contents of the vial with 2 to 3ml D5W, or sterile water, (NO OTHER DILUENT SHOULD BE USED) After reconstitution, nitroprusside is not suitable for direct injection. The reconstituted solution must be further diluted in D5W before infusion. (1)

If properly protected from light, the infusion solution is stable for 24 hours (1).

Nitroprusside Sodium (Nipride, Nitropress)

Indications and use:

Severe hypertension and hypertension crisis, congestive heart failure, congenital heart lesions that have resulted in pulmonary hypertension with increased pulmonary vascular resistance.

Actions: Direct-acting vasodilator (arterial and venous) that reduces peripheral vascular resistance (afterload). Venous return is reduced (preload). Acts within seconds to lower blood pressure; when discontinued, the effect dissipates within minutes. Rapidly metabolized to thiocyanate, which is eliminated by the kidneys.

Route: Continuous IV infusion.

Dosage: 0.5-8 mcg/kg/min (titrate to desired response) by IV infusion.

Adverse effects: Generally related to too-rapid reduction in blood pressure. Thiocyanate may accumulate, especially in patients receiving high doses or those who have impaired renal function. Cyanide toxicity can develop abruptly if large doses are administered rapidly. Cyanide causes early persistent acidosis. Thiocyanate toxicity appears at plasma levels of ~ 5-10 mg/dL; levels of 20 mg/dL have been associated with death. Thiocyanate levels should be monitored in any patient receiving 5 mcg/kg/min or more of nitroprusside, especially patients with renal impairment. Toxicity is treated with 20% sodium thiosulfate (10 mg/kg/min for 15 min).

Comments: Contraindicated with increased intracranial pressure, hypertension secondary to arteriovenous shunts, or coarctation of the aorta. Reconstitute contents of 50-mg vial in 2-3 mL D_5W, then further dilute in D_5W for infusion. Protect from light.

(Gomella: Neonatology 1999, pp. 580-581)

Nitroprusside

THERAPY FOR ACUTE CONGESTIVE CARDIAC FAILURE

Nitroprusside is administered by continuous intravenous infusion, from 0.5 to 8 μg/kg/minute. Typical dose regimens are in the range of 1 to 3 μg/kg/minute. Nitroprusside is light-sensitive, and substantial photochemical degradation may occur within 6 hours. Exposure to light increases the free cyanide concentration, which increases the risk of toxicity and reduces the vasodilating capacity. When given intravenously, its effects occur within 2 to 3 minutes and are reversed minutes after the drug is discontinued.

Toxicity is an important issue with nitroprusside. Sodium nitroprusside contains cyanide. Red blood cells convert nitroprusside to cyanide, which is converted to thiocyanate by rhodanese in the liver. Thiocyanate is excreted by the kidney. toxicity generally occurs with 40 μM (1 mg/L) of cyanide or 8 mg/L of thiocyanate. Toxicity may result from accumulation of either cyanide or thiocyanate, and is more likely with hepatic or renal dysfunction. Cyanide toxicity results in metabolic acidosis, a rise in mixed venous oxygen tension, and a fall in arterial-mixed venous oxygen content differences. The decrease in oxygen uptake and metabolic acidosis is probably related to cyanide intoxication of cellular cytochrome oxidases. Cyanide toxicity also produces CNS dysfunction characterized by disorientation agitation, lethargy, convulsions, and coma. Thiocyanate toxicity produces fatigue, gastrointestinal symptoms, hypothyroidism, and CNS dysfunction similar to cyanide toxicity, but does not cause metabolic acidosis. Nitroprusside also reduces oxygen transport by formation of cyanmethemoglobin in red cells and by inhibition of red cell carbonic anhydrase. If toxicity occurs, nitroprusside should be discontinued, and thiosulfate, sodium nitrite, and oxygen should be administered. Thiosulfate accelerated the conversion of cyanide to thiocyanide. To prevent this toxicity, we routinely add 10% sodium thiosulfate to the nitroprusside so that they are infused simultaneously at a ration of 10:1 (w:w). The mixtures are stable for up to 7 days if they are protected from sunlight. Although we have essentially eliminated the metabolic toxicity with this approach, we rarely use nitroprusside for more than 1 to 2 days. We have found that nitroprusside is preferable for afterload reduction in fresh non-steady-state post-operative patients who experience significant shifts in the intravascular volume and require frequent titration of this therapy. The short half-life of this agent allows us to make rapid titrations of the dose. However, we prefer milrinone for more long-term afterload reduction of the very sick patient who remains in the ICU with limited oxygen transport because in this setting we have experienced fewer episodes of hypotension with low cardiac output during administration of milrinone than of nitroprusside. It should be noted that these are strictly observational data.

(Garson: The science and practice of pediatric cardiology 1998, pp.2329-2341)

Nitroprusside (Nipride)

Dose: 0.5-6 μg/kg/min IV

Mode of Action: Mixed vasodilator

Adverse Effects: Hypotension, cyanide toxicity (headache, vomiting, tachypnea, tachycardia, change in consciousness)

Comments: Same as nitroglycerin; also check thiocyanate levels (<5%); light-sensitive in solution

(Garson: The science and practice of pediatric cardiology 1998, p.2951)

Nitroprusside (Nipride)

THERAPY FOR ACUTE CONGESTIVE CARDIAC FAILURE

Dose and Route of Administration: 0.5 to 8.0 µg/kg/minute i.v.

Hemodynamic Effects:

Mixed vasodilation. Increases cardiac output if preload is normal or increased.

Complications and Comments Regarding Use:

Hypotension: hemodynamic monitoring required
Thiocyanate toxicity
Cyanide toxicity
Light-sensitive

(Garson: The science and practice of pediatric cardiology 1998, pp.2329-2341)

Nitroprusside

Dosage: i.v. infusion: 0.5-5 µg/kg/min

Comments: Maximum 10 µg/kg/min

(Allen: Moss and Adam's Heart Disease in Infants, children and Adolescents 2001, pp.1460-1468)

Nitroprusside

Dose & Route: Children: IV, continuous infusion

Dose: Start at 0.3-0.5 mcg/kg/min, titrate to effect. Usual dose is 3-4 mcg/kg/min. **Max dose**: 10 mcg/kg/min.

Remarks: **Contraindicated** in patients with decreased cerebral perfusion and in situations of compensatory hypertension (increased ICP). Monitor for hypotension and acidosis, Dilute with D5W and protect from light.

Nitroprusside is nonenzymatically converted to cyanide, which is converted to thiocyanate. Cyanide may produce metabolic acidosis and methemoglobinemia. Thiocyanate may produce psychosis and seizures. Monitor thiocyanate levels if used for >48 hrs or if dose ≥4 mcg/kg/min. **Thiocyanate levels should be <50 mg/L.** Monitor **cyanide levels (toxic levels >2 mcg/ml)** in patients with hepatic dysfunction and thiocyanate levels in patients with renal dysfunction.

(Siberry: The Harriet Lane Handbook 2000, p.791)

NOREPINEPHRINE (Levophed)

Supplied: Injection 1mg/mL in 4mL amps

Administration: IV infusion

Administer as infusion in D5W or D5NS. Fluids containing dextrose are protection against significant loss of potency due to oxidation. Administration in saline solutions alone is not recommended (1).

Dilute in D5W to a concentration of 4 mcg/mL to 16mcg/mL (1).

For treatment of EXTRAVASATION, see phentolamine monograph.

Norepinephrine Bitartrate (Levarterenol Bitartrate) (Levophed)

Indications and use: Vasoconstriction and cardiac stimulation as adjunctive therapy to correct shock after fluid volume replacement. Prolongation of local anesthetics by decreasing vascular absorption.

Actions: Direct effect on α-adrenergic receptors and β-adrenergic receptors of the heart (β_1) but not those of the bronchi or peripheral blood vessels (β_2). Norepinephrine has less effect on β_1 receptors than does epinephrine or isoproterenol.

Route: IV infusion.

Dosage: 0.02-0.1 mcg/kg/min initially, titrated to attain desired perfusion.

Adverse effects: Respiratory distress, arrhythmias, bradycardia or tachycardia, hypertension, and vomiting.

Comments: In case of extravasation, use phentolamine 0.1-0.2 mg/kg SC infiltrated into the area of extravasation within 12 h.

(Gomella: Neonatology 199, p.581)

Norepinephrine

Dose: 0.1-2 µg/kg/min

Mode of Action: $B_1 >> B_2$, mild α-agonist

Adverse Effects: Hypertension; similar to epinephrine

(Garson: The science and practice of pediatric cardiology 1998, p.2950)

Norepinephrine

THERAPY FOR ACUTE CONGESTIVE CARDIAC FAILURE

Norepinephrine is rarely considered for its inotropic effects in the clinical setting because of the profound deleterious effect on systemic afterload and renal blood flow, and the significant increase in myocardial oxygen demand. The infusion rate is initiated at 0.05 to 0.1 µg/kg/minute. side effects from norepinephrine are essentially the same as those seen with epinephrine. Intravenous extravasations should be treated with phentolamine, and α-adrenergic blocking agent, which is used to avoid local tissue necrosis. Depending on the child's body size, 1 to 5 mg of phentolamine should be diluted in 1 to 5 mL of normal saline and injected locally at the site of extravasation.

(Garson: The science and practice of pediatric cardiology 1998, pp.2329-2341)

Norepinephrine Bitartrate

Dose & Route: Children: Continuous IV infusion doses as norepinephrine base. Start at 0.05-0.1 mcg/kg/min. Titrate to effect. Max dose: 2 mcg/kg/min.

Remarks: May cause cardiac arrhythmias, hypertension, hypersensitivity, headaches, vomiting, uterine contractions, and organ ischemia. May cause decreased renal blood flow and urine output. Avoid extravasation into tissues; may cause severe tissue necrosis. If this occurs, treat locally with phentolamine.

(Siberry: The Harriet Lane Handbook 2000, p.791)

NYSTATIN (Mycostatin, Nilstat)

Supplied: Oral suspension 100,000 units/ml in 5ml, 60ml, 480ml 100,000 units/gm topical as a cream, ointment 15 grams and 30 grams, powder 15 grams

Administration: PO, Topical

Nystatin (Mycolog, Mycostatin)

Recommended Doses of Parenteral and Oral Antifungal Drugs

Route: PO

Dose (per day): Infants: 200 000 U, 4 times a day, after meals

Adverse Reactions: Gastrointestinal tract symptoms, rash

Topical Drugs for Superficial Fungal Infections

Strength: 100 000 U/mL or 100 000 U/g

Applications per day 2-3

Adverse Reactions/Notes:

Rare adverse reactions; effective against yeast only

(American Academy of Pediatrics: Report of the Committee on Infectious Diseases. Red Book 2000, pp.671,673)

Nystatin

Nystatin has been used successfully in patients with mucocutaneous and dermal infections with *Candida*. The oral suspension contains 100,000 units of nystatin per ml; in infants with thrush, 1 ml should be slowly instilled into each side of the mouth every 6 hours and should be continued for several days after lesions have disappeared. Nystatin ointment, which contains 100,000 units per g, may be used liberally for cutaneous or oral candidiasis. In moist, intertriginous areas, nystatin powder is the preparation of choice; it may be used four times a day until skin infection has cleared. Occasional failures occur when *Candida* persists, resulting in a relapse 1 week to 1 month late. In such cases, therapy should be reinstituted and continued until smears or cultures are negative. In infants with gastrointestinal candidiasis, oral nystatin suspension, 400,000 to 1.6 million units per day in four to six divided doses, has been shown to be effective in eradicating *Candida* from feces within 3 days of initiation of therapy. However, it is recommended that treatment be continued for 7 to 10 days. Diarrhea in the reported infants disappeared concomitant with eradication of the organism.

Nystatin may be used as an irrigating solution in patients with saprophytic or localized infection with *Aspergillus* at a concentration of 500 units per ml of sterile water.

(Remington: Infectious Diseases of the Fetus and Newborn Infant 2001, p.837)

<u>Nystatin</u>

Route: PO (not swallowed)
Dosage: Infants 2 ml/dose, children 4-6 ml or 1 tab/dose
Interval: q6h
NON-NEWBORN SECTION

(Nelson: Pocket Book of Pediatric Antimicrobial Therapy 2000-2001, p.81)

<u>Nystatin</u> (Mycostatin, Nilstat)

Action and spectrum:
Fungistatic and fungicidal in vitro against a wide variety of yeasts and yeastlike fungi. Acts by disrupting cell membranes. Neonatal indications include oral candidiasis (thrush), Candida diaper rash, and benign mucocutaneous candidiasis.

Route: PO, topical.

Dosage: Oral thrush: 0.5-1mL to each side of the mouth qid after feedings for 7-10 days.
Diaper rash: Topical cream applied tid-qid for 7-10 days.

Elimination and metabolism:
Poorly absorbed. Most is passed unchanged in the stool.

Adverse effects: Side effects uncommon, but may cause diarrhea.

(Gomella: Neonatology 1999, p.581)

<u>Nystatin</u>

Dose & Route: Oral:
Preterm infants: 0.5 ml (50,000 U) to each side of mouth QID

Term infants: 1 ml (100,000 U) to each side of mouth QID

Topical: Apply BID-QID

Remarks: May produce diarrhea and GI side effects. Treat until 48-72 hr after resolution of symptoms. Drug is poorly absorbed through the GI tract. Do **not** swallow troches whole.

(Siberry: The Harriet Lane Handbook 2000, p.793)

OCTREOTIDE ACETATE (Sandostatin, Sandostatin LAR Depot)

Supplied: Injection: 0.05 mg/ml, 0.1 mg/ml, 0.5 mg/ml, 1 mg/ml, in 1 ml amps

Depot: injection: 10 mg/5 ml, 20 mg/5 ml, 30 mg/5 ml

Administration: Octreotide may be administered SC or IV. SC is the usual route of administration. (1)

Sandostatin LAR Depot administration: Do not administer IV or SC. Administer immediately after mixing. Administer intragluteally at 4-week intervals. Avoid deltoid injections because of significant discomfort at the injection site. (1)

Octreotide acetate is a long-acting octapeptide with pharmacologic actions mimicking those of the natural hormone somatostatin.

Usage in children: The youngest patient to receive the drug was 1 month old. Doses of 1 to 10 mcg/kg body weight are well tolerated in young patients.

A single case of an infant (nesidioblastosis) was complicated by a seizure thought to be independent of octreotide acetate therapy (1).

<u>Octreotide</u> (Sandostatin)

Indications and use:

Short-term management of persistent hyperinsulinemic hypoglycemia of nesidioblastosis. A few patients have been treated for as long as 5 years. Has also been used to treat hypersecretory diarrhea and fistulas in infants. Significant reductions in stool or ileal output were achieved with this drug.

Actions: A long-acting analog of somatostatin that suppresses pancreatic insulin release. Inhibits serotonin, glucagon, and growth hormone release. Reduces splanchnic blood flow and both exocrine and hormonal GI secretions. Duration of action is 6-12 h.

Route: Continuous IV infusion, SC. Continuous SC infusion using a portable pump has been used in two infants with nesidioblastosis.

Dosage: Hypoglycemia: Starting dose is 2-10 mcg/kg/day divided q6-8h, up to 40 mcg/kg/day divided q 4-8h. Adjust the dose to maintain symptomatic control.

Continuous SC infusion: 2-10 mcg/kg/day

Diarrhea: 1-10 mcg/kg/dose given q12h. Adjust the dose to maintain symptomatic control.

Adverse effects: Possible growth retardation during long-term treatment; gallbladder microlithiasis reported in adolescents; flushing, hypertension, insomnia, fever, chills, seizures, Bell's palsy, hair loss, bruising, rash, hypoglycemia, hyperglycemia, galactorrhea, hypothyroidism, diarrhea, abdominal distention, constipation, hepatitis, jaundice, local injection site pain, thrombophlebitis, muscle weakness, increased creatine kinase, muscle spasm, tremor, oliguria, shortness of breath, and rhinorrhea.

Comments: Tachyphylaxis may occur.
(Gomella: Neonatology 1999, pp.581-582)

<u>Octreotide</u>

Dose: Hypoglycemia:

- Intermittent IV or SC: Starting dose: 2-10 mcg/kg/day divided every 6-8 hours, up to 40 mcg/kg/day divided every 4-8 hours. Adjust dose to maintain symptomatic control.
- Continuous SC Infusion: 2-10 mcg/kg/day. (Continuous SC infusion using a portable pump has been used in two infants with nesidioblastosis).

Antidiarrheal: 2-20 mcg/kg/day divided every 12 hours. Adjust dose to maintain symptomatic control.

Administration: SC: May give undiluted or may dilute with NS or D_5W. Continuous SC Infusion: May dilute with NS or D_5W in an amount based on the dose and fluid requirements of the infant.

IV—Rate: Infuse over at least 3 minutes in emergencies; however, infusion over 30 minutes is preferred.

IV—Concentration: Mau give undiluted in emergencies; however, it si preferred to give diluted with NS or D_5W in an amount based on the fluid requirements of the infant for a 30-minute infusion.

IV—Compatibility: Not compatible with parenteral nutrition because of the formation of a glycosyl octreotide conjugate, which may decrease the effectiveness of octreotide.

Storage: Refrigerate for long-term storage; however, stable at room temperature for 14 days if protected from light. Protect from light.

Adverse Effects: Tachyphylaxis may occur.

Cardiovascular: Flushing, hypertension.

CNS/Muscle: Insomnia, fever, chills, seizures, Bell's palsy, muscle weakness, increased creatine phosphokinase, muscle spasm, tremor.

Dermatologic: Hair loss, bruising, rash.

Endocrine: Possible growth retardation (suppresses growth hormone) during long-term treatment; however, in most studies, growth and development were within normal range. May also cause hypoglycemia, hyperglycemia, galactorrhea, hypothyroidism (suppresses thyroid-stimulating hormone).

GI: Nausea, diarrhea, abdominal distension, abdominal pain, flatulence, constipation. Scheduling injections of octreotide between meals and at bedtime reduces the occurrence of GI side effects. Rare: GI bleed.

GU: Oliguria.

Hepatic: Gallbladder microlithiasis (reported in adolescents), hepatitis, jaundice.

Local: Local injection-site pain, stinging with redness and swelling; thrombophlebitis. Local reactions may be reduced by allowing the solution to reach room temperature before administration (do not heat artificially) and injecting slowly.

Respiratory: Shortness of breath, rhinorrhea.

Nursing Implications:
Monitor blood glucose.
Monitor for thrombophlebitis.
Rotate injection sites.
Consider dose increase if tachyphylaxis occurs.

Comments: Interactions: Concurrent use of glucagon, growth hormone, or insulin may result in hypo- or hyperglycemia; monitoring and dose adjustments may be necessary.

(Zenk: Neonatal Medications & Nutrition. A Comprehensive Guide 2000; pp:367-369)

Octreotide

Dose/kg: 1-10 µg
Route & frequency: IV, SC q12h-q24h
Comments: Start treatment using lower end of dosage range. Causes growth hormone suppression.

(Avery: Neonatology Pathophysiology and Management of the Newborn 1999, p.1559)

Somatostatin

An enteric fistula developed 3 days after ostomy closure. The baby was started on total parenteral nutrition and 7 days later the fistual output remained constant. Somatostatin was then given intravenously (3.0 µg/kg/hr) and the fistula closed on the third day of treatment.

(Julia: Treatment of an enteric fistula with somatostatin in a premature. Clin Pediatr 1989;28:149-150)

Octreotide Acetate

Dose: Infants and Children:
Diarrhea (IV/SC): 1-10 mcg/kg/24 hr ÷ Q12-24 hr. Dose may be increased within the recommended range by 0.3 mcg/kg/dose every 3 days as needed.

Comments: Cholelithiasis, hyperglycemia, hypoglycemia, nausea, diarrhea, abdominal discomfort, headache, pain at injection site may occur. Growth hormone suppression may occur with long-term use. Cyclosporine levels may be reduced in patients receiving this drug.

(Siberry: The Harriet Lane Handbook 2000, p.793)

OMPERAZOLE (Prilosec)

Supplied: 10, 20mg Sustained Release Capsules

Administration: PO

Take before eating

Swallow capsule whole; do not open, chew, or crush (1).

Extemporaneous Compounding (Recipe)

Dosage form: Oral suspension

Made from: Capsules

Concentration: 2 mg/ml

Stability: 30 days

Store: Refrigerate

Label: Shake well

Ingredient	Strength	Quantity
Omeprazole capsules	20 mg	20
Sodium Bicarbonate	8.4%	qs 200 mL

Instructions: Empty the contents of the capsules in a mortar and crush to a fine powder. Add the finely ground powder to an amber bottle, add the sodium bicarbonate. Shake well, Refrigerate. Stable for 30 days at 5°C.

Alternative method: Add the contents of the capsules to an amber bottle. Add the sodium bicarbonate. Shake vigorously until dissolved.

Omeprazole

Therapy for Reflux

Common doses: 0.7-3.3 mg/kg/dose qd or divided bid; adult 20 mg HS or bid

(Wyllie: Pediatric Gastrointestinal Disease 1999, p.180)

Omeprazole

Dose & Route: Children: Start at 0.6-0.7 mg/kg/dose PO QD. Dose may be increased to 0.6-0.7 mg/kg/dose PO BID if needed. Effective dosage range of 0.3-3.3 mg/kg/24 hr has been reported.

Remarks: Common side effects: headache, diarrhea, nausea, and vomiting.

Administer all doses before meals.

(Siberry: The Harriet Lane Handbook 2000, p.795)

Omeprazole

Omeprazole, a potent inhibitor of acid secretion, is effective in adults with severe gastroesophageal reflux, but no such data are available on children. We studied 15 children in whom treatment with histamine (type 2)

blockers and prokinetic agents had failed; 4 had also had one or more fundoplications. Their ages were 0.8 to 17 years (mean, 8.1 years) and weights were 7.5 to 30.7 kg (mean, 18.6 kg)....Patients were initially given omeprazole at 10 to 20 mg; the dose was titrated upward until results of a subsequent 24-hour intraesophageal pH study was normal. Symptoms and signs abated and evidence of esophagitis diminished in all patients ...The dosage range was 0.7 to 3.3 to mg/kg per day (mean, 1.9 mg/kg)....We found omeprazole to be highly effective in this group of patients with severe esophagitis refractory to other measures. We recommend a starting dose of 0.7 mg/kg as a single morning dose; and adequacy of reflux control is then determined by follow-up 24 hour intraesophageal pH studies. Omeprazole appears to be safe for short-term use, but further studies are needed to assess long-term safety because the significance of chronically elevated gastrin levels in children is unknown.

(Gunasekaran: Efficacy and safety of omeprazole for severe gastroesophageal reflux in children. J Pediatr 1993;123:148-154)

OPIUM TINCTURE DEODORIZED

Supplied: Liquid 10% opium in 120ml

Administration: PO

Opium tincture 0.6ml is equivalent to 6mg morphine. Contains 19% alcohol.

Opium tincture contains 25 times more morphine than does paregoric and should never be confused with paregoric.

Opium, Tincture of

Indication: Drug therapy for withdrawal syndrome in infants.

Tincture of opium can be utilized instead of paregoric. Tincture of opium (0.4 mg/ml of morphine equivalent) is administered in a dose of 0.1 ml/kg given orally. the dose can be increased by 0.05 to 0.10 ml increments every 3 to 4 hours until the symptoms are controlled. The usual dose for infants ranges from 0.2 to 0.5 ml every 3 to 4 hours. Tincture of opium, unlike paregoric, does not contain camphor, a central nervous system stimulant.

At the present time we recommend *tincture of opium as the drug of first choice* in therapy. *Phenobarbital* should be added if central nervous system phenomena are particularly marked and are not controlled by the narcotic agent alone, an unusual occurrence in may experience.

(Volpe: Neurology of the Newborn 2001, p.882)

Opium Tincture

Use: Treatment of diarrhea or relief of pain; **a 25-fold dilution with water** (final concentration 0.4 mg/mL morphine) can be used to treat neonatal abstinence syndrome (opiate withdrawal)

Adverse Reactions:

Cardiovascular: Hypotension, bradycardia, peripheral vasodilation

Central nervous system: CNS depression, increased intracranial pressure, drowsiness, dizziness, sedation

Dermatologic: Pruritus

Endocrine & metabolic: Antidiuretic hormone release

Gastrointestinal: Nausea, vomiting, constipation

Genitourinary: Urinary tract spasm, urinary retention

Hepatic: Biliary tract spasm

Ocular: Miosis

Respiratory: Respiratory depression

Miscellaneous: Physical and psychological dependence, histamine release

Stability: Protect from light and excessive heat; do not refrigerate, decreased solubility and precipitation may occur

Usual Dosage: Oral:

Neonates, (full-term): Neonatal abstinence syndrome (opiate withdrawal): **Use a 25-fold dilution of opium tincture** (final concentration: 0.4 mg/mL morphine); Initial: Give 0.2 mL of the 25-fold dilution per dose every 3 hours; increase as needed by 0.05-0.1 mL of the 25-fold dilution every 3 hours until withdrawal symptoms are controlled; usual dose: 0.2-0.5 mL of the 25-fold dilution per dose given every 3-4 hours; it is rare to exceed 0.7 mL of the 25-fold dilution per dose; stabilize withdrawal symptoms for 3-5 days, then gradually decrease dosage over a 2- to 4-week period

Administration: Oral: May administer with food to decrease GI upset

Monitoring Parameters:

Respiratory rate, blood pressure, heart rate, resolution of diarrhea or pain, mental status; if using a 25-fold dilution to treat neonatal abstinence syndrome, monitor for resolution of withdrawal symptoms (such as irritability, high-pitched cry, stuffy nose, rhinorrhea, vomiting, poor feeding, diarrhea, sneezing, yawning etc), and signs of overtreatment (such as bradycardia, lethargy, hypotonia, irregular respirations, respiratory depression etc). An abstinence scoring system (eg, Finnegan abstinence scoring system) can be used to more objectively assess neonatal opiate withdrawal symptoms and the need for dosage adjustment. Monitor fluid and electrolyte balance in young children being treated for prolonged or severe diarrhea.

Nursing Implications:

Observe patient for excessive sedation, respiratory depression; implement safety measures; assist with ambulation; do not abruptly discontinue after prolonged use.

(Taketomo: Pediatric dosage Handbook 1998-1999, pp.808-809)

Opium Tincture

Dose & Route: **Dilute 25-fold with water to make a** final concentration of 0.4 mg/ml morphine equivalent. Dose for the **dilution** is equivalent to paregoric doses. (see paregoric).

Use 25 fold dilution to treat neonatal abstinence syndrome (NAS). Doses for the **dilution** are equivalent to paregoric doses. Morphine may also be used to treat NAS. May cause respiratory depression, hypotension, bradycardia, and CNS depression.

(Siberry: The Harriet Lane Handbook 2000, p.796)

OXACILLIN (Bactocill, Prostaphlin)

Supplied: Oral solution, powder for 250mg/5ml in 100ml
Injection, powder for 250mg, 500mg, 1gm vial (contains 3.1mEq Na/gm).

Administration: IV, IM, PO
For DIRECT IV INJECTION, add 5ml, 5ml, 10ml NS or SWFI to the 250mg, 500mg, or 1 gm vial to yield approximately a 50mg, 100mg/ml concentration respectively. The appropriate dose should then be injected slowly over 10 minutes to avoid vein irritation. (1)

For INTERMITTENT INFUSION DILUTE TO A CONCENTRATION of 0.5-40mg/mL (3).

Oral solutions, once reconstituted, are stable for 3 days at room temperature, or 14 days refrigerated (3).

Oxacillin

Antibacterial Drugs for Newborn Infants
Dose (mg/kg or Units [U]/kg} and Frequency of Administration
Route: IV, IM

Dose: Infants 0 - 4 wk
BW <1200 g: 25 every 12 h

Infants < wk old
BW ≤1200-2000 g: 25-50 every 12 h
BW >2000 g: 25-50 every 8 h

Infants ≥1 wk old
BW ≤2000-2000 g: 25-50 every 8 h
BW >2000 g: 25-50 every 6 h

Note: For meningitis, the larger dosage is recommended.

Antibacterial Drugs for Pediatric Patients Beyond the Newborn Period
Dosage per kg/d
Route: IV, IM

Mild to Moderate Infections: 100-150 mg in 4 doses

Severe Infections: 150-200 mg in 4-6 doses

Note: In patients with history of allergy to penicillin or one of its many congeners, alternative drugs are recommended. In some circumstances, a cephalosporin or other β-lactam class drug may be acceptable. However, these drugs should not be used in patients with an immediate hypersensitivity (anaphylaxis) to penicillin because approximately 5% to 15% of penicillin-allergic patients will also be allergic to the cephalosporins.

(American Academy of Pediatrics: Report of the Committee on Infectious Diseases. Red Book 2000, pp.651-652,660,662)

Oxacillin

Route: IV, IM

Dosage (mg/kg) and Interval of Administration:

Weight <1200 g
Age 0-4 wk: 25 q12h

Weight 1200-2000 g
Age 0-7 days: 25 q12h
Age >7 days: 25 q8h

Weight >2000 g
Age 0-7 days: 25 q8h
Age >7 days: 37.5 q6h

(Remington: Infectious Diseases of the Fetus and Newborn Infant 2001, p.1454)

Oxacillin

Route: IV, IM

Dosages (mg/kg/day) and Intervals of Administration:

Body weight < 2000 g
0-7 days old: 50 div q12h
8-28 days old: 75 div q8h

Body weight > 2000 g
0-7 days old: 75 div q8h
8-28 days old: 150 div q6h

>28 days old: 150 div q6

(Nelson: Pocket Book of Pediatric Antimicrobial Therapy 2000-2001, p.16)

Oxacillin Sodium (Bactocill, Prostaphlin)

Classification: Semisynthetic penicillinase-resistant penicillin.

Action and spectrum: Mechanism of action is identical to that of other ß-lactam antibiotics. Spectrum of activity is identical to that of nafcillin sodium and methicillin sodium.

Route: IM, IV (infuse over 30 min).

Dosage: <2000 g and 0-7 days old: 50 mg/kg/day divided q12h.
<2000 g and >7 days old: 100 mg/kg/day divided q8h.
>2000 g and 0-7 days old: 75 mg/kg/day divided q8h.
>2000 g and >7 days old: 150 mg/kg/day divided q6h.

Elimination and metabolism:
Metabolized chiefly in the liver and excreted in bile. Renal excretion is substantial but requires no adjustment in renal failure.

Adverse effects: Hypersensitivity reactions (rash), thrombophlebitis, mild leukopenia, elevation in AST (SGOT).

Comments: Avoid IM injection. Contains 2.8 meq sodium per gram.
(Gomella: Neonatology 1999, p.582)

Oxacillin Sodium

Dose/kg: 25 mg
Route & Frequency: IV, IM ≤2 kg ≤7 d: q12h

Dose/kg: 33 mg
Route & Frequency: IV, IM ≤2 kg >7 d: q8h

Dose/kg: 25 mg
Route & Frequency: IV, IM >2 kg ≤7 d: q8h

Dose/kg: 37.5 mg
Route & Frequency: IV, IM >2 kg >7 d: q6h

Comments: Contraindicated in patients allergic to penicillins. May cause thrombophlebitis and colstridium difficile colitis. Monitor live function.
(Avery: Neonatology Pathophysiology and Management of the Newborn 1999, p.1559)

OXYBUTYNIN (Ditropan)

Supplied: Syrup 5mg/5ml, Tablet 5mg

Administration: PO

Oxybutynin exerts direct antispasmodic effect on smooth muscle and inhibits the muscarinic action of acetylcholine on smooth muscle. It exhibits one-fifth the anticholinergic activity of atropine, but 4 to 10 times the antispasmodic activity (1).

Oxybutynin

Indication: Newborns and infants with myelodysplasia.

When oxybutynin therapy was begun, the dose used was 1.0 ml per year of age after age 1 year administered twice daily and proportionately less for infants younger than age 1 year.
(Kasabian: The prophylactic value of clean intermittent catheterization and anticholinergic medication in newborns and infants with myelodysplasia at risk of developing urinary tract deterioration. AJDC 1992;146:840-843)

Oxybutynin Chloride

Dose & Route: Child ≤5 yr: 0.2 mg/kg/dose BID-QID PO

Remarks: Anticholinergic side effects may occur, including drowsiness and hallucinations. **Contraindicated** in glaucoma, GI obstruction, megacolon, myasthenia gravis, severe colitis, hypovolemia, and GU obstruction.

(Siberry: The Harriet Lane Handbook 2000, p.797)

Oxybutynin

Usual Dosage: Oral: Children: 1-5 years: 0.2 mg/kg/dose 2-4 times/day

Administration: Oral: May administer with food or milk to decrease GI distress

(Taketomo: Pediatric Dosage Handbook 1998-1999, pp.813-814)

OXYMETHOLONE (Anadrol - 50)

Supplied: Tablets 50mg

Administration: PO

Comment: Possess a high anabolic, low androgenic activity ratio, the dissociation of anabolic from androgenic effects is incomplete and variable (1).

Oxymetholone

Route: PO

Neonatal Dose: 0.175 mg/kg/24h given once daily

Pediatric Dose: 1-2 mg/kg/24h given once daily

Discussion: Do not use in patients with severe renal or hepatic impairment

(Rudolph: Rudolph's Pediatrics 1996, p.2197)

PALIVIZUMAB (Synagis)

Supplied: Injection; lypophilized: 50 mg, 100 mg vials. Preservative free.

Administration: Preparation for administration: slowly add sterile water for injection to vial. Gently swirl the vial for 30 seconds to avoid foaming. Do not shake vial. Reconstituted palivizumab should stand at room temperature for a minimum of 20 minutes until the solution clarifies. Reconstituted palivizumab does not contain a preservative; administer within 6 hours of reconstitution. (1)

<u>Palivizumab</u> (Synagis)

Children were eligible if they were either: 1) 35 weeks gestation or less and 6 months of age or younger; or 2) 24 months old or younger and had a clinical diagnosis of BPD requiring ongoing medical treatment (ie, supplemental oxygen, steroids, bronchodilators, or diuretics within the past 6 months).

Children were excluded if they had any of the following: hospitalization at the time of entry that was anticipated to last more than 30 days; mechanical ventilation at the time of entry; life expectancy less than 6 months; active or recent RSV infection; known hepatic or renal dysfunction, seizure disorder, immunodeficiency, allergy to IgG products; receipt of RSV immune globulin within the past 3 months; or previous receipt of palivizumab, other monoclonal antibodies, RSV vaccines, or other investigational agents. Children with congenital heart disease were excluded, except for those with a patent ductus arteriosus or a septal defect that was uncomplicated and hemodynamically insignificant.

A randomized, double-blind, placebo-controlled trial was conducted at 139 centers in the United States, the United Kingdom, and Canada. During the 1996 to 1997 RSV season, 1502 children with prematurity (≤35 weeks) or bronchopulmonary dysplasia (BPD) were randomized to receive 5 injections of either palivizumab (15 mg/kg) or an equivalent volume of placebo by intramuscular injection every 30 days. The primary endpoint was hospitalization with confirmed RSV infection. Children were followed for 150 days (30 days from the last injection). Those with hospitalization as a result of RSV infection were evaluated for total number of days in the hospital, total days with increased supplemental oxygen, total days with moderate or severe lower respiratory tract illness, and incidence and total days of intensive care and mechanical ventilation. The incidence of hospitalization for respiratory illness not caused by RSV and the incidence of otitis media were also evaluated. The placebo and palivizumab groups were balanced at entry for demographics and RSV risk factors.

Ninety-nine percent of children in both groups completed the protocol and ~93% received all five scheduled injections.

Participants were randomized to receive either palivizumab (15 mg/kg) or an equal volume of identically appearing placebo (same formulation, except without antibody and with 0.02% Tween-80 added) by intramuscular injection every 30 days for a total of 5 doses.

In summary, palivizumab is safe and effective for prevention of serious RSV illness in premature infants (≤35 weeks gestation), including those with BPD. Monthly intramuscular administration is well tolerated. Prophylaxis with this monoclonal antibody results in a significant (55%) reduction in RSV hospitalization in children at high risk for severe RSV infection.

(The IMpact-RSV Study Group: Palivizumab, a Humanized Respiratory Syncytial Virus Monoclonal Antibody, Reduces Hospitalization From Respiratory Syncytial Virus Infection in High-risk Infants. Pediatrics 1998;102:531-537)

<u>Synagis</u>

Dose/kg: 15 mg

Route & frequency: IM; monthly during RSV season

Comments: Typically RSV season begins in November and lasts through April. Inject in the anterolateral aspect of the thigh. Gluteal injections may damage the sciatic nerve.

(Avery: Neonatology Pathophysiology and Management of the Newborn 1999, p.1560)

<u>Palivizumab</u> (Synagis)

Dose: 15 mg/kg/dose once per month throughout respiratory syncytial virus (RSV) season. (RSV season is usually November through April, but may very. Check with local Health Department.)

Give monthly even if RSV infection develops.

Consider use for a second RSV season in patients with severe chronic lung disease (CLD), especially those requiring continuing medical therapy.

Administration: Intramuscular to anterolateral thigh. Give dose volumes >1 ml as a divided dose.

Storage: Refrigerate. Do not freeze. Opened vials should be used within 6 hours.

Cost-Saving Tip: The American Academy of Pediatrics recommends that, to minimize waste, physicians should schedule administration so that 2 or more eligible patients can receive the vaccine within the 6-hour period after a vial is opened.

Cautions/Contraindications:

Palivizumab has not been studied in infants and children with congenital heart disease and is not licensed by the FDA for these patients.

As with all IM injections, do not use in patients with thrombocytopenia (platelets <40,000/mm) or coagulation disorders.

Adverse Effects: Well tolerated.

May cause mild and transient erythremia, pain, and induration at injection site (2.7 percent patients).

Mild or moderate elevations of the enzyme aspartate aminotransferase occurred in 3.6 percent of those who received palivizumab versus 1.6 percent of those receiving a placebo.

Nursing Implications:

Advise parents that palivizumab should be accompanied by a program to prevent RSV transmission:

- Eliminate exposure to cigarette smoke
- Limit exposure to contagious settings such as chid care centers
- Emphasize hand washing

(Zenk: Neonatal Medications & Nutrition. A Comprehensive Guide 2000; pp:371-373)

PANCREATIC ENZYMES (Pancrelipase)

Supplied: Capsules: Cotazym, KuZymeHP
Capsules, delayed release: Pancrease MT 4, MT 10, MT 16, Pancrease, Cotazym 5 (containing enteric-coated spheres, microspheres, or microtablets)
Powder: Viokase
Tablets: Viokase, Ilozyme

To protect the enteric coating, do not crush or chew the microspheres/tablets.

<u>Pancreatic Enzymes</u> (Pancrease, Cotazyme)

Dose & Route: Initial doses: (actual requirements are patient specific)

Enteric-coated microspheres and microtabs:
Infants: 2000-4000 U lipase per 120 ml formula or per breast feeding
Children <4 yr: 1000 U lipase/kg/meal
Children ≥4 yr: 500 U lipase/kg/meal

The total daily dose should include approximately three meals and two to three snacks per day. Snack doses are approximately 1/2-meal doses.

Remarks: May cause occult GI bleeding, allergic reactions to porcine proteins, hyperuricemia, and hyperuricosuria with high doses. Dose should be titrated to eliminate diarrhea and to minimize steatorrhea. Do not chew microspheres or microtabs. Concurrent administration with H_2 antagonists or gastric acid pump inhibitors may enhance enzyme efficacy. Doses higher than 6000 U lipase/kg/meal have been associated with colonic strictures in children <12 years of age. Powder dosage form is not preferred due to potential GI mucosal ulceration.

(Siberry: The Harriet Lane Handbook 2000, p.800)

PANCREATIN

Supplied: Capsules: Creon containing delayed release, Creon 10, 20
Tablets: Donnazyme, Pancreatin 4x, 8x.

Administration: PO
Pancreatin preparations should not be held in the mouth prior to swallowing, since the drug may irritate the oral mucosa (3).

To protect the enteric coating, do not crush or chew the microspheres/tablets.

Pancreatin

Route & Dose: PO: 2000 units of lipase with each feeding.
PR and into colostomy: 0.3-0.5 gm in sufficient liquid (for meconium ileus)

(Taeusch: Avery's Diseases of the Newborn 1998, p.1346)

Pancreatin

Usual Dosage: Infants: 2000-4000 lipase units/120 mL (4 ounce) formula

Administration: (use mixture immediately, do not make ahead of time). Place mixture onto the middle of the infant's tongue and then give bottle or breast. As an alternative, the parent may dip a clean finger into the food/enzyme mixture and then place finger into the infant's mouth and allow infant to suck on. Check infant's mouth after eating for lodged enzyme beads and remove.

(Taketomo: Pediatric Dosage Handbook 1999-2000, pp.723-724)

PANCURONIUM BROMIDE (Pavulon)

Supplied: Injection 1 mg/ml in 10 ml; 2 mg/ml in 2 ml, 5 ml

Administration: IV
Stable in D5W or NS for 48 hours (1).
Neonates are especially sensitive to this drug class during the first month of life. Give a test dose of 0.02 mg/kg to assess responsiveness. (1)

Storage/Stability: Refrigerate at 2° - 8° C (36-46° F) to maintain potency for 18 months. If stored at 18-22° C (65-72° F), potency is maintained for 6 months. (1)

Pancuronium Bromide (Pavulon)

Indications and use: To increase pulmonary compliance in an uncooperative neonate during mechanical ventilation. To produce skeletal muscle relaxation during surgery.

Actions: Nondepolarizing neuromuscular blocking agent that produces skeletal muscle paralysis mainly by causing a decreased response to acetylcholine at the myoneural junction. Pancuronium may cause an increase in heart rate. The onset of action is generally 30-60 s, with a duration of action of ~ 40-60 min, but may be much longer in neonates.

Route: IV

Dosage: Initial dosage: 0.03 mg/kg IV; repeat prn.
Maintenance dosage: 0.03-0.09 mg/kg IV q1-4h prn to maintain paralysis.

Adverse effects: Tachycardia may occur.

Comments: Neonates are particularly sensitive to the actions; prolonged paralysis may be noted. Ventilation must be supported during neuromuscular blockade. Many centers place a sign over patient's bedside to alert all medical personnel that the infant is paralyzed. Neostigmine methylsulfate and atropine sulfate are used for reversal.

(Gomella: Neonatology 1999, p.582)

Pancuronium

Indication: Protocol for inborn infants with Congenital Diaphragmatic Hernia

Pancuronium bromide (100 µg/kg) was given every 60 to 90 minutes

(Finer: Congenital diaphragmatic Hernia: Developing a Protocolized Approach. J Pediatr Surg 1998;33:1331-1337)

Pancuronium (Pavulon)

Dose: 0.02-0.09 mg/kg every 1-4 hours. Begin with lowest dose and titrate upward, if needed.

Dose Titration: Administration at intervals of 2 hours or less should prompt an increase in dose. Paralysis lasting beyond 4-6 hours suggests excessive dosing.

Administration: Rate: Over at least 1 minute IV push, or by continuous infusion.
Concentration May give undiluted or may dilute with sodium chloride, dextrose, or lactated Ringer's.

Use: A long-acting neuromuscular blocking agent for skeletal muscle relaxation (paralysis) during surgical procedures such as PDA ligation.

Also used for severe, unresponsive seizures such as neonatal tetany.

Nursing Implications:
Refrigerate drug. When taken on transport, refrigerate immediately upon return. Have reversal agents at bedside.

All paralyzed infants need analgesia and/or sedation in conjunction with paralyzation. Consider concomitant infusion of fentanyl, morphine, or midazolam.

Provide range of motion, position changes, and eye lubrication to avoid side effects of paralysis.

Consider need for bladder catheterization or Crede" if urine output decreases. Monitor for movement and side effects, including hypertension and tachycardia.

Comments: Mechanical ventilation must be provided during use. Drug does not produce analgesia or sedation, only paralysis.

Reversal of Neuromuscular Blockade:

- Mechanism of Reversal: Neostigmine inhibits acetylcholinesterase at the neuromuscular junction, allowing the accumulation of acetylcholine, which can successfully compete with the neuromuscular blocker at the neuromuscular junction, thus restoring muscle activity. Atropine is also given to avert the nonneuromuscular effects of neostigmine, such as increased secretions, bronchoconstriction, and bradycardia.
- Reversal Dose: Neostigmine 0.06 mg/kg IV plus atropine 0.02 mg/kg IV.
- Onset of Reversal: Approximately 10 minutes.

(Zenk: Neonatal Medications & Nutrition. A Comprehensive Guide 2000; pp:374-375)

Pancuronium Bromide (Pavulon)

Dose/kg: 0.04-0.1 mg

Route & Frequency: IV q1h-q4h prn movement

Comments: Short half-life; titrate close based on clinical response. Aminoglycosides increase the action of pancuronium

(Avery: Neonatology Pathophysiology and Management of the Newborn 1999, p.1559)

Pancuronium Bromide

PB (100 µg/kg) was usually given every 60 to 90 minutes and according to the discretion of physician for continuous muscle paralysis (assessed clinically and not by nerve stimulation). Muscle paralysis was continued during ECMO.

In summary, in our CDH population with a frequency of 62% of SNHL among the survivors, we found an unexpected association between childhood SNHL in the survivors of CDH and the prolonged use of PB during the neonatal period, but not with the studied ototoxic drugs (aminoglycosides, vancomycin, and furosemide).

Although the association of PB administration and SNHL justifies further investigation, the retrospective nature and small sample size in our study demand cautious interpretation of negative findings. Multicenter studies are required to evaluate the possible adverse audiologic effects of prolonged use of PB and to identify the mechanism of the development of SNHL in these survivors.

SNHL: Sensorineural hearing loss
CDH: congential diaphragmatic hernia

(Cheung: Prolonged use of pancuronium bromide and sensorineural hearing loss in childhood survivors of congential diaphragmatic hernia. J Pediatr 1999;135:233-9)

<u>Pancuronium</u> (Pavulon)

Dose: 0.1-0.2 mg/kg IV

Mode of Action: Competitive neuromuscular blockade

Adverse Effects: Tachycardia

(Garson: The science and practice of pediatric cardiology 1998, p.2955)

<u>Pancuronium Bromide</u> (Pavulon)

Dose & Route: Neonate:
Initial: 0.02 mg/kg/dose IV.
Maintenance: 0.05-0.1 mg/kg/dose Q 0.5-4 hr PRN

1 mo-adult:
Initial: 0.04-0.1 mg/kg/dose IV
Maintenance: 0.015-0.1 mg/kg/dose IV Q30-60 min.
Continuous IV infusion: 0.1 mg/kg/hr

Remarks: Onset of action is 1-2 minutes. Drug effects may be accentuated by hypothermia, acidosis, neonatal age, decreased renal function, halothane, succinylcholine, hypokalemia, clindamycin, tetracycline, and aminoglycoside antibiotics. May cause tachycardia, salivation, and wheezing. Antidote is neostigmine (with atropine or glycopyrrolate). **Avoid** use in severe renal impairment (CrCl <10 ml/min).

(Siberry: The Harriet Lane Handbook 2000, p.801)

PAPAVERINE HCL

Supplied: Injectable 30 mg/ml in 2 ml, 10 ml

<u>Papaverine Hydrochloride</u>

Indications and use: Peripheral arterial spasms.

Actions: Directly relaxes vascular smooth muscle and results in vasodilation.

Route: PO, IM, IV (infuse over 1-2 min).
Dosage: 6 mg/kg/24h in 4 divided doses.

Comments: IV infusion should be performed under a physician's supervision, since arrhythmias and fatal apnea may result from rapid injection.

Note: Limited experience in neonates.

(Gomella: Neonatology 1999, p.582)

PARALDEHYDE (Paral)

Supplied: Liquid (oral, rectal): 1g/mL in 30mL

Administration: Paraldehyde 1ml is essentially equivalent to 1gm.

A parenteral dosage form is no longer available in the United States.

Paraldehyde is irritating to mucous membranes and must be well diluted. Esophagitis, hemorrhagic gastritis and proctitis have occurred.

Oral: Mix in milk or fruit juice to mask the taste and odor.

Rectal: Dissolve in oil as a retention enema. Mix with 1-2 parts of olive oil or isotonic sodium chloride solution to avoid rectal irritation.

Storage/Stability: Upon exposure to light and air, paraldehyde decomposes to acetaldehyde and oxidizes to acetic acid. Do not use if liquid is brownish color or sharp odor of acetic acid is present. Discard unused portion. Do not use paraldehyde from a container that has been opened for longer than 24 hours (1).

Paraldehyde

Indication: For Neonatal Seizures
Paraldehyde administered as an intravenous bolus and then continuous infusion has been effective as adjunctive therapy in approximately 50% of the infants studied. However, the intravenous form of this drug is no longer available in the Untied States. Moreover, the potential side effects of respiratory disturbance, secondary to pulmonary excretion of paraldehyde, and of hypotension make this drug not highly desirable in the newborn.

(Volpe: Neurology of the Newborn 2001, p.206)

Paraldehyde (Paral)

Indications and use: Status epilepticus resistant to conventional therapy (i.e. phenobarbital, phenytoin, diazepam, lorazepam).

Actions: A rapid-acting hypnotic agent effective against all types of seizures when administered in large doses. Precise mechanism of action is unknown.

Route: PO, PR.

Dosage: 0.3 mL/kg/dose q4-6h if needed. For rectal use: Dilute in equal volume of olive oil or mineral oil.
For oral use, dilute in infant formula.

Adverse effects: Side effects severely limit use. May cause pulmonary edema and hemorrhage, severe coughing, irritation to GI mucosa, and thrombophlebitis. Overdose may cause cardiac and respiratory depression. Rectal administration may cause proctitis.

Comments: Routine use in infants is discouraged. Contraindicated in pulmonary or hepatic disease.

Note: Dissolves plastic and reacts with rubber stoppers in bottles and syringes. Do not use plastic equipment for administration. For rectal administration, use glass syringes. Discard a container opened >24h, discolored solution, or solution smelling of acetic acid (vinegar), as it may be toxic.

(Gomella: Neonatology 1999, pp.582-583)

<u>Paraldehyde</u>

Route & Dose: PR: 0.3 ml/kg q 4-6 h

Adverse Effects, Cautions:
Reserve for refractory status epilepticus. Local irritation, pulmonary edema, hemorrhage. Hepatic dysfunction decreases clearance. Avoid IM if possible. Do not give by arterial catheter. Avoid plastic containers.

(Taeusch: Avery's Diseases of the Newborn 1998, p.1346)

<u>Paraldehyde</u>

Dosage: 0.3 ml/kg/dose per rectum every 4-6 hr

(Fanaroff: Neonatal-Perinatal Medicine 1997, p.1747)

PAREGORIC (Opium Tincture Camphorated)

Supplied: Liquid in 60 ml, pints

Administration: PO

Paregoric liquid contains 2 mg morphine equivalent per 5 ml. Contains 45% alcohol (1).

Note: DO NOT confuse paregoric with opium tincture.

<u>Paregoric</u>

Indication: Drug therapy for withdrawal syndrome in infants.

Paregoric is a commonly used drug in this context. It is highly effective in treating both the central nervous system and gastrointestinal disturbances. The dose range needed is three to six drops, administered every 4 to 6 hours.

(Volpe: Neurology of the Newborn 2001, p882)

<u>Paregoric</u>

Dose: 0.2 ml (equivalent to 80 mcg morphine) every 3 hours. Increase dose by 0.05 ml (equivalent to 20 mcg morphine) every 3 hours until symptoms are under control

Maximum: 0.7 ml/dose (equivalent to 280 mcg morphine/dose).

Tapering the Dose: Begin tapering when symptoms have been under control for 3-5 days, and taper gradually over 2-4 weeks, as tolerated.

The Neonatal Withdrawal Score Sheet in Appendix K facilitates objective assessment of the infant's symptoms.

Cautions/Contraindications:

See Use for Components of this drug that are potentially hazardous to infants.

Opium tincture contains 25 times more morphine than does paregoric (camphorated opium tincture); it is vital that these two products not be confused. If opium tincture is used, prepare a 1:25 dilution in water before use. A 1:25 dilution of opium tincture may be given at the doses shown above.

Use: Neonatal narcotic withdrawal. Consider use if GI symptoms such as diarrhea occur. However, other agents are preferred (see below).

The 1996 USP DI states that paregoric is not recommended for ameliorating withdrawal symptoms in opioid-dependent neonates. Paregoric contains substances that are potentially hazardous to infants: camphor (a CNS stimulant), benzoic acid (a potent displacer of bilirubin from albumin binding sites and one of the metabolic products of benzyl alcohol, a preservative that has caused deaths in preterm infants), and 45 percent alcohol (a gastric irritant, a CNS depressant, may cause hepatic damage and hypoglycemia). Paregoric has been replaced for this purpose by other opioid drugs with fewer or no hazardous additional ingredients, such as morphine oral solution, benzodiazepines, barbiturates, or diluted opium tincture. Methadone has also been used, but tapering is difficult due to its long elimination half-life. These other medications should be used, whenever possible, instead of paregoric.

Adverse Effects: Hold dose if excessive drowsiness or respiratory depression appears. **Antidote**: Naloxone 0.1 mg/kg/dose IV. See Appendix J: Antidotes for Drugs That Cause Loss of Respiratory Effort. Note: Naloxone administration may precipitate withdrawal.

To rapid tapering of dose may lead to recurrence of symptoms.

Opium has all the toxic potentials of narcotic agonists.

May cause respiratory depression, constipation, hypotension, bradycardia, CNS depression, increased intracranial pressure, sedation, release of antidiuretic hormone, urine retention, urinary tract spasm, histamine release, physical dependence, and tolerance.

Nursing Implications: Monitor for respiratory depression, lethargy.
Utilize the Neonatal Withdrawal Score Sheet in Appendix K to determine effectiveness of therapy and timing of titration.

(Zenk: Neonatal Medications & Nutrition. A Comprehensive Guide 2000; pp.376-377)

Paregoric (Camphorated Opium Tincture)

Dose & Route: Analgesia/Antidiarrheal:
Children: 0.25-0.5 ml/kg/dose PO QD-QID

Neonatal opiate withdrawal:
Start with 0.2-0.3 ml/dose Q3-4 hr, increase dose by 0.05 ml/dose Q3-4 hr until symptoms abate; **max dose** 0.7 ml/dose

Remarks: Each 5 ml paregoric contains 2 mg morphine equivalent, 0.02 ml anise oil, 20 mg benzoic acid, 20 mg camphor, 0.2 ml glycerin, and alcohol. The final concentration of morphine equivalent is 0.4 mg/ml. This is 25-fold less potent than undiluted deodorized tincture of opium (DTO: 10 mg morphine equivalent/ml). **If using DTO to treat neonatal abstinence, must dilute 25-fold prior to use**. Similar side effects to morphine. After symptoms are controlled for several days, dose for opiate withdrawal should be decreased gradually over a 2- to 4-week period (e.g., by 10% Q2-3 days).

(Siberry: The Harriet Lane Handbook 2000, p.801)

PAROMOMYCIN SULFATE (Humatin)

Supplied: Capsules, 250 mg
Administration: Oral

Paromomycin (Humatin)

Antibacterial Drugs for pediatric Patients Beyond the Newborn Period
Dosage per kg/d
Route: PO
Mild to Moderate Infections: 30 mg in 3 doses
Severe Infections: Inappropriate
Note: Dosages for the aminoglycosides may differ from those recommended by the manufacturers (see package insert)

(American Academy of Pediatrics: Report of the Committee on Infectious Diseases. Red Book 2000, pp.653,662)

PENICILLIN G AQUEOUS 'Na' and 'K' (Aqueous Penicillin)

Supplied: Powder for injection:
Na 5 million unit vial
K 1 and 5 million unit vials

Administration: IV, IM
Penicillin G 'Na' contains 2 mEq of Na/1 million units.
Penicillin G 'K' contains 1.7 mEq of K and 0.3 mEq of Na/1 million units (1).
Infuse of 15-30 minutes (1).

Penicillin G

Antibacterial Drugs for Newborn Infants
Dose (mg/kg or Units [U]/kg) and Frequency of Administration
Route: IV, IM
Dose: Infants 0-4 wk
BW <1200 g: 25 000-50 000 U every 12 h

Infants <1 wk old
BW ≤1200-2000 g: 25 000-50 000 U every 12 h
BW >2000 g: 25 000-50 000 U every 8 h

Infants ≥1 wk old
BW ≤2000-2000 g: 25 000-50 000 U every 8 h
BW >2000 g: 25 000-50 000 U every 6 h

Note: For meningitis, the larger dosage is recommended

High doses are recommended for the treatment of group B streptococcal meningitis.

Antibacterial Drugs for Pediatric Patients Beyond the Newborn Period
Dosage per kg/d
Route: IV, IM
Mild to Moderate Infections: 25 000-50 000 U in 4 doses
Severe Infections: 250 000-400 000 U in 4-6 doses

Comments; Larger dosage appropriate for central nervous system infections

Note: In patients with history of allergy to penicillin or one of its many congeners, alternative drugs are recommended. In some circumstances, a cephalosporin or other β-lactam class drug may be acceptable. However, these drugs should not be used in patients with an immediate hypersensitivity (anaphylaxis) to penicillin because approximately 5% to 15% of penicillin-allergic patients will also be allergic to the cephalosporins.

Patients with a history of allergy to penicillin G or V should be considered for subsequent skin testing. Many such patients can be treated safely with penicillin, since only 10% of children with such history are proven allergic when skin tested.

(American Academy of Pediatrics: Report of the Committee on Infectious Diseases. Red Book 2000, pp.652,659,662)

Penicillin G

Route: IV
Dosage (mg/kg) and Interval of Administration:
(units)
Meningitis:

Weight <1200 g
Age 0-4 WK: 50,000 q12h

Weight 1200-2000 g
Age 0-7 Days: 50,000 q12h
Age >7 Days: 50,000 q8h

Weight >2000 g
Age 0-7 Days: 50,000 q8h
Age >7 Days: 50,000 q6h

Other infections:

Weight <1200 g
Age 0-4 Wk: 25,000 q12h

<u>Weight 1200-2000 g</u>
Age 0-7 Days; 25,000 q12h
Age >7 Days: 25,000 q8h

<u>Weight >2000 g</u>
Age 0-7 Days: 25,000 q8h
Age >7 Days; 25,000 q6h

(Remington: Infectious Diseases of the Fetus and Newborn Infant 2001, p.1454)

<u>Penicillin</u>

Indication: Therapy for congenital syphilis

Penicillin is the drug of choice in the treatment of congenital syphilis. The major questions faced in the neonatal period are *whom to treat and how to treat.* Detection of the infants with congenital syphilis requires a high index of suspicion and a careful evaluation. Particularly important are historical data related to the mother, maternal serology at delivery, and careful clinical radiographic, metabolic, and serological studies of the infant. Because maternal antibody response may occur so late in pregnancy that the infant's VDRL test is negative, positive maternal serology should provoke careful evaluation of the infant and consideration for treatment as outlined in Table. the mode of penicillin therapy depends largely on the adequacy of treatment of the mother during pregnancy (see table below). When the mother has had no or inadequate treatment during pregnancy, the infant is treated with a full 10- to 14-day course of either crystalline or procaine penicillin G in the doses shown in the table, whether the infant is asymptomatic or symptomatic and whether infection of the infant is confirmed or not. The dose schedule described in table results in adequate spirocheticidal levels in CSF, although some data indicate that crystalline penicillin G is superior to procaine penicillin. The importance of treating all confirmed or presumptive cases of congenital syphilis with the higher doses relates to the fact that the CNS may be infected without demonstrable abnormalities of CSF and may serve as an incubating reservoir of infection that culminates in relapse and neurosyphilis.

For infants who are asymptomatic, who have normal physical examinations and laboratory evaluations, and whose mothers have been adequately treated, the risk of congenital syphilis is very low. Treatment is not compulsory if close follow-up can be ensured. However, if follow-up cannot be ensured, administration of a single dose of benzathine penicillin G is recommended. Whether follow-up can be ensured or not, the CSF should be examined, and if there is any suspicion of CNS involvement, a 10- to 14-day course of crystalline or procaine penicillin G should be carried out.

TABLE
Treatment of Infants Born to Mothers with Syphilis

MATERNAL TREATMENT	NEONATAL CLINICAL FINDINGS	PENICILLIN G	DOSE AND DURATION
None or inadequate	Present or absent	Crystalline	100,000-150,000 units/kg/day IV every 8-12 hr for 10-14 days
		Procaine	50,000 units/kg/day IM once daily for 10-14 days
Adequate	Absent	Benzathine	500,000 units/kg IM, one dose (only if follow-up cannot be ensured and cerebrospinal fluid is normal)

(Volpe: Neurology of the Newborn 2001, pp.750-751)

Penicillin G

Route: IV

Dosages (mg/kg/day)[sic] and Intervals of Administration:

Body weight: < 2000g
0-7 days old: 100,000 U div q12h
8-28 days old: 225,000 U div q8h

Body weight: >2000g
0-7 days old: 150,000 U div q8h
8-28 days old: 200,000 U div q6h

>28 days old: 200,000 U div q6h

(Nelson: Pocket Book of Pediatric Antimicrobial Therapy 2000-2001, p.16)

Penicillin G

Condition: Congenital syphilis

Therapy: Aqueous penicillin G 50,000 U/kg q12h (day of life 1-7), q8h (>7 days) IV OR procaine penicillin G 50,000 U/kg IM once daily; x 10-14 days; Optional alternative for asymptomatic infant or when infant's nontreponemal test is negative: benzathine penicillin G 50,000 U/kg IM, single dose

Comment: Obtain follow-up serology at 3, 6, and 12 mos until nontreponemal test nonreactive or decreased fourfold

(Nelson: Pocket Book of Pediatric Antimicrobial Therapy 2000-2001, p.8)

Penicillin G (Aqueous), Parenteral

Action & spectrum:

Mechanism of action is identical to that of other β-lactam antibiotics. Effective mainly against streptococci, some community-acquired staphylococci (except methicillin-resistant and penicillinase-producing strains), *Neisseria gonorrhoeae*, *Neisseria meningitides*, *Bacillus anthracis*, *Clostridium tetani*, *Clostridium perfringens*, *Bacteroides* (oropharyngeal strains), *Leptospira* spp, and *Treponema pallidum*.

Route: IM or IV (infuse over 30 min).

Dosage:

Meningitis:
<2000 g and 0-7 days old: 100,000 units/kg/day divided q12h
<2000 g and >7 days old: 150,000 units/kg/day divided q8h.
>2000 g and 0-7 days old: 150,000 units/kg/day divided q8h.
>2000 g and >7 days old: 200,000 units/kg/day divided q6h.

Other indications:
<2000 g and 0-7 days old: 50,000 units/kg/day divided q12h.
<2000 g and >7 days old: 75,000 units/kg/day divided q8h.
>2000 g and 0-7 days old: 50,000 units/kg/day divided q8h.
>2000 g and >7 day old: 100,000 units/kg/day divided q6h.

Elimination and metabolism: Renal

Adverse effects: Allergic reactions, rash, fever, change in bowel flora, *Candida* superinfection, diarrhea, hemolytic anemia. Very large doses may cause seizures. Rapid IV push of potassium penicillin G may cause cardiac arrhythmias and arrest because of potassium content. Infuse slowly over 30 min.

Comments: 1600 units = 1 mg. Some strains of group B streptococci are penicillinase producers, thus requiring the addition of an aminoglycoside antibiotic for synergistic bactericidal effect. Good activity against anaerobes. Drug of choice for tetanus neonatorum. Contains 1.7 meq of sodium or potassium per million unit.

(Gomella: Neonatology 1999 p.583)

PENICILLIN G BENZATHINE (Bicillin LA, Permapen)

Supplied: 300,000 U/ml in 10 ml.
600,000 U/dose in 1 ml tubex.

Administration: IM only. 1,200,000 units/dose in 2ml
2,400,000 units/dose in 4ml
Do not administer IV

Penicillin G Benzathine

Antibacterial Drugs for Pediatric Patients Beyond the Newborn Period:

Dosage per kg/d

Route: IM

Mild to Moderate Infections:
<27.3 kg (60 lb): 600,000 U
≥27.3 kg: 1,200,000 U

Severe Infections: Inappropriate

Comments: Major use is prevention of rheumatic fever by treatment and prophylaxis of streptococcal infections

Note: In patients with history of allergy to penicillin or one of its many congeners, alternative drugs are recommended. In some circumstances, a cephalosporin or other β-lactam class drug may be acceptable. However, these drugs should not be used in patients with an immediate hypersensitivity (anaphylaxis) to penicillin because approximately 5% to 15% of penicillin-allergic patients will also be allergic to the cephalosporins.

Patients with a history of allergy to penicillin G or V should be considered for subsequent skin testing. Many such patients can be treated safely with penicillin, since only 10% of children with such history are proven allergic when skin-tested

(American Academy of Pediatrics: Report of the Committee on Infectious Diseases. Red Book 2000, pp.659,662)

Penicillin benzathine

Route: IM

Dosage (mg/kg) and Interval of Administration:
(units)

Weight 1200-2000 g
Age 0-7 Days: 50,000 (one dose)
Age >7 Days: 50,000 (one dose)

Weight >2000 g
Age 0-7 Days: 50,000 (one dose)
Age >7 Days: 50,000 (one dose)

(Remington: Infectious Diseases of the Fetus and Newborn Infant 2001, p.1454)

Penicillin G Benzathine (Bicillin L-A, Permapen)

Action & spectrum:
See Penicillin G (Aqueous), Parenteral. A drug of choice in the treatment of asymptomatic congenital syphilis.

Route: IM only. (Viscosity requires ≥ 23-gauge needle.)
Dosage: 50,000 units/kg once.

Elimination and metabolism:
Renally excreted over a prolonged interval owing to slow absorption from the injection site.

Adverse effects & Comments:
See Penicillin G (Aqueous), Parenteral. 1211 units = 1 mg. Not often used.

(Gomella: Neonatology 1999, p.583)

Penicillin G, Benzathine

Route: IM
Dosages (units/kg/day) and Intervals of Administration:

Weight 1200-2000g
Age 0-7 days: 50,000 units/kg (One dose)
Age > 7 days: 50,000 units/kg (One dose)

Weight: >2000g
Age 0-7 days: 50,000 units/kg (One dose)
Age > 7 days: 50,000 units/kg (One dose)

(Nelson: Pocket Book of Pediatric Antimicrobial Therapy 2000-2001, p.82)

PENICILLIN G PROCAINE (Wycillin)

Supplied: Wycillin 600,000 U in 1ml and 1,200,000 U/dose, in 2ml, 2,400,000 units/dose in 4ml

Administration: IM only, Do not inject into or near an artery or nerve. Penicillin G Procaine must never be used IV. (1)

Penicillin G Procaine

Antibacterial Drugs for Newborn Infants

Dose (mg/kg or Units [U]/kg) and Frequency of Administration

Route: IM

Dose: Infants <1 wk old
BW ≤1200-2000 g: 50 000 U every 24 h
BW >2000 g: 50 000 U every 24 h

Infants ≥1 wk old
BW ≤2000-2000 g: 50 000 U every 24 h
BW >2000 g: 50 000 U every 24 h

Antibacterial Drugs for Pediatric patients Beyond the Newborn Period

Dosage per kg/d

Route: IM

Mild to Moderate Infections: 25 000-50 000 U in 1-2 doses

Severe Infections: Inappropriate

Comments: Contraindicated in procaine allergy

Note: In patients with history of allergy to penicillin or one of its many congeners, alternative drugs are recommended. In some circumstances, a cephalosporin or other β-lactam class drug may be acceptable. However, these drugs should not be used in patients with an immediate hypersensitivity (anaphylaxis) to penicillin because approximately 5% to 15% of penicillin-allergic patients will also be allergic to the cephalosporins.

Patients with a history of allergy to penicillin G or V should be considered for subsequent skin testing. Many such patients can be treated safely with penicillin, since only 10% of children with such history are proven allergic when skin-tested.

(American Academy of Pediatrics: Report of the Committee on Infectious Diseases. Red Book 2000, pp.652,659,662)

Penicillin procaine

Route: IM

Dosage (mg/kg) and Interval of Administration:

(units) Weight 1200-2000 g
Age 0-7 Days: 50,000 q24h
Age >7 Days: 50,000 q24h

Weight >2000 g
Age 0-7 Days: 50,000 q24h
Age >7 Days: 50,000 q24h

(Remington: Infectious Diseases of the Fetus and Newborn Infant 2001, p.1454)

Penicillin G, Procaine

Route: IM

Dosages (mg/kg/dose)[sic] and Intervals of Administration:

Body weight: < 2000g
0-7 days old: 50,000 U q24h
8-28 days old: 50,000 U q24h

Body weight: >2000g
0-7 days old: 50,000 U q24h
8-28 days old: 50,000 U q24h

> 28 days old: 50,000 U q24h

(Nelson: Pocket Book of Pediatric Antimicrobial Therapy 2000-2001, p.16)

Penicillin G Procaine

Condition: Congenital syphilis

Therapy: Aqueous penicillin G 50,000 U/kg q12h (day of life 1-7), q8h (>7 days) IV OR procaine penicillin G 50,000 U/kg IM once daily; x 10-14 days; Optional alternative for asymptomatic infant or when infant's nontreponemal test is negative: benzathine penicillin G 50,000 U/kg IM, single dose

Comment: Obtain follow-up serology at 3, 6, and 12 mos until nontreponemal test nonreactive or decreased fourfold

(Nelson: Pocket Book of Pediatric Antimicrobial Therapy 2000-2001, p.8)

Penicillin G Procaine (Wycillin)

Action & spectrum:
See Penicillin G (Aqueous), Parenteral. A drug of choice in the treatment of symptomatic or asymptomatic congenital syphilis.

Route: IM only. (Viscosity requires ≥ 23-gauge needle.)

Dosage: 50,000 units/kg/dose q24h.

Elimination and metabolism: See Penicillin G (Aqueous), Parenteral.

Adverse effects: See Penicillin G (Aqueous), Parenteral. May also cause sterile abscess formation at injection site. Contains 120 mg procaine per 300,000 units, which may cause allergic reactions, myocardial depression, or systemic vasodilatation. There is cause for much greater concern about these effects in the neonate than in older patients.

Comments: 1000 units = 1 mg. Not often used.

(Gomella: Neonatology 1994, pp. 583-584)

PENICILLIN V POTASSIUM (PenVeeK)

Supplied: Suspension, powder for 125 mg, 250 mg/5ml in 80, 100, 150, 200 ml.

Administration: PO.
Following reconstitution, oral solutions must be refrigerated. Unused portion should be discarded after 14 days (3).

Penicillin V

Antibacterial Drugs for Pediatric Patients Beyond the Newborn Period
Dosage per kg/d
Route: PO
Mild to Moderate Infections: 25 000-50 000 U in 3 or 4 doses
Severe Infections: Inappropriate

Comments: Optimal to administer on an empty stomach

Note: In patients with history of allergy to penicillin or one of its many congeners, alternative drugs are recommended. In some circumstances, a cephalosporin or other β-lactam class drug may be acceptable. However, these drugs should not be used in patients with an immediate hypersensitivity (anaphylaxis) to penicillin because approximately 5% to 15% of penicillin-allergic patients will also be allergic to the cephalosporins.

Patients with a history of allergy to penicillin G or V should be considered for subsequent skin testing. Many such patients can be treated safely with penicillin, since only 10% of children with such history are proven allergic when skin-tested.

(American Academy of Pediatrics: Report of the Committee on Infectious Diseases. Red Book 2000, pp.659,662)

Penicillin V

Condition: Otitis Media, Streptococcus
Therapy: Penicillin V 30 mg/kg/day PO div q8h x 10 days
Comment: May be given IV

(Nelson: Pocket Book of Pediatric Antimicrobial Therapy 2000-2001, p.11)

PENTAMIDINE (Pentam 300, NebuPent)

Supplied: Injection 300mg/vial
Aerosol 300mg
Administration: IM, IV, Aerosol

Pentamidine

Indication: Infection, Pneumocystis carinii pneumonia

Dosage: 3-4 mg/kg IV daily x 14-21 days

Adverse Effects: Frequent:
Hypotension; hypoglycemia often followed by diabetes mellitus; vomiting; blood dyscrasias; renal damage; pain at injection site; GI disturbances

Occasional:
May aggravate diabetes; shock; hypocalcemia; liver damage; cardiotoxicity; delirium; rash

Rare:
Herxheimer-type reaction; anaphylaxis; acute pancreatitis; hyperkalemia and vomiting with amoxicillin/clavulanic acid in children

For Treatment of Pneumocystis Carinii Infection:

The drug of choice is trimethoprim-sulfamethoxazole (15 to 20 mg/kg per day of trimethoprim; 75 to 100 mg/kg of sulfamethoxazole daily in divided doses every 6 hours), usually given intravenously. Oral therapy should be reserved for patients with mild disease who do not have malabsorption or diarrhea. The rate of adverse reactions is higher in HIV-infected patients than in patients without HIV infection; the incidence in HIV-infected children treated with trimethoprim-sulfamethoxazole is approximately 15% but may be as high as 60% in adults with HIV infection. If the adverse reaction is not severe, continuation of therapy is recommended, because 50% of patients with adverse reactions subsequently have been treated successfully with trimethoprim-sulfamethoxazole.

Parenterally administered pentamidine (4 mg/kg per day of salt given once a day) is an alternative drug for children and adults who cannot tolerate trimethoprim-sulfamethoxazole or who have severe disease and who have not responded to trimethoprim-sulfamethoxazole after 5 to 7 days of therapy. the therapeutic efficacy of parenteral pentamidine in adults with PCP has been similar to that of trimethoprim-sulfamethoxazole. However, pentamidine is associated with a high incidence of adverse reactions, including pancreatitis, renal dysfunction, hypoglycemia, hyperglycemia, hypotension, fever, and neutropenia. Pentamidine should not be used concomitantly with didanosine, since both drugs can cause pancreatitis. If a recipient of didanosine develops PCP and requires pentamidine, didanosine should be discontinued until 1 week after the pentamidine therapy has been discontinued.

Atovaquone is approved for the oral treatment of mild to moderate PCP in adults who are intolerant of trimethoprim-sulfamethoxazole. Experience with the use of atovaquone in children is limited.

Other potentially useful drugs identified by in vitro studies, animal models, and clinical trials in adults include dapsone with trimethoprim, trimetrexate with leucovorin, and clindamycin with primaquine. Experience with the use of these combinations in children is limited.

A minimum duration of 2 weeks of therapy is recommended; many experts advise 3 weeks of therapy for patients with AIDS. In patients with AIDS, continuous lifelong prophylaxis should be initiated at the end of therapy for acute infection.

Corticosteroids seem to be beneficial in the treatment of HIV-infected adults with moderate to severe PCP (as defined by an arterial oxygen pressure [PaO_2] of less than

70 mm Hg or an arterial-alveolar gradient of more than 35 mm Hg).

Although no controlled studies of the use of corticosteroids in young children have been performed, most experts would include corticosteroids as part of therapy for children with moderate to severe PCP. The optimal dose and duration of corticosteroid therapy for children have not been determined, but most experts suggest 2 mg/kg per day of prednisone or its equivalent for 7 to 10 days, followed by a tapering dose during the next 10 to 14 days.

(American Academy of Pediatrics: Report of the Committee on Infectious Diseases. Red Book 2000, pp.712,722462-463)

<u>Pentamidine Isethionate</u>

Infection: Pneumocystis carinii pneumonia

Therapy: Trimethoprim-sulfamethoxazole 15-20 mg <u>OR</u> pentamidine isethionate 4 mg base/kg/day IV daily x 10-14 days; Alternatives: trimethoprim and dapsone; primaquine and clindamycin; trimetrexate and folinic acid; atovaquone for nonsevere disease

Comments: Prophylaxis: 5 mg TMP, 25 daily or three times weekly <u>OR</u> dapsone 1 mg/kg PO once daily

(Nelson: Pocket Book of Pediatric Antimicrobial Therapy 2000-2001, p.58)

PENTOBARBITAL (Nembutal)

Supplied: Injectable 50mg/ml
Elixir 20mg/5ml
Suppository 30mg, 60mg, 120mg, 200mg

Administration: IV, IM, PO, PR

Comment: IM: Inject deeply into a large muscle mass. May cause tissue irritation.
Parenteral: Pentobarbital solutions are highly alkaline. Therefore, exercise extreme care to avoid perivascular extravasation or intra-arterial injection. (1)

<u>Pentobarbital Sodium</u> (Nembutal)

Indications and use: Sedative/hypnotic. Used for agitation, for preprocedure sedation, or as an anticonvulsant.

Actions: Short-acting barbiturate.

Route: PO, PR, IM, IV.

Dosage: Sedative:
2-6 mg/kg/day divided tid. Maximum:100 mg/day.

Hypnotic and anticonvulsant:
3-5 mg/kg/dose. Maximum: 100 mg/dose.

Adverse effects: Inject the IV dose slowly in fractional doses. Observe the IV site closely during administration, as this drug may cause extravasation injury. Tolerance and physical dependence may occur with continued use. May cause somnolence, apnea, bradycardia, rash, pain on IM injection, thrombophlebitis, osteomalacia from prolonged use (rare), and excitability. May increase reaction to painful stimuli. Rapid IV administration may cause hypotension and apnea.

(Gomella: Neonatology 1999, p.584)

Pentobarbital

Route & Dose: Maintain q 12 h for 4 wk for <1200 mg
PO, IM, IV: 2-6 mg/kg prn

Adverse Effects and Cautions:
Blood level monitoring helpful (sedative level 0.5-3 μg/ml). Higher doses may depress respirations. Monitor blood pressure

(Taeusch: Avery's Diseases of the Newborn 1998, p.1346)

PETROLATUM WHITE OINTMENT

Supplied: In 430 gm jars. Available as jelly or ointment in various sizes.

Petrolatum Ointment

Conclusions: We conclude that the use of topical petrolatum ointment (TPO) promoted an increase in the incidence of SC (Systemic Candidiasis) in ELBW infants. Additional investigation of potential infectious risks for ELBW infants receiving TPO skin care is warranted.

(Campbell: Systemic Candidiasis in Extremely Low Birth Weight Infants Receiving Topical Petrolatum Ointment for Skin Care: A Case-Control Study. Pediatrics 2000;105:1041-1045)

PHENOBARBITAL

Supplied: Elixir 20 mg/5 ml in 120 ml and 480 ml, 15mg/5ml
Injection 30 mg, 60 mg, 65 mg, 130 mg/ml in 1 ml

Administration: IV, IM, PO

Compatible with D5W, NS (5).

For DIRECT IV INJECTION, administer by slow IV push not greater than 1 mg/kg/minute (2,4).

The commercial injection is highly alkaline and may cause local tissue damage (1).

Phenobarbital

Indications and use:
Tonic-clonic and partial seizures, neonatal withdrawal syndrome, and neonatal jaundice.

Actions: Anticonvulsant that limits the spread of seizure activity and increases the threshold for electrical stimulation of the motor cortex. In neonates, the initial half-life is 100-120 h or longer, gradually declining to 60-70 h at about 3-4 weeks of age. Reduction in serum bilirubin levels is attributed to increased levels of glucuronyl transferase and intracellular Y-binding protein. More effective in reducing bilirubin levels in full-term infants than premature infants and must be administered at least 2 or 3 days before detectable reductions can be observed. Effective in controlling symptoms of neonatal withdrawal syndrome with the exception of vomiting and diarrhea.

Route: IV, IM, PO.

Dosage: Seizures:

Loading dose: 20-30 mg/kg IV or IM over 15-30 min. May give in 2 divided doses.

Maintenance dose: 2.5-4 mg/kg/day as single dose or divided q12h. For neonates <30 weeks start 1-3 mg/kg/day.

Hyperbilirubinemia: Dose not clearly established. Generally 4-5 mg/kg/day.

Neonatal withdrawal syndrome: 5-10 mg/kg/day in 4 divided doses. Monitor serum phenobarbital concentrations and withdrawal score.

Adverse effects: Sedation, lethargy, paradoxical excitement, GI distress, ataxia, and rash.

Comments: Contraindicated in porphyria. Monitor serum levels and adjust dosage to maintain between 15 and 40 mcg/mL for anticonvulsant activity.

(Gomella: Neonatology 1999, p.584)

Phenobarbital

Indication: For Neonatal Seizures

If hypoglycemia is not present, I administer phenobarbital intravenously in a loading dose of 20 mg/kg, delivered over approximately 10 to 15 minutes. Careful surveillance of respiratory effort is important under these circumstances. The work of Painter and co-workers has shown clearly that this dose is necessary to achieve a blood level of approximately 20 μg/ml. This level is necessary to achieve a clearly measurable anticonvulsant effect in the newborn. Weight or gestational age does not appear to influence the dose-blood level relationship appreciably, although infants less than 30 weeks' gestation may require slightly lower doses to achieve the same blood level. to achieve the same blood level, the intramuscular dose must be approximately 10% to 15% greater than the intravenous dose. I prefer the intravenous route because of the more rapid onset of action and the more reproducible effect on the blood level of phenobarbital.

If the initial 20 mg/kg dose of phenobarbital is not effective in controlling the seizures, I administer additional doses of

5 mg/kg until seizures have ceased or a total dose of 40 mg/kg has been reached. Utilizing phenobarbital in approximately this manner, Gilman and co-workers and Gal and co-workers attained control of seizures in approximately 70% of 71 infants. Approximately similar doses were utilized ina more recent study of 59 infants, and the drug controlled the seizures in 43%. These data indicate that phenobarbital is effective as a single drug in control of neonatal seizures in 43% to 70% of infants, if adequate amounts are administered. It is particularly noteworthy that definite worsening of respiratory function by such relatively high blood levels of phenobarbital has not been observed.

In my experience, however, total loading doses in excess of 40 mg/kg generally do not provide additional anticonvulsant benefit. Moreover, I have been impressed in severely asphyxiated infants, often with evidence for accompanying hepatic or renal dysfunction or both, that a total loading dose of phenobarbital of 40 mg/kg not infrequently results in blood levels of approximately 50 µg/ml or more. These levels appreciably sedate the infants for several days, thereby impairing neurological analysis, and may lead to toxic effects on the cardiovascular system. Thus as an alternative to the use of the additional phenobarbital, the clinician may wish to precede directly to phenytoin (see later discussion) after the initial 20 mg/kg dose of phenobarbital, in selected severely asphyxiated infants in whom clearance may be impaired.

Certain pharmacological properties of phenobarbital are beneficial in the treatment of neonatal seizures. Thus the drug enters CSF (and presumably brain) rapidly and with high efficiency (e.g., in one series, 30 minutes after an intravenous loading dose was administered, the CSF to blood ratio was 0.58 ± 0.07); the blood level is largely predictable from the dose administered; the agent can be administered intramuscularly as well as intravenously (preferably the latter) for acute therapy; and maintenance therapy is accomplished easily with oral therapy (see later discussion). Moreover, experimental data suggest that entrance of phenobarbital into brain is accelerated by the local acidosis associated with seizures. Protein binding is lower in the newborn (33%) than in the older child and adult (41%), and thus free levels of the drug are relatively higher. Because binding may be decreased further by hyperbilirubinemia and apparently other factors, still to be defined, routine monitoring of free phenobarbital levels ultimately will be optimal for management of the infant with seizures.

(Volpe: Neurology of the Newborn 2001, pp.203-204)

Phenobarbital

Acute Treatment of Neonatal Seizures

Dose: Loading dose: 20 mg/kg IV

Additional doses: 5 mg/kg IV (10 to 15 min) to maximum of 20 mg/kg

(Hill: Neonatal Seizures Pediatrics in Review 2000;21:117-121)

Phenobarbital

For Neonatal Seizures

The choice of antiepileptic drugs in neonates is based on tradition rather than proven efficacy. No studies demonstrate the superiority of phenobarbital, phenytoin, or the benzodiazepines, but, at present, phenobarbital is the initial drug chosen in almost all neonatal units [Boer and Gal, 1982]. Loading doses of at least 20 mg/kg of phenobarbital should be given intravenously to achieve efficacious but nontoxic levels [Jalling, 1975; Lockman et al., 1979; Painter et al,. 1978; 1981; 1983]. Seizure control is attained in 85% of newborns when loading doses of up to 40 mg/kg are used [Gal et al., 1982]. The study of Gal et al. [1982], however, reported seizure control in a much higher proportion of neonates with plasma levels of approximately 20 μg/ml of phenobarbital. Comparison of series is hampered by inadequate control for population differences, unspecified diagnostic criteria, and particularly the lack of EEG confirmation and monitoring.

Although data regarding the effects of plasma levels of phenobarbital above 40 μg/ml on the newborn are limited, significant cardiovascular compromise and impaired cerebral blood flow are a concern. Because the therapeutic and toxic component of phenobarbital is the unbound or free plasma concentration, it would appear appropriate to concentrate on this level rather than total phenobarbital concentrations. Limited data are available on the neonate; however, in one study, marked variability of protein binding of phenobarbital was noted. A formula based on in vitro binding profiles of phenobarbital can be used to accurately calculate a loading dose and achieve predetermined plasma concentrations.

Because the half-life of phenobarbital is relatively long in newborns, maintenance doses of 2 to 4 mg/kg/day are sufficient. After 2 weeks, metabolism and/or clearance of phenobarbital increases, and maintenance doses must be increased to approximately 5 mg/kg/day. Seizure control is unusual below a level of 16 μg/ml [Lockman et al., 1979].

Swainman: Pediatric Neurology 1999; p.188)

Phenobarbital

Indication: Drug therapy for withdrawal syndrome in infants

Phenobarbital is effective in treating the central nervous system phenomena. A loading dose of 20 mg/kg is administered and followed by a dose of approximately 5 mg/kg/day, although the clinical response should determine the maintenance dose. Most patients exhibit marked improvement within 24 hours, and the duration of therapy is usually somewhat shorter than for paregoric. More important, however, vomiting and diarrhea are *not* benefited by this drug, and poor sucking and feeding may, in fact, be made worse. Thus, if gastrointestinal phenomena are prominent, phenobarbital is not the appropriate drug.

(Volpe: Neurology of the Newborn 2001, p.882)

Phenobarbital

Usual Dosage: Anticonvulsant: Status epilepticus: **Loading dose**: I.V.:
Neonates: 15-20 mg/kg in a single or divided dose
Infants, Children: 15-18 mg/kg in a single or divided dose; usual maximum loading dose 20 mg/kg
Note: In select patients, may give additional 5 mg/kg/dose every 15-30 minutes until seizure is controlled or a total dose of 30 mg/kg is reached; be prepared to support respirations.

Anticonvulsant **maintenance dose**: Oral, I.V. (**Note**: Maintenance dose usually starts 12 hours after loading dose):
Neonates: 3-4 mg/kg/day given once daily; assess serum concentrations; increase to 5 mg/kg/day if needed (usually be second week of therapy)
Infants: 5-6 mg/kg/day in 1-2 divided doses

Administration: Oral: Administer elixir with water, milk, or juice
Parenteral: do not inject I.V. faster than 1 mg/kg/minute with a maximum of 30 mg/minute for infants and children and 60 mg/minute for adults >60kg; do not administer intra-arterially; avoid extravasation; use only powder for injection for S.C. use, not solutions for injection

Reference Range:
Therapeutic: 15-40 µg/mL (SI: 65-172 µmol/L)
Potentially toxic: >40 µg/mL (SI: 172 µmol/L)
Coma: >50 µg/mL (SI: >215 µmol/L)
Potentially lethal: >80 µg/mL (SI: >344 µmol/L)

Patient Information:
Avoid alcohol; limit caffeine; may be habit-forming; may cause dizziness or drowsiness and impair ability to perform activities requiring mental alertness or physical coordination; do not abruptly discontinue

Nursing Implications: Parenteral solutions are very alkaline

Additional Information: Injectable solutions contain propylene glycol

(Taketomo: Pediatric Dosage Handbook 1999-2000, pp.711-713)

Phenobarbital

Infants in the treatment group received 40 mg/kg phenobarbital administered over one hour as soon as possible following admission to the NICU. (Control infants received phenobarbital (initial dose 20 mg/kg intravenously) only if clinical seizures appeared....Phenobarbital administered in a dose of 40 mg/kg intravenously over one hour in term, severely asphyxiated newborn infants appeared to be safe and was associated with a 27% reduction in the incidence of seizures and a significant improvement in neurologic outcome at 3 years of age. Results of the present study are encouraging but should not be construed as definitive evidence of efficacy.

(Hall: High Dose Phenobarbital Therapy In Term Newborn Infants With Severe Perinatal Asphyxia: A Randomized, Prospective Study With Three Year Follow-Up. Pediatrics 1996;98(3):582)

SEE ALSO: THERAPY FOR NEONATAL SEIZURES p.657

PHENOXYBENZAMINE HCL (Dibenzyline)

Supplied: Capsule 10 mg (contains benzyl alcohol)
Administration: PO.
Approved indication:

For the control of hypertension and sweating in adult with pheochromocytoma.

Has shown in vitro mutagenic activity in the Ames test and in the mouse lymphoma assay (1).

Phenoxybenzamine

Dosage: 0.1-5 μg/kg/min.
Comments: Vasodilator for long-term IV therapy; long half-life

(Fanaroff: Neonatal-Perinatal Medicine 1997, p.1743)

PHENTOLAMINE (Regitine)

Supplied: Injection, powder for 5 mg/vial
Administration: IV, and for tissue infiltration

For prevention and treatment of dermal necrosis and sloughing following IV administration or extravasation of norepinephrine or dopamine (1).

For treatment, inject 5 mg to 10 mg in 10 ml 0.9% NaCl into the area of extravasation within 12 hours. FOR CHILDREN, use 0.1 to 0.2 mg/kg up to a maximum of 10 mg (1).

Phentolamine (Regitine)

Dose: SC:

Treatment of extravasation of α-adrenergic drugs: 0.1-0.2 mg/kg/dose SC.

Physician's Order: "Regitine ___ mg SC to IV extravasation site, per unit protocol."

IV:

Afterload Reduction in congestive Heart Failure/Pulmonary Hypertension: 2.5-15 mcg/kg/minute by IV continuous infusion.

Pheochromocytoma:

- Diagnosis: 0.05-0.1 mg/kg/dose IV, IM (See warning under Cautions/Contraindications.)
- Hypertension (prior to surgery for pheochromocytoma): 0.05-0.1 mg/kg/dose given 1-2 hours prior to pheochromocytomectomy; repeat as needed to control blood pressure. Titrate the dose to control or prevent hypertension. Maximum: 5 mg/dose.

Administration: SC—Treatment of Extravasation of α-adrenergic Drugs Concentration: 0.5 mg/ml.

Preparation of Dilution: Dilute 0.1 ml of commercially available phentolamine 5 mg/ml with 0.9 ml normal saline (=0.5 mg/ml, 1 ml).

Administration Procedure:

- Stop the intravenous infusion and remove the needle.
- Cleanse the site and surrounding area with a povidone-iodine solution.
- Inject phentolamine (0.5 mg/ml) locally into area of extravasation in divided increments of approximately 0.2 ml using a 25-gauge needle. Change needle between each dose increment.

IV—Rate: Infuse over at least 1 minute. May also be given by continuous infusion.

IV—Concentration: 5 mg/ml. May give undiluted or dilute with normal saline.

Cautions/Contraindications:
Warning Regarding the Phentolamine Test: Although phentolamine is indicated as an aid in the diagnosis of pheochromocytoma, determinations of blood and urine catecholamine concentrations are considered safer and more reliable.

- Deaths have occurred after IV administration of phentolamine for the diagnosis of pheochromocytoma. The phentolamine test may be considered when additional confirmatory evidence of pheochromocytoma is required and the potential benefits of the test outweigh the possible risks.
- The test is more reliable in detecting pheochromocytomas in patients with sustained hypertension than in those with paroxysmal hypertension. It is of no value if the patient is not hypertensive at the time of the test.
- False-negative response may occur with a pheochromocytoma which is not secreting enough epinephrine or norepinephrine to elevate the blood pressure or to sustain an elevation.
- False-positive responses to the test have occurred in patients with essential hypertension, in patients

receiving sedatives, opiates, or antihypertensives, and in patients with uremia.

Use: Used to treat extravasation of α-adrenergic drugs (norepinephrine, phenylephrine, dopamine, epinephrine). These drugs can sometimes cause severe tissue blanching, gangrene, and sloughing on infiltration.

Small areas of blanching, such as those following the vein and blanching limited locally at the insertion site into which dopamine is infusing, are not harmful and will usually reverse without treatment. It may be necessary to alternate the lines into which dopamine is infusing. If blanching extends more than approximately ¼ inch (=1/2 inch diameter) past the insertion site and is spreading, it should alert the nurse to a potential extravasation. Assess the entire clinical picture: Is the area large, cold, hard, edematous, or severely blanched?

May be used up to 12 hours after the extravasation occurred.

A short-acting drug, it is particularly effective for IV use when rapid and precise control of blood pressure is necessary. Phentolamine has little effect on the blood pressure of healthy individuals or patients with essential hypertension.

Pheochromocytoma. Controls or prevents paroxysmal hypertension immediately prior to or during pheochromocytomectomy. Although indicated as an aid in the diagnosis of pheochromocytoma, determinations of blood and urine catecholamine concentrations are considered safer and more reliable.

Peripheral Vasospastic Disorders: Used as an adjunctive therapy in the treatment of peripheral vasospastic disorders, although efficacy has not been established.

Congestive Heart Failure. Used for afterload reduction in congestive heart failure.

Adverse Effects: Marked hypotension, cardiac arrhythmias, tachycardia, and nasal congestion.

Although local SC injection is usually well tolerated, the infant should be monitored for hypertension. Blood pressure decrease may result from administration of phentolamine in addition to the temporary discontinuation of the drug that infiltrated *e.g., dopamine).

Treatment of Hypotension: Use supportive measures such as IV fluids. If drug treatment is needed, use norepinephrine. **Do not treat hypotension with epinephrine** because that drug may exacerbate the hypotension. (Epinephrine stimulates both α and β receptors. Because phentolamine is blocking the α receptors, the resultant effect is a β-effect of vasodilation and further decrease in blood pressure.)

Nursing Implications:

Subcutaneous Treatment of Extravasation of α-adrenergic Drugs:

- Document site condition and treatment in the medical record.
- Observe site carefully. Area should become hyperemic, then return to normal skin color.
- Monitor for hypotension.

IV:

- Monitor blood pressure, vital signs.

(Zenk: Neonatal Medications & Nutrition. A Comprehensive Guide 2000; pp:393-395)

Phentolamine (Regitine)

Indications and use: Treatment of extravasation from IV dopamine or norepinephrine bitartrate (levarterenol bitartrate [Levophed]). Helps prevent dermal necrosis and sloughing.

Actions: Phentolamine is an α-adrenergic blocking drug that works to reverse the severe vasoconstriction from extravasation of vasopressors such as dopamine.

Route: SC.

Dosage: 0.1-0.2 mg/kg diluted to 1 mL of saline injected into the area of extravasation within 12 h.

Adverse effects: Hypotension, tachycardia, cardiac arrhythmias, flushing, and GI upset.

(Gomella: Neonatology 1999, pp.584-585)

Phentolamine

THERAPY FOR ACUTE CONGESTIVE CARDIAC FAILURE

Phentolamine may be given orally or parenterally. Experience in children is limited to intravenous administration. The drug has been started at 2.5 μg/kg/minute and increased to 15 μg/kg/minute. Adverse effects include tachycardia, arrhythmia, and increased gastric acid secretion.

(Garson: The science and practice of pediatric cardiology 1998, pp.2329-2341)

Phentolamine (Regitine)

Dose: 2.5-15 μg/kg/min IV

Mode of Action: Competitive α_1 and α_2 receptor blockade

Adverse Effects: Hypotension, tachycardia, arrhythmia, abdominal pain

Comments; Postop low cardiac output

(Garson: The science and practice of pediatric cardiology 1998, p.2951)

Phentolamine

Use: Diagnosis of pheochromocytoma; treatment of hypertension associated with pheochromocytoma or other causes of excess sympathomimetic amines; local treatment of dermal necrosis after extravasation of drugs with alpha-adrenergic effects (dobutamine, dopamine, epinephrine, metaraminol, norepinephrine, phenylephrine)

Usual Dosage: Treatment of alpha-adrenergic drug extravasation: S.C.: Neonates: infiltrate area with a small amount (eg 1 mL) of solution (made by diluting 2.5-5 mg in 10 mL of preservative free NS) within 12 hours of extravasation; do not exceed 0.1 mg/kg or 2.5 mg total

Nursing Implications:
When drugs with alpha-adrenergic effects extravasate, they cause local vasoconstriction which causes blanching of the skin and a pale, cold, hard appearance; S.C. phentolamine blocks the alpha-adrenergic receptors and reverses the vasoconstriction; the extravasation area should "pink up" and return to normal skin color; monitor the site of extravasation closely, as repeat doses of S.C. phentolamine may be needed.

(Taketomo: Pediatric Dosage Handbook 1999-2000, pp.714-715)

Phentolamine Mesylate

Dose & Route: Treatment of alpha adrenergic drug extravasation (most effective within 12 hr of extravasation)
Neonates: Make a solution of 0.25-0.5 mg/ml with normal saline. Inject 1 ml (in 5 divided doses of 0.2 ml) SC around site of extravasation: **max total dose**: 0.1 mg/kg or 2.5 mg total.
Infants, Children: Make a solution of 0.5-1 mg/ml with normal saline. Inject 1-5 ml (in 5 divided doses) SC around site of extravasation; **max total dose**: 0.1-0.2 mg/kg or 5 mg total.

Diagnosis of pheochromocytoma, IM/IV:
Children: 0.05-0.1 mg/kg/dose up to a **max** of 5 mg

Hypertension, prior to surgery for pheochromocytoma, IM/IV:
Children: 0.05-0.1 mg/kg/dose up to a **max** of 5 mg 1-2 hrs prior to surgery, repeat Q2-4 hr PRN

Remarks: For diagnosis of pheochromocytoma, patient should be resting in a supine position. A blood pressure reduction of more than 35 mm Hg systolic and 24 mm Hg diastolic is considered a positive test for pheochromocytoma. For treatment of extravasation, use 27- to 30-gauge needle with multiple small injections and monitor site closely as repeat doses may be necessary.

(Siberry: The Harriet Lane Handbook 2000, pp.811-812)

PHENYLACETATE

Orphan Drug Status

Sodium Phenylacetate

Definitions: CPS = Carbamyl phosphate synthetase I

OTC = Ornithine transcarbamylase
UCD = Urea Cycle Disorder

Recommendation:
The labeling for intravenous sodium benzoate and sodium phenylacetate should be modified to include a new indication for the treatment of patients with argininosuccinic aciduria.

Rationale: Clinical experience indicates that these drugs are helpful in reducing ammonia in this condition, acting by a mechanism different from that of arginine.

Recommendation:
Intravenous arginine-HCL and sodium benzoate/sodium phenylacetate should be available in hospitals where patients with UCD are treated.

Rationale: These medications are not routinely available and may be required on an emergency basis to treat patients with acute hyperammonemia.

Recommendation:
Where available, plasma levels of ammonia scavenging drugs should be monitored to avoid toxicity.

Rationale: Variable drug excretion may cause toxicity. In the absence of drug levels, a serum anion gap of >15 mEq/L and an anion gap that has risen >6 mEq/L could indicate drug accumulation and increased risk for toxicity.

(The Urea Cycle Disorders Conference Group: Consensus statement from a conference for the Management of Patients with Urea cycle Disorders. J Pediatr 2001;138:S1-S5)

PHENYLEPHRINE HCL (NeoSynephrine)

Supplied: Injection 1% (10mg/ml) in 1ml, 5ml
Ophthalmic 0.12%, 2.5%, 10%

Administration: IV, Ophthalmic
For CONTINUOUS INFUSION, dilute to 0.02 to 0.1mg/ml in D5W (preferred) or NS, and infuse at a rate of 0.01 to 0.5mcg/kg/minute (2).

Extravasation may cause necrosis and sloughing of surrounding tissue. For extravasation, treat with phentolamine.

<u>Phenylephrine</u>
Intravenous antiarrhythmic agent:

Dosage: 0.02 mg/kg IV slowly

Comments: Used for raising blood pressure and eliciting a baroreceptor vagal reflex.

(Fanaroff: Neonatal-Perinatal Medicine 1997, p.1176)

<u>Phenylephrine</u>

Dosage: 0.04-50.0 μg/kg/min IV

Comments: This is a specific α-adrenergic agonist, a pressor agent; dosage should be adjusted with continuous blood pressure monitoring to target effect.

(Fanaroff: Neonatal-Perinatal Medicine 1997, p.1743)

Phenylephrine

Uses: PSVT

Dosing: 0.01 mg/kg; double q 5 min until Systolic blood pressure (SBP) twice baseline or paroxysmal supraventricular tachycardia (PSVT) termination

Acute Side Effects:
Sinus bradycardia; atrioventricular (AV) block; hypertension

Other Considerations:
Atropine for excessive vagal response; less effective in infants

---

PSVT, paroxysmal supraventricular tachycardia.

(Gillette: Clinical Pediatric Arrhythmias 1999, p.153)

Phenylephrine HCL (Neo-Synephrine)

Dose & Route: Hypotension:
Children:
IM/SC: 0.1 mg/kg/dose Q1-2 hr PRN: **max dose**: 5 mg
IV bolus: 5-20 mcg/kg/dose Q10-15 min PRN
IV drip: 0.1-0.5 mcg/kg/min, titrate to effect

Pupillary Dilation: 2.5% sol; 1 drop in each eye 15 min before exam.

Remarks: Use **cautiously** in presence of arrhythmias, hyperthyroidism, or hyperglycemia. May cause tremor, insomnia, palpitations. Metabolized by MAO. **Contraindicated** in pheochromocytoma and severe hypertension. Nasal decongestants may cause rebound congestion with excessive use (>3 days). Injectable product may contain sulfites. Note: Phenylephrine is found in a variety of combination cough and cold products.

(Siberry: The Harriet Lane Handbook 2000, pp.813-814)

PHENYTOIN (Dilantin)

Supplied: Oral suspension 125 mg/5ml in 240 ml
Injection 50mg/ml in 2ml

Administration: IV, PO
Administer IV PUSH not greater than 50mg/min in adults or 1-3mg/kg/minute in neonates (1). Monitor ECG and blood pressure continuously (1).

Although intramuscular injection can be used, erratic or delayed absorption may occur. Subcutaneous injection should be avoided because of the possibility of local tissue damage (3).

The drug has generally not been recommended for use in IV infusions because of the possibility that precipitation may occur. However, some clinicians suggest that IV infusions are feasible PROVIDED that appropriate precautions are taken, such as using a suitable infusion solution (e.g., 0.9% NaCl), using a sufficiently diluted solution (e.g., less than 6.7mg/ml), starting the infusion immediately after preparation and completing administration within a relatively short period, using a 0.22 MICRON IN-LINE FILTER, and carefully observing the admixture (3).

Phenytoin (Dilantin)

Indications and use: Seizures unresponsive to phenobarbital.

Actions: Raises seizure threshold of the motor cortex to electrical or chemical stimuli. Precise mechanism of anticonvulsant activity has not been determined. Bilirubin displaces phenytoin from albumin binding sites, increasing the percentage of unbound drug; this may complicate the interpretation of serum levels. Follows zero-order pharmacokinetics, where small dosage adjustments may result in large changes in serum drug concentrations. Neonates and other infants absorb phenytoin poorly from the GI tract. Use in the long-term management of seizures in neonates in questionable owing to the difficulty in appropriate dosing.

Route: PO, IV.

Dosage: IV: 15-20 mg/kg as loading dose at a rate not greater than 0.5 mg/kg/min, followed by maintenance dose of 5-8 mg/kg/day divided q12-24h

PO: Highly variable, from 5-8 mg/kg/day up to 8 mg/kg/dose q12h.

Adverse effects: Few reports of toxicity in neonates, probably because of the difficulty of physically assessing the common toxic manifestations. In adults and children, adverse effects include nystagmus, ataxia, lethargy, slurred speech, diplopia, headache, hirsutism, behavioral changes, and gum hyperplasia. Hypotension occurs with rapid IV administration.

Comment: Therapeutic levels between 10 and 20 mcg/mL (may be lower in preterm infants.) Multiple drug interactions.

(Gomella: Neonatology 1999, p.585)

Phenytoin

Acute Treatment of Neonatal Seizures

Dose: 20 mg/kg (1 mg/kg minute)

(Hill: Neonatal Seizures Pediatrics in Review 2000;21:117-121)

Phenytoin

For Neonatal Seizures

Phenytoin is the second agent selected when phenobarbital fails. As with phenobarbital, loading doses of 20 mg/kg must be used to obtain plasma levels in the 15 to

20 μg/ml range. Intravenous maintenance dosages are within the range of 4 to 6 mg/kg/day. Careful monitoring is necessary when plasma levels of 20 mg/ml are achieved because drug accumulation may begin at these levels. As with phenobarbital, the active component of phenytoin is the unbound concentration. Unlike phenobarbital, this component is very highly protein-bound anticonvulsant. Small change in binding capacity would be expected to cause dramatic changes in plasma free concentrations and result in clinical effects. However, like phenobarbital, in vitro binding can be used to carefully and accurately achieve predetermined free plasma concentrations.

The brain/plasma ratios reflecting distribution of phenobarbital and phenytoin to brain are approximately 1.0 and 1.2 respectively, values comparable with those reported in adults [Sherwin et al., 1973; Vajda et al., 1974].

(Swainman: Pediatric Neurology 1999; p.188)

Phenytoin

Class: IB

Uses: Chronic ventricular arrhythmias, digitalis intoxication

Dose (Level): PO: 4 mg/kg/dose q6hr x 1 day, then 5-6 mg/kg/day divided q12hr
IV: bolus 15 mg/kg over 1 hr (q5min pushes) (15-20 μg/mL)

Mode of Action: Similar to lidocaine; weak Ca^{++} channel blockade, suppresses digitalis-induced delayed afterdepolarizations, central sympathetic inhibition

ECG/EP Changes: Slight ↓ QTc, decreases VERP, ↓ AH only in digitalis intoxication

Side Effects: Hypotension (V), rash, gingival hyperplasia, ataxia; warfarin-↑ PT; verapamil-↑ verapamil effect (displaced from protein)

(Garson: The science and practice of pediatric cardiology 1998, p.2952)

Phenytoin

Dosing: PO: 15 mg/kg load, chronic 5-6 mg/kg/day
Warnings: CNS gingival hyperplasia

Dosing: IV: 1-3 mg/kg load
Warnings: Hypotension

Oral Administration:

Peak serum concentrations are very variable, occurring 3 to 12 hours after dose administration. Dairy products may decrease absorption, whereas high protein or fatty diets can enhance absorption.

Phenytoin has a unique metabolic feature among the antiarrhythmic agents: it saturates its metabolism at high doses, usually when doses are greater than 10 mg/kg/day.

This is an important point, because levels can rise precipitously with small dose increases at the saturation point.

Despite more extensive metabolism in young patients, infants have a prolonged elimination $t_{1/2}$ of phenytoin, up to 24 hours. In patients older than 1 year this drops to 8 hours an then rises again in the adult toward 24 hours. The usual therapeutic serum level range is 10 to 20 mg/ml.

Intravenous Administration:

Intravenous loading with phenytoin must be done carefully to avoid hypotension. The loading dose is on the order of 1 to 3 mg/kg given over 15 to 30 minutes, with a maximum daily load of 10 to 15 mg/kg.

Oral Dosing and Interactions:

Oral loading with phenytoin avoids the risk of hypotension. The total loading dose (TLD) is 15 mg/kg, divided every 6 hours. Maintenance doses vary with age; those beyond the newborn period up to 5 to 6 years receive the drug every 12 hours, with a total daily dosage of 5 to 6 mg/kg.

One of the more important drug interactions with phenytoin involves warfarin, with an increase in the prothrombin time and INR.

Side Effects: The most frequent side effect of phenytoin is hypotension associated with intravenous administration.

Skin rashes are also common and may progress to Stevens-Johnson syndrome.

(Gillette: Clinical Pediatric Arrhythmias 1999,pp.231-248)

Phenytoin

Uses: VT from digoxin intoxication; occasionally other VTs

Dosing: 15 mg/kg over 60 min (q 5 min pushes)

Acute Side Effects: Hypotension

Other Considerations: Increases verapamil effect

VT, ventricular tachycardia.

(Gillette: Clinical Pediatric Arrhythmias 1999, p.152)

Phenytoin

Dose & Route: Status epilepticus:

- Loading dose (all ages): 15-20 mg/kg IV
  Max dose: 1500 mg/24 hr

Maintenance for seizure disorders:

- Neonates: start with 5 mg/kg/24 hr PO/IV ÷ Q12 hr; usual range 5-8 mg/kg/24 hr PO/IV ÷ Q8-12 hr
- Infants/Children: start with 5 mg/kg/24 hr ÷ BID-TID PO/IV; usual dose range (doses divided BID-TID):
- 6 mo-3 yr: 8-10 mg/kg/24 hr

Anti-arrhythmic (secondary to digitalis intoxication):

- Load (all ages): 1.25 mg/kg IV Q5 min up to a total of 15 mg/kg

- Maintenance:
  Children: IV/PO: 5-10 mg/kg/24 hr ÷ Q12 hr

Remarks: Contraindicated inpatients with heart block or sinus bradycardia, IM administration is not recommended because of erratic absorption and pain at injection site. Side effects: gingival hyperplasia, hirsutism, dermatitis, blood dyscrasia, ataxia, SLE-like and Stevens-Johnson syndromes, lymphadenopathy, liver damage, and nystagmus. Many drug interactions: levels may be increased by cimetidine, chloramphenicol, INH, sulfonamides, trimethoprim, etc. Levels may be decreased by some antineoplastic agents. Phenytoin induces hepatic microsomal enzymes (CYP 450 3A4) leading to decreased effectiveness of oral contraceptives, quinidine, valproic acid, and theophylline.

Oral absorption reduced in neonate. $T_{1/2}$ is variable (7-42 hr) and dose-dependent. Drug is highly protein-bound; free fraction of drug will be increased n patients with hypoalbuminemia. IV push/infusion rate: not to exceed 0.5 mg/kg/min in neonates, or 1 mg/kg/min infants, children and adults with max: 50 mg/min; may cause cardiovascular collapse.

For seizure disorders, therapeutic levels: 10-20 mg/L (free and bound phenytoin) OR, 1-2 mg/L (free only). Recommended serum sampling times: trough level (PO/IV) within 30 minutes prior to the next scheduled dose; peak or post load level (IV) 1 hour after the end of IV infusion. Steady state is usually achieved after 5-10 days of continuous dosing. For routine monitoring, measure trough.

(Siberry: The Harriet Lane Handbook 2000, pp.813-814)

<u>Phenytoin</u>

Usual Dosage: Status epilepticus: I.V.:
Loading dose:
Neonates: 15-20 mg/kg in a single or divided dose;
Infants, Children: 15-18 mg/kg in a single or divided dose
Maintenance dose: anticonvulsant (**Note**: Maintenance dose usually starts 12 hours after the loading dose):
Neonates: Initial: 5 mg/kg/day in 2 divided doses; usual: 5-8 mg/kg/day in 2 divided doses; some patients may require dosing every 8 hours
Infants and Children: Initial: 5 mg/kg/day in 2-3 divided doses: 0.5-3 years: 8-10mg/kg/day

Administration: Oral: May administer with food or milk to decrease GI upset; but to ensure consistent absorption, phenytoin should be administered at the same time with regards to meals

Parenteral: I.V.: Neonates: Do not exceed I.V. infusion rate of 0.5 mg/kg minute; Infants, Children, Adults: do not exceed I.V. infusion rate of 1-3 mg/kg/minute, maximum rate: 50 mg/minute; I.V. injections should be followed by NS flushes through the same needle or I.V. catheter to avoid local irritation of the vein; I.V. intermittent infusion: Dilute with NS to a concentration <6 mg/mL, use an in-line 0.22 micron filter; avoid extravasation; avoid I.M. use due to erratic absorption, pain on injection, and precipitation of drug at injection site

Monitoring Parameters:
Serum concentrations, CBC with differential, liver enzymes; blood pressure with I.V use; free and total serum concentrations in patients with hyperbilirubinemia, hypoalbuminemia, renal dysfunction, or uremia

Reference Range: Neonates: Therapeutic 8-15 µg/mL

Nursing Implications: Separate administration of antacids or tube feedings and oral phenytoin by 2 hours

Additional Information:
The 30 mg/5 mL oral suspension is no longer made; injection contains propylene glycol and benzyl alcohol; possible permanent cerebellum damage may occur with chronic toxic serum concentrations

(Taketomo: Pediatric Dosage Handbook 1999-2000, pp.719-921)

PHOSPHOROUS REPLACEMENT PRODUCTS

Phosphorus Replacement Preparations

Product	Potassium (mEq)	Sodium (mEq)	Phosphorus (mmol)	Phosphorus (mg)
Neutra-Phos powder**	7	7	8	250
K Phos Neutral Tablets	1.1	13	8	250
Neutra-Phos K powder**	14.25	0	8	250
Fleets Phosphosoda per mL	0	4.8	4.1	128
K Phosphate IV (per mL)	4.4	0	3	94
Na Phosphate IV (per mL)	0	4	3	94
Whole milk (cup)	9	5.3	7.3	228
Skim milk (cup)	9.1	5.5	7.5	234

* Phosphorus content after mixing 1 capsule in 75 mL water
** Phosphorus content (per 75 mL) after mixing with 1 gallon of water

Phosphate, sodium, or potassium

Route & Dose: PO: 1-3 mmol/kg/day in divided doses or supplement formula phosphorus intake to 75 mg/kg/day; diluted solution contains 3.3 mg phosphorus/ml; 1 packet of potassium PO_4 contains 250 mg (8 mmol) of phosphorus

Adverse Effects and Cautions:
Large amounts may cause catharsis; increase gradually to full supplementation

(Taeusch: Avery's Diseases of the Newborn 1998, p.1347)

Phosphorus Supplements

Dose & Route: Acute hypophosphatemia: 5-10 mg/kg/dose IV over 6 hr
Maintenance/Replacement:
Children:
IV: 15-45 mg/kg over 24 hr
PO: 30-90 mg/kg/24 hr ÷ TID-QID
Recommended infusion rate: ≤3.1 mg/kg/hr (0.1 mM/kg/hr) of phosphate. When potassium salt is used, the rate will be limited by the maximum potassium infusion fate. Do not co-infuse with calcium containing products.

Remarks: May cause tetany, hyperphosphatemia, hyperkalemia, hypocalcemia. Use with caution in patients with renal impairment. Be aware of sodium and/or potassium load when supplementing phosphate. IV administration may cause hypotension, renal failure; or arrhythmias, heart block, cardiac arrest with potassium salt. PO dosing may cause nausea, vomiting, abdominal pain, or diarrhea.

(Siberry: The Harriet Lane Handbook 2000, p.815)

Phosphorus

Indications and use:
Treatment of hypophosphatemia, provision of maintenance phosphorus in parenteral nutrition solutions, and treatment of nutritional rickets of prematurity.

Actions: Phosphorus is an intracellular ion required for formation of energy-transfer enzymes such as ADP and ATP. Phosphorus is also needed for bone metabolism and mineralization.

Route: IV, PO.

Dosage: Severe hypophosphatemia:
0.15-0.3 mmol/kg/dose (= 5-9 mg of elemental phosphorus per kilogram per dose). Infuse slowly over several hours or dilute in daily 24-h maintenance IV solution (preferred).

Maintenance: 0.5 -2 mmol/kg/day (= 16-63 mg of elemental phosphorus per kilogram per day). For oral use, may use parental form and give PO in divided doses, diluted in infant's feedings.

Adverse effects: Hyperphosphatemia, hypocalcemia, and hypotension. GI discomfort may occur with oral administration. Rapid IV bolus of potassium phosphates can cause cardiac arrhythmias.

(Gomella: Neonatology 1999, p.585)

PIPERACILLIN (Pipracil)

Supplied: Injection, powder for 2gm, 3gm, 4gm vial (contains 1.85 mEq Na/gm).

Administration: IV, IM.

IM administration: Reconstitute each gram of piperacillin with 2ml of diluent for a concentration of 400 mg/ml. Administer this concentration IM. Stable 24 hours at room temperature, 7 days refrigerated.

IV administration:

For INTERMITTENT IV INFUSION: Withdraw the appropriate dose from the above dilution (400 mg/ml), and further dilute in NS, D5W to a concentration of 40 mg/ml and administer over 30 minutes.

For DIRECT INTERMITTENT IV INJECTION: Withdraw the appropriate dose from the above dilution (400 mg/ml), and further dilute to a concentration of 100 mg/ml and administer directly into a vein over a period of 3-5 minutes (1,3).

Piperacillin (Pipracil)

Antibacterial Drugs for Pediatric Patients Beyond the Newborn Period

Dosage per kg/d

Route: IV, IM

Mild to Moderate Infections: 100-150 mg in 4 doses

Severe Infections: 200-300 mg in 4-6 doses

Notes: In patients with history of allergy to penicillin or one of its many congeners, alternative drugs are recommended. In some circumstances, a cephalosporin or other β-lactam class drug may be acceptable. However, these drugs should not be used in patients with an immediate hypersensitivity (anaphylaxis) to penicillin because approximately 5% to 15% of penicillin-allergic patients will also be allergic to the cephalosporins.

Patients with a history of allergy to penicillin G or V should be considered for subsequent skin testing. Many such patients can be treated safely with penicillin, since only 10% of children with such history are proven allergic when skin-tested.

(American Academy of Pediatrics: Report of the Committee on Infectious Diseases. Red Book 2000, pp.658,662)

Piperacillin

Route: IV, IM

Dosage (mg/kg) and Interval of Administration:

Weight 1200-2000 g

Age 0-7 days: 50-75 q12h

Age >7 days: 50-75 q8h

Weight >2000 g
Age 0-7 days: 50-75 q8h
Age >7 days: 50-75 q6h

(Remington: Infectious Diseases of the Fetus and Newborn Infant 2001, p.1454)

Piperacillin

Route: IV

Dosage: 200-300 mg/kg/day q4-6h (not approved for children).

(Nelson: Pocket Book of Pediatric Antimicrobial Therapy 2000-2001, p.82)

Piperacillin Sodium (Pipracil)

Classification: Semisynthetic extended-spectrum penicillin.

Action and spectrum: See Mezlocillin Sodium. Good in vivo activity against *Pseudomonas aeruginosa*.

Route: IM, IV (infuse over 30 min).

Dosage:
< 2000 g and 0-7 days old: 150 mg/kg/day divided q12h
< 2000 g and > 7 days old: 225 mg/kg/day divided q8h
> 2000 g and 0-7 days old: 225 mg/kg/day divided q8h
> 2000 g and > 7 days old: 300 mg/kg/day divided q6h

Elimination and metabolism: Excreted unchanged in the urine.

Adverse effects: See Mezlocillin. Hypokalemia and leukopenia are less pronounced.

Comments : Avoid IM use where possible. Should be reserved for cases resistant to ticarcillin disodium. Contains 1.85 meq (42.5 mg) sodium per gram.

(Gomella: Neonatology 1999, pp.585-586)

PIPERACILLIN/TAZOBACTAM (Zosyn)

Supplied: 2g piperacillin/0.25g tazobactam in vials
Contains 2.35 mEg sodium per gm of piperacillin (5).

Administration: IV infusion over 30 minutes (1).

Reconstitute conventional vials with 5ml of compatible diluent per gram of piperacillin. Discard any unused portion after 24 hours if stored at room temperature or after 48 hours if stored at refrigerated temperature (1).

Piperacillin / tazobactam

Antibacterial Drugs for Pediatric Patients Beyond the Newborn Period
Dosage per kg/d
Route: IV
Mild to Moderate Infections: Inappropriate
Severe Infections: 240 mg of piperacillin in 3 doses

Comments: Not approved for children

Note: In patients with history of allergy to penicillin or one of its many congeners, alternative drugs are recommended. In some circumstances, a cephalosporin or other β-lactam class drug may be acceptable. However, these drugs should not be used in patients with an immediate hypersensitivity (anaphylaxis) to penicillin because approximately 5% to 15% of penicillin-allergic patients will also be allergic to the cephalosporins.

Patients with a history of allergy to penicillin G or V should be considered for subsequent skin testing. Many such patients can be treated safely with penicillin, since only 10% of children with such history are proven allergic when skin-tested.

(American Academy of Pediatrics: Report of the Committee on Infectious Diseases. Red Book 2000, pp.658,662)

Piperacillin/Tazobactam

Route: IV
Dosage: 240mg PIP/kg/day (not approved for children)
Interval: q4-6h

(Nelson: Pocket Book of Pediatric Antimicrobial Therapy 2000-2001, p.82)

Piperacillin/Tazobactam

Dose & Route: All doses based on piperacillin component
Infant <6 mo: 150-300 mg/kg/24 hr IV ÷ Q6-8 hr
Infants >6 mo and Children:
300-400 mg/kg/24 hr IV ÷ Q6-8 hr
Cystic Fibrosis: see piperacillin

Remarks: Tazobactam is a beta-lactamase inhibitor, thus extending the spectrum of piperacillin. Like other penicillins, CSF penetration occurs only with inflamed meninges. **Adjust dose in renal impairment**. See Piperacillin and Penicillin for other comments.

(Siberry: The Harriet Lane Handbook 2000, p.817)

PLECONARIL

Not available in the United States.

Pleconaril

Indication: Anti-enteroviral agent

Subjects. Subjects were eligible for enrollment if they were ≥32 weeks gestational age; were between 0 and 30 days postnatal age; weighed ≥1200 g; had presumptive viral sepsis associated with fever, poor feeding, vomiting, diarrhea, irritability and/or somnolence; demonstrated clinical and biochemical evidence of normal gastrointestinal, hepatic and renal function; had normal fluid and electrolyte status; and were receiving no other systemic antiviral agents.

Study design: Study medication was supplied as a single lot by the sponsor (ViroPharma, Inc., Exton, PA) as an oral liquid containing 40 mg/ml active ingredient. Pleconaril (5.0 or 7.5 mg/kg) was administered to each infant via an oral dosing syringe or through an existing nasogastric tube mixed in a 1:1 (v/v) ratio with either breast milk or infant formula.

In conclusion pleconaril has the potential to become the first orally active anti-enteroviral agent suitable for therapeutic use in neonates, infants, adolescents and adults. Our pharmacokinetic data suggest that doses of pleconaril oral solution ranging form 5.0 to 7.5 mg/kg given every 8 to 12 h should produce steady state plasma and tissue concentrations which will exceed those required to inhibit the growth of nonpolio enteroviruses. Accordingly clinical investigations of pleconaril in neonates and infants with enteroviral disease are warranted to define its potential place in therapy.

(Kearns: Single dose pharmacokinetics of pleconaril in neonates. Pediatr Infect Dis J, 2000;19:833-9)

PNEUMOCOCCAL 7-VALENT CONJUGATE VACCINE

(DIPHTHERIA CRM_{197}PROTEIN) (Prevnar)

Supplied: Injection: 2 mcg each of 6 polysaccharide isolates; 4 mcg of 1 polysaccharide isolate per 0.5 ml dose in 0.5 ml dose vials

Preparation: Since this product is a suspension containing an aluminum phosphate adjuvant shake vigorously immediately prior to use to obtain a uniform suspension prior to withdrawing the dose. Do not use the vaccine if it cannot be resuspended. After shaking, the vaccine appears as a homogeneous, white suspension.

Pneumococcal Conjugate Vaccine (Prevnar)

The PCV7 vaccine is recommended for routine administration to all children 23 months and younger at 2, 4, 6, and 12 to 15 months (Table 1). Each .5 mL dose of PCV7 should be administered intramuscularly. The initial 2-month dose should be given no earlier than 6 weeks of age. Infants of very low birth weight (≤1500 g) should be immunized at the time that they attain a chronological age of 6 to 8 weeks, regardless of their calculated gestational age.

(Policy Statement: Recommendations for the Prevention of Pneumococcal Infections, Including the Use of Pneumococcal Conjugate Vaccine (Prevnar), Pneumococcal Polysaccharide Vaccine, and Antibiotic Prophylaxis. American Academy of Pediatrics. Committee on Infectious Disease: 2000;106:362-366)

POLYMYXIN B SULFATE (Aerosporin)

Supplied: Injection, powder for 500,000 units vial

Administration: IV, intrathecal

For IV administration, polymyxin B sulfate is reconstituted by dissolving 500,000 units of the drug in 300ml to 500ml of D5W. The drug is administered as an IV infusion, usually over a period of 60 to 90 minutes.

For intrathecal administration, it is reconstituted by adding 10ml of 0.9% NaCl to the vial, with a resultant concentration of 50,000 units/ml of polymyxin B.

Although it may be administered by deep intramuscular injection in the upper outer quadrant of the gluteal muscles, this route is generally not recommended, because severe pain at the injection site results. (5)

Each mg of polymyxin B is equivalent to 10,000 units of polymyxin B activity (3).

Solutions for parenteral use should be stored under refrigeration and discarded after 72 hours (3).

Polymyxin B

For newborns with EPEC gastroenteritis

On the basis of these data, there appears to be sufficient evidence to recommend oral administration of nonabsorbable antibiotics in the treatment of severely or moderately ill newborns with EPEC gastroenteritis. The drug most frequently used for initial therapy is neomycin sulfate in a dosage of 100 mg/kg per day administered PO every 8 hours in three divided doses. In communities in which neomycin-resistant EPEC has been prevalent, treatment should be started with colistin sulfate or polymyxin B in a dosage of 15 to 20 mg/kg PO daily, divided into three equal doses.

(Remington: Infectious Diseases of the Fetus and Newborn Infant 2001, p.1264)

Polymyxin B Sulfate (Aerosporin)

Action and spectrum:

Acts by disrupting the integrity of the bacterial cell wall. Bactericidal against most aerobic Gram-negative bacilli. Chiefly useful against *Pseudomonas* spp. Effective also against *Escherichia coli*, *Enterobacter* spp, and *Klebsiella* spp. Not active against *Proteus* spp. This drug has been replaced by other safer agents, but is still used treating organisms resistant to other drugs.

Route: PO, IV (dilute to final concentration of 1000-2000 units/mL in D_5W and infuse over 1-2 h).

Dosage: IV: 30,000-40,000 units/kg/day divided q8h
PO: 10-20 mg/kg/day divided q6-8h for up to 5 days.

Elimination and metabolism: Slow renal excretion.

Adverse effects: May cause reversible renal injury (proteinuria, hematuria, azotemia), rash, fever, thrombophlebitis at the injection site, and rarely neuromuscular blockade.

Comments: Poor tissue penetration. Does not cross blood-brain barrier. Not absorbed orally. Not often used.

(Gomella: Neonatology 1999, p.586)

Polymyxin

Indication: Ventriculitis

Ventriculostomy (with intermittent intraventricular instillation of an antibiotic, usually through a reservoir) is indicated when the ventricular tap demonstrates purulent fluid with persistent infection. Antibiotics should be instilled in concentrations that generally exceed those usually sought in serum. Table shows the commonly used intraventricular antibiotics and the concentrations sought. Serial measurements of the CSF concentrations of the antibiotics are important. the best approach is to administer the agent at a dose calculated to produce a concentration approximately 20-fold greater than the measured minimal bactericidal concentration.

Ventriculostomy, with external drainage, may be required in neonatal bacterial meningitis when ventriculitis has caused obstruction to CSF flow and acute hydrocephalus, manifested by increased intracranial pressure and dilated lateral ventriculus. This condition may develop despite eradication of the ventricular infection by the systemic antibiotics and therefore with a sterile ventricular CSF. In such a circumstance, intraventricular instillation of antibiotic is not needed, and the task is management of the intracranial hypertension by CSF drainage, as described in Chapter 11 in relation to rapidly progressive posthemorrhagic hydrocephalus.

TABLE
Intraventricular Antibiotics for Ventriculitis

Antibiotic	Dose (mg)	Desired Peak Cerebrospinal Fluid concentration (µg/ml)
Gentamicin	1-5	80-120*
Vancomycin	4-5	80-100
Polymyxin	1-2	Unknown

*Histological change in white matter observed with concentrations >150 µg/ml.

(Volpe: Neurology of the Newborn 2001, p.798)

POTASSIUM SUPPLEMENTS

POTASSIUM CHLORIDE
Supplied: Oral solution 10% (20 mEq/15ml) 20% (40 mEq/15ml)
Injection 2 mEq/ml
Administration: IV, PO, DILUTE PRIOR TO USE

POTASSIUM GLUCONATE
Supplied: Kaon Liquid 20mEq/15ml
Administration: PO, DILUTE PRIOR TO USE, contains 5% alcohol

POTASSIUM TRIKATES
Supplied: 45mEq/15ml (as K -acetate, -bicarbonate, -citrate)
Administration: PO, DILUTE PRIOR TO USE

POTASSIUM PHOSPHATES

Supplied: 4.4mEq K/ml and 3 mMol PO4/ml

Administration: IV, DILUTE PRIOR TO USE

Potassium (Chloride, Acetate)

Dose: Maintenance: 2-6 mEq/kg/day (usually 2-3 mEq/kg/day) diluted in 24-hour maintenance IV solution. Higher doses are required in infants receiving diuretics. titrate dose with previous day's requirements and potassium serum levels.

Intermittent: 1 mEq/kg/dose.

Oral Potassium Supplement: 2-6 mEq/kg/day (usually 2-3 mEq/kg/day) divided every 6 hours and diluted in feedings.

Administration: IV—Rate:

- <0.3 mEq/kg/hour IV, cardiac monitor not required.
- 0.3-0.5 mEq/kg/hour IV, cardiac monitor required.
- Maximum IV infusion rate: 0.5 mEq/kg/hour.

Do not give by IV push. Intermittent doses should be administered over 6-8 hours or, preferably, diluted in the entire day's maintenance IV solution.

IV—Concentration:

- Peripheral line preferred: <40 mEq/liter (=0.04 mEq/ml). Maximum: 80 mEq/liter (=0.08 mEq/ml). Concentrations >80 mEq/liter (=0.08 mEq/ml) should be infused via a central line because of the potential for severe vein irritation and risk of IV extravasation injury.
- Central line: >80 mEq/liter (=0.08 mEq/ml). One investigator recommended a maximum of 150 mEq/liter (=0.15 mEq/ml) in a central line and, in severely fluid restricted patients with central lines, 200 mEq/liter (=0.2 mEq/ml).
- Vials of KCl are commercially available at a concentration of 2 mEq/ml (=2,000 mEq/liter). **This must be diluted**. It cannot be infused full strength particularly via a peripheral line because of the extremely high osmolality.
- In the infant whose IV rate is minimal, potassium added to the IV fluid in the volumetric chamber may take several hours to travel through the tubing. Mix well with solution in chamber to avoid layering, which would result in infusion of concentrated potassium. Administer via pump (at the appropriate rate and concentration) at a port close to patient if urgently needed.

Cautions/Contraindications:

Do not keep potassium chloride on floor stock because of the toxicity of this drug and to protect against inadvertent overdose, which could be fatal. Doses should be prepared by pharmacy whenever possible.

Do not use the word "bolus" to refer to intermittent potassium doses because "bolus" implies an IV push, which could cause arrhythmias and cardiac arrest.

Do not give to anuric or severely oliguric patients. Be sure patient is urinating before giving potassium.

Changes in the potassium concentrations of an IV solution should be made in the pharmacy, rather than on the ward. Prevent potassium layering by agitating the bag or bottle before infusion.

Adverse Effects: If inadequately diluted, severe vein irritation with extravasation injury. Hyperkalemia, hyperchloremia (chloride salt), alkalosis (acetate salt). Potassium accumulation with renal dysfunction.

Cardiac arrhythmias (peaked T waves, widened QRS, flattened P waves, bradycardia, heat block), respiratory paralysis, hypotension if infused too rapidly.

Oral potassium and/or sodium citrates may cause diarrhea. Oral KCl may cause gastric irritation.

Treatment of Overdose:

- Stop potassium infusion and monitor EKG. Infuse dextrose and insulin at a ration of 3-4 gm dextrose to 1 unit regular insulin IV to shift potassium into the cells.
- Give sodium bicarbonate 1 mEq/kg IV to reverse acidosis and produce shift of potassium into cells.
- Give calcium gluconate 10 percent, 100 mg/kg IV to reverse EKG changes.
- Give sodium polystyrene sulfonate (Kayexalate)1 gm/kg per rectum to remove potassium from the body.
- Hemodialysis or peritoneal dialysis is effective.

Nursing Implications:

Monitor IV site carefully because infiltration causes severe tissue damage.

Continuous cardiac monitoring is required during intermittent IV infusion.

Oral dosing may cause feeding intolerance.

Comments: Correction of serum potassium concentrations of ≥3 mEq/liter is not an emergency and can be done in the next day's IV solution. There is usually cause for concern only if the infant has a serum potassium <3 mEq/liter with a normal pH, is symptomatic with marked weakness or paralysis, and is having arrhythmias on EKG.

(Zenk: Neonatal Medications & Nutrition. A Comprehensive Guide 2000; pp.406-408)

<u>Potassium Chloride</u> (KCl) (Various)

Indications and use:

To correct hypokalemia and as maintenance potassium provision. Also corrects hypochloremia.

Actions: Potassium is essential for maintaining intracellular tonicity; transmission of nerve impulses; contraction of cardiac, skeletal, and smooth muscle; and maintenance of normal renal function.

Route: IV, PO.

Dosage: Maintenance: 2-3 meq/kg/day diluted in 24-h maintenance IV solution. Higher doses are often required in infants receiving diuretics. Titrate the dose with the previous day's requirements and daily serum potassium determination. Maximum rate: Infants on a cardiac monitor; 0.5 meq/kg/h; infants not on a cardiac monitor: 0.3 meq/kg/h. Dilute bolus doses in 6-8 h of IV solution if possible. For oral use, the injectable form of the drug may be given in divided doses PO and diluted in the infant's formula.

Adverse effects: Avoid rapid IV injection. Excessive dose or rate may cause cardiac arrhythmias (peaked T waves, widened QRS, flattened P waves, bradycardia, and heart block), respiratory paralysis, and hypotension with rapid infusion. Potassium accumulates with renal dysfunction. Causes severe vein irritation; do not give undiluted in a peripheral vein. Dilute to 0.08 meq/mL if possible.

(Gomella: Neonatology 1999, p.586)

<u>Potassium chloride</u> (50 mg/100 mL)

Dose: 0.5 mg/kg/hr IV
1-2 mEq/kg/day PO

Comments: Useful in digoxin toxicity

(Garson: The science and practice of pediatric cardiology 1998, p.2956)

<u>Potassium Supplements</u>

Dose & Route: Replacement: Determine based on maintenance requirements, deficit and ongoing losses.
Hypokalemia:
Oral: Children: 1-4 mEq/kg/24 hr ÷ BID-QID. Monitor serum potassium.
IV: MONITOR SERUM **K** CLOSELY
Children: 0.5-1 mEq/kg/dose given as an infusion of 0.5 mEq/kg/hr x 1-2 hr. **Max** IV infusion rate: 1 mEq-kg/hr. This may be used in critical situations (i.e. hypokalemia with arrhythmia).

Remarks: PO administration may cause GI disturbance and ulceration. Oral liquid supplements should be diluted in water or fruit juice prior to administration. Sustained-release tablets must be swallowed whole, and not dissolved in the mouth or chewed.

Do **not** administer IV potassium undiluted. IV administration may cause irritation, pain, phlebitis at the infusion site. **Rapid or central IV infusion may cause cardiac arrhythmias**. Patients receiving infusion >0.5 mEq/kg/hr should be placed on an ECG monitor.

(Siberry: The Harriet Lane Handbook 2000, pp.821-822)

POVIDONE-IODINE (Betadine)

Supplied: Ointment: 5%, 10% in 30 grams and lb.
Solution: 7.5%, 10%, in pt and gal
Liquid: in pt.
Also available in many different application forms.

Povidone-iodine 2.5%

Gonococcal Ophthalmia.

For newborn infants, topical 1% silver nitrate solution, 0.5% erythromycin ointment, and 1% tetracycline ointment are considered equally effective for prophylaxis of ocular gonorrheal infection. Each is available in single-dose tubes. **Povidone-iodine in a 2.5% solution** also might be useful for preventing gonococcal ophthalmia, but more studies are required, and a product for this purpose currently is not available in the United States. Silver nitrate causes more chemical conjunctivitis than other agents but is recommended in areas where the incidence of penicillinase-producing *Neisseria gonorrhoeae* (PPNG) is appreciable. The efficacy of erythromycin or povidone-iodine prophylaxis against PPNG is not known; 1 study has demonstrated tetracycline to be effective for prophylaxis of PPNG infections. Infants born to women with untreated gonococcal infection should receive 1 dose of ceftriaxone (25-50 mg/kg) or cefotaxime (100 mg/kg), as well as topical prophylaxis. Infants who have gonococcal ophthalmia should be hospitalized and evaluated for signs of disseminated infection.

Chlamydial Ophthalmia.

Neonatal ophthalmia due to *Chlamydia trachomatis*, although not as severe as gonococcal conjunctivitis, is common in the United States. Results of studies on the clinical efficacy of erythromycin and of tetracycline ointment for prophylaxis of chlamydial conjunctivitis have been conflicting. Topical antibiotics and silver nitrate do not have proven efficacy in preventing conjunctivitis or nasopharyngeal colonization. One study has shown that **2.5% povidone-iodine** is likely to be more effective than either topical erythromycin or silver nitrate for preventing chlamydial conjunctivitis but does not prevent nasopharyngeal colonization and subsequent risk of pneumonia. Infants with ophthalmia neonatorum caused by *C trachomatis* should be evaluated and treated

(American Academy of Pediatrics: Report of the Committee on Infectious Diseases. Red Book 2000, pp.737-736)

Povidone-iodine

...multicenter, nonrandomized prospective study in a tertiary neonatal intensive care setting in which povidone-iodine and chlorhexidine gluconate were each used as antiseptic skin preparations over sequential 6-month periods. During the first 6 months of the study when povidone-iodine was in use 9.3% (38 or 408) of catheters were colonized. During the second 6 months of the study when chlorhexidine gluconate was in use, catheter colonization occurred in 4.7% (20 of 418, $P = 0.01$). Catheter-related bacteremia occurred during only 0.2% (2 of 826) of all catheterizations.

We concluded that 0.5% chlorhexidine gluconate in 70% isopropyl alcohol appears to be more efficacious than 10% povidone-iodine for the prevention of peripheral intravenous catheter colonization in neonates.

(Garland: Comparison of 10% povidone-iodine and 0.5% chlorhexidine gluconate for the prevention of peripheral intravenous catheter colonization in neonates: a prospective trail. Pediatr Infect Dis J 1995;14:510-516)

Povidone-Iodine

All infants in the study received one of three ophthalmic preparations in both eyes within 20 minutes of birth, after the eyes and face were cleaned: a drop of 2.5 percent povidone-iodine solution, a 1-cm strip of 0.5 percent erythromycin ophthalmic ointment, or a drop of 1 percent silver nitrate ophthalmic solution.

A 2.5 percent ophthalmic solution of povidone-iodine as prophylaxis against ophthalmic neonatorum is more effective than treatment with silver nitrate or erythromycin, and it is less toxic and costs less.

(Isenberg: A controlled Trial Of Povidone-Iodine As Prophylaxis Against Ophthalmia Neonatorum. N Engl J Med 1995;332:562-566)

PRAZOSIN HCL (Minipress)

Supplied: Capsules 1 mg, 2 mg, 5 mg
Administration: PO

Prazosin Hydrochloride (Minipress)

Indications and use: Hypertension and congestive heart failure. Experimental in infants and should be used only when traditional therapy has failed.

Actions: Postsynaptic α-adrenergic blocking agent that reduces peripheral vascular resistance and blood pressure.

Route: PO

Dosage: Test dose: 5-10 mcg/kg PO.
Maintenance dosage: Up to 25 mcg/kg/dose q6h.

Adverse effects: Dizziness, weakness, fatigue, palpitations, headache, and nausea. The most severe adverse effect in adults is the "first-dose phenomenon," in which severe orthostatic hypotension occurs.

(Gomella: Neonatology 1999, pp. 586-587)

Prazosin

Vasodilator Therapy in Children with CHF

Dose/Route of Administration:

0.01-0.05 mg/kg/dose PO q 6-8 hr
0.1 mg/kg/dose max

Disadvantages: "First pass" hypotensive effect

Clinical Use of Orally Available Vasodilators

Prazosin hydrochloride is an oral agent that has a vasodilatory effect on both the arterial and the venous bed. It acts as a postsynaptic –adrenergic blocking agent. It is well absorbed from the gastrointestinal tract, with peak plasma concentrations observed within 2 to 3 hours of administration. The drug has relatively few side effects. Reflex tachycardia is uncommon. Patients may experience a "first-dose effect," with dizziness or syncope within 30 to 90 minutes of the initial dose, and therefore should be closely observed for this first dose or have the first dose administered at bedtime.

(Garson: The science and practice of pediatric cardiology 1998, pp.2309-2323)

Prazosin

THERAPY FOR AUCTE CONGESTIVE CARDIAC FAILURE

Prazosin typically is started at a dose of 10 mg/kg orally. If hypotension does not develop, it should be increased to the full dose of 25 mg/kg every 6hours. The drug is well absorbed orally, peaks in the plasma in 2 to 3 hours, and has a half-life of 2 to 4 hours. It is metabolized by the liver and excreted in the bile. The most significant adverse effect is the first-dose phenomenon; the initial development of severe orthostatic hypotension. This problem does not persist after the first dose. A further problem with chronic therapy is tachyphylaxis. Other adverse effects noted in adult patients include polyarthralgias, headache, nausea, urinary incontinence, rashes, depression, and dry mouth. Although efficacious, prazosin is not used very much for management of acute congestive cardiac failure because of the availability of i.v. milrinone, nitroprusside, hydralazine, and angiotensin-converting enzyme inhibitors such as intravenous enalaprilat.

(Garson: The science and practice of pediatric cardiology 1998, pp.2329-2341)

Prazosin

Dose: 0.01-0.05 mg/kg/dose PO q6-8hr; max. 0.1 mg/kg/dose

Mode of Action: Competitive α_1 receptor blockade

Adverse Effects: Hypotension (first-dose phenomenon, 30-90 min after dose), dry mouth, stuffy nose

Comments: Tachyphylaxis

(Garson: The science and practice of pediatric cardiology 1998, p.2951)

Prazosin HCl

Dose & Route: Children:
Initial: 5 mcg/kg PO test dose
Maintenance: 25-150 mcg/kg/ 24 hr ÷ Q6 hr
Max dose: 15 mg/24 hr or 0.4 mg/kg/24 hr

Remarks: May cause syncope, tachycardia, hypotension, dizziness, nausea, headache, drowsiness, fatigue, anticholinergic effects. Marked orthostatic hypotension, syncope, and loss of consciousness may occur with first dose.

(Siberry: The Harriet Lane Handbook 2000, p.823)

PREDNISOLONE (Prelone, Pediapred, Key-Pred-SP)

Supplied: Syrup: 5mg/5ml, 15mg/5ml (as Prelone)
Oral liquid: 5mg/5ml (as Pediapred)
Injection: 20mg/ml (as Key-Pred-SP)
Ophthalmic solution: (as Prednisolone Sodium Phosphate)
0.125%; in 5 ml, 10 ml, 15 ml
1%; in 3 ml, 5 ml, 10 ml, 15 ml
Suspension: (as Prednisolone Acetate)
0.12%; in 5ml, 10 ml
0.125%; in 5 ml, 10 ml
1%; in 1ml, 5 ml, 10 ml, 15 ml

Administration: PO, IM, IV

Prednisolone

Dose/kg: Antiinflammatory: 0.5-1 mg
Route and frequency: PO q12h

Comments: May cause hypertension, GI irritation, and adrenal suppression

(Avery: Neonatology Pathophysiology and Management of the Newborn 1999, p.1559)

Prednisolone

Route: IV, IM, PO

Neonatal Dose: 0.5-2 mg/kg/24 h q6-8h

Pediatric Dose: 0.5-2 mg/kg/24 h q6-8h

Discussion: Prednisolone 5 mg is equivalent to hydrocortisone 20 mg; doses 4-10 times greater are used to treat cerebral edema.

(Rudolph: Rudolph's Pediatrics 1996, p.2200)

Prednisolone

Dose & Route: See Prednisone (equivalent dosing)
Ophthalmic:
Children: Start with 1-2 drops Q1 hr during the day and Q2 hr during the night until favorable response, then reduce dose to 1 drop Q4 hr. Dose may be further reduced to 1 drop TID-QID.

(Siberry: The Harriet Lane Handbook 2000, p.824)

PREDNISONE (Liquid Pred, oral intensol solution)

Supplied: Oral Intensol solution 5 mg/ml in 30 ml (contains 30% alcohol)
Liquid Pred 5 mg/5 ml in 120 ml and 240 ml (contains 5% alcohol)
Tablets available in 1mg, 2.5mg, 5mg, 10mg, 20mg, 50mg. May be crushed and mixed in feeding.

Administration: PO

Prednisone

(Liquid Pred, Prednisone Intensol Concentrate)

Indications and use:
Resistant neonatal hypoglycemia, airway edema, and weaning of infants with BPD from the ventilator. Used chiefly as an anti-inflammatory or immunosuppressive agent. Not indicated for adrenocortical insufficiency because of minimal mineralocorticoid activity.

Actions: An intermediate-acting glucocorticoid. Prednisone has four times the anti-inflammatory potency of hydrocortisone, and 1/2 the mineralocorticoid potency.

Route: PO.

Dosage: 0.1-2 mg/kg/day qd or divided q 12h.

Adverse effects: Cataracts, leukocytosis, peptic ulcer, nephrocalcinosis, myopathy, osteoporosis, diabetes, growth failure, hyperlipidemia, hypocalcemia, hypokalemic alkalosis, sodium retention and hypertension, and increased susceptibility to infection. Withdraw the dose gradually after prolonged therapy to prevent acute adrenal insufficiency.

(Gomella: Neonatology 1999, p.587)

Prednisone

Dose: As an Anti-inflammatory and Immunosuppressive: 0.5-2 mg/kg/day given as a single daily dose or divided every 6-12 hours. Base dose on severity of disease and response of patient. Reduce dose gradually to lowest effective level.

Administration: For oral use only.
Supplied as:

- Oral Liquid: 1 mg/ml (5 percent alcohol content). **Avoid the 5 mg/ml product because of its high (30 percent) alcohol content**.
- Tablets: 1, 2.5, 5 and 10 mg for those doses that equal these tablet or half-tablet (most are scored) sizes. Use of the solid dosage form may be preferred for fluid-restricted infants. Crush tablet and dilute in a small amount of feeding immediately prior to administration.

Use: Glucocorticoids have been used in neonates for congenital adrenal hyperplasia, for hypoglycemia, for BPD to shorten weaning from respirator, for hemangiomatosis, and prior to extubation to reduce laryngeal edema and stridor.

Nursing Implications:

Monitor blood pressure, serum electrolytes, and fluid status and for hyperglycemia after dose.

Monitor for signs and symptoms of infections.

Monitor growth parameters such as head circumference, length, and weight weekly and plot on growth curve.

Monitor for glucose spillage in urine.

(Zenk: Neonatal Medications & Nutrition. A Comprehensive Guide 2000; pp.409-410)

Prednisone (Corticosteroids)

Congenital *Toxoplasma* infection in the infant

(Remington: Infectious Diseases of the Fetus and Newborn Infant 2001)

SEE ALSO: CONGENITAL TOXOPLASMA INFECTION p.656

Prednisone

Dose & Route: Children:

Anti-inflammatory/immunosuppressive: 0.5-2 mg/kg/24 hr PO ÷ QD-QID

Nephrotic Syndrome: Starting doses of 2 mg/kg/24 hr PO (**Max dose**: 80 mg/24 hr) are recommended. Further treatment plans are individualized. Consult a nephrologist.

Remarks: Methylprednisolone is preferable in hepatic disease because prednisone must be converted to methylprednisolone in the liver. Side effects may include: mood changes, seizures, hyperglycemia, diarrhea, nausea, abdominal distension, GI bleeding, and HPA axis suppression, cushingoid effects, cataracts with prolonged use. Barbiturates, carbamazepine, phenytoin, rifampin, isoniazid, may reduce the effects of prednisone; whereas estrogens may enhance the effects.

(Siberry: The Harriet Lane Handbook 200, p.824)

Prednisone

5 mg/kg per day in four divided doses, with the total daily dose not exceeding 40.... After 2 weeks of treatment the dose was tapered gradually and discontinued after 6 to 8 weeks in most patients, in some patients after 10 weeks, and in one patient after 12 weeks.

(Sadan: Treatment of hemangiomas of infants with high doses of prednisone. J Pediatr 1996;128:141-146)

PRIMAQUINE

SEE CHLOROQUINE (Nelson: Pocket Book of Pediatric Antimicrobial Therapy 1998-1999, pp.63-64)

PRIMIDONE (Mysoline)

Supplied: Oral suspension 250 mg/5 ml in 240 ml

Administration: PO

Primidone and its two major metabolites, phenobarbital and phenylethylmalonamide, (PEMA) have anticonvulsant activity (1).

PEMA is the major metabolite and is less active than primidone. Phenobarbital formation ranges from 15% to 25%, the plasma half-life of primidone is 5-15 hours. PEMA and phenobarbital have longer half-lives (10–18 hours and 53-140 hours respectively) and accumulate with chronic use. About 40% of primidone is excreted unchanged in the urine, the remainder of the drug is excreted as unconjugated PEMA and as phenobarbital and its metabolites (1).

Primidone

Indication: For Neonatal Seizures

The potential value of primidone as an anticonvulsant drug in the neonatal period is suggested by two reports. In the initial study, primidone was administered orally to 24 infants with neonatal seizures in whom the seizures had recurred despite high levels of phenobarbital (15 to 40 µg/ml) and phenytoin (10 to 20 µg/ml). Seizure control was achieved within 48 hours in 50% of patients, but 34% of infants required 9 days for seizure control. The minimum primidone level at which a response occurred was approximately 6 µg/ml. However, there was marked interpatient variability in blood levels of primidone, and phenobarbital clearance was prolonged after addition of primidone. In a second report 10 infants were treated with oral primidone after discontinuation of previously ineffective anticonvulsant drugs (primarily phenobarbital or phenytoin or both). Eight achieved seizure control within 1 to 5 days of onset of therapy. Blood levels varied between 5 to 16 µg/ml. More data are needed.

(Volpe: Neurology of the Newborn 2001, pp.205-206)

Primidone

For Neonatal Seizures

Primidone may be of value in treating newborns whose seizures are refractory to phenobarbital and phenytoin [Powell et al., 1984]. Primidone is not converted to phenobarbital as in older children but does impair phenobarbital clearance and may cause a precipitous rise in phenobarbital levels after primidone loading. Primidone loading doses of 15 to 20 mg/kg and maintenance doses of 12 to 20 mg/kg/day are recommended. The lowest effective primidone level is 6 µg/ml.

(Swainman: Pediatric Neurology 1999; p.188)

PROCAINAMIDE HCL (Pronestyl)

Supplied: Capsules 250 mg, 375 mg, 500 mg
Injection 100 mg/ml in 10 ml
Injection 500 mg/ml in 2 ml

Administration: PO, IV

Extemporaneous Compounding (Recipe)

Dosage form: Oral suspension
Made from: Capsules
Concentration: 50 mg/mL
Stability: 60 days
Store: Refrigerate
Label: Shake well

Ingredient	Strength	Quantity
Procainamide capsules	250 mg	24
Ora-Sweet or Ora-Sweet SF		
Ora-plus		aa qs 120 mL

Instructions: Open the capsules and place the powder in a mortar. Reduce to a fine powder. Add approximately 20 mL of vehicle and mix to a uniform paste. Add vehicle in geometric portions to almost desired volume while mixing. Transfer to a graduate and qs to volume with vehicle. Mix well. (11)

Procainamide Hydrochloride (Various)

Indications and use: As prophylaxis to maintain normal sinus rhythm in paroxysmal atrial tachycardia, atrial fibrillation, premature atrial and ventricular contractions, and ventricular tachycardia.

Action: Class I antiarrhythmic agent similar to quinidine sulfate. Partially metabolized by the liver to the active metabolite N-acetylprocainamide (NAPA).

Route: PO, IM, IV.

Dosage: IV (monitor the electrocardiogram and blood pressure): 1.5-2 mg/kg (dilute to 10 mg/mL) over 10-30 min. Repeat as needed to maximum dose of 10-15 mg/kg; then continuous infusion of 20-60 mcg/kg/min.
PO: 5-15 mg/kg q4-6h.

Therapeutic levels:
Procainamide: 3-10 mcg/mL: Toxicity associated with levels > 12 mcg/mL.
NAPA: 10-20 mcg/mL; toxicity associated with levels >30 mcg/mL.

Adverse effects: Serious toxic effects if given rapidly IV, including asystole, myocardial depression, ventricular fibrillation, hypotension, and reversible lupus-like syndrome. May cause nausea, vomiting, diarrhea, anorexia, skin rash, tachycardia, agranulocytosis, and hepatic toxicity.

Comments: Contraindicated in second- or third-degree heart block, bundle branch block, digitalis intoxication, and allergy to procaine. Do not use in atrial fibrillation or flutter until ventricular rate is adequately controlled, to avoid a possible paradoxic increase in ventricular rate. Quinidine Sulfate is generally used for long-term therapy because it has less associated toxicity. Phenylephrine should be available to treat severe hypotension caused by IV procainamide. QRS or Q-T prolongation >35% of baseline is an indication to withhold further doses of procainamide.

(Gomella: Neonatology 1999, p.587)

Procainamide

Dosing: PO: 40-100 mg/kg/day
Warnings: Lupus-like syndrome

Dosing: IV: 7-15 mg/kg load, 40-100 mcg/kg/min infusion
Warning: Hypotension

Oral Administration:

Procainamide levels are in the range of 4 to 8 µg/ml. Infants often require slightly higher plasma levels.

After intravenous administration, procainamide is very rapidly distributed.

Dosing and Interactions:

Chronic oral dosages range from 40 to 100 mg/kg/day. The amount is divided into six doses for administration every 4 hours in small patients and may be every 6 hours in most patients older than 1 to 2 years. In teenage patients, a schedule of every 8 hours is often possible.

Intravenous administration of procainamide is somewhat more predictable. In patients younger than 1 year, a loading dose of 7 to 10 mg/kg, given over 30 to 45 minutes, is generally used. In older patients, the bolus dose is 15 mg/kg. The bolus is then followed by an infusion of procainamide, usually starting at 40 to 50 µg/kg/min. Top infusion rates of up to 100 µg/kg/min are occasionally necessary to maintain levels in infants. Plasma levels are obtained 4 hours after bolus during maintenance infusion. Procainamide does not elevate digoxin levels. Amiodarone, however, can elevate both procainamide levels and NAPA levels. Cimetidine will reduce renal clearance of procainamide and increase its $t_{1/2}$ by 25%.

Side Effects: The most common side effect is a drug-induced lupus-like syndrome. Fever, pericardial fluid accumulation, and arthralgia can be observed. During long-term procainamide therapy, more than half of patients will convert to a positive antinuclear antibody, but only 20% may show symptoms. During intravenous administration, procainamide can have negative inotropic effects. Drug-induced ventricular arrhythmia is less common than sinus bradycardia as a result of procainamide administration.

(Gillette: Clinical Pediatric Arrhythmia 1999,pp.231-248)

Procainamide

Uses: AFl, PSVT, VT, JET

Dosing: 10-15 mg/kg over 15-60 min (load); 20-60 μg/kg/min (infusion)

Acute Side Effects:
Hypotension; more rapid ventricular response during atrial flutter (AFl)

Other Considerations:
Additional atrioventricular (AV) node blockade for atrial flutter (AFl)

AFl, atrial flutter; JET, junctional ectopic tachycardia; PSVT, paroxysmal supraventricular tachycardia; VT, ventricular tachycardia.

(Gillette: Clinical Pediatric Arrhythmias 1999, p.152)

Procainamide

Class: IA

Uses: Conversion of AFL if on digoxin, conversion of SVT, multiform PVC, couplets, VT unresponsive to lidocaine, predict PO quinidine effect

Dose (Level): IV: <1 year old: 7 mg/kg over 1 hr, then 3.5 mg/kg per dose q4hr; >1 year old: 15 mg/kg over 1 hr, then 7 mg/kg per dose q4hr; if effect lasts <4 hr, infusion 1-4 mg/kg/hr
PO: 15-50 mg/kg/day divided q4hr (PA, 5-10 μg/mL)

Mode of Action: Similar to quinidine

ECG/EP Changes: Similar to quinidine

Side Effects: Similar to quinidine; lupuslike syndrome in slow acetylators
Amiodarone-↑ PA

(Garson: The science and practice of pediatric cardiology 1998, p.2952)

Procainamide

Guidelines for Dosage: Antidysrhythmics

Dosage: 10 -15 mg/kg slow i.v, (over 30 min) loading dose; then 20-80 μg/kg/min continuous I.V.

p.o.: 20-40 mg/kg/24 h in 6 divided doses (maximum = 60 mg/kg/24 h or 4 g/24 h)

Comments: during i.v. infusion, carefully monitor ECG and BP (may cause hypotension)

(Allen: Moss and Adam's Heart Disease in Infants, children and Adolescents 2001, pp.1460-1468)

Procainamide

Dose & Route: Children:
IM: 20-30 mg/kg/24 hr ÷ Q4-6 hr; **max dose**: 4 g/24 hr (peak effect in 1 hr).
IV: Load: 2-6 mg/kg/dose over 5 min (max dose: 100 mg/dose); repeat dose Q5-10 min PRN up to a total **maximum** of 15 mg/kg. Do not exceed 500 mg in 30 minutes.
Maintenance: 20-80 mcg/kg/min by continuous infusion; **max dose**: 2 g/24 hr

PO: 15-50 mg/kg/24 hr ÷ Q3-6 hr; **max dose**: 4 g/24 hr

Remarks: **Contraindicated** in myasthenia gravis, complete heart block, SLE, torsade de pointes. Use with **caution** in asymptomatic premature ventricular contractions, digitalis intoxication, CHF, renal or hepatic dysfunction. **Adjust dose in renal failure**

May cause lupus-like syndrome, positive Coombs' test, thrombocytopenia, arrhythmias, GI complaints, confusion. Monitor BP's ECG when using IV. QRS widening by >0.02 sec suggests toxicity.

Cimetidine, ranitidine, amiodarone, beta-blockers, trimethoprim may increase procainamide levels. Procainamide may enhance the effects of skeletal muscle relaxants and anticholinergic agents. Therapeutic levels: 4-10 mg/L of procainamide or 10-30 mg/L of procainamide and NAPA levels combined. Recommended serum sampling times: M/PO intermittent dosing: trough level within 30 minutes prior to the next scheduled dose after 2 days of continuous dosing (steady-state). IV continuous infusion: 2 and 12 hours after start of infusion and at 24 hour interval thereafter.

(Siberry: The Harriet Lane Handbook 2000, pp.826-827)

PROMETHAZINE (Phenergan)

Supplied: Injection 25 mg/ml
Syrup 6.25 mg/5 ml
Syrup Fortis 25 mg/5 ml
Suppositories: 12.5 mg, 25 mg, 50 mg

Administration: IV, IM, PO, PR
Injection: Use only 25 mg/ml concentration for IV administration. Caution in children with dehydration due to increased susceptibility of dystonias. IV administration should be ≤25mg/ml at a rate ≤25mg/min. Avoid SQ and intra-arterial injection because tissue necrosis and gangrene can result (1).

Promethazine

Dosage: 0.25-1.0 mg/kg/dose divided every 6-8 hr as needed PO, IM.

(Fanaroff: Neonatal-Perinatal Medicine 1997, p.1752)

Promethazine

Dosage: 0.5-1 mg/kg/dose p.o., i.m., i.v., p.r.; may repeat every 6 h p.r.n.

(Allen: Moss and Adam's Heart Disease in Infants, children and Adolescents 2001, pp.1460-1468)

PROPAFENONE (Rythmol)

Supplied: Tablets 150mg, 225mg, 300mg

Administration: PO

Propafenone

Guidelines for Dosage: Antidysrhythmics

Dosage: 0.2 mg/kg i.v. every 10 min; may repeat up to maximum total dose of 2 mg/kg i.v.;
4-8 μg/kg/min continuous infusion i.v.;
10 mg/kg/day p.o. (divided t.i.d.)

Comments: May be useful in managing postoperative junctional ectopic tachycardia

(Allen: Moss and Adam's Heart Disease in Infants, children and Adolescents 2001, pp.1460-1468)

Propafenone

Dosing: PO: 150-600 mg/m^2/day
Warning: Avoid in abnormal hearts

Oral Administration, Kinetics, Metabolites:
Most patients required levels of at least 150 to 200 ng/ml for clinical effect.

Dosing and Interactions:
The oral preparation is dosed on the basis of body surface area, starting at approximately 150 to 200 mg/m^2/day on a schedule of every 8 hours.

The intravenous preparation has been used in a dose of 0.2 to 1.0 mg/kg boluses, given slowly over 5 to 10 minutes each to a maximum of 2 mg/kg total load.

An infusion of 4 to 10 μg/kg/min has been used.

Side Effects: Like flecainide, propafenone should be provided with caution, if at all, in patients with a structurally abnormal heart.
Conduction system disturbances are relatively common.

(Gillette: Clinical Pediatric Arrhythmias 1999,pp.231-248)

Propafenone

Class: IC

Uses: Same as flecainide

Dose (Level): PO: 150-300 mg/m^2/day divided q8h

Mode of Action: Diffuse slowing of conduction; negative inotropism; mild β- and Ca^{++} blockade; prolongs both A and V refractoriness

ECG/EP Charges: Increases PR, QRS, QTc

Side Effects: Hypotension, decreases contractility, ? hepatic toxicity, paresthesia, headache

(Garson: The science and practice of pediatric cardiology 1998, p.2953)

PROPOFOL (Diprivan)

Supplied: Injection 10mg/mL in 20mL
Administration: IV

Propofol

Dosage: 1-2 mg/kg/h i.v. (may use initial dose of 0.5-1 mg/kg i.v. over 2-5 min)

Comments: short acting anesthetic; often produces transient hypotension (responds to fluid administration)

(Allen: Moss and Adam's Heart Disease in Infants, children and Adolescents 2001, pp.1460-1468)

Propofol

Propofol is a short-acting hypnotic, the administration of which is followed by a very rapid pleasant recovery. Propofol is an emulsion in soybean oil, a vehicle that supports bacterial growth; hence extreme caution with asepsis is required and all unused solutions should be discarded promptly. The dose required for induction of anesthesia is 3.5 mg/kg in the young infant and 2.5 mg/kg in the older child. The respiratory and cardiovascular effects of a sleep dose (2.5 - 3.5 mg/kg) are similar to those of thiopentone, a short period of apnea may occur, and there is a slight decline in blood pressure.

Propofol has been used for prolonged sedation in the ICU. This is no longer recommended in children, as prolonged dosage may have been associated with myocardial failure and also with post-infusion neurologic dysfunction.

(Steward: Manual of Pediatric Anesthesia 1995, pp.52-53)

PROPRANOLOL (Inderal)

Supplied: Oral solution 4 mg/ml and 8 mg/ml in 500 ml
Oral intensol solution 80 mg/ml in 30 ml with dropper
Injection 1 mg/ml in 1 ml

Administration: IV, PO
IV administration over 10 minutes (3, and Klaus. Care of the High Risk Neonate, p. 399, 1986)

Propranolol (Inderal)

Indications and use:
Hypertension, supraventricular tachycardia, premature ventricular contractions, tachycardia, and tetralogy spells.

Actions: Nonselective β-adrenergic blocking agent. Inhibits adrenergic stimuli by competitively blocking β-adrenergic receptors within the myocardium and bronchial and vascular smooth muscle. Decreases heart rate, myocardial contractility, and cardiac output.

Route: PO, IV.

Dosage: Arrhythmias:
IV: 0.025-0.15 mg/kg/dose to a maximum of 1 mg/dose as slow push.

PO: 0.5-2 mg/kg/day q6-8h. May increase to 1 mg/kg q6h or more as tolerated.

Hypertension:
0.5-2 mg/kg/day PO divided q6-12h. May increase as tolerated.

Tetralogy spells:
0.15-0.25 mg/kg/dose slow IV. May repeat q15min prn, or 1-2 mg/kg/dose PO q6h prn.

Adverse effects: Generally dose-related hypotension, nausea, vomiting, bronchospasm, heart block, depression, hypoglycemia, and depressed myocardial contractility.

Comments: Contraindicated in obstructive pulmonary disease, asthma, heart failure, shock, second- or third-degree heart block, hypoglycemia. Use with caution in renal or hepatic failure.

(Gomella: Neonatology 1999, pp.587-588)

Propranolol

Propranolol is the most commonly used beta-blocking agent. It is one of the few antiarrhythmic agents with a marketed liquid solution. There are at least two different concentrations: 20 mg/5ml and 10 mg/ml. This lack of uniformity can result in erroneous overdosing or underdosing. The 20 mg/5ml preparation is the more common of the two, and it is probably wise to make this concentration the standard, avoiding the 10 mg/ml solution.

Dosing: PO: 1-2 mg/kg/day
Warning: Fatigue, nightmares, bradycardia

Dosing: IV: 0.1-0.2 mg/kg
Warning: Bradycardia, hypotension

Drug Action: Propranolol is the classic nonselective beta blocker.

Oral Administration:
The plasma levels of propranolol range from 50 to 150 µg/ml, but appear helpful more in assaying absorption and compliance than in assessing therapeutic efficacy.

Dosing and Interactions:
Oral propranolol can be given as a liquid preparation, pill, or sustained-release preparation. Generally, the total daily doses are the same: starting dosages usually range from 1 to 2 mg/kg/day. In infants, the total dose is divided on a schedule of every 6 hours until age 6 to 8 months. By the time young children can swallow pills, a three times daily schedule of the standard propranolol is often effective.

Intravenous propranolol is given as a 0.1 to 0.2 mg/kg dose over 1 to 5 minutes. Significant caution is advised, as discussed next.

Side Effects: With intravenous administration, there can be bradycardia and hypotension. This finding is particularly true in children younger than 1 year, and the drug probably needs to be avoided in intravenous form in these young patients. Tachyarrhythmias may be eliminated with a resultant sinus arrest and loss of vascular tone. The exception to this advice may be the use of intravenous propranolol in the young child with hypercyanotic spells, in whom the drug may be given with caution.

Propranolol has a number of potential adverse side effects besides bradycardia, AV block, and worsening congestive heart failure. The drug crosses the blood-brain barrier and can cause fatigue, depression, and nightmares. Because it is a beta blocker, it can exacerbate bronchospasm and increase the risk of hypoglycemia. A peripheral vasoreactive condition can cause discoloration and cool extremities.

(Gillette: Clinical Pediatric Arrhythmias 1999,pp.231-248)

Propranolol

Class:	β-Blockers
Uses:	SVT-WPW: alone or with quinidine SVT-non WPW: alone or with digoxin Tetralogy spells, prolonged QT, VT, thyrotoxicosis
Dose (Level):	PO: 1-5 mg/kg/day divided q6hr (50-150 ng/mL) IV: 0.05-0.15 mg/kg Increased t1/2 if cyanotic
Mode of Action:	Nonselective β-blockade; some local anesthetic effect at high doses. Suppress renin-aldosterone-angiotensin axis; nonpolar, so crosses blood-brain barrier
ECG/EP Changes:	Slow HR, may ↓ QT; ↑ CSNRT, SACT, AH, AVNERP; no change in HV
Side Effects:	Bronchospasm, depression, nightmares, sinus arrest, AV block, CHF, hypoglycemia; May ↑ LDL, VLDL; decrease contractility; contraindicated with verapamil

(Garson: The science and practice of pediatric cardiology 1998, p.2953)

Propranolol

Dosage:	Pediatrics: 0.01 mg/kg i.v. initially; 3-5 mg/kg/day p.o. (divided t.i.d.)
Comments:	Pediatrics: May cautiously increase to maximum of 0.10 mg/kg/dose i.v.

(Allen: Moss and Adam's Heart Disease in Infants, children and Adolescents 2001, pp.1460-1468)

Propranolol

Guidelines for Dosage: Antidysrhythmics

Dosage:	0.5-1 mg/kg/day divided q.i.d. or t.i.d.; may increase to maximum of 6-8 mg/kg/day

(Allen: Moss and Adam's Heart Disease in Infants, children and Adolescents 2001, pp.1460-1468)

Propranolol

Usual Dosage: Neonates:

Oral: Initial: 0.25 mg/kg/dose every 6-8 hours; increase slowly as needed to maximum of 5 mg/kg/day

I.V.: Initial: 0.01 mg/kg slow I.V. push over 10 minutes; may repeat every 6-8 hours as needed; increase slowly to maximum of 0.15 mg/kg/dose every 6-8 hours

Tetralogy spells: Infants and Children:
Oral: Usual: 1-2 mg/kg/dose every 6 hours, may initiate at ½ the usual dose; may increase by 1 mg/kg/day every 24 hours to maximum of 5 mg/kg/day; if refractory may increase slowly to a maximum of 10-15 mg/kg/day but must carefully monitor heart rate, heart size, and cardiac contractility (Garson, 1981)
I.V.: 0.15-0.25 mg/kg/dose slow I.V.: may repeat in 15 minutes

Thyrotoxicosis:
Neonates: Oral: 2 mg/kg/day in divided doses every 6-12 hours; occasionally higher doses may be required

Administration: Oral: Administer with food; sustained action capsules should be swallowed whole, not chewed or crushed; ;mix concentrated oral solution with water, fruit juice, liquid, or semisolid food before administration

Parenteral: I.V. administration should not exceed 1 mg/minute; administer slow I.V. over 10 minutes in children; maximum concentration for injection: 1 mg/mL

Monitoring Parameters: EKG, blood pressure

Nursing Implications: The I.V. dose is much smaller than oral dose

Additional Information:

Not indicated for hypertensive emergencies; do not abruptly discontinue therapy, taper dosage gradually over 2 weeks

(Taketomo: Pediatric Dosage Handbook 1999-2000, pp.771-773)

Propranolol

Dose & Route: Arrhythmias: Children:

IV: 0.01-0.1 mg/kg/dose IV push over 10 minutes, repeat Q6-8 hr PRN. **Max dose**: 1 mg/dose for infants; **Max dose**: 3 mg/dose in children.

PO: Start at 0.5-1 mg/kg/24 hr ÷ Q6-8 hr; increase dosage Q3-5 days PRN. Usual dosage range: 2-4 mg/kg/24 hr ÷ Q6-8 hr. **Max dose**: 60 mg/24 hr or 16 mg/kg/24 hr.

Hypertension: Children:
PO: Initial: 0.5-1 mg/kg/24 hr ÷ Q6-12 hr. May increase dose Q3-5 days PRN; **max dose**: 8 mg/kg/24 hr.

Tetralogy Spells:
IV: 0.15-0.25 mg/kg/dose slow IV push. May repeat in 15 min x 1.

PO: Start at 2-4 mg/kg/24 hr ÷ Q6 hr PRN. Usual dose range: 4-8 mg/kg/24 hr ÷ Q6 hr PRN. Doses as high as 15 mg/kg/24 hr have been used with careful monitoring.

Thyrotoxicosis:
Neonates: 2 mg/kg/24 hr PO ÷ Q6-12 hr.

Remarks: **Contraindicated** in asthma, Raynaud's syndrome, heart failure, and heart block. Use with **caution** in presence of obstructive lung disease, diabetes mellitus, renal or hepatic disease. May cause hypoglycemia, hypotension, nausea, vomiting, depression, weakness, impotence, bronchospasm, and heart block.

Therapeutic levels: 30-100 ng/ml. Drug is metabolized by multiple CYP 450 isoenzymes. Concurrent administration with barbiturates, indomethacin, or rifampin may cause decreased activity of propranolol. Concurrent administration with cimetidine, hydralazine, flecainide, quinidine, chlorpromazine, or verapamil may lead to increased activity of propranolol. Avoid IV use of propranolol with calcium channel blocker.

Note: Oral bioavailability is 30%-60% of dose (may be increased in Down syndrome).

(Siberry: The Harriet Lane Handbook 2000, p.829)

PROPYLTHIOURACIL (PTU)

Supplied: Tablets 50mg
Administration: PO

Propylthiouracil

Route & Dose: PO: 2-4 mg/kg q 8 h. Increase to max of 10 mg/kg/dose. Onset of action may be delayed days to weeks

(Taeusch: Avery's Diseases of the Newborn 1998, p.1347)

Propylthiouracil Triiodothyronine (T_3)

Dosage: 5-10 mg/kg/day divided every 8 hr
Comments: Dosage for infants not well established.

(Fanaroff: Neonatal-Perinatal Medicine 1997, p.1750)

PROSTAGLANDIN E_1 (Prostin VR Pediatric, Alprostadil)

Supplied: Injection 500 mcg/ml in 1 ml amps
Administration: IV continuous infusion
Administer by IV continuous infusion into a large vein. Alternatively, the drug may be administered through an umbilical artery catheter placed at the ductal opening. Increases in pO2 have been the same in neonates who received the drug by either route of administration.

Dilute the 1 ml Prostin VR Pediatric to a volume appropriate for the pump delivery system available.

Discard and prepare fresh infusion solutions every 24 hours (1).

Comment: Apnea occurs in about 10% to 12% of neonates with congential heart defects treated with alprostadil (1).

<u>Prostaglandin E_1</u> (Alprostadil) (Prostin VR)

Indications and use: Any state in which blood flow must be maintained through the ductus arteriosus to sustain either pulmonary or systemic circulation until corrective or palliative surgery can be performed. Examples are pulmonary atresia, pulmonary stenosis, tricuspid atresia, transposition of the great arteries, aortic arch interruption, coarctation of the aorta, and severe tetralogy of Fallot.

Actions: Vasodilator, platelet aggregation inhibitor. Smooth muscle of the ductus arteriosus is especially sensitive to its effects, responding to the drug with marked dilatation. Decreased response after 96 h of infusion. Maximal improvement in $Pa0_2$, usually within 30 min in cyanotic infants, 1.5-3 h in acyanotic infants.

Route: IV

Dosage: 0.05 mcg/kg/min. Decrease to lowest rate that will maintain response.

Adverse effects: Cutaneous vasodilation, seizure-like activity, jitteriness, temperature elevation, hypocalcemia, apnea, thrombocytopenia, hypotension. May cause apnea. Have an intubation kit at the bedside if the patient is not already intubated.

Comments: Use cautiously in infants with bleeding tendencies.

(Gomella: Neonatology 1999, pp.551-552)

<u>Prostaglandin E_1</u>

Dosage: Initial dose 0.05 μg/kg/min; may increase to 0.1-0.15 μg/kg/min

Comments: Lower does (as low as 0.01 μg/kg/min) may be effective; tapering to lowest effective dose is recommended; may cause apneas or hypotension

(Allen: Moss and Adam's Heart Disease in Infants, children and Adolescents 2001, pp.1460-1468)

<u>Prostaglandin E_1</u> (Prostin)

Dose: 0.025-0.1 μg/kg/min IV

Mode of Action: Ductal, smooth muscle relaxation

Adverse Effects: Hypotension, apnea, fever, irritability, lethargy, NEC

Comments: Apnea

(Garson: The science and practice of pediatric cardiology 1998, p.2954)

Prostaglandin E_1, alprostodil

Route & Dose: IV: 0.05-0.1 µg/kg/min. Often, dose may be reduced by ½ after initial response. Intra-arterial infusion offers no advantage

Adverse Effects and Cautions:
Apnea, seizures, fever, disseminated intravascular coagulation, diarrhea, cutaneous vasodilatation, decreased platelet aggregation, cortical bone proliferation during prolonged infusion

(Taeusch: Avery's Diseases of the Newborn 1998, p.1347)

Prostaglandin E_1

Dose & Route: Neonates:
Initial: 0.05=0.1 mcg/kg/min. Advance to 0.2 mcg/kg/min if necessary

Maintenance: When increase in PaO_2 is noted, decrease immediately to lowest effective dose. Usual dosage range: 0.01-0.4 mcg/kg/min; doses above 0.4 mcg/kg/min not likely to produce additional benefit.

Remarks: For palliation only. Continuous vital sign monitoring essential. **May cause apnea**, fever, seizures, flushing, bradycardia, hypotension, diarrhea, gastric outlet obstruction, and reversible cortical proliferation of long bones (with prolonged use). Decreases platelet aggregation.

(Siberry: The Harriet Lane Handbook 2000, p.830)

PROTAMINE SULFATE

Supplied: Injection 10 mg/ml in 5 ml, 25ml

Administration: IV: Give very slowly IV over 10 minutes in doses not to exceed 50mg.

The following discussion relates to ADULT PROTAMINE DOSES.

Protamine sulfate 1mg neutralizes approximately 90 units of heparin activity derived from lung tissue or approximately 115 units from intestinal mucosa.

Because heparin disappears rapidly from circulation, the protamine dose required also decreases rapidly with time elapsed since IV heparin injection. For example, if protamine is give 30 minutes after heparin, half the usually dose may be sufficient (1).

Protamine Sulfate

Indications and use: Reversal of heparin; heparin overdose.

Actions: Combines with heparin, forming a stable salt complex. Devoid of anticoagulant activity. Effect on heparin is almost immediate and persists for ~2 hours.

Route: IV.

Dosage: For every 100 units of heparin estimated to remain in patient, give 1 mg by slow infusion over 3-5 min or not >5 mg/min. Maximum 50 mg.

Adverse effects: May cause fall in blood pressure, bradycardia, dyspnea, anaphylaxis. Excessive administration beyond that needed to reverse heparin effect may have anticoagulant effect.

(Gomella: Neonatology 1999, p.588)

Protamine

Dose: 1 mg for each 115 units of intestinal heparin or each 90 units of lung heparin.
Maximum: 50 mg.

If time has elapsed since IV heparin injection, use a smaller dose because heparin has a short half-life (i.e., give half the usual dose if 30 minutes have elapsed since the heparin was given; give one-quarter the usual dose if more than 2 hours have elapsed). The half-life of heparin is 1-3 hours; half-life is shorter in preterm infants and in infants with thrombosis.
Repeat doses may be needed (see Nursing Implications).

Administration: IV—Rate: May be given slowly IV over 3 minutes, but infusion over 10 minutes is preferred. Monitor blood pressure during infusion; slow infusion if hypotension occurs.

IV—Concentration: May give undiluted (10 mg/ml), or may dilute further in D_5W or NS.

Compatible with: Dextrose 5 percent, sodium chloride.
Storage: Must be refrigerated.

Nursing Implications: Monitor for hypotension and bradycardia.

Monitor for reversal of heparin effects using activated PTT.

Continue to monitor the infant's coagulation status for 24 hours after protamine has been given. Recurrence of bleeding has occurred 30 minutes to 18 hours after cardiac surgery despite complete neutralization of heparin with protamine. Repeat dosing may be required.

(Zenk: Neonatal Medications & Nutrition. A Comprehensive Guide 2000; pp.411-412)

Protamine Sulfate

Dose & Route. Heparin antidote, IV:
1 mg protamine will neutralize 115 U porcine intestinal or 90 U beef lung heparin.
Consider time of heparin and antidote administration:
If protamine given immediately after heparin: give 1-1.5 x doses above.
If within 0.5-1 hr: give 50% of above dose
If ≥2 hr: give 25% of above dose
Max dose: 50 mg IV
Max rate: 5 mg/min

Remarks:	May cause hypotension, bradycardia, dyspnea, and anaphylaxis. Monitor APTT or ACT. Heparin rebound with bleeding has been reported to occur 8-18 hours later.

(Siberry: The Harriet Lane Handbook 2000, p.831)

Protamine

Usual Dosage:	I.V.: Protamine dosage is determined by the most recent dosage of heparin or low molecular weight heparin (LMWH); 1 mg of protamine neutralizes 90 USP units of heparin (lung), 115 USP units of heparin (intestinal), and 1 mg (100 units) LMWH; maximum dose: 50 mg
Administration:	Parenteral: Reconstitute vial with 5 mL sterile water; if using protamine in neonates, reconstitute with preservative free sterile water for injection; resulting solution equals 10 mg/mL; inject without further dilution over 10 minutes; maximum of 50 mg in any 10-minute period

(Taketomo: Pediatric Dosage Handbook 1999-2000, pp.774-775)

PYRAZINAMIDE

Supplied:	Tablets 500 mg
Administration:	PO (1).

Extemporaneous Compounding (Recipe)

Dosage form:	Oral suspension
Made from:	Tablets
Concentration:	100 mg/mL
Stability:	90 days
Store:	Refrigerate

Ingredient	Strength	Quantity
Pyrazinamide tablets	500 mg	20
Citrucel	2.5 g/water	qs 50 mL
Syrup		50 mL

Instructions: Crush the tablets in a mortar and triturate to a fine powder. Mix the Citrucel powder with water and stir until uniform. Mix the Citrucel suspension and syrup. Add water to the pyrazinamide powder in the mortar to make a paste. Add the Citrucel syrup mixture to this paste gradually while stirring. When a fluid mixture results, transfer to a graduate and qs to volume with the Citrucel syrup mixture. Dispense in an amber glass bottle. (11)

Pyrazinamide

Antituberculosis Drugs in Children

Daily Dose (mg/kg)	Twice Weekly Dose (mg/kg/per dose)
20-40	50-70

The usual adult daily dose is 30 to 40 mg/kg. The optimal dose for infants and childrn has not been established firmly because no formal pharmacokinetic studies have been reported. The adult dose is tolerated well by infants and chidren, results in high cerebrospinal fluid concentrations, and clearly is effective in therapy trials for active tuberculosis in children. PZA appears to exert its maximum effect during the first 2 months of therapy. Hepatotoxicity can occur at high doses but is rare at the usual dose.

(Remington: Infectious Diseases of the Fetus and Newborn Infant 2001, p.1188)

<u>Pyrazinamide</u>

Usual Dosage: Oral: Neonates: 5 mg every 4-6 hours
I.M., I.V.: Neonates and Children:
0.05-0.15 mg/kg/dose (maximum single dose: 10 mg)

(Taketomo: Pediatric dosage Handbook 1999-2000, pp.780-781)

PYRIDOSTIGMINE (Mestinon, Regonol)

Supplied: Oral syrup 60 mg/5 ml
Injection 5 mg/ml in 2 ml, 5 ml

Administration: IV, IM, PO

<u>Pyridostigmine</u>

Dosage: 1-2 mg every 4-12 hr PO
0.05-0.15 mg every 4-8 hr IM

(Fanaroff: Neonatal-Perinatal Medicine 1997, p.1747)

<u>Pyridostigmine Bromide</u>

Dose & Route: Myasthenia Gravis:
Neonates:
PO: 5 mg/dose Q4-6 hr
IM/IV: 0.05-0.15 mg/kg/dose Q4-6 hr; **max single IM/IV dose**: 10 mg

Remarks: Changes in oral dosages may take several days to show results. Use with **caution** in patients with epilepsy, asthma, bradycardia, hyperthyroidism, arrhythmias, or peptic ulcer. May cause nausea, vomiting, diarrhea, rash, headache, and muscle cramps. Atropine is the antidote for autonomic.

(Siberry: The Harriet Lane Handbook 2000, p.834)

<u>Pyridostigmine</u>

Usual Dosage: Myasthenia gravis (dosage should be adjusted so patient takes large doses prior to time of greatest fatigue)
Oral: Neonates: 5 mg every 4-6 hours
I.M., I.V.: Neonates and Children: 0.05-0.15 mg/kg/dose (maximum single dose: 10 mg)

(Taketomo: Pediatric Dosage Handbook 1999-2000, pp.780-781)

PYRIDOXINE

Supplied: Tablets: 25 mg, 50 mg, 100 mg, 250 mg, 500 mg
Tablets, enteric coated: 20 mg (also contains 5 mg chorobutanol anhydrous)
Injection: 100 mg/ml; 1 ml vials

In infants with seizures, pyridoxine should be administered by IM or IV injection (3).

Pyridoxine

Reemphasis should be made of recurrent seizures that are not accompanied by any obvious associated findings to aid in diagnosis. This situation should raise the possibility of pyridoxine dependency. As noted previously, the best means of diagnosis is a therapeutic trail of pyridoxine, administered intravenously in a dose of 50 to 100 mg (or higher), accompanied by simultaneous monitoring of EEG. In the true case this trail is accompanied by cessation of seizure within minutes and normalization of the EEG within minutes or hours. In evaluating the response to pyridoxine, one should not consider as significant a transient attenuation of seizure discharges that may accompany infusion of essentially any material. This "arousal" response should last only a few seconds. Any question in the mind of the operator should provoke a second infusion of pyridoxine, a trial of oral pyridoxine, or both. In addition, it should be recognized that infants with pyridoxine dependency may exhibit hypotonia or even apnea after pyridoxine infusion, perhaps because of an abrupt increase of synthesis of GABA in brain.

(Volpe: Neurology of the Newborn 2001, p.208)

SEE ALSO: THERAPY FOR NEONATAL SEIZURES p.657

Pyridoxine (vitamin B_6)

Dose/kg: Deficiency: 5-10 mg total dose

Route and frequency:

PO, IV, IM

q24h

Dose/kg: B_6-dependent seizure: 50-100 mg total dose

Route and frequency:

PO, IV, IM

q24h

Comments: Decreases serum levels of phenobarbital, phenytoin, and folic acid; may cause hypersensitivity reactions, respiratory distress, and burning at site of injection

(Avery: Neonatology Pathophysiology and Management of the Newborn 1999, p.1560)

Pyridoxine (Vitamin B_6)

Indications and use:

For treatment of pyridoxine-dependent seizures and to prevent or treat vitamin B_6 deficiency.

Actions: Vitamin B_6 is essential in the synthesis of GABA, an inhibitory neurotransmitter in the CNS; GABA increases the seizure threshold. Vitamin B_6 is also required for heme synthesis and amino acid, carbohydrate, and lipid metabolism.

Route: PO, IM, IV.

Dosage: For vitamin B_6 - dependent seizures, give 100 mg IV as a single test dose, followed by a 30 min observation period. If a definite response is seen, begin maintenance of 50 - 100 mg PO daily.

(Gomella: Neonatology 1999, p.588)

<u>Pyridoxine</u>

Acute Treatment of Neonatal Seizures

Dose: 50 to 100 mg IV

(Hill: Neonatal Seizures Pediatrics in Review 2000;21:117-121)

<u>Pyridoxine</u> (Beesix)

Dose: Pyridoxine-Dependent Epilepsy:

- Initial: 100 mg/dose IV (preferred) or IM.
- Maintenance: 50-100 mg/dose PO given once daily. (the daily maintenance dose ranges from 2 to 200 mg PO, with an average of 50 mg.) Lifelong oral administration of pyridoxine is often required. the dose may need to be increased with age or during illnesses.

Diagnosis of Pyridoxine-Dependent Seizures:

1. Administer pyridoxine 100 mg/dose IV slowly.
2. Observe the infant for 30 minutes or up to 1 hour if seizures have not stopped. Seizures typically stop within 10 minutes, although it can take up to 1 hours after the dose for seizures to end.
3. If severe seizures do not stop during the 30-minute test period, administer anticonvulsants.
4. If possible, monitor the EEG with the first dose. The EEG readings will normalize within minutes to several weeks after the dose.
5. If a definite response to pyridoxine occurs, continue pyridoxine 50-100 mg/dose PO once daily. The dose may need to be increased during intercurrent illnesses.
6. To confirm the diagnosis, stop the pyridoxine and monitor the EEG. Seizures usually recur within 1 week in neonate and after 2-14 days in older infants and children.

Treatment of Acute Isoniazid (INH) Overdose: Give a dose of pyridoxine equal to the amount of INH ingested. Administer IM or IV in divided doses together with other anticonvulsants.

Prevention of Drug-Induced Neuritis (caused by isoniazid, hydralazine): 1-2 mg/kg/day.

Parenteral Nutrition: 0.18 mg/kg/day.
Recommended Daily Allowance: Birth to 3 years: 0.3-1 mg/day.

Administration: Supplied as: Injection: 100 mg/ml. Tablet: 25 mg. Storage: Protect from light.
IV—Rate: Infuse slowly over 2 minutes or more.

IV—Concentration: May give undiluted or diluted with saline or dextrose.

IM: May give undiluted

PO: Give with feedings.

Nursing Implications:

Monitor respiratory rate, heart rate, and blood pressure during IV administration of large doses.

Comments: Infant oral multivitamin drops (Poly-Vi-Sol) contain 0.4 mg vitamin B_6/ml.

Interactions: May decrease serum levels of phenobarbital and phenytoin.

Benzyl Alcohol Content: Pyridoxine injection contains benzyl alcohol 1.5 percent (=15 mg/ml or 15 mg/100 mg pyridoxine). Oral, rather than IV, administration is preferred for maintenance doses to reduce risk of benzyl alcohol toxicity and other adverse effects, particularly in preterm infants. Benzyl alcohol is associated with the fatal gasping syndrome of metabolic acidosis, as well as with central nervous system, respiratory, circulatory, and renal impairment. A toxic benzyl alcohol dose is approximately 100-400 mg/kg/day.

(Zenk: Neonatal Medications & Nutrition. A Comprehensive Guide 2000; pp.413-418)

PYRIMETHAMINE (Daraprim)

Supplied: Tablet 25 mg
Administration: PO

Extemporaneous Compounding (Recipe)

Dosage form: Oral suspension
Made from: Tablets
Concentration: 2 mg/mL
Stability: 91 days
Store: Refrigerate
Label: Shake well

Ingredient	Strength	Quantity
Pyrimethamine tablets	25 mg	2
Sorbitol	70%	qs ad 25 mL

Instructions: Crush the tablets in a mortar and reduce to a fine powder. Add a small amount of sorbitol and mix to a fine paste. Then qs with sorbitol solution. (11)

Pyrimethamine

Concentration: 2mg/ml*
Dispense: 25ml
Dosage: Sig: half baby's current weight in Kg equals number of ml

given once each day. eg. If baby weighs 5Kg give 2.5ml daily.

*Suspended in 2% sugar solution. Suspension at usual concentration must be made up each week. Store refrigerated.

(Remington: Infectious Diseases of the Fetus and Newborn Infant 2001, pp.292-294)

Pyrimethamine

Oral Suspension Formulations for Pyrimethamine and Sulfadiazine in the United States.

Pyrimethamine, 2 mg/ml suspension;

1. Crush four 25-mg pyrimethamine tablets in a mortar to a fine powder.
2. Add 10 ml of syrup vehicle.
3. Transfer mixture to an amber bottle.
4. Rinse mortar with 10 ml of sterile water and transfer.
5. Add enough of the serum vehicle to q.s. to 50 ml final volume.
6. Shake very well until this is a fine suspension.
7. Label and give a 7-day expiration.
8. Store refrigerated.

Note: Pyrimethamine: 25-mg tablets (Daraprim, Glaxo Wellcome Inc.) NDC # 0173-0201-55

Syrup vehicle: suggest 2% sugar suspension for pyrimethamine. If the infant is not lactose intolerant, 2% sugar suspension can be 2 g lactose per 100 ml distilled water. Suggest simple syrup or alternatively cherry syrup for sulfadiazine suspension.

(Remington: Infectious Diseases of the Fetus and Newborn Infant 2001, pp.292-294)

Pyrimethamine

Congenital *Toxoplasma* infection in the infant

(Remington: Infectious Diseases of the Fetus and Newborn Infant 2001)

SEE ALSO: CONGENITAL TOXOPLASMA INFECTION p.656

Pyrimethamine

Indication: For treatment of toxoplasmosis

Although significant injury has already occurred in many cases of congenital toxoplasmosis by the time of birth, there is good evidence that some of this injury is reversible and that continuing postnatal injury is preventable by therapy directed against the organism.

The drugs of choice are pyrimethamine and sulfadiazine with the addition of folinic acid to counteract the folic acid antagonistic effect of pyrimethamine on the bone marrow. Pyrimethamine is highly effective in experimental infection with *Toxoplasma* and, because of its high lipid solubility, appears to be concentrated in brain. Sulfadiazine acts synergistically with pyrimethamine, such that their combined activity is eight times that expected if additive effects were operative. Caution must be exercised with sulfadiazine, particularly in infants with hyperbilirubinemia. Thrombocytopenia is a particularly early manifestation of pyrimethamine toxicity, and folinic acid is particularly effective in correcting this phenomenon. These antimicrobials kill actively multiplying parasites but not resistant cyst stages. Therefore treatment must begin promptly and continue until the infant's immune system has matured sufficiently to control the infection. Total recommended duration of therapy in both symptomatic and asymptomatic disease is 1 year. In infants with evidence for severe inflammation, manifested by markedly elevated CSF protein (≥1 g/dl) or by severe chorioretinitis, corticosteroids have been recommended.

(Volpe: Neurology of the Newborn 2001, pp.732-733)

Pyrimethamine

Condition: Congenital toxoplasmosis

Therapy: Sulfadiazine 100 mg/kg/day PO div q6-12hr AND pyrimethamine 2 mg/kg PO daily x 2 (loading dose), then 1 mg/kg PO once daily for 6 wks, then 3 times weekly up to 1 year; Alternative: pyrimethamine (as above) AND clindamycin

Comment: Supplemental folinic acid 5-10 mg 3 times weekly; Steroids if chorioretinitis of CSF protein > 1 g/dl

(Nelson: Pocket Book of Pediatric Antimicrobial Therapy 2000-2001, p.8)

Pyrimethamine (Daraprim)

Action and spectrum:

Folic acid antagonist selective for plasmodial dihydrofolate reductase. Activity highly selective for plasmodia (cidal) and *Toxoplasma gondii*.

Route: PO.

Dosage: For toxoplasmosis, give 1 mg/kg/day divided q12h for 4 weeks. Combine with sulfadiazine.

Elimination and metabolism: Hepatic metabolism

Adverse effects: Anorexia, vomiting, megaloblastic anemia, leukopenia, thrombocytopenia, pancytopenia, atrophic glossitis, rash, seizures, shock.

Comments: Give folinic acid (leucovorin), 1 mg PO daily or 3 mg twice weekly, if leukopenia or thrombocytopenia occurs. Administer with feedings if vomiting persists. Give sulfadiazine alone in empirical therapy of toxoplasmosis until the diagnosis is ruled out. Reduced dosage in hepatic dysfunction.

(Gomella: Neonatology 1999, p.588)

SEE ALSO: CHLOROQUINE

(Nelson: Pocket Book of Pediatric Antimicrobial Therapy 2000-2001, pp.64-65)

QUINIDINE SULFATE

Supplied: Tablets (sulfate) 200mg, 300 mg
Injection (gluconate) 80mg/ml in 10ml (50 mg/ml quinidine)

Administration: IM, PO
Quinidine sulfate tablets contain 83% quinidine.

Extemporaneous Compounding (Recipe)
Dosage form: Oral suspension
Made from: Capsules
Concentration: 50 mg/5 mL
Stability: 30 days
Store: Refrigerate

Ingredient	Strength	Quantity
Quinidine capsules	200 mg	6
Alcohol USP		15 mL
Citric acid syrup		qs ad 120 mL

Instructions: Add the contents of the capsules and alcohol to a calibrated 120-mL bottle and shake well. Then qs to volume with syrup.

Note: If this preparation is filtered, varying concentrations of quinidine may result. Although this formula contains alcohol, typical dosages should not result in alcohol intoxication.

Note: Citric acid syrup contains 1% citric acid and lemon flavor in syrup base. (11)

Quinidine (Various)

Indications and use:
Restoration of normal sinus rhythm in atrial flutter or fibrillation once the ventricular rate is controlled by digoxin. Prevention of atrial and ventricular arrhythmias.

Actions: Group 1 antiarrhythmic agent with cardiac effects similar to those of procainamide hydrochloride. Direct depressant effect on myocardial contractility, conduction velocity, and excitability. Causes increase in P-R, QRS and Q-T intervals.

Route: PO, IM (IV not recommended).

Dosage: 5-15 mg/kg q6h PO or 2-4 mg/kg q2-4h IM. Total daily dose: 10-30 mg/kg.

Therapeutic levels: 3-7 mcg/mL.

Adverse effects: Severe hypotension with IV use. Adverse reactions in ~30% of patients include nausea, vomiting, diarrhea, blood dyscrasias, and drug fever.
Overdose may cause cinchonism or respiratory depression.

Comments: Contraindicated with AV nodal block.
(Gomella: Neonatology 1999, p.588)

Quinidine

Dosing: PO: 30-60 mg/kg/day
Warning: Torsades de pointes, "cinchonism"

Oral Administration:

Quinidine is administered orally as quinidine sulfate or gluconate. In adults, the gluconate form is absorbed slowly, with a peak serum level 3 to 4 hours after administration. Its dosing schedule is generally every 8 hours. Quinidine sulfate reaches a serum peak concentration in 1 to 2 hours and is usually given every 6 hours.

The presumed therapeutic range of quinidine at steady state is 2 to 6 μg/ml.

Side Effects: Side effects with quinidine are common: 25 to 30% of patients experience some difficulty. The most common problems are gastrointestinal. *Cinchonism* refers to central nervous system effects, including tinnitus, visual changes, headaches, and mental status changes. Other noncardiac side effects are predominantly hematologic: thrombocytopenia, anemia, and agranulocytosis.

Cardiac side effects are those that may be expected and those that are unwanted and mostly proarrhythmic. Electrocardiographic effects include prolongation of the PR, QRS, and QT intervals, which need to be monitored at drug initiation in particular. Bradycardia can appear de novo or can be exacerbated. Bundle branch blocks may occur, and with high levels of drug, AV block may result. The most dangerous side effect is drug-induced torsades de pointes ventricular tachycardia (VT), resulting in syncope and potential sudden death. This phenomenon often occurs in the first several days of dosing and may be accompanied by slightly low serum potassium levels and by electrocardiographic evidence of significant QT prolongation. This possibility argues strongly for in-hospital initiation of quinidine. The drug may also be a negative inotropic agent and can worsen congestive heart failure.

Dosing and Interaction:

Quinidine dosing depends on whether the sulfate or gluconate form is used. Quinidine sulfate is given in a dosage of 30 to 60 mg/kg/day, divided into a three or four times daily dose. Quinidine gluconate has 20% less quinidine base and needs to have the dose adjusted upward to compensate.

Drugs that increase microsomal enzyme activity, such as phenytoin, phenobarbital, and rifampin, can increase quinidine metabolism. In patients older than 5 years, administration of digoxin with quinidine has been shown to potentially increase digoxin levels. Coadministration of warfarin with quinidine can result in prolongation of the prothrombin time, but effects on international ratio (INR) are unknown.

(Gillette: Clinical Pediatric Arrhythmias 1999,pp.231-248)

Quinidine

Class:	IA Inhibit Na^+ fast channel Prolong repolarization Marked Na^+ channel inhibition with fast rate
Uses:	AFL with digoxin, SVT-WPW with propranolol, resistant PVC/VT
Dose (Level):	PO only, 15-60 mg/kg/day, divided q6hr for sulfate, q8hr for gluconate (2-6 µg/mL)
Mode of Action:	Depress conduction and prolong refractoriness in A, HP, V; peripheral α-block, vagolytic, negative inotrope, decrease phase 4 and automaticity (high dose)
ECG/EP Changes:	Increase Pr, QRS, ? toxicity if QTc increases by 30% or QT 0.5 sec; increased CSNRT, HRALSRA, HV, ERP-Kent; decreased AH
Side Effects:	Hypotension, SAN exit block, AV block (below His bundle), VT, CHF, headache, rash, tinnitus, nausea, thrombocytopenia; digoxin-↑ dig level, phenytoin-↓ DPA t1/2, warfarin-↑ PT

(Garson: The science and practice of pediatric cardiology 1998, p.2952)

Quinidine

Dose & Route:	All doses expressed as salt forms Antiarrhythmia: Children (Give PO as sulfate. Give IM/IV as gluconate): Test dose: 2 mg/kg x 1 IM/PO; **max dose**: 200 mg Therapeutic dose: IV (as gluconate): 2-10 mg/kg/dose Q3-6 hr PRN PO (as sulfate): 15-60 mg/kg/24 hr ÷ Q6 hr
Remarks:	Test doe is given to assess for idiosyncratic reaction to quinidine. Toxicity indicated by increase of QRS interval by ≥0.02 sec (skip dose or stop drug). May cause GI symptoms, hypotension, tinnitus, TTP, rash, heart block, blood dyscrasias. When used alone, may cause 1:1 conduction in atrial flutter leading to ventricular fibrillation. May get idiosyncratic ventricular tachycardia with low levels, especially when initiating therapy. Can cause increase in digoxin levels. Quinidine potentiates the effect of neuromuscular blocking agents, beta-blockers, anticholinergics, and warfarin. Amiodarone,

antacids, delavirdine, saquinavir, ritonavir, verapamil, or cimetidine may enhance the drug's effect. Barbiturates, phenytoin, cholinergic drugs, nifedipine, sucralfate, or rifampin may reduce quinidine's effect. Use with **caution** in renal insufficiency (15-25% of drug is eliminated unchanged in the urine). **Adjust dose in renal failure**.

Therapeutic levels: 3-7 mg/L.

Recommended serum sampling times at steady-state: trough level obtained within 30 minutes prior to the next scheduled dose after 1-2 days of continuous dosing (steady-state).

(Siberry: The Harriet Lane Handbook 2000, p.836)

RADIOPAQUE AGENTS

BARIUM SULFATE SUSPENSION:

Indications for contrast examinations of the GI tract are discussed subsequently in the appropriate sections.

There are two relative contraindications to using barium as a contrast agent: suspected bowel perforation or a predisposition for pulmonary aspiration of barium. Neither one is an absolute contraindication: Barium in the retroperitoneum, mediastinum, or peritoneal cavity that is removed shortly after entering these spaces holds only a minimal risk for sequelae such as granuloma formation, adhesions, or peritonitis. Likewise, aspirated barium provokes a cough reflex. Thus when routine care is taken, barium constitutes a most useful and safe contrast agent in pediatric age group.

WATER-SOLUBLE CONTRAST AGENTS:

The most commonly used of the water-soluble contrast agents are diatrizoate meglumine/sodium (Gastrografin) and diatrizoate meglumine (Hypaque). Iothalamate meglumine (Conray; Cysto-Conray) is also used. These agents are hyperosmolar water-soluble media and should not be used routinely in the upper GI tract. There is a serious risk of pulmonary edema or death when these agents are aspirated because the aspirated contrast medium causes a release of histamine or histamine-like substances in the lung. In addition, hyperosmolar agents can be toxic to the bowel mucosa, and their hydrophilic nature can result in massive fluid shifts, especially in neonates. These hyperosmolar contrast agents also draw fluid into the GI lumen, often resulting in their marked dilution, sometimes as early as the third portion of the duodenum, thus severely limiting their diagnostic use for the rest of the GI tract. In the large bowel, on the other hand, these agents can be used in an enema to exploit their hyperosmolar quality (e.g., to facilitate meconium plug evacuation by absorbing fluid into the bowel lumen, thus having a "lubrication" effect).

CONTRAST/SEDATION SUGGESTIONS

Oral: The contrast material commonly used to opacify the GI tract is 5 ml of Gastrografin in 6 oz (180 ml) of orange juice. Orange juice is preferred because Gastrografin's taste in water is not pleasant.

Suggested Dosage:
Neonates: one 6-oz cup of the prepared contrast agent when the infant is on the CT table (upon entering the CT suite)

Intravenous (informed consent varies from institution to institution):

It is strongly suggested to use low-osmolar water-soluble contrast agents (physician-administered or physician-supervised) because contrast reactions and discomfort in case of extravasation are much less than those experienced with hyperosmolar water-soluble contrast agents.

Child's Weight (lb)	Suggested Dose
Up to 12	2 ml/lb
13-25	25 ml

Sedation (Informed consent mandatory)

Monitoring sedated patients with a pulse oximeter and a trained pediatric nursing staff and having the radiologist perform the study are highly recommended, if not mandatory.

Suggested Dose:
Chloral hydrate 50-75 mg/kg PO or PR
(75% effective in 30 min)
Pentobarbital or Thiopental 0.5 mg/kg IV as a second line.

CONTRAST

Oral: To opacify the bowel, newborns and infants undergoing abdominal or pelvic examinations may be given a bottle of formula with a high iron (Enfamil) content 2 hours before imaging. If patients are to undergo general anesthesia, the stomach should be evacuated before induction. If oral contrast is given, glucagon 0.2 ml IV should be given before imaging to minimize motion artifacts.

Intravenous: Gd DTPA 0.1 mM/kg is the usual pediatric dose. It necessitates written consent from the parents.

Common pediatric gastrointestinal nuclear medicine procedures

Procedure	Radioisotope	Dose
Meckel scan	$^{99m}TcO^{4}$	1-5 mCi IV
Liver or spleen scan	^{99m}Tc sulfur colloid	0.5-5 mCi IV
Biliary scan	^{99m}Tc diSIDA	0.1-1 mCi IV
Milk scan	^{99m}Tc sulfur colloid	1 mCi PO or per NG tube
Gastric emptying study	^{111}In DTPA	<1 mCi PO or per NG tube

(Blickman: Pediatric Radiology 1998; pp.78-80)

<u>Radiopaque Agents</u>

Line Angiogram: A line angiogram is performed using 2 to 3 mL of contrast, which is rapidly injected through the line to be assessed. A line angiogram differs from a line-o-gram in that the volume of contrast used is larger.

(Calhoun: Consistent approaches to procedures and practices in neonatal hematology. Clinics in Perinatology 2000,27:733-753)

RANITIDINE (Zantac)

Supplied: Injection 25mg/ml
Syrup 15mg/ml

Administration: IV, PO
For direct IV injection dilute to a concentration not greater than 2.5mg/ml and inject over ≥5 minutes (1).

For intermittent IV infusion dilute to a concentration not greater than 0.5mg/ml and infuse over 15-20 minutes (1).

Stable in D5W, NS, D10W for 48 hours at room temperature (1).

Ranitidine (Zantac)

Indications and use: Duodenal and gastric ulcers, gastroesophageal reflux, and hypersecretory conditions (et, Zollinger-Ellison syndrome).

Actions: Histamine (H_2) receptor antagonist; competitively inhibits the action of histamine on the parietal cells, decreasing gastric acid.

Route: PO, IV

Dosage: 1-2 mg/kg/dose divided q8h IV; 3-4 mg/kg/day divided q12h PO.
Maximum: 6 mg/kg/day.
Continuous IV infusion: 1.5 mg/kg/day. Reduce dose in renal dysfunction.

Adverse effects: Constipation, diarrhea, sedation, tachycardia rarely.

Notes: Does not interact with other drugs. Injection contains 0.5% phenol. No short-term toxicity noted. May add daily dose to the total parenteral nutrition regimen and infuse over 24h to avoid need for separate q8h dosing.

(Gomella: Neonatology 1999, p.589)

Ranitidine (Zantac)

Dose: PO: 2-4 mg/kg/day divided every 8-12 hours.
Maximum PO dose: 6 mg/kg/day divided every 6 hours.

IV (Preferred) or IM: 1-2 mg/kg/day divided every 6-8 hours.
Maximum IV dose: 6 mg/kg/day divided every 6 hours.

- Wiest and associates recommend 0.7 mg/kg/dose IV every 6 hours (=2.8 mg/kg/day) infused over 20 minutes. They found a large degree of variability in pharmacokinetic parameters in their patients.

Continuous IV Infusion (preferred over intermittent dosing): 0.06-0.17 mg/kg/hour (=1.44-4 mg/kg/day).
Maximum: 6 mg/kg/day.

- Kelly and associates found that an IV infusion of 0.063 mg/kg/hour (=1.5 mg/kg/day) was sufficient to increase and maintain gastric pH above 4 in preterm infants receiving dexamethasone. There was no benefit from a higher dose of 0.125 mg/kg/hour (=3 mg/kg/day).

- Fontana and associates estimate that a continuous IV infusion of 0.03-0.06 mg/kg/hour (=0.7-1.44 mg/kg/day) in term newborns will achieve serum concentrations greater than 100-200 ng/ml.
- A dose of 0.2 mg/kg/hour stopped GI hemorrhage in a 30-week-gestational-age newborn with anuria.

Reduce dose or prolong interval in renal impairment.

Adjust to lowest dose that will maintain pH of gastric secretions above 4.

Continuous intragastric monitoring of gastric pH with a pH-sensitive electrode avoids problems associated with variability of gastric pH, changes in serum concentrations of H_2 blockers, and other problems associated with intermittent pH determinations.

Administration: IV—Rate: May infuse IV over at least 5 minutes, but infusion over 15-30 minutes is preferred.

IV—Concentration: Dilute to at least 2.5 mg/ml. Continuous Infusion: May infuse continuously over 24 hours. May also be given by continuous infusion by syringe pump or added to parenteral nutrition solution.

IV—Compatibility: May admix IV dose with parenteral nutrition solution for infusion over 24 hours. Be sure that intermittent IV does of ranitidine are not also being given. See Appendix E: Y-Site Compatibility of Common NICU Drugs.

IM: May give undiluted.

PO: Oral liquid available at 15 mg/ml (7.5 percent alcohol).

Use: For treatment of gastroesophageal reflux, gastric hypersecretory states, and upper GI mucosal lesions. Also used for prophylaxis of stress-induced gastric mucosal injury.

Comparison with Cimetidine: Ranitidine is more potent than cimetidine and longer acting. Unlike cimetidine, ranitidine has been associated with effects on hepatic drug metabolism, endocrine function, the immune system, or the central nervous system and therefore has fewer adverse effects and drug interactions. Ranitidine is not likely to increase theophylline levels as cimetidine does.

Adverse Effects: Usually well tolerated.

May cause abdominal symptoms such as diarrhea or constipation, rash, and dizziness.

Uncommonly, causes a decrease in white blood cell and platelet count and increased transaminase levels.

Hypotension may occur with IV infusion over less than 5 minutes.

Tolerance to the acid-inhibiting effects of ranitidine after 2-6 weeks of continuous IV therapy has been reported in infants treated for gastric hypersecretion associated with short-bowel syndrome.

Nursing Implications:

Monitor for response to therapy, including decreased irritability from reflux and prevention of stress ulcer.

Monitor hepatic and renal function.

Comments: Ranitidine is usually not needed when the infant is receiving approximately 90 ml/kg/day or more of feedings, because of the buffering effect of milk.

Consider converting from IV to PO ranitidine as soon as the infant is able to take oral medications, to reduce cost of therapy.

Unlike cimetidine, ranitidine is not likely to increase the half-life and serum concentrations of theophylline, caffeine, and other drugs metabolized in the liver, although idiosyncratic reactions have occurred in some patients.

Interactions: Absorption of ranitidine is decreased slightly when it is given with antacids; doses should be staggered. Food does not affect ranitidine absorption.

(Zenk: Neonatal Medications & Nutrition. A Comprehensive Guide 2000; pp.419-421)

<u>Ranitidine</u>
Therapy for Reflux

Common doses: 4-5 mg/kg/day divided bid to tid

Partial list of side effects:

similar to cimetidine, less gynecomastia, more hepatitis

(Wyllie: Pediatric Gastrointestinal Disease 1999, p.180)

<u>Ranitidine</u>

Usual Dosage: Premature and Term Infants <2 weeks:
Oral: 2 mg/kg/day divided every 12 hours

I.V.: 1.5 mg/kg/dose as loading dose, then 12 hours later maintenance dose of 1.5 mg/kg/day divided every 12 hours

Continuous infusion: 1.5 mg/kg/dose as loading dose followed by 0.04 mg/kg/hour infusion (or 1 mg/kg/day)

(Taketomo: Pediatric Dosage Handbook 1999-2000, pp.788-790)

<u>Ranitidine HCl</u> (Zantac)

Dose & Route: Neonates:
PO: 2-4 mg/kg/24 hr ÷ Q8-12 hr
IV: 2 mg/kg/24 hr ÷ Q6-8 hr

Infants and Children:
PO: 4-5 mg/kg/24 hr ÷ Q8-12 hr
Max dose: 6 mg/kg/24 hr
IM/IV: 2-4 mg/kg/24 hr ÷ Q6-8 hr

Continuous infusion, all ages: Administer daily IV dosage over 24 hr (may be added to parenteral nutrition solutions)

Remarks: May cause headache and GI disturbance, malaise, insomnia, sedation, arthralgia, hepatotoxicity, May increase levels of nifedipine. May decrease levels of ketoconazole, itraconazole, delavirdine. Extemporaneously compounded carbohydrate-free oral solution dosage form useful for patients receiving the ketogenic diet. **Adjust dose in renal failure**.

(Siberry: The Harriet Lane Handbook 2000, p.837)

RESPIRATORY SYNCYTIAL VIRUS IMMUNE GLOBULIN INTRAVENOUS (HUMAN) [RSV-IGIV] (RespiGam)

Supplied: Injection 2500 mg RSV Immunoglobulin
Administration: IV infusion
The maximum recommended total dosage per monthly infusion is 750 mg/kg, administered according to the following schedule.

RSV-IGIV Infusion Schedule	
Time after start of infusion	Rate of infusion (mL/kg of body mass per hour)
0-15 minutes	1.5 mL/kg/hr
15-30 minutes	3 mL/kg/hr
30 minutes to end of infusion	6 mL/kg/hr

Incompatibility: It is recommended that RSV-IGIV be administered separately from other drugs or medications that the patient may be receiving (1).

<u>Respiratory Syncytial Immune Globulin Intravenous</u> (RSV-IGIV)
Prevention of RSV Infections.
Two products are available to prevent RSV infection: Respiratory Syncytial Virus Immune Globulin Intravenous (RSV-IGIV), prepared from donors selected for high serum titers of RSV neutralizing antibody, and palivizumab, a humanized mouse monoclonal antibody that is given intramuscularly. Both have been approved for prevention of RSV disease in children younger than 24 months of age with bronchopulmonary dysplasia or with a history of premature birth (<35 weeks' gestation). Neither RSV-IGIV nor palivizumab has been approved for treatment of RSV infection. RSV-IGIV is given once per month just before

the monthly throughout the RSV season at a dose of 15 mL/kg (750 mg/kg). Palivizumab is administered intramuscularly in a dose of 15 mg/kg once a month during RSV season.

Recommendations by the American Academy of Pediatrics for the use of palivizumab and RSV-IGIV are as follows:

- Palivizumab or RSV-IGIV prophylaxis should be considered for infants and children younger than 2 years of age with chronic lung disease (CLD) who have required medical therapy for CLD within 6 months before the anticipated RSV season. Palivizumab is preferred for most high-risk children because of its ease of administration, safety, and effectiveness. Patients with more severe CLD may benefit from prophylaxis for 2 RSV seasons, especially those who require medical therapy. Decisions about individual patients may need additional consultation from neonatologists, intensivists, or pulmonologists. There are limited data on the efficacy of palivizumab during the second year of age; risk of severe RSV disease exists for children with CLD who require medical therapy. Although children with less severe underlying disease may receive some benefit for the second season, immunoprophylaxis may not be necessary.

- Infants born at 32 weeks of gestation or earlier without CLD or who do not meet the aforementioned criteria also may benefit from RSV prophylaxis. For these infants, major risk factors to consider are gestational age and chronologic age at the start of the RSV season. Infants born at 28 weeks of gestation or earlier may benefit from prophylaxis up to 12 months of age. Infants born at 29 to 32 weeks of gestation may benefit most from prophylaxis up to 6 months of age. Decisions about duration of prophylaxis should be individualized according to the duration of the RSV season. Pediatricians may wish to use RSV rehospitalization data from their own region to assist in the decision-making process.

- Given the large number of patients born between 32 and 35 weeks of gestation and the cost of the drug, the use of palivizumab and RSV IGIV in this population should be reserved for infants with additional risk factors until more data are available.

- Palivizumab and RSV-IGIV are not licensed by the US Food and Drug Administration for patients with congenital heart disease. (CHD). Available data indicate that RSV-IGIV is contraindicated in patients with cyanotic CHD. However, patients with CLD, who were born prematurely, or both, who meet the criteria in the first and second recommendations and who also have asymptomatic acyanotic CHD (eg, patent ductus arteriosus or ventricular septal defect) may benefit from prophylaxis.

- Palivizumab or RSV-IGIV prophylaxis has not been evaluated in randomized trials in immunocompromised children. Although specific recommendations for immunocompromised patients cannot be made, children with severe immunodeficiencies (eg, severe combined immunodeficiency or severe acquired immunodeficiency syndrome) may benefit from prophylaxis. If these infants and children are receiving standard IGIV monthly, physicians may consider substituting RSV-IGIV during the RSV season.
- Prophylaxis for RSV should be initiated at the onset of the RSV season and terminated at the end of the RSV season. In most areas of the United States, the usual time for the Beginning of RSV outbreaks is October to December, and termination is March to May, but regional differences occur. Physicians should consult with health departments or diagnostic virology laboratories in their area or the Centers for Disease Control and Prevention if such information is not available locally.
- The RSV is know to be transmitted in the hospital setting and to cause serious disease in high-risk infants. In high-risk hospitalized infants, the major means to prevent RSV disease is strict observance of infection control practices, including the use of rapid means to identify and segregate RSV-infected infants. If an RSV outbreak is documented in a high-risk unit (eg, pediatric intensive care unit), primary emphasis should be placed on proper infection control practices. The need for and efficacy of prophylaxis in these situations has not been evaluated.
- Palivizumab does not interfere with the response to vaccines.
    - In contrast, in infants and children receiving RSV-IGIV prophylaxis, immunization with measles-mumps-rubella and varicella vaccines should be deferred for 9 months after the last dose. The use of RSV-IGIV should not alter the primary immunization schedule for other routinely recommended vaccines. The manufacturer of RSV-IGIV has suggested that an additional dose of vaccine may be needed to assure an adequate immune response to DTaP (diphtheria and tetanus toxoids and acellular pertussis), *Haemophilus influenzae* b conjugate, and oral poliovirus vaccine, but more information is needed before recommendations can be made. The available data at this time do not support the need for

supplemental doses of any of these routinely administered vaccines.

(American Academy of Pediatrics: Report of the committee on Infectious Diseases. Red Book 2000, pp.485-487)

<u>Respiratory Syncytial Virus Immune Globulin</u>
(RSV-IVIG) (RespiGam)

Indications and use:
Prevention of serious lower respiratory tract infection from RSV. Consider prophylactic use of RSV-IGIV in patients <2 years old who have BPD and are receiving oxygen therapy or have received oxygen in the past 6 months, and infants with a gestational age of ≤32 weeks, even if there is no BPD. RSV-IGIV should not be given to infants with cyanotic congential heart disease because of safety concerns. Immunization with measles-containing vaccines should be delayed for 9 months after the last dose of RSV-IGIV, but no changes need to be made in all other routinely given vaccines (American Academy of Pediatrics: Respiratory syncytial virus immune globulin intravenous: indications for use. *Pediatrics* 1997;99:645). RSV-IGIV may be substituted for IGIV during the RSV season for severely immunocompromised infants and children who receive IGIV monthly.

Actions: Passive immunization to RSV. RSV-IGIV contains immunoglobulin G (IgG) that contains antibody to neutralize RSV pooled from adult human plasma having high titers of neutralizing antibody against RSV. Reduces the number of RSV hospitalizations. Reduces the frequency and severity of RSV infections by 40-60%

Pharmacokinetics: Mean half-life is 22-28 days.

Route: IV.

Dosage: 750 mg/kg (= 15 mL/kg) once per month during flu season (November-April). Infuse at 1.5 mL/kg/h for the first 15 min, then at 3 mL/kg/h for the next 15 min, then increase the rate to 6 mL/kg/h until the end of the infusion.

Monitor vital signs frequently during administration for increases in heart rate, respiratory rate, retractions, and rales; observe for fluid overload or allergic reaction during infusion. Furosemide should be available for management of fluid overload. If severe allergic reaction occurs, discontinue infusion and consider epinephrine.

Adverse effects: Many adverse effects relate to the rate of infusion. Respiratory distress, tachycardia, fever, allergic reactions, rash, gastroenteritis, local site inflammation, and fluid overload in fluid-sensitive patients. Aseptic meningitis syndrome may occur (rare). Do not use in patients who previously had severe reactions to human immunoglobulin preparations or in those with IgA deficiency or allergy to any component in the product.

(Gomella: Neonatology 1999, p.589)

RSV immune globulin

Dose/kg: 750 mg (15 mL)

Route & frequency: IV, monthly during RSV season
Administration guidelines:
1.5 mL/kg/h x 15 min
3 mL/kg/h x 15 min
6 mL/kg/h until finished

Comments: Not recommended for use in patients with cyanotic heart disease. Some patients may develop respiratory distress due to excessive fluid. Live vaccines should be delayed for 9 mo after administration.

(Avery: Neonatology Pathophysiology and Management of the Newborn 1999, p.1560)

Respiratory Syncytial Virus Immune Globulin

Dose & Route: RSV Prophylaxis:
Children <2 yrs: 750 mg/kg/dose IV Q monthly during the RSV season (typically November through April in the northern hemisphere but may begin earlier or persist later in certain communities).

Remarks: Although this product has a broad indication for use in children <2 yrs old with BPD or history of prematurity (<35 weeks' gestation), see latest version of the AAP Redbook for specific use recommendations. **Contraindicated** in Ig A deficiency. Should **not** be used in patients with cyanotic heart disease. Use with **caution** in patients with fluid restrictions. Frequent side effects include fever, respiratory distress, vomiting, and wheezing. Monitor heart rate, blood pressure, temperature, respiratory rate. Parenteral live virus vaccines (i.e., MMR, measles, varicella) should be deferred for 9-10 months after the last dose of RSVIG. Gradually increase IV infusion (if tolerated) by starting at 1.5 ml/kg/hr for 15 minutes, increase to 3 ml/kg/hr the next 15 minutes, then to 6 ml/kg/hr to the end of infusion.

(Siberry: The Harriet Lane Handbook 2000, pp.837-838)

Respiratory Syncytial Virus Immune Globulin

Usual Dosage: I.V. infusion: Infants and Young Children: 750 mg/kg once monthly during RSV season (starting November with the last infusion in April)

Administration: Infusion should start within 6 hours and be completed by 12 hours after vial entry; an in-line filter is not necessary, but if one issued, the pore size should be larger than 15 µM; if dilution is needed, a dilution of no greater than 1:2 should be used.

Monitoring Parameters:
Heart rate, blood pressure, temperature, respiratory rate observed for retractions and rales

Additional Information:
PREVENT (Prophylaxis of RSV in elevated-risk neonates trial) was a multicenter, randomized, double-blind, placebo-

controlled trial (n=250 RSV-IGIV, n=260 placebo) among infants ≤24 months, born prematurely (≤35 weeks gestation), or children with BPD and a requirement for supplemental oxygen within the past 6 months. Each patient received a monthly infusion from November through April. The trial showed that children treated with RSV-IGIV had less RSV hospitalizations (20 days vs. 35 days, p=0.047); fewer RSV hospital days per 100 days (60 days vs. 129 days, p=0.045); fewer RSV hospital days with supplemental oxygen (34 days vs. 85 days, p=0.007). There was no difference between the two groups for ICU admissions, RSV ICU days per 100 children, RSV mechanical ventilation or days of ventilation per 100 children. (Groothius, 1993)

(Taketomo: Pediatric Dosage Handbook 1999-2000, pp.791-792)

RIBAVIRIN (Virazole)

Supplied: Aerosol, powder for reconstitution; 6 gm 100ml vial
Administration: Aerosol administration

Contraindications: Pregnancy: Category X: Ribavirin has demonstrated significant teratogenic (malformation of skull, palate, eye, jaw, limbs, skeleton and GI tract) or embryocidal potential in all animal species in which adequate studies have been conducted. Ribavirin is toxic to lactating animals and their offspring. (1)

Ribavirin

Clinical Diagnosis: Respiratory syncytial virus infection (bronchiolitis, pneumonia)

Therapy: Ribavirin 6-g vial (20 mg/ml in sterile water) aerosolized by SPAG-2 generator over 18- to 20-hr period daily x 3-5 days

Comments: Treat only for severe disease or patients with underlying cardiopulmonary disease

(Nelson: Pocket Book of Pediatric Antimicrobial Therapy 2000-2001, p.30)

Ribavirin

Route & Dose: 6 g nebulized in hood with a solution of 20 mg/ml 12-18 h/day for 3-7 days

Adverse Effects and Cautions:
May precipitate in endotracheal tube; avoid exposure of pregnant staff; possible teratogenic effects

(Taeusch: Avery's Diseases of the Newborn 1998, p.1347)

Ribavirin

Dose & Route: Inhalation:
Continuous: Administer 6 g by aerosol over 12-18 hr QD for 3-7 days. The 6 g ribavirin vial is diluted in 300 ml preservative-free sterile water to a final concentration of 20 mg/ml. Must be administered with Viratek Small Particle Aerosol Generator (SPAG-2).

Intermittent (For non-ventilated patients): Administer 2 g by aerosol over 2 hours TID for 3-7 days. The 6 g ribavirin vial is diluted in 100 ml preservative-free sterile water to a final concentration of 60 mg/ml. Use not recommended in patients with endotracheal tubes.

Remarks: Use of ribavirin in RSV is controversial. Ribavirin aerosol therapy is a consideration for selected infants and young children at high risk for serious RSV disease (see Redbook for details). Most effective if begun early in course of RSV infection; generally in the first 3 days. May cause worsening respiratory distress, rash, conjunctivitis, mild bronchospasm, hypotension, anemia, and cardiac arrest. Respiratory therapy and nursing personnel should be trained in ribavirin administration because of it teratogenic effects in animals. Drug can precipitate in the respiratory equipment.

(Siberry: The Harriet Lane Handbook 2000, p.839)

<u>Ribavirin</u>

Usual Dosage: Infants, Children: Aerosol inhalation:

Use with Viratek small particle aerosol generator (SPAG-2) at a concentration of 20 mg/mL (6 g reconstituted with 300 mL of sterile water without preservatives); 6 g ribavirin vial has also been diluted with 300 mL of sterile 0.9% sodium chloride solution rather than sterile water to achieve a near isotonic solution.

Note: Dose actually delivered to the patient will depend on patient's minute ventilation

Continuous aerosolization: 12-18 hours/day for 3 days, or up to 7 days in length

Intermittent aerosolization (high dose, short-duration aerosol): 2 g over 2 hours 3 times/day at a concentration of 60 mg/mL (6 g reconstituted with 100 mL of sterile water without preservatives) in **non-mechanically ventilated** patients for 3-7 days has been used to permit easier accessibility for patient care and limit environmental exposure of healthcare worker. Due to apparent increased potential for crystallization of the high-dose 60 mg/mL solution around areas of turbulent flow such as bends in tubing or connector pieces, use of high-dose therapy in individuals with an endotracheal tube in place is **not** recommended.

Administration: Mechanically ventilated patients: Ribavirin can potentially be deposited in the ventilator delivery system depending on temperature, humidity, and electrostatic forces; this deposition can lead to malfunction or obstruction of the expiratory valve, resulting in inadvertently high positive end-expiratory pressures. The use of on-way valves in the inspiratory lines, a breathing circuit filter in the expiratory line, and frequent monitoring and filter replacement have been effective in preventing these problems.

Monitoring Parameters: Respiratory function, hemoglobin, reticulocyte count, CBC, I & O

Nursing Implications:

Healthcare workers who are pregnant or who may become pregnant should be advised of the potential risks of exposure and counseled about risk reduction strategies including alternate job responsibilities; limit contact by visitors with patients receiving ribavirin, ribavirin may adsorb to contact lenses

Additional Information:

RSV season is usually December to April; viral shedding period for RSV is usually 3-8 days

(Taketomo: Pediatric Dosage Handbook 1999-2000, pp.795-797)

RIFAMPIN (Rifadin, Rimactane)

Supplied: Capsules 150mg, 300mg
Injection, Powder for 600mg vial

Administration: PO, IV

PREPARATION of extemporaneous oral suspension: (Hoechst Marion Roussel Pharmaceuticals) Content 10mg/ml. Empty contents of 4 rifampin 300mg (or 8 rifampin 150mg) capsules into a 4-ounce amber bottle and add 20ml Simple Syrup (Syrup, NF). Shake vigorously. Add 100ml of Simple Syrup. Shake again. This suspension is stable for 4 weeks when stored at room temperature or in refrigerator (1).

IV injection is stable at room temperature for 24 hours at a concentration of 60 mg/ml. Dilute further with D5W. Sterile saline may be used when dextrose is contraindicated, but the stability of rifampin is slightly reduced (1).

<u>Extemporaneous Compounding (Recipe)</u>

Dosage form: Oral suspension
Made from: Capsules
Concentration: 10 mg/mL
Stability: 56 days
Store: Refrigerate
Label: Shake well

Ingredient	Strength	Quantity
Rifampin capsules	300 mg	4
Syrup		qs ad 120 mL

Instructions: Mix the contents of the capsules with a small amount of syrup in a mortar. Then qs to volume with syrup in a graduate. (11)

Rifampin

Antibacterial Drugs for Pediatric Patients Beyond the Newborn Period

Dosage per kg/d

Route: PO

Mild to Moderate Infections: 10-20 mg in 1-2 doses

Severe Infections: 20 mg in 2 doses

Comments: Should not be used as monotherapy except when given for prophylaxis

Route: IV

Mild to Moderate Infections: 10-20 mg in 1-2 doses

Severe Infections: 20 mg in 2 doses

(American Academy of Pediatrics: Report of the Committee on Infectious Diseases. Red Book 2000, p.660)

Rifampin

Route: PO, IV

Dosage (mg/kg) and Interval of Administration:

Weight 1200-2000 g

Age 0-7 Days: 10 q24h

Age >7 Days: 10 q24h

Weight >2000 g

Age 0-7 Days: 10 q24h

Age >7 Days: 10 q24h

(Remington: Infectious Diseases of the Fetus and Newborn Infant 2001, p.1454)

Rifampin

Antituberculosis Drugs in Children

Daily Dose (mg/kg)	Twice Weekly Dose (mg/kg/per dose)
10-20	10-20

In many patients receiving RIF treatment, the tears, saliva, urine, and stool turn orange as a result of a harmless metabolite, and the patient and parents always must be warned of this in advance. RIF can be made into a suspension easily for use in children. RIF is very well tolerated by neonates and infants. The incidences of hepatitis, leukopenia, and thrombocytopenia are extremely low. RIF should be used alone only when treating *M. tuberculosis* infection due to an INH-resistant organism. If one uses INH, 20 mg/kg, and RIF, 15 to 20 mg/kg, there is an appreciable incidence of hepatoxicity. Therefore, when using the two together, one would be wise to approximate INH, 10 mg/kg, and RIF, 15 to 20 mg/kg.

(Remington: Infectious Diseases of the Fetus and Newborn Infant 2001, p.1188)

Rifampin

Route: PO, IV

Dosage: 10-20 mg/kg/day q12-24h (max 600 mg)

NON-NEWBORN SECTION

(Nelson: Pocket Book of Pediatric Antimicrobial Therapy 2000-2001, p.83)

Rifampin (Rifadin, Rimactane)

Action and spectrum:
A broad-spectrum antibiotic that exerts its bacteriostatic action by inhibiting DNA-dependent RNA polymerase activity. Effective against mycobacteria, *Neisseria* spp, and Gram-positive cocci (eg, staphylococci). Resistance develops rapidly, so the drug should always be used in combination with other agents for synergistic effect.

Route: PO, IV

Dosage: 10-20 mg/kg/day divided q12h

Elimination and metabolism: Hepatic. Half-life is ~3 hours.

Adverse effects: GI irritation (anorexia, vomiting, diarrhea), hypersensitivity (rash, pruritus, eosinophilia), drowsiness, ataxia, blood dyscrasias (leukopenia, thrombocytopenia, hemolytic anemia), hepatitis (rare), elevation of serum urea nitrogen and uric acid levels. Causes pink to red discoloration of urine.

Comments: Crosses into CSF. When used, it should always be used in combination with other agents to provide synergistic effect (eg, vancomycin hydrochloride plus gentamicin sulfate, with or without rifampin, for infection with vancomycin-resistant or tolerant staphylococci).

Note: A potent enzyme inducer of hepatic metabolism. Patients receiving phenytoin, phenobarbital, or theophylline may have a substantial decrease in serum concentration of these drugs after starting rifampin. Careful monitoring of serum drug concentrations is necessary.

(Gomella: Neonatology 1999, p.590)

Rifampin (Rimactane, Rifadin)

Dose & Route: Tuberculosis:
Twice weekly therapy may be used after 1-2 months of daily therapy
Children:
Daily therapy: 10-20 mg/kg/24 hr ÷ Q12-24 hr IV/PO
Twice weekly therapy: 10-20 mg/kg/24 hr PO twice weekly
Max daily dose: 600 mg/24 hr

Prophylaxis for N. meningitidis:
0-1 mo: 10 mg/kg/24 hr ÷ Q12 hr PO x 2 days
>1 mo: 20 mg/kg/24 hr ÷ Q12 hr PO x 2 days
Max dose (all ages): 1200 mg/24 hr

Prophylaxis for H. influenzae:
0-1 mo: 10 mg/kg/dose PO QD x 4 days
>1 mo: 20 mg/kg/dose PO QD x 4 days
Max dose (all ages): 600 mg/24 hr

Remarks: May cause GI irritation, allergy, headache, fatigue, ataxia, confusion, fever, hepatitis, blood dyscrasias, interstitial nephritis, and elevated BUN and uric acid. Causes red discoloration of body secretions such as urine, saliva, and tears (which can permanently stain contact lenses). Induces hepatic enzymes (CYP 450 2C9, 2C19, and 3A4) which may decrease plasma concentration of digoxin, corticosteroids, benzodiazepines, calcium channel blockers, beta-blockers, cyclosporine, oral anticoagulants, barbiturates, and theophylline. May reduce the effectiveness of oral contraceptives. Reduce dose in hepatic impairment. Give 1 hour before or 2 hour after meals. **Adjust dose in renal failure**.

(Siberry: The Harriet Lane Handbook 2000, 841)

ROCURONIUM BROMIDE (Zemuron)

Supplied: Injection 10 mg/ml in 5 ml vials

Administration: For IV use only, direct IV injection, continuous infusion Rocuronium injection is a nondepolarizing neuromuscular blocking agent with a rapid to intermediate onset (depending on dose) and intermediate duration (1).

The use of rocuronium in children < 3 months of age has not been studied (1).

Children administration: Initial doses of 0.6 mg/kg in children under halothane anesthesia produces excellent to good intubating conditions within 1 minute. This dose will provide a median time of clinical relaxation of 41 minutes (range, 24-68) in 3 months to 1 year old children and 27 minutes (range, 17-41) in 1-12 year-old children. Maintenance doses of 0.075 mg to 0.125 mg/kg administered upon return of T1 to 25% of control, provide clinical relaxation for 7-10 min (1).

<u>Rocuronium</u>

Dose & Route: Children:
IV: Start with 0.6-1.2 mg/kg/dose x 1 if needed, maintenance doses at 0.1-0.2 mg/kg/dose Q 20-30 min.

Continuous IV Infusion: Start at 10-12 mcg/kg/min and titrate to effect.

Remarks: Hypertension, hypotension, arrhythmia, tachycardia, nausea, vomiting, bronchospasm, wheezing, hiccups, rash and edema at the injection site may occur. Increased neuromuscular blockade may occur with concomitant use of aminoglycosides, clindamycin, tetracycline, magnesium sulfate, quinine, quinidine, succinylcholine, and inhalation anesthetics. Carbamazepine, phenytoin, phenylephrine, azathioprine, and theophylline may reduce neuromuscular blocking effects.

Peak effects occur in 0.5-1 min for children and in 1-3.7 min for adults. Duration of action: 30-40 minutes in children and 20-94 minutes in adults (longer in geriatrics). Recovery time in children 3 months to 1 year is similar to adults. In obese patients, use actual body weight for dosage calculation.

(Siberry: The Harriet Lane handbook 2000, pp.843-844)

<u>Rocuronium</u>

Neuromuscular Blocking Drug:

Initial dose 0.6 mg/kg, incremental doses 0.15 mg/kg.
Infusion rate 10-12 μg/kg/min.

(Steward: Manual of Pediatric Anesthesia 1995, p.512)

SAFFLOWER OIL

Modular component for supplementing neonatal feeds:

Calories: 8.3 cal/ml
Fat: 0.93 gm/ml
Provides essential fatty acids and fat soluble vitamin. Will not increase osmolarity. Excessive amounts may cause steatorrhea. 1 Tbsp = 15 ml = 14 gm = 124 cal.

(Ohio Neonatal Nutritionists: Nutritional Care for High Risk Newborns 1985, p.40)

SECOBARBITAL (Seconal)

Supplied: 100 mg capsule
Administration: PO

<u>Secobarbital</u>

Dosage: 2-5 mg/kg/dose every 6-8 hr as needed IV
(Fanaroff: Neonatal-Perinatal Medicine 1997, p.1752)

<u>Secobarbital</u>

Usual Dosage: Neonates: Sedation for neonates receiving mechanical ventilation: Limited information is available; one study (Nahata, 1991) assessed secobarbital dosing and prolonged sedation (sedation >24 hours after the last dose) in 17 ventilated infants (GA 30-40 weeks; PNA 0-3 days) who received secobarbital 4-14 mg/kg/day I.V. for 1-10 days for sedation; duration of sedation after the last dose increased with higher daily doses and with the total cumulative dose; the authors recommend that initial daily doses should not exceed 7 mg/kg/day to avoid prolonged sedation; further studies are needed.

Administration: I.V.: Administer undiluted or diluted with SWI, NS or Ringer's injection; maximum infusion rate: 50 mg/15 seconds; avoid intra-arterial injection.

Rectal: Commercial rectal formulations are no longer available in the U.S.; the I.V. product has been diluted with water to a concentration of 10-15 mg/mL and administered rectally.

Monitoring Parameters:
Blood pressure, heart rate, respiratory rate, pulse oximetry, CNS status.

(Taketomo: Pediatric Dosage Handbook 2000-2001; pp.861-863)

SELENIUM

Supplied: Injection 40 mcg/ml, in 10 ml, 30* ml, vials
* with benzyl alcohol

<u>Selenium</u>

Infants were eligible for study if they had a birth weight < 1500 g, were born in or were transferred to the participating center by 72 hours of age, and had no major congenital abnormalities. In a double-blinded fashion infants randomized to treatment received 7 µg/kg/d of sodium selenate added to the amino acid solution when fed parenterally and 5 µg/kg/d of sodium selenite (0.5 mL/kg of a colorless 10 µg/mL solution) when fed enterally. Infants randomized to P received no parenteral supplement and 0.5 mL/kg of sterile water when fed enterally. Infants changed from parenteral to oral SE supplements when tolerating 3 mL/h or equivalent feeds. Supplements were continued until 36 weeks' postmenstrual age or discharge home, if earlier. SE solutions and placebo were supplied by Biomed, Auckland, New Zealand.

Conclusion: Postnatal SE supplementation in very low birth weight infants did not improve neonatal outcome. Further investigation of SE supplementation of mothers from the second half of pregnancy is warranted.

(Darlow: The effect of selenium supplementation on outcome in very low birth weight infants: A randomized controlled trial. J Pediatr 2000;136:473-80)

SILVER NITRATE

Supplied: Ophthalmic solution 1% in wax ampules

Administration: Ophthalmic

Immediately after birth, clean the child's eyelids with sterile absorbent cotton or gauze, and sterile water. Use a separate pledget for each eye; wash unopened lids from the nose outward until free of blood, mucus, or meconium. Next, separate the lids and instill 2 drops of 1% solution. Elevate lids away from the eyeball so that a lake of silver nitrate may lie for ≥ 30 seconds between them, contacting the entire conjunctival sac. The American Academy of Pediatrics has endorsed a statement from the Committee on Opthalmia Neonatorum of the National Society for the Prevention of Blindness, which does not recommend irrigation of the eyes following instillation of the silver nitrate(1).

Staining: handle solutions carefully because they tend to stain skin and utensils. Stains may be removed from linen by applications of iodine tincture followed by sodium thiosulfate solution.

Silver Nitrate

Prevention of Neonatal Ophthalmia

Gonococcal Ophthalmia.

For newborn infants, topical **1% silver nitrate solution**, 0.5% erythromycin ointment, and 1% tetracycline ointment are considered equally effective for prophylaxis of ocular gonorrheal infection. Each is available in single-dose tubes. Povidone-iodine in a 2.5% solution also might be useful for preventing gonococcal ophthalmia, but more studies are required, and a product for this purpose currently is not available in the United States. Silver nitrate causes more chemical conjunctivitis than other agents but is recommended in areas where the incidence of penicillinase-producing *Neisseria gonorrhoeae* (PPNG) is appreciable. The efficacy of erythromycin or povidone-iodine prophylaxis against PPNG is not known; 1 study has demonstrated tetracycline to be effective for prophylaxis of PPNG infections. Infants born to women with untreated gonococcal infection should receive 1 dose of ceftriaxone (25-50 mg/kg) or cefotaxime (100 mg/kg), as well as topical prophylaxis. Infants who have gonococcal ophthalmia should be hospitalized and evaluated for signs of disseminated infection.

Chlamydial Ophthalmia.
Neonatal ophthalmia due to *Chlamydia trachomatis*, although not as severe as gonococcal conjunctivitis, is common in the United States. Results of studies on the clinical efficacy of erythromycin and of tetracycline ointment for prophylaxis of chlamydial conjunctivitis have been conflicting. Topical antibiotics and **silver nitrate** do not have proven efficacy in preventing conjunctivitis or nasopharyngeal colonization. One study has shown that 2.5% povidone-iodine is likely to be more effective than either topical erythromycin or **silver nitrate** for preventing chlamydial conjunctivitis but does not prevent nasopharyngeal colonization and subsequent risk of pneumonia. Infants with ophthalmia neonatorum caused by *C trachomatis* should be evaluated and treated.

(American Academy of Pediatrics: Report of the Committee on Infectious Diseases. Red Book 2000, pp.735-736)

Silver nitrate (1% solution)

Route & Dose: Prophylaxis: 1 or 2 drops each eye
Adverse Effects and Cautions: Chemical conjunctivitis
(Taeusch: Avery's Diseases of the Newborn 1998, p. 1347)

Silver Nitrate

Use: Prevention of gonococcal ophthalmia neonatorum; cauterization of wounds and sluggish ulcers, removal of granulation tissue and warts

Usual Dosage: Neonates: Ophthalmic: Instill 2 drops immediately after birth into conjunctival sac of each eye as a single dose; do not irrigate eyes following instillation of eye drops; silver nitrate prophylaxis should be administered immediately after delivery or no later than 1 hours after delivery

(Taketomo: Pediatric Dosage Handbook 1999-2000, p.820)

Silver Nitrate, 1% Solution

Route: Topical

Neonatal Dose: 2 drops in each eye prophylactically.

Discussion: Rinsing eyes with water or NS does not reduce chemical conjunctivitis; but may reduce effectiveness.

(Rudolph: Rudolph's Pediatrics 1996, p.2203)

SILVER SULFADIAZINE (Silvadene Cream)

Supplied: Cream 1% in 20, 50, 400 gm.
Administration: Topical.

Silver Sulfadiazine

Dose & Route: Cover affected areas completely QD-BID. Apply cream to a thickness of 1/16" using sterile technique.

Remarks: **Contraindicated** in premature infants and infant ≤ to 2 months of age due to concerns of kernicterus. Discard product if cream has darkened. Adverse effects include pruritus, rash, bone marrow suppression, and hemolytic anemia, as well as interstitial nephritis.

(Siberry: The Harriet Lane Handbook 2000, p.848)

Silver Sulfadiazine (Silvadene Cream)

Silver sulfadiazine is bacterial against both gram-negative and gram-positive organisms. It is used primarily as an adjunct in the prevention and treatment of infection in burn patients. In addition, it does not bind with chloride ions, thereby eliminating potential electrolyte and acid-base disturbances. Transient leukopenia, occurring after 2 to 3 days of treatment, has been seen in many patients treated with silver sulfadiazine. Despite continued use, the leukopenia generally resolves in a few days.

(Yeh: Neonatal Therapeutics 1991, p.377)

SEE ALSO: CORD CARE

SIMETHICONE (Mylicon)

Supplied: Drops 40mg/0.6ml, in 30ml with calibrated dropper.
Administration: PO

Simethicone (Mylicon)

Dose: 20 mg/0.3 ml with each feeding every 3-6 hours

Use: For relief of intestinal gas and painful symptoms of gastric bloating.

Infantile Colic: Results of investigations of the efficacy of simethicone in treating infantile colic are mixed. A placebo-controlled, multicenter trial found simethicone to be no better than placebo in the treatment of infantile colic. Two other studies also showed no improvement in symptoms. However, Sethi and Sethi did find efficacy in its use, as did Becker and colleagues, who reported efficacy in 44 of 51 infants treated.

Nursing Implications:

Shake well before use.

Monitor for a decrease in symptoms such as crying, fussiness, and intestinal gas.

Discontinue if there is no improvement after about 48 hours.

(Zenk: Neonatal Medications & Nutrition. A Comprehensive Guide 2000; pp.435-436)

Simethicone

Dose & Route: Infants and Children <2 yrs: 20 mg PO QID; **max dose**: 240 mg/24 hr

Remarks: Avoid carbonated beverage and gas-forming foods. Oral liquid may be mixed with water, infant formula, or other suitable liquids for ease of oral administration.

(Siberry: The Harriet Lane Handbook 2000, pp.848-849)

Simethicone

Route: PO

Neonatal Dose: Colic: 20 mg/dose 3-4 times daily 30 min before feedings; may increase to 40-80 mg/dose if no response

Pediatric Dose: 40-80 mg/dose 4 times daily after meals and at bedtime

Discussion: There are no reported adverse effects, contraindications, or warnings for simethicone

(Rudolph: Rudolph's Pediatrics 1996, p.2203)

SKIN and CORD CARE

Skin and Cord Care

Every effort should be made to promote colonization of the newborn with normal flora and to impede colonization with nosocomial pathogens. This is easier said than done, especially in the NICU. To do so, multiple methods of skin and cord care have been evaluated. These practices are divided into measures taken in the delivery room and daily routines in the nursery. Several approaches to skin and cord care have been used, but no optimal procedures have been recommended until recently. Lund and colleagues reviewed the literature addressing the care of neonatal skin and created a new and comprehensive practice guideline for clinicians, which is in the process of being evaluated in 58 sites in the United States. Excessive drying, manipulation, exposure to irritating chemicals, or other trauma (e.g., adhesive tape) should be avoided to reduce the risk of damage to newborn skin. The skin of the premature infant is particularly fragile. Bathing should be postponed until the neonate's thermal stability is ensured.

After initial observation and stabilization of the newborn, meconium and blood may be wiped off with sterile cotton sponges soaked with warm water to remove potential blood-borne pathogens such as HBV or HIV and other contaminating microorganisms such as HSV. Personnel should wear gloves until cleaning is complete. The skin should be carefully dried to minimize further heat loss. Except for cleaning and bathing as needed with water alone or a mild soap, the skin and cord may be kept dry for the rest of the hospital stay. The gelatinous skin of extremely immature neonates should be cleaned with sterile water and only when necessary. The effectiveness of Aquafor ointment (Beiersdorf, Norwalk, Conn) in protecting neonatal skin and reducing nosocomial infections is being studied.

Whole-body bathing and antiseptic soaps are not necessary for routine care, but they may be indicated in outbreaks or when the endemic rate of infection is high. Various antiseptic compounds for skin care have been studied to determine their safety and efficacy in preventing colonization and infection in neonates. The most frequently used compounds capable of reducing bacterial colonization of the skin are iodophors, hexachlorophene, and chlorhexidine. Hexachlorophene, although relatively effective against gram-positive bacteria, is no longer recommended for routine daily bathing of newborns and is now seldom used in any circumstance in premature neonates because of its neurotoxicity when absorbed. It may be useful as an alternative for term infants for control of *S. aureus* outbreaks. It should be used for limited number of baths at a concentration of no more than 3% and should be carefully rinsed off after bathing.

Preparations containing chlorhexidine, a compound that is poorly absorbed through intact skin, may be less toxic than hexachlorophene and have been found to be useful for bathing or for localized skin care. Chlorhexidine has also been used in outbreak control. It is less effective than hexachlorophene for *S. aureus* but more effective for gram-negative bacilli. Iodophor detergents, widely used for surgical scrubs and nursery hand washing, are not recommended for routine bathing or cord care. Staining of the infant's skin with iodine is unattractive, and iodine-containing compounds may suppress neonatal thyroid function. The benefits of using an antiseptic agent for bathing should be weighed against the risk of toxicity.

No single method of cord care has proved to be superior in preventing colonization and disease. The cord should be cut and tied using aseptic technique. Dry cord care is an acceptable regimen. A number of studies have evaluated the effectiveness of antimicrobial agents in cord care. Isopropyl alcohol, which is often applied daily or even more frequently during the hospitalization and after discharge, may accelerate drying and separation of the cord but does not affect colonization. Triple dye (2.29 g of brilliant green, 1.14 g of proflavine hemisulfate, and 2.29 g of crystal violet per liter in an aqueous solution) delays drying and cord separation for 7 to 10 days and inhibits colonization, but colonization of the cord after discontinuation of its use can, of course, occur. In one NICU study, triple dye was shown to delay but not prevent colonization with MRSA, but in another report, application of triple dye after umbilical vessel catheterization in the first 12 hours after birth was instrumental in controlling a prolonged MRSA outbreak. Chlorhexidine cord care has been reported to be effective in reducing colonization and infection. Topical mupirocin was shown to be effective in an outbreak of MRSA when applied to the cord and nares of infants in a special care unit. Short-term use of mupirocin ointment for control of an outbreak associated with susceptible *S. aureus* or MRSA may be considered, but prolonged use has been associated with the emergence of resistant strains. Other agents that have been studied include bacitracin ointment and silver sulfadiazine cream. The literature on cord care is confusing and inconsistent, as pointed out by a recent meta-analysis.

(Remington: Infectious Diseases of the Fetus and Newborn Infant 2001, pp.1392-1393)

<u>Skin Care</u>

Skin care, including bathing, may be important for the health and appearance of the individual neonate and for infection control within the nursery. The first bath should be postponed until the neonate's thermal stability is ensured. The medical and nursing services of each hospital should develop guidelines regarding the time of the first bath, circumstances and method of skin cleansing, and the roles of personnel and parents.

Effects on the neonate's skin should be considered in selecting skin care techniques. Some agents are absorbed and may be toxic; others change skin flora and may increase the risk of infection. Whole-body bathing of the neonate may not be necessary. Localized skin care or techniques that minimize exposure to water may reduce the neonate's heat loss. Sterile cotton sponges (not gauze) soaked with warm water may be used to remove blood and meconium from the neonate's face, head, and body. Alternatively, the baby can be cleaned with a mild, nonmedicated soap and then rinsed with water. Careful drying of the neonate's skin and removal of blood after birth may minimize the risk of infection with potentially contaminating microorganisms, such as hepatitis B virus, herpes simplex virus, and HIV. If the neonate's skin is not grossly soiled, it may not require much cleansing.

For the remainder of the neonate's stay in the hospital nursery, the buttocks and perianal regions should be cleansed with fresh water and cotton, with a mild soap and water, at diaper changes. The gelatinous skin of extremely immature neonates should be cleaned with sterile water and only when necessary. Ideally, agents used on the newborn's skin should be dispensed in single-use containers, or each neonate should have a personal dispenser.

Various antiseptic compounds for skin care have been studied to determine their safety and effectiveness in preventing colonization and infection in neonates. Hexachlorophene, although relatively effective against gram-positive bacteria, particularly Staphylococcus aureus, should not be used routinely for bathing neonates because of its potential for neurotoxic effects in neonates. Although iodophores are good antiseptics, they have not been proved both safe and effective for routine skin care. Chlorhexidine gluconate, a compound that is poorly absorbed through intact skin, is useful for bathing or for localized skin care.

(AAP/ACOG: Guidelines for Perinatal Care 1997, pp.158-159)

Cord Care

No single method of cord care has proved to be superior in preventing colonization and disease. Current methods include the local application of antimicrobial agents, such as bacitracin, or of triple dye agents. The skin absorption and toxicity of triple dye agents in newborns have not been carefully studied. Alcohol is probably not effective in preventing cord colonization and omphalitis.

(AAP/ACOG: Guidelines for Perinatal Care 1997, p.159)

SEE ALSO: PETROLATUM OINTMENT

SODIUM ACETATE

Supplied: Injection 2 mEq/ml and 4 mEq/ml

Administration: IV (Dilute prior to use).
The acetate ion is metabolized to bicarbonate almost on an equimolar basis. Metabolism occurs outside the liver (1).

Sodium Acetate

Use: Sodium salt replacement; correction of acidosis through conversion of acetate to bicarbonate

Adverse Reactions:

Cardiovascular: Thrombosis, hypervolemia, edema, cerebral hemorrhage
Endocrine & metabolic: Hypernatremia, hypokalemic metabolic alkalosis, hypocalcemia
Local: Extravasant, local cellulitis
Respiratory: Pulmonary edema

Usual Dosage: Sodium acetate is metabolized to bicarbonate on an equimolar basis outside the liver; administer in large volume I.V. fluids as a sodium source. Dosage is dependent upon the clinical condition, fluid, electrolytes and acid-base balance of the patient.

Maintenance sodium requirements: I.V.:
Neonates, Infants, and Children: 3-4 mEq/kg/day; maximum dose: 100-150 mEq/day

Metabolic acidosis: if sodium acetate is desired over sodium bicarbonate, the amount of acetate may be dosed utilizing the equation found in the sodium bicarbonate monograph as each mEq acetate is converted to a mEq of HCO_3

Administration: Parenteral: Must be diluted prior to I.V. administration; infuse hypertonic solutions (>154 mEq/L) via a central line; maximum rate of administration: 1 mEq/kg/hour

Monitoring Parameters:
Serum electrolytes including calcium, arterial blood gases (if indicated)

(Taketomo: Pediatric Dosage Handbook 2000-2001; p.869)

Sodium Acetate

The continuous infusion of sodium acetate appears to be suitable for the slow correction of metabolic acidosis, and the daily sodium supply of 3 mEq/kg gives a stable serum sodium concentration in the premature infant with a gestational age of no more than 34 weeks.

(Ekblad: Slow sodium acetate infusion in the correction of metabolic acidosis in premature infants. Am J Dis Child 1985;139:708-710)

SODIUM BENZOATE

Supplied: Powder

Sodium Benzoate

Use: Adjunctive therapy for the prevention and treatment of hyperammonemia due to suspected or proven urea cycle defects

Adverse Reactions:
Endocrine & metabolic: Metabolic acidosis
Gastrointestinal: Nausea, vomiting

Usual Dosage: Investigational use (not FDA approved): Children; Oral, I.V.: 0.25 g/kg bolus followed by 0.25-0.5 g/kg/day as continuous infusion or divided every 6-8 hours

Monitoring Parameters: Serum ammonia level

Additional Information:
Used to treat urea cycle enzyme deficiency in combination with arginine; not available commercially; oral solutions must be compounded using chemical powder form; I.V. solutions must also be compounded and tested for sterility and pyrogenicity prior to use

(Taketomo: Pediatric Dosage Handbook 1999-2000, p.823)

Sodium Benzoate

Definitions:
CPS = Carbamyl phosphate synthetase I
OTC = Ornithine transcarbamylase
UCD = Urea Cycle Disorder

Recommendation:

The labeling for intravenous sodium benzoate and sodium phenylacetate should be modified to include a new indication for the treatment of patients with argininosuccinic aciduria.

Rationale: Clinical experience indicates that these drugs are helpful in reducing ammonia in this condition, acting by a mechanism different from that of arginine.

Recommendation:

Intravenous arginine-HCL and sodium benzoate/sodium phenylacetate should be available in hospitals where patients with UCD are treated.

Rationale: These medications are not routinely available and may be required on an emergency basis to treat patients with acute hyperammonemia.

Recommendation:

Where available, plasma levels of ammonia scavenging drugs should be monitored to avoid toxicity.

Rationale: Variable drug excretion may cause toxicity. In the absence of drug levels, a serum anion gap of >15 mEq/L and an anion gap that has risen >6 mEq/L could indicate drug accumulation and increased risk for toxicity.

(The Urea Cycle Disorders Conference Group: Consensus statement from a conference for the Management of Patients with Urea cycle Disorders. J Pediatr 2001;138:S1-S5)

Benzoate

For Nonketotic hyperglycinemia:

On day 12, after informed consent of the parents and with the approval of the institutional review board, treatment with DM (Delsym) was instituted. A single dose of 7.5 mg/kg resulted in profound sedation. On day of life 15, a dosage of 7.5 mg/kg per day in three divided doses was initiated and tolerated. Attempts at higher doses resulted in somnolence, agitation, and involuntary movements. At approximately day 70, the patient became increasingly agitated and inconsolable, prompting reduction of the DM dose to 5 mg/kg per day. Ultimately a regimen of 5 days of DM therapy followed by 2 days of no therapy appeared to eliminate the episodes of agitation.

At 9 months of age the patient had intermittent vomiting. Evaluation by barium radiologic studies and upper gastrointestinal tract endoscopy revealed diffuse gastritis, esophagitis, and duodenitis, possibly related to high-dose benzoate therapy. Our results indicate that sodium benzoate at a dose of 750 mg/kg per day normalizes plasma glycerine levels and substantially reduces but does not normalize CSF glycine levels. Reduction of the benzoate dose was associated with increased CSF and plasma glycine concentrations. Dextromethorphan at a dose of 5 mg/kg per day, on a regimen of 5 days of therapy followed by 2 days of no therapy, appeared to be well tolerated by our patient. Higher doses were associated with increased somnolence and agitation and with involuntary movements when awake. Therapy with benzoate, 500 mg/kg per day, was started on day 5, and the dosage was increased to 750 mg/kg per day on day 8, with prompt normalization of the neurologic and electroencephalographic findings. The glycine concentrations in both plasma and cerebrospinal fluid were substantially reduced. Dextromethorphan was added to the regimen on day 12.

(Hamosh: Dextromethorphan and high-dose benzoate therapy for nonketotic hyperglycinemia in an infant. J Pediatr 1992;121:131-135)

Sodium Benzoate

For management of seizures in nonketotic hyperglycinemia:

0.25-0.75 gm/kg/day PO

Vomiting, anorexia.

(Wolff: The effectiveness of benzoate in the management of seizures in nonketotic hyperglycinemia. Am J Dis Child 1986;140:596-602)

SEE ALSO: DEXTROMETHORPHAN

SODIUM BICARBONATE

Supplied: Injection 4.2% (0.5mEq/ml) in 2.5ml, 5ml, 10ml, 8.4% (1mEq/ml) in 10ml, 50ml

Administration: IV

Use 4.2% (0.5mEq/ml) concentration (2,3) or 1:4 solution diluted with sterile water (0.25 mEq/ml - ~450 mOsm/L)(see Papille: J Pediatr 1978;93:834-836)

Comment: Neonates and children <2 yrs old: Rapid injection (10ml/min) of hypertonic sodium bicarbonate solutions may produce hypernatremia, a decrease in cerebrospinal fluid pressure and possible intracranial hemorrhage. DO NOT administer >8mEq/kg/day. A 4.2% solution is preferred for such slow administration (1).

Bicarbonate

There is insufficient data to recommend routine use of bicarbonate in resuscitation of the newly born. In fact, the hyperosmolarity and CO_2-generating properties of sodium bicarbonate may be detrimental to myocardial or cerebral function. Use of Sodium bicarbonate is discouraged during brief CPR. If it is used during prolonged arrests unresponsive other therapy, it should be given only after establishment of adequate ventilation and circulation. Later use of bicarbonate for treatment of persistent metabolic acidosis or hyperkalemia should be directed by arterial blood gas levels or serum chemistries, among other evaluations. A dose of 1 to 2 mEq/kg of a 0.5 mEq/mL solution maybe given by slow intravenous push (over at least 2 minutes) after adequate ventilation and perfusion have been established.

Medications Drugs are rarely indicated in resuscitation of the newly born infant. Bradycardia in the newly born infant is usually the result of inadequate lung inflation or profound hypoxia, and adequate ventilation is the most important step in correcting bradycardia. Administer medications if, despite adequate ventilation with 100% oxygen and chest compressions, the heart rate remains <60 bpm.

Routes of Medication Administration.

The tracheal route is generally the most rapidly accessible route for drug administration during resuscitation. It maybe used for administration of epinephrine and naloxone, but it should not be used during resuscitation for administration of caustic agents such as sodium bicarbonate. The tracheal route of administration may result in a more variable response to epinephrine than the intravenous route; however, neonatal data is insufficient to recommend a higher dose of epinephrine for tracheal administration.

Attempt to establish intravenous access in neonates who fail to respond to tracheally administered epinephrine. The umbilical vein is the most rapidly accessible venous route; it may be used for epinephrine or naloxone administration as well as for administration of volume expanders and bicarbonate. Insert a 3.5F or 5F radiopaque catheter so that the tip is just below skin level and a free flow of blood returns on aspiration. Deep insertion poses the risk of infusion of hypertonic and vasoactive medications into the liver. Take care to avoid introduction of air emboli into the umbilical vein.

Peripheral sites for venous access (scalp or peripheral vein) may be adequate but are usually more difficult to cannulate. Naloxone may be given intramuscularly or subcutaneously but only after effective assisted ventilation has been established and only if the infant's peripheral circulation is adequate. We do not recommend administration of resuscitation drugs through the umbilical artery because the artery is often not rapidly accessible and complications may result if vasoactive or hypertonic drugs (eg, epinephrine or bicarbonate) are given by this route.

Intraosseous lines are not commonly used in newly born infants because the umbilical vein is more accessible, the small bones are fragile, and the intraosseous space is small in a premature infant. Intraosseous access has been shown to be useful in the neonate and older infant when vascular access is difficult to achieve.[82] Intraosseous access can be used as an alternative route for medications/volume expansion if umbilical or other direct venous access is not readily attainable (Clas IIb. LOE 5).

(American Heart Association: Part 11: Neonatal Resuscitation 2000;102:I-343-I-357)

Sodium Bicarbonate (Various)

Indications and use:
Metabolic acidosis. Treatment of certain intoxications (eg, salicylates, phenothiazines) and renal tubular acidosis. Adjunctive treatment of hyperkalemia.

Actions: Alkalinizing agent that dissociates to provide bicarbonate ion.

Route: PO, IV.

Dosage: Cardiac arrest (no longer recommended for routine use):
Initial dose: 1-2 meq/kg IV slowly over 2 min.
Subsequent doses: Number of milliequivalents = 0.3 x weight (kg) x base deficit.

Renal tubular acidosis:
Distal: 2-3 meq/kg/day.
Proximal: 5-10 meq/kg/day as initial dose; adjust prn for maintenance.

Adverse effects: Rapid correction of metabolic acidosis with sodium bicarbonate can lead to intraventricular hemorrhage, hyperosmolality, metabolic alkalosis, hypernatremia, and hypokalemia.

Comments: Use with close monitoring of arterial blood pH.
(Gomella: Neonatology 1999, p.590)

Sodium Bicarbonate

Dose: Metabolic Acidosis: 1-2 mEq/kg/dose initially, then 0.5 mEq/kg/dose IV.
Maximum Dose: 8 mEq/kg/day IV. Alternatively, use the following formula to calculate the dose:

Weight (in kg) x 0.3 base deficit (in mEq/liter) = dose (in mEq HCO_3)

- Complete correction is not recommended. Give half the calculated dose to minimize fluid and sodium load. Give over 8-12 hours added to the IV solution (incompatible with calcium).

Cardiac Resuscitation: Not for routine use (see comments under Use). 0.5-1 mEq/kg/dose IV. May repeat every 10 minutes or as needed as determined by arterial blood gases.

Renal Tubular Acidosis: 3-15 mEq/kg/day PO in 3 or 4 divided doses given with feedings. Adjust dose according to urine pH. (sodium and/or potassium citrate can be used instead. See monograph on potassium.)

- Individualize dose.

Clearing Occluded Central Venous Catheters: (See Appendix F: Restoring Patency to Occluded Central Venous Catheters.) Sodium bicarbonate is one alternative for clearing occluded central lines. It may dissolve occlusions caused by drugs that are soluble in an alkaline pH.

Administration: IV, PO, NG. May also be given intraosseous (IO).

IV—Rate: Usually over 20-30 minutes. If the infant is unstable, may infuse at 1 mEq/kg/hour or more slowly to minimize sudden changes in serum osmolality. Maximum rate of administration in emergencies: 1 mEq/kg/minute of 4.2 percent (0.5 mEq/ml).

IV—Concentration: 4.2 percent (0.5 mEq/ml). Use the 8.4 percent (1 mEq/ml)for central line administration in fluid-restricted infants.

IV-compatibility: Incompatible with IV solutions containing calcium (precipitation will occur). See Appendix E: Y-Site Compatibility of Common NICU Drugs.

PO: Sodium bicarbonate injection may be administered PO or NG. Dilute in feedings or with water prior to administration. For renal problems, sodium and/or potassium citrate solutions are often used.

Use: For correction of persistent and severe metabolic acidosis (pH <7.15) despite maximum cardiorespiratory support.

Also used for urinary alkalinization, replacement in bicarbonate deficit as in severe diarrhea, and to treat hyperkalemia.

For cardiac resuscitation, use only after adequate alveolar ventilation has been established and effective cardiac compressions have been provided. Not for brief CPR, but may be beneficial during prolonged arrests that do not respond to other therapy. There is no evidence that sodium bicarbonate is useful in the acute phase of neonatal resuscitation in the delivery room.

For pulmonary hypertension, use to adjust pH >7.4 as an adjunct to other therapies to reduce pulmonary vascular resistance.

Adverse Effects: May cause hypernatremia, metabolic alkalosis, elevation in $PaCO_2$

May cause nausea with oral use.

Sodium bicarbonate, particularly 8.4 percent (1 mEq/ml), is extremely hypertonic. It may cause vein erosion, which can result in IV extravasation and lead to severe tissue damage.

Rapid administration of concentrated sodium bicarbonate produces sudden increases in serum osmolality, increasing the risk of intracranial hemorrhage. The critical variables are concentration, rate, and dose. The anatomy of the immature brain includes a fragile subependymal germinal matrix, which is particularly vulnerable to bleeding when subjected to hypoxia or rapid changes in vascular pressure and osmolarity. A dose of 4 mEq/kg given over 30 seconds raises the serum osmolality about 25 mOsm/kg water.

Overdose from Too-Rapid or Excessive Administration: Symptoms are tetany (as a result of decreased ionized calcium), hypokalemia (as K enters the cell), and irritability.

Treatment of Overdose: Rebreathe expired air; give calcium gluconate for tetany and hyperexcitability. Treat alkalosis with chloride salts (ammonium, potassium, or sodium) as medical condition warrants.

Nursing Implications:

Use only 4.2 percent solution (0.5 mEq/ml) for peripheral administration because of hyperosmolar content. Severe tissue injury is likely with infiltration.

Monitor acid-base balance carefully and ensure that infant has established adequate ventilation to avoid CO_2 retention.

Comments: Sodium bicarbonate 8.4 percent (1 mEq/ml) is not recommended for floor stock in the NICU; stock the 4.2 percent (0.5 mEq/ml) solution.

(Zenk: Neonatal Medications & Nutrition. A Comprehensive Guide 2000; pp.437-439)

<u>Sodium Bicarbonate</u>

Use: Management of metabolic acidosis; antacid; alkalinization of urine; stabilization of acid base status in cardiac arrest and treatment of life-threatening hyperkalemia

Usual Dosage: Cardiac arrest: Patient should be adequately ventilated before administering $NaHCO_3$

Infants: 1 mEq/kg slow IVP initially; may repeat with 0.5 mEq/kg in 10 minutes one time, or as indicated by the patient's acid-base status

Metabolic acidosis: Dosage should be based on the following formula if blood gases and pH measurements are available:

Neonates, Infants and Children: HCO_3 (mEq) = 0.3 x weight (kg) x base deficit (mEq/L) **or** HCO_3 (mEq) = 0.5 x weight (kg) x [24 - serum HCO_3 (mEq/L)]

Administration: Parenteral: For direct I.V. administration: in neonates and infants, use the 0.5 mEq/mL solution or dilute the 1 mEq/mL solution 1:1 with **sterile water**; in children and adults, the 1 mEq/mL solution may be used; administer slowly (maximum rate in neonates and infants: 10 mEq/minute); for infusion, dilute to a maximum concentration of 0.5 mEq/mL in dextrose solution and infuse over 2 hours (maximum rate of administration: 1 mEq/kg/hour)

(Taketomo: Pediatric Dosage Handbook 1999-2000, pp823-825)

Sodium bicarbonate

Dose: 1-2 mEq/kg IV

Comments: Alkalosis increases Na^+

(Garson: The science and practice of pediatric cardiology 1998, p.2956)

SODIUM CHLORIDE, HYPERTONIC

Supplied: 3%, 5% in 500 ml

Administration: IV infusion
3% = 513 mEq Na/Cl per Liter (1030 mOsm/L)
5% = 855 mEq Na/Cl per Liter (1710 mOsm/L) (2).

Sodium Chloride (NaCl)

Dose: Maintenance (term and preterm infants): 3-4 mEq/kg/day. Range for preterm infants: 2-8 mEq/kg/day.

Replacement of Deficit: Use the following formula to calculate how much sodium to give to correct acute, serious hyponatremia:

Weight (in kg) x 0.6 x (CD-CA) = dose (in mEq Na)

where: CD = desired serum sodium concentration in mEq/liter

CA = infant's actual, current serum sodium concentration in mEq/liter

Replace sodium gradually. Usually only half of this amount is given over 12-24 hours.

Administration: IV—Rate: Infuse at 1 mEq/kg/hour or less to minimize sudden changes in serum osmolality.

IV—Concentration:

- NaCl 23.4 percent: Dilute in maintenance IV solution. Not for direct IV push or retrograde administration.
- NaCl 3 percent: May be used for retrograde or direct IV push administration. For emergency treatment of severe hyponatremia only.
- NaCl 0.9 percent "normal saline" (isotonic): For direct IV, retrograde, or maintenance fluid administration. This concentration is preferred, except in fluid-restricted infants.
- NaCl 0.45 percent ("half-normal" saline): For flushing IV lines. Use heparinized saline flush solutions only for heparin locks and to start IVs; use NaCl 0.45 percent without heparin for all other flushing indications.

PO: NaCl injection may be administered PO or NG. When NaCl 23.4 percent is used to minimize fluid volume/dose, dilute in feedings or in water prior to administration.

Nursing Implications:

In th low birth weight infants, consider sodium chloride flushes as a source of sodium and fluid. Monitor electrolytes carefully.

(Zenk: Neonatal Medications & Nutrition. A Comprehensive Guide 2000; pp.440-441)

Sodium Chloride

Usual Dosage: Dosage depends upon clinical condition, fluid, electrolyte and acid-base balance of patient; hypertonic solutions (>0.9%) should only be used for the initial treatment of acute serious symptomatic hyponatremia

Maintenance sodium requirements: Oral, I.V.:
Premature neonates: 2-8 mEq/kg/day
Term neonates: 1-4 mEq/kg/day
Infants, and Children: 3-4 mEq/kg/day; maximum dose; 100-150 mEq/day

To correct acute, serious hyponatremia: mEq sodium = [desired sodium (mEq/L) actual sodium (mEq/L)] x 0.6 x wt (kg); for acute correction use 125 mEq/L as the desired serum sodium; acutely correct serum sodium in 5 mEq/L/dose increments; more gradual correction in increments of 10 mEq/L/day is indicated in the asymptomatic patient

Administration: Parenteral: Infuse hypertonic solutions (>0.9% saline) via central line only; maximum rate of administration: 1 mEq/kg/hour

Monitoring Parameters: Serum sodium, chloride, I & O, weight

Reference Range: Serum/plasma sodium levels:
Premature neonates: 132-140 mEq/L
Full-term neonates: 133-142 mEq/L
Infants ≥2 months to Adults: 135-145 mEq/L

Nursing Implications:
Bacteriostatic NS should not be used for diluting or reconstituting drugs for administration in neonates

(Taketomo: Pediatric Dosage Handbook 2000-2001, pp.871-872)

Sodium Chloride

For Treatment of Congenital Adrenal Hyperplasia:
Treatment: Administration of glucocorticoids inhibits excessive production of androgens and prevents progressive virilization. A variety of glucocorticoids (hydrocortisone, prednisone, dexamethasone) and dosage schedules have been used for this purpose. Most often, hydrocortisone (10-20 mg/m^2 per 24 hours) is administered orally in 3 divided doses. There have been recent problems with consistent dosing with the liquid formulation of hydrocortisone. Tablets may give more reliable levels. Infants usually require 2.5 to 5 mg 3 times daily and children, 5 to 10 mg 3 times daily. The morning dose should be given as early as possible to blunt the early morning corticotropin increase that begins during the predawn hours. Doses must be individualized by

monitoring growth, bone age, and hormonal levels. Patients with disturbances of electrolyte regulation (salt losers) and elevated plasma renin activity require a mineralocorticoid and sodium supplementation in addition to the glucocorticoid. Maintenance therapy with fludrocortisone acetate (Florinef) (0.05-0.3 mg daily) and sodium chloride (1-3 g) is usually sufficient to normalize plasma renin activity. Increased doses of glucocorticoid are indicated during periods of stress, such as infection or surgery, for salt-losing and non-salt-losing patients.

ABSTRACT. The Section on Endocrinology and the Committee on Genetics of the American Academy of Pediatrics, in collaboration with experts from the fields of pediatric endocrinology and genetics, developed this policy statement as a means of providing up-to-date information for the practicing pediatrician about current practice and controversial issues in congenital adrenal hyperplasia (CAH), including the current status of pre-natal diagnosis and treatment, the benefits and problem areas of neonatal screening programs, and the management of children with nonclassic CAH. The reference list is designed to allow physicians who wish more information to research the topic more thoroughly.

(American Academy Of Pediatrics: Section on Endocrinology and Committee on Genetics. Technical Report: Congenital Adrenal Hyperplasia. Pediatrics 2000;106:1511-1518)

SOTALOL (Betapace)

Supplied: Tablets 80mg, 120mg, 160mg, 240mg

Administration: PO

Marketed by Berlex Lab. Intravenous form not available.

Sotalol

In pediatrics, it is being given for a number of postoperative tachyarrhythmias that are difficult to control.

Dosing: PO: 90-200 mg/m^2/day

Warnings: Bradycardia, torsades de pointes

Dosing and Interactions:

The starting sotalol dosage is generally 90 mg/m^2/day and can be given on a schedule of two or three times daily, up to 200 mg/m^2/day. The smallest unit dose is 80 mg, so that suspensions must be made up for small children. A concentration of 5 mg/ml is common. An intravenous preparation is available outside the United States, and doses are in the range of 0.2 to 1.5 mg/kg.

Side Effects: Sotalol has the usual side effect profile of beta-blocking agents, with mild negative inotropic effects. Unlike standard beta-blocking drugs, sotalol will prolong the QT interval because of its class III effects. The most serious adverse cardiovascular side effect is a drug-induced torsades de pointes, with an incidence approximating that of quinidine-induced torsades.

(Gillette: Clinical Pediatric Arrhythmias 1999,pp.231-248)

Sotalol

Class: III

Uses: WPW
AFL
Vent. ectopy
Post-op hearts

Dose (Level): 90-200 $mg/m^2/day$ divided BID

Mode of Action: Prolongs repolarization and β-blocker (~ 1/3 as potent as propranolol)

ECG/EP Changes: May prolong QTc; HR

Side Effects: Orthostatic hypotension; torsade de pointes

(Garson: The science and practice of pediatric cardiology 1998, p.2953)

Sotalol

Guidelines for Dosage: Antidysrhythmics

Dosage: 2-8 mg/kg/day p.o. (divided b.i.d.);
maximum dose = 160 mg/day

Comments: May prolong QT interval. β-adrenergic blocking effects

(Allen: Moss and Adam's Heart Disease in Infants, Children, and Adolescents 2001, pp.1460-1468)

SPIRAMYCIN

Spiramycin

Spiramycin, a macrolide antibiotic that is available to physicians in the United States only by request to the U.S. Food and Drug Administration, has an antibacterial spectrum comparable to that of erythromycin and is active against *T. gondii*, as demonstrated in animal experiments.

Spiramycin is supplied as a syrup and in capsules. The usual dose in adults is 1 g three times a day daily in three divided doses.

Because the optimal dose and route of administration of spiramycin in infants and adults have never been established for toxoplasmosis, the study by Back and co-workers on the pharmacology of parenteral spiramycin as an antineoplastic agent is pertinent. Twelve patients with various types of far-advanced neoplastic diseases were treated intravenously with daily doses ranging from 5 to 160 mg/kg. Doses above 35 mg/kg produced local vasospasm, a feeling of coolness, strange taste, vertigo, dizziness, flushing of the face, tearing of the eyes, nausea, vomiting, diarrhea, and anorexia. No hematologic toxicity, electrocardiographic change, or impairment of liver or kidney function was noticed. However, QT interval prolongation and life-threatening arrhythmias (cardiac arrest) have been reported in two neonates being treated with spiramycin (300,000 IU/kg per day by mouth). The infants recovered completely after immediate cardiopulmonary resuscitation maneuvers.

(Remington: Infectious Diseases of the Fetus and Newborn Infant 2001, pp.295-296)

SPIRONOLACTONE (Aldactone)

Supplied: Tablets 25 mg, 50 mg, 100 mg

Administration: PO

Oral suspensions of spironolactone (prepared by pulverizing commercially available tablets of the drug and adding them to cherry syrup) have been reported to be stable for one month refrigerated (3).

Warning: Spironolactone has been shown to be a tumorigen in chronic toxicity studies in rats. At 25 to 250 time the usual human dose, there was a significant dose related increase in benign adenomas of the thyroid and testes, in malignant mammary tumors and in proliferative changes in the liver.

Extemporaneous Compounding (Recipe)

Dosage form: Oral suspension
Made from: Tablets
Concentration: 1 mg/mL
Stability: 90 days
Store: Refrigerate
Label: Shake well

Ingredient	Strength	Quantity
Spironolactone tablets	25 mg	10
Carboxymethylcellulose	1.5%	50 mL
Syrup		100 mL
Purified water USP		qs ad 250 mL

Instructions: Put the tablets and a small amount of water ina blender and allow to soak for 5 min. Add carboxymethylcellulose and syrup to the blender and mix. Transfer to a graduate and qs to volume with water. (11)

Spironolactone (Aldactone)

Indications and use:
Primarily used in conjunction with a thiazide diuretic in the treatment of hypertension, congestive heart failure, and edema when prolonged diuresis is desirable.

Actions: Mild diuretic with potassium-sparing effects. Competitive antagonist of aldosterone.

Route: PO

Dosage: 1-3 mg/kg/day divided q12h.

Adverse effects: Hyperkalemia, dehydration, hyponatremia, and gynecomastia (usually reversible).

Comments: Contraindicated in hyperkalemia, anuria, and rapidly deteriorating renal function. Monitor potassium closely when giving potassium supplements. More expensive but more effective than potassium supplements. Peak effect after 2-3 days.

(Gomella: Neonatology 1999, pp. 590-591)

Spironolactone (Aldactone)

Dose: 1-3.5 mg/kg/day PO divided BID-TID
Mode of Action: Potent loop diuretic
Adverse Effects: Hypokalemia, hyponatremia, alkalosis
Comments: Limited experience in young children

(Garson: The science and practice of pediatric cardiology 1998, p.2951)

Spironolactone

Route and Dose: PO: 1-3 mg/kg/day q 8-24 h
Adverse Effects and Cautions:
Contraindicated with hyperkalemia; onset of action delayed; drowsiness; nausea; vomiting; diarrhea; androgenic effects in females; gynecomastia in males.

(Taeusch: Avery's Diseases of the Newborn 1998, p.1347)

STAVUDINE (Zerit) d4T

Supplied: Powder for oral solution: 1mg/ml in 200ml
15, 20, 30, 40 mg capsules
Route: PO

Stavudine

Route: PO
Dosage: 2 mg/kg/day
Interval: q12h
NON-NEWBORN SECTION

(Nelson: Pocket Book of Pediatric Antimicrobial Therapy 2000-2001, p.84)

STREPTOKINASE (Kabikinase, Streptase)

Supplied: 250,000 I.U.; 600,000 I.U.; 750,000 I.U. in 5 ml or 1,500,000 I.U. in 10ml vials
Administration: IV infusion
Slowly add 5 ml 0.9% NaCl or D5W directing the diluent at the side of the bottle or vial rather than into the drug powder. Roll and tilt gently to reconstitute. Avoid shaking to prevent foaming. Dilute to appropriate volume for specific indication (1).

Streptokinase (Kabikinase, Streptase)

Indications and use:
Deep venous thrombosis and femoral artery thrombosis following cardiac catheterization.

Actions: Thrombolytic enzyme that converts plasminogen to the enzyme plasmin (fibrinolysin). Plasmin degrades fibrin, fibrinogen, and other plasma procoagulant proteins.

Route: IV.

Dosage: Loading dose: 1500-2000 units/kg infused over 30-60 min. Maintenance dosage: 1000 units/kg/h as continuous infusion for 24-72 h. Titrate the dose to maintain thrombin time at 2-5 times the normal control value.

Adverse effects: May cause severe spontaneous bleeding, hypersensitivity and anaphylactic reactions, fever (common), and chills.

Comments: Before starting therapy, obtain baseline for thrombin time, activated partial thromboplastin time, prothrombin time, hematocrit, and platelet count; repeat all tests q12h. It is desired to maintain thrombin time at 2-5 times normal and prothrombin time and activated partial thromboplastin time as 1.5-2.0 times normal. Prepare final infusion solution to concentration of 1000 units/mL in D_5W. At the end of streptokinase therapy, begin IV heparin. Antidote: Aminocaproic acid (loading dose 200 mg/kg IV or PO stat followed by maintenance dose of 100 mg/kg/dose IV or PO q6h for up to 10 days after the procedure.
Note: Limited experience in neonates.

(Gomella: Neonatology 1999, p.591)

Streptokinase

Usual Dosage: Children: Safety and efficacy not established; limited studies have used the following doses:

Thromboses: I.V.: *Chest*, 1998 recommendations: Initial (loading dose): 2000 units/kg followed by 2000 units/kg/hour for 6-12 hours **or** initial (loading dose): 3500-4000 units/kg over 30 minutes followed by I.V. continuous infusion: 1000-1500 units/kg/hour; dose should be individualized based on response

Clotted catheter: **Note**: Not recommended due to possibility of allergic reactions with repeated doses: 10,000-25,000 units diluted in NS to a final volume equivalent to catheter volume; instill into catheter and leave in place for 1 hour, then aspirate contents out of catheter and flush catheter with NS

Administration: Parenteral: I.V.: Dilute in NS (preferred) or D_5W maximum concentration: 1.5 million units/50 mL

Monitoring Parameters:
For systemic therapy: Blood pressure, TT, PTT, APTT, fibrinogen level, fibrin/fibrinogen degradation products, D-dimers, platelet count, hemoglobin, hematocrit, signs of bleeding

Nursing Implications:
For intravenous or intracoronary use only; avoid I.M. injections

Additional Information:

Best results are realized if used within 5-6 hours of MI; antibodies to streptokinase remain for 3-6 months after initial dose, use another thrombolytic enzyme (ie, urokinase) if repeat thrombolytic therapy is indicated

Failure of thrombolytic agents in newborns/neonates may occur due to the low plasminogen concentrations (~50% to 70% of adult levels), streptokinase-induced clot lysis my be more impaired than urokinase or TPA in these patients, supplementing plasminogen (via administration of fresh frozen plasma) may possibly help

(Takemoto: Pediatric Dosage Handbook 1999-2000, pp.835-836)

Streptokinase

Dose & Route: DVT: **Should be used in consultation with a hematologist.** Duration of therapy will depend on clinical response and generally does not exceed 3 days. Children: 3500-4000 U/kg over 30 min, followed by 1000-1500 U/kg/hr; OR 2000 U/kg load over 30 min followed by 2000 U/kg/hr. Duration of infusion is individualized based on response.

Remarks: **Contraindicated** with intracranial or intraspinal surgery, hx of internal bleeding, recent streptococcus infection, CVA within 2 months. May cause hemorrhage, urticaria, itching, flushing, musculoskeletal pain, bronchospasm, and anaphylaxis. Pediatric safety and efficacy information is limited.

(Siberry: The Harriet Lane Handbook 2000, pp.851-852)

Streptokinase

Local infusion of intra-arterial streptokinase (50 U/kg/h) directly into the clot for 36 hours resulted in resolution of ischemic symptoms. No complications were encountered with the use of this protocol.

(Richardson: Effective thrombolytic therapy of aortic thrombosis in the small premature infant. J. Pediatr Surg 1988;23:137-141)

STREPTOMYCIN

Supplied: Injection, 400 mg/mL in 2.5 mL amps.
Administration: IM

Streptomycin

Commonly Used Drugs for the Treatment of Tuberculosis in Infants, Children, and Adolescents

Route: IM

Daily Dosage, mg/kg per day: 20-40

Twice Weekly Dose, mg/kg per day: 20-40

Maximum dose: 1 g

Adverse Reactions:

Auditory and vestibular toxic effects, nephrotoxic effects, rash

(American Academy of Pediatrics: Report of the Committee on Infectious Diseases. Red Book 2000, p.602)

Streptomycin

Antituberculosis Drugs in Children

Daily Dose (mg/kg)	Twice Weekly Dose (mg/kg/per dose)
20-40 (IM)	20-40 (IM)

Streptomycin (STM) is a valuable drug to be used in conjunction with INH and RIF in life-threatening forms of tuberculosis. It is bactericidal and tolerated well by children in the usual dose of 20 to 40 mg/kg per day intramuscularly up to 1 g. Usually, STM can be discontinued within 1 to 3 months if clinical improvement is definite, whereas the other two or three drugs are continued with oral administration.

(Remington: Infectious Diseases of the Fetus and Newborn Infant 2001, pp.1188-1189)

Streptomycin sulfate

Route: IM
Dosage: 20-30 mg/kg/day
Interval: q12h
NON-NEWBORN SECTION

(Nelson: Pocket Book of Pediatric Antimicrobial Therapy 2000-2001, p.84)

Streptomycin Sulfate

Dose & Route: Tuberculosis:
Children:
Daily therapy: 20-40 mg/kg/24 hr IM QD
Max daily dose: 1 g/24 hr

Twice weekly therapy: 20-40 mg/kg/dose IM twice weekly
Max daily dose: 1.5 g/24 hr

Remarks: Use with caution in pre-existing vertigo, tinnitus, hearing loss, neuromuscular disorders. **Adjust dose in renal insufficiency**. Drug is administered via deep IM injection only. Follow auditory status. May cause CNS depression or other neurologic problems, myocarditis, serum sickness.

Therapeutic levels: peak 15-40 mg/L, trough: <5 mg/L. Recommended serum sampling time at steady-state: trough within 30 minutes prior to the 3rd consecutive dose and peak 30-60 minutes after the administration of the 3rd consecutive dose. Therapeutic levels are not achieved in CSF.

(Siberry: The Harriet Lane Handbook 2000, p.853)

SUCCINYLCHOLINE (Anectine, Quelicin)

Supplied:	Injection 20 mg, 50 mg, 100 mg/ml
Administration:	IV, IM
Comment:	Refrigerate at 2°-8° C. (36°-46° F.) Succinylcholine is incompatible with alkaline solutions and will precipitate if mixed or administered simultaneously.

<u>Succinylcholine</u> (Anectine)

Dose: IV: 1-2 mg/kg initially, then 0.3-0.6 mg/kg every 5-10 minutes as needed. Tachyphylaxis (rapid appearance of a progressive decrease in response) occurs with repeated dosing. An initial test dose of 0.1 mg/kg may determine patient's sensitivity and recovery time.

IM: Up to 3-4 mg/kg

Administration: Usually given IV, but may be given IM in infants.

IV—Rate: May be infused IV push over 10-30 seconds.

IV—Concentration: May give undiluted or diluted in D_5W or sodium chloride injection to 1-2 mg/ml. Discard diluted solution after 24 hours.

IV—Compatibility: Do not mix with alkaline solutions such as sodium bicarbonate or thiopental sodium. Flush line and change needle between alkaline solutions and succinylcholine to avoid inactivation and precipitation.

Adverse Effects: Hypoxemia resulting from inadequate ventilation. Bradycardia is common; asystole occurs rarely. Pretreatment with atropine (0.02 mg/kg) eliminates bradycardia.

Increase or decrease in blood pressure may occur. Succinylcholine has weak histamine-releasing effects.

As with other neuromuscular blockers, continuous administration over a prolonged period may result in irreversible blockade.

Myoglobinemia and myoglobinuria may occur.

Masseter muscle rigidity, defined as a transient contraction of the muscles of mastication that limits mouth opening, may indicate a susceptibility to malignant hyperthermia.

Hyperkalemia.

Increases intraocular pressure.

Nursing Implications:

Monitor for bradycardia.

Monitor vital signs continuously before, during, and after administration. Drug produces only paralysis. Collaborate with physician to provide analgesia and/or sedation (e.g., fentanyl or morphine).

Refrigerate drug. When taken on transport, refrigerate immediately upon return.

Comments: Mechanical ventilation must be provided during use. Does not produce analgesia or sedation, only paralysis.

Neonates are relatively resistant to the relaxant effects of succinylcholine, requiring up to 4 times the adult does.

(Zenk: Neonatal Medications & Nutrition. A Comprehensive Guide 2000; pp.449-450)

Succinylcholine (Anectine, Quelicin)

Dose & Route: Paralysis for intubation:
Infants and Children:
Initial:
IV: 1-2 mg/kg/dose x 1
IM: 3-4 mg/kg/dose x 1
Max dose: 150 mg/dose
Maintenance: 0.3-0.6 mg/kg/dose IV Q5-10 min PRN.
Continuous infusion not recommended.

Remarks: Pretreatment with atropine is recommended to reduce incidence of bradycardia. May cause malignant hyperthermia, bradycardia, hypotension, arrhythmia, and hyperkalemia. Use with **caution** in patients with severe burns, paraplegia, or crush injuries and in patients with preexisting hyperkalemia. Beware of prolonged depression in patients with liver disease, malnutrition, pseudocholinesterase deficiency, hypothermia, and those receiving aminoglycosides, phenothiazines, quinidine, beta-blockers, amphotericin b, cyclophosphamide, diuretics, lithium, acetylcholine, and anticholinesterases. Diazepam may decrease neuromuscular blocking effects. Duration of action 4-6 minutes

IV, 10-30 minutes IM. Must be prepared to intubate within 1 minute.

(Siberry: The Harriet Lane Handbook 2000, pp.853-854)

SUCRALFATE (Carafate)

Supplied: Suspension 1gm/10mL
Tablets 1 gm

Administration: PO

Sucralfate slurry

Therapy for Reflux

Common doses: 1 g in 5 to 15-mL solution, qid PC, HS-protects against bile salts, trypsin, acid

Partial list of side effects:
constipation, gastric concretions, potential binding of other medications

(Wyllie: Pediatric Gastrointestinal Disease 1999, p.180)

Sucralfate

Dose & Route: Children: 40-80 mg/kg/24 hr ÷ Q6 hr PO

Remarks: May cause vertigo, constipation, dry mouth. Aluminum may accumulate in patients with renal failure. This may be augmented by the use of aluminum-containing antacids. Decreases absorption of phenytoin, digoxin, theophylline, cimetidine, fat soluble vitamins, ketoconazole, quinolones, and oral anticoagulants. Administer these drugs at least 2 hours before or after sucralfate doses.

(Siberry: The Harriet Lane Handbook 2000, p.854)

<u>Sucralfate</u> (Carafate)

Therapeutic Category:
Gastrointestinal Agent, Gastric or Duodenal Ulcer Treatment

Usual Dosage: Oral:
Children: Dose not established; doses of 40-80 mg/kg/day divided every 6 hours have been used

(Takemoto: Pediatric dosage Handbook 1999-2000, pp.840-841)

SUCROSE

<u>Intraoral Sucrose</u>

Fifteen infants of 32-34 weeks postmenstrual age were tested in a blind crossover manner on two separate occasions no more than two days apart. Either 1 ml of 25% sucrose solution or sterile water was syringed into the baby's mouth 2 minutes before routine heel lancing. Response to the painful stimuli was measured by duration of cry and by facial expression (pain score).

There was a significant reduction in the duration of first cry, the percentage of time spent crying in the 5 minutes after heel prick, and the pain score in the sucrose treated group. It is concluded that sucrose has analgesic effects in healthy premature infants.

(Ramenghi: Reduction of pain response in premature infants using intraoral sucrose. Arch Dis Child 1996;74:F126-F128)

<u>Sucrose</u> (artificial sweetener)

A substance commercially described as 'sugar free,' used as a sweetener for paracetamol suspension, was evaluated on measures of neonatal pain. Sixty infants were randomly allocated to receive one of four solutions before heel stab blood sampling: sterile water (placebo); 25 or 50% sucrose (weight/volume); and the commercial sweet-tasting solution. There was a significant reduction in crying time and pain score 3 minutes after the painful stimulus in all groups compared with the controls.

It is concluded that this sweet-tasting solution has analgesic effects as potent as those of concentrated sucrose solutions.

(Ramenghi: Effect of non-sucrose sweet tasting solution on neonatal heel prick responses. Arch Dis Child 1996;74:F129-F131)

SUFENTANIL (Sufenta)

Supplied: Injection 50 mcg/ml in 1 ml, 2 ml, 5 ml
Administration: IV

Sufentanyl

Indication: Protocol for inborn infants with Congenital Diaphragmatic Hernia

Postoperatively sedation or analgesia was provided via a sufentanyl infusion, 2 µg/kg/hr for the first 24 hours and the dose gradually weaned.

(Finer: Congenital diaphragmatic Hernia: Developing a Protocolized Approach. J Pediatr Surg 1998;33:1331-1337)

Sufentanil

Usual Dosage: Doses should be titrated to appropriate effects; wide range of doses, dependent upon desired degree of analgesia or anesthesia, use lean body weight to dose patients who are >20% above ideal body weight

Children <12 years: Anesthesia: I.V.: Initial: 10-25 mcg/kg; maintenance; Up to 25-50 mcg as needed

Administration: Parenteral: I.V.: Slow I.V. injection or by infusion

Monitoring Parameters:

Respiratory rate, blood pressure, heart rate, oxygen saturation, neurological status (for degree of analgesia/anesthesia)

Nursing Implications:

Patient may develop rebound respiratory depression postoperatively

(Taketomo: Pediatric Dosage handbook 1999-200, pp.841-842)

Sufentanil

When 10 or 20 µg/kg of sufentanil was used as the sole induction agent for anesthesia, systolic and diastolic arterial blood pressures increased significantly with tracheal intubation and surgical incision. Heart rate increased in patients receiving 5 or 10 µg/kg but decreased in patients receiving 20 µg/kg. Sufentanil 20 µg/kg prolonged the pre-ejection period and pre-ejection period/left ventricle ejection time ration, suggesting that higher doses of sufentanil have a mild negative inotropic effect. Children receiving sufentanil 20 µg/kg had lower serum epinephrine concentrations than children receiving 5 or 10 µ/kg.

Infants given sufentanil 5 or 10 µg/kg for cardiac surgery had small decreases in heart rate and arterial blood pressure with the induction of anesthesia and a return to baseline with tracheal intubation. A small rise in arterial pressure occurred with sternotomy. This finding differs from that seen with fentanyl 50 or 75 µg/kg, in which sternotomy increased systolic blood pressure by about 20 percent.

(Gregory: Pediatric Anesthesia 1994, p.32)

SULFACETAMIDE EYE DROPS, EYE OINTMENT

(Sulamyd, Bleph-10)

Supplied: Ophthalmic solution 10%, 15%, 30%
Ophthalmic ointment 10% 3.5 gm
Administration: Ophthalmic

Sulfacetamide Sodium (Isopto Cetamide, Sodium Sulamyd, Others)

Action and spectrum:
Mechanism, see Sulfadiazine. Indicated in acute conjunctivitis. Spectrum includes *Staphylococcus aureus*, *Streptococcus pneumoniae*, *Haemophilus influenzae* and *Moraxella* spp.

Route: Topical
Dosage: Instill 1-2 drops in each eye q2h initially, then increase time interval as condition responds or ointment in each eye q4-6h for 7-10 days.

Comments: For adverse effects, see Sulfadiazine. May cause local irritation. Ophthalmic solution preferred over neomycin-containing ophthalmic preparation because of decreased incidence of local irritation and allergic response.

(Gomella: Neonatology 1999, p.591)

Sulfacetamide Sodium

Route: Ophthalmic
Neonatal Dose: Apply ointment or instill 1-2 drops to affected eye 3-4 times daily.
Pediatric Dose: Apply ointment to affected eye 2-4 times daily or instill 1-2 drops 3-4 times daily.
Discussion: Ointment may interfere with vision for short periods of time; may cause sulfa skin allergy.

(Rudolph: Rudolph's Pediatrics 1996, p.2204)

SULFADIAZINE

Supplied: Tablets 500 mg
Administration: PO
Clinicians interested in additional information on the commercial availability of sulfadiazine should contact EON Laboratories at (800) 366-1595 or (800) 526-0225 (3).

Sulfadiazine

For Treatment of Toxoplasmosis
Concentration: 100mg/ml
Dispense: 50ml
Dosage: Sig: half baby's current weight equals number of ml given in AM and PM. eg. if baby weighs 5Kg give 2.5ml at 7AM and 2.5 ml at 7PM

Note: Suspended in 2% sugar solution suspension at usual concentration must be made up each week. Store refrigerated.

(Remington: Infectious Diseases of the Fetus and Newborn Infant 2001, pp.292-294)

Sulfadiazine

Oral Suspension Formulations for Pyrimethamine and Sulfadiazine in the United States.

Sulfadiazine, 100 mg/ml suspension

1. Crush ten 500-mg sulfadiazine tablets in a mortar to a fine powder.
2. Add enough sterile water to make a smooth paste.
3. Slowly triturate the syrup vehicle close to the final volume of 50 ml.
4. Transfer the suspension to a larger amber bottle.
5. Add sufficient syrup vehicle to q.s. to 50 ml final volume.
6. Shake well.
7. Label and give a 7-day expiration.
8. Store refrigerated.

Note: Pyrimethamine: 25-mg tablets (Daraprim, Glaxo Wellcome Inc.) NDC #0173-0201-55

Sulfadiazine: 500-mg tablets (Eon Labs Manufacturing, Inc.) NDC #00185-0757-01

Syrup vehicle: suggest 2% sugar suspension for pyrimethamine. If the infant is not lactose intolerant, 2% sugar suspension can be 2 g lactose per 100 ml distilled water. Suggest simple syrup or alternatively cherry syrup for sulfadiazine suspension

(Remington: Infectious diseases of the Fetus and Newborn Infant, 2001, pp.292-294

Sulfadiazine

Congenital *Toxoplasma* infection in the infant

(Remington: Infectious Diseases of the Fetus and Newborn Infant 2001)

SEE ALSO: CONGENITAL TOXOPLASMA INFECTION p.656

Sulfadiazine

Condition: Congenital toxoplasmosis

Therapy: Sulfadiazine 100 mg/kg/day PO div q6-12hr AND pyrimethamine 2 mg/kg PO daily x 2 (loading dose), then 1 mg/kg PO once daily for 6 wks, then 3 times weekly up to 1 year; Alternative: pyrimethamine (as above) AND clindamycin

Comment: Supplemental folinic acid 5-10 mg 3 times weekly; Steroids if chorioretinitis or CSF protein > 1 g/dl

(Nelson: Pocket Book of Pediatric Antimicrobial Therapy 2000-2001, p.8)

Sulfadiazine

Action and spectrum:

Acts via competitive antagonism of *p*-aminobenzoic acid, an essential factor in folic acid synthesis. Spectrum of action includes both Gram-positive and Gram-negative organisms. In neonatology, used chiefly against *Toxoplasma gondii* in combination with pyrimethamine.

Route: PO

Dosage: For toxoplasmosis, give 120 mg/kg/day divided q6h for 4 weeks. Combine with pyrimethamine.

Elimination and metabolism: Rapid renal excretion.

Adverse effects: Hypersensitivity (fever, rash, hepatitis, vasculitis, lupus-like syndrome), neutropenia, agranulocytosis, thrombocytopenia, aplastic anemia, Stevens-Johnson syndrome, and crystalluria (keep urine alkaline and output high). Kernicterus may occur.

Comments: Avoid use in neonates except for treatment of congenital toxoplasmosis. See comments under pyrimethamine regarding folinic acid use.

(Gomella: Neonatology 1999, pp. 591-592)

Sulfadiazine

Indication: For treatment of toxoplasmosis

Although significant injury has already occurred in many cases of congenital toxoplasmosis by the time of birth, there is good evidence that some of this injury is reversible and that continuing postnatal injury is preventable by therapy directed against the organism.

The drugs of choice are pyrimethamine and sulfadiazine with the addition of folinic acid to counteract the folic acid antagonistic effect of pyrimethamine on the bone marrow. Pyrimethamine is highly effective in experimental infection with *Toxoplasma* and, because of its high lipid solubility, appears to be concentrated in brain. Sulfadiazine acts synergistically with pyrimethamine, such that their combined activity is eight times that expected if additive effects were operative. Caution must be exercised with sulfadiazine, particularly in infants with hyperbilirubinemia. Thrombocytopenia is a particularly early manifestation of pyrimethamine toxicity, and folinic acid is particularly effective in correcting this phenomenon. These antimicrobials kill actively multiplying parasites but not resistant cyst stages. Therefore treatment must begin promptly and continue until the infant's immune system has matured sufficiently to control the infection. Total recommended duration of therapy in both symptomatic and asymptomatic disease is 1 year. In infants with evidence for severe inflammation, manifested by markedly elevated CSF protein (≥1 g/dl) or by severe chorioretinitis, corticosteroids have been recommended.

(Volpe: Neurology of the Newborn 2001, pp.732-733)

Sulfadiazine

Dose & Route: Congenital toxoplasmosis (administer with pyrimethamine and folinic acid) (From Clin Infect Dis 18:38, 1994)
Infants: 100 mg/kg/24 hr PO ÷ BID x 12 months

Toxoplasmosis (administer with pyrimethamine and folinic acid)
Children: 100-200 mg/kg/24 hr ÷ Q6 hr PO x 3-4 weeks.

Remarks: **Contraindicated** in porphyria and hypersensitivity to sulfonamides. Use with **caution** in premature infants and infants <2 mo because of risk of hyperbilirubinemia; and in hepatic or renal dysfunction (30-44% eliminated in urine). Maintain hydration, May cause increased effects of warfarin, methotrexate, and sulfonylureas due to drug displacement from protein binding sites. May cause fever, rash, hepatitis, SLE-like syndrome, vasculitis, bone marrow suppression, hemolysis in patients with G6PD deficiency, and Steven-Johnson syndrome.

(Siberry: The Harriet Lane Handbook 2000, p.855)

SULFISOXAZOLE (Gantrisin)

Supplied: Pediatric suspension 500 mg/5 ml, 500mg tablets
Administration: PO

Sulfisoxazole (Gantrisin)

Antibacterial Drugs for Pediatric Patients Beyond the Newborn Period
Dosage per kg/d
Route: PO
Mild to Moderate Infections: 120-150 mg in 4-6 doses
Severe Infections: 120-150 mg in 4-6 doses

(American Academy of Pediatrics: Report of the Committee on Infectious Diseases. Red Book 2000, p.661)

Sulfisoxazole

Route: IV, SC
Neonatal Dose: >2wk: 100 mg/kg/24 h q6-8h
Pediatric Dose: 100 mg/kg/24 h q6-8h

Route: PO
Neonatal Dose: 100-150 mg/kg/24 h q6h
Pediatric Dose: 150 mg/kg/24 h q6h

Discussion: Do not use with severe renal impairment; use in <2 wk olds may cause kernicterus due to displacement of bilirubin from albumin sites.

(Rudolph: Rudolph's Pediatrics 1991, p.2000)

SULFONAMIDES

Sulfonamides

Indications: Contraindicated in newborns.
Toxicity: Displaces bilirubin from albumin-binding sites.

(Fanaroff: Neonatal-Perinatal Medicine 1997, p.730)

SUNFLOWER SEED OIL

Supplied: Oil
Administration: Topical

Sunflower Seed Oil

Route: Topical
Neonatal Dose: 1400 mg/kg/24 h q8h
Discussion: Rubbing into skin may allow absorption of essential fatty acids.

(Rudolph: Rudolph's Pediatrics 1996, p.2204)

SUPEROXIDE DISMUTASE

Recombinant Human Superoxide Dismutase

The two separate dosages of rhSOD were provided as 1 mg (for the 0.5-mg/kg dose group) or 10 mg (for the 5-mg/kg dose group) in 2 mL of saline. The first group of infants received IT saline (1 mL/kg total volume), the next group of patients received 0.5 mg/kg rhSOD IT (suspended in 1 mL/kg), and the final group received 5 mg/kg (1 mL/kg) of rhSOD. Drug or placebo was administered in two IT 0.5-mL/kg aliquots over a 1- to 2-minute period 30 to 60 minutes after surfactant administration (because of potential drug-drug interactions when combining the two agents, the surfactant and rhSOD were given separately).

BPD has become the major sequela of neonatal intensive care. Its cost in terms of mortality, morbidity, and the expenditure of health care dollars is great. Previous interventions for the prevention of BPD have not proved to be efficacious. A new direction in treatment, augmentation of antioxidant defenses, needs to be studied further. This preliminary phase I study provides the basis for theses additional investigations. The ability to increase antioxidant activity may also be important in the treatment of other disease processes in premature infants where free radical injury has also been implicated, such as intraventricular hemorrhage. Prophylactic treatment with antioxidants may also help reduce the incidence of this significant neonatal problem.

(Rosenfeld: Safety and Pharmacokinetics of Recombinant Human Superoxide Dismutase Administered Itratracheally to Premature Neonates With Respiratory Distress Syndrome. Pediatrics 1996;97:811-817)

SURFACTANT

Surfactant

ABSTRACT. Respiratory failure secondary to surfactant deficiency is a major cause of morbidity and mortality in low birth weight immature infants. Surfactant therapy substantially reduces mortality and respiratory morbidity for this population. The statement summarizes the indications for surfactant replacement therapy.

Because respiratory insufficiency may be a component of multiorgan dysfunction in sick infants, surfactant should be administered only at institutions with qualified personnel and facilities for the comprehensive care of sick infants.

(American Academy Of Pediatrics: Committee on Fetus and Newborn. Surfactant Replacement Therapy for Respiratory Distress Syndrome. Pediatrics 1999;103:684-865)

Surfactant

The value of the Herting article is to demonstrate clearly that there should be no concerns about treating preterm or term infants with sepsis/pneumonia syndromes and respiratory failure with surfactant-the treatment will not hurt and it will help about 70% of the time.

(Jobe: Commentary on Surfactant Treatment of Neonates With Respiratory Failure and Group B Streptococcal Infection. Pediatrics 2000; 106:1135-1136)

Surfactant

Conclusion: Surfactant therapy improves gas exchange in the majority of patients with GBS pneumonia. The response to surfactant is slower than in infants with RDS, and repeated surfactant doses are often needed. The mortality and morbidity are substantial, considering the relatively high mean birth weight of the treated infants.

(Herting: Surfactant Treatment of Neonates With Respiratory Failure and Group B Streptococcal Infections. Pediatrics 2000;106:957-964)

BERACTANT (Survanta, Natural Lung Surfactant)

Supplied: Suspension 25mg phospholipid /ml suspended in 0.9% NaCl - 8ml suspension - single use.

Administration: Intratracheal administration

Survanta

The color of beractant is off-white to light brown. Store unopened vials at refrigeration temperature 2-8°C. Protect from light. Store vials in carton until ready for use. Vials are for single use only. Upon opening, discard unused drug.

Indications and Usage: SURVANTA is indicated for prevention and treatment ("rescue") of Respiratory Distress Syndrome (RDS) (hyaline membrane disease) in premature infants. SURVANTA significantly reduces the incidence of RDS, mortality due to RDS and air leak complications.

Prevention: In premature infants less than 1250 g birth weight or with evidence of surfactant deficiency, give SURVANTA as soon as possible, preferably within 15 minutes of birth.

Rescue: To treat infants with RDS confirmed by x-ray and requiring mechanical ventilation, give SURVANTA as soon as possible, preferably by 8 hours of age.

Contraindications: None known.

Warnings: Survanta is intended for intratracheal use only. Survanta can rapidly affect oxygenation and lung compliance.

Dosage: Each dose of SURVANTA is 100 mg of phospholipids/kg birth weight (4 mL/kg).

Repeat Doses: The dosage of SURVANTA for repeat doses is also 100mg phospholipids/kg and is based on the infant's birth weight.

Four doses of SURVANTA can be administered in the first 48 hours of life. Doses should be given no more frequently than every 6 hours.

Dosing Procedures

General: SURVANTA is administered intratracheally by instillation through a 5 French end-hole catheter inserted into the infant's endotracheal tube with the tip of the catheter protruding just beyond the end of the endotracheal tube above the infant's carina. Before inserting the catheter through the endotracheal tube, the length of the catheter should be shortened. SURVANTA should not be instilled into a main-stem bronchus.

It is important to ensure homogenous distribution of SURVANTA through the lungs. In the controlled clinical trials, each dose was divided into four quarter doses. Each quarter-dose was administered with the infant in a different position. The sequence of positions was:

- Head and body inclined slightly down, head turned to the right.
- Head and body inclined slightly down, head turned to the left.
- Head and body inclined slightly up, head turned to the right.
- Head and body inclined slightly up, head turned to the left.

(Ross Laboratories, Columbus, Ohio 43216, Printed June, 1991)

Beractant (Survanta): See also Surfactant

Indications and use: Prevention and treatment of respiratory distress syndrome of preterm infants.

Actions: A natural bovine lung extract containing phospholipids, neutral lipids, fatty acids, and surfactant-associated proteins to which dipalmitoylphosphatidylcholine (DPPC), palmitic acid, and tripalmitin are added to mimic the surface tension-lowering properties of natural lung surfactant. Surfactant lowers surface tension on alveolar surfaces during respiration and stabilizes the alveoli against collapse.

Route: Intratracheal using a No. 5 French end –hole catheter.

Dosage: 4 mL/kg (100 mg of phospholipids per kilogram) birth weight. Give in 4 increments, repositioning the infant with each dose. Inject each ¼ dose gently into the catheter over 2-3 s. Ventilate the infant after each ¼ dose for at least 30 s or until stable. Four doses of 4 mL/kg can be given in the first 48 h of life, no more frequently than q 6h. Wean ventilator settings rapidly after administration.

Adverse effects: Most adverse effects are associated while administering the beractant to the infant: transient bradycardia and oxygen desaturation. *Less frequent adverse effects:* Endotracheal tube (ET) reflux, pallor, vasoconstriction, hypotension, ET blockage, hypertension, hypocarbia, hypercarbia, and apnea. In two studies, the rate of intracranial hemorrhage was significantly higher in infants who received beractant than in controls. When all study results were pooled, however, there was no difference in intracranial hemorrhage rates.

(Gomella: Neonatology 1999, pp.554-555)

Survanta (beractant)

Dose/kg: 4 mL

Route & frequency: Endotracheal rescue treatment:
One dose as soon as RDS diagnosis is confirmed. May repeat q6h to a total of four doses

Comments: Adverse effects include pulmonary hemorrhage, apnea, and mucous plugging. Adjust ventilatory parameters to prevent hyperoxia and hypocarbia.

Route & frequency: Prophylaxis:
First dose given as soon as possible after birth; may give a total of four doses during first 48 h or life, no more frequently than 6 h apart

Comments: May open ductus

(Avery: Neonatology Pathophysiology and Management of the Newborn 1999, p.1560)

Beractant

Route & Dose: IT: for prophylactic treatment: Give 4 ml/kg as soon as possible; may repeat at 6-h intervals to a maximum of 4 doses in 48 hours

IT: for rescue treatment: Give 4 ml/kg as soon as respiratory distress syndrome diagnosed; may repeat at 6-h intervals to a maximum of 4 doses in 48 h

Adverse Effects and Cautions:
May give additional doses if infant still has respiratory distress, or is intubated and needed >30% FIO_2 to keep $PA0_2$ ≤80 torr. Administer each dose as 4 doses of 1 ml/kg each, giving each dose over 2-3 seconds and turning newborn to a different position after each dose

(Taeusch: Avery's Diseases of the Newborn 1998, p.1343)

Beractant

Use: Prevention and treatment of respiratory distress syndrome (RDS) in premature infants.
Prophylactic therapy: Infants with body weight <1250 g who are at risk for developing or with evidence of surfactant deficiency.

Rescue therapy: Treatment of infants with RDS confirmed by x-ray and requiring mechanical ventilation.

Warnings: Rapidly affects oxygenation and lung compliance and should be restricted to a highly supervised use in a clinical setting with immediate availability of clinicians experienced with intubation and ventilatory management of premature infants. If transient episodes of bradycardia and decreased oxygen saturation occur, discontinue the dosing procedure and initiate measures to alleviate the condition; produces rapid improvements in lung oxygenation and compliance that may require immediate reductions in ventilator settings and FiO_2.

Precautions: Use of beractant in infants <600 g birth weight or >1750 g birth weight has not been evaluated

Adverse Reactions: During the dosing procedure:
Cardiovascular: Transient bradycardia, vasoconstriction, hypotension, hypertension, pallor

Respiratory: Oxygen desaturation, endotracheal tube blockage, hypocarbia, hypercarbia, apnea, pulmonary air leaks, pulmonary interstitial emphysema

Miscellaneous: Increased probability of post-treatment nosocomial sepsis

Stability: Refrigerate; protect from light; prior to administration warm by standing at room temperature for 20 minutes or hold in hand for 8 minutes; artificial warming methods should not be used; unused, unopened vials warmed to room temperature may be returned to the refrigerator within 8 hours of warming only once.

Mechanism of Action:
Replaces deficient or ineffective endogenous lung surfactant in neonates with respiratory distress syndrome (RDS) or in neonates at risk of developing RDS. Surfactant prevents the alveoli from collapsing during expiration by lowering surface tension between air and alveolar surfaces.

Usual Dosage: Intratracheal: Neonates:
Prophylactic treatment: Give 4 mL/kg as soon as possible; as many as 4 doses may be administered during the first 48 hours of life, no more frequently than 6 hours apart. The need for additional doses is determined by evidence of continuing respiratory distress or if the infant is still

intubated and requiring at least 30% inspired oxygen to maintain a $PaO_2 \leq 80$ torr.

Rescue treatment: Give 4 mL/kg as soon as the diagnosis of RDS is made; may repeat if needed, no more frequently than every 6 hours to a maximum of 4 doses

Administration: Intratracheal: For intratracheal administration only. Suction infant prior to administration; inspect solution to verify complete mixing of the suspension. Administer intratracheally by instillation through a 5-French end-hole catheter inserted into the infant's endotracheal tube. Administer the dose in four 1 mL/kg aliquots. Each quarter-dose is instilled over 2-3 seconds; each quarter-dose is administered with the infant in a different position; slightly downward inclination with head turned to the right, then repeat with head turned to the left; then slightly upward inclination with head turned to the right, then repeat with head turned to the left.

Monitoring Parameters:

Continuous heart rate and transcutaneous O_2 saturation should be monitored during administration; frequent ABG sampling is necessary to prevent postdosing hyperoxia and hypocarbia.

Nursing Implications:

Do not shake; if settling occurs during storage, gently swirl

(Taketomo: Pediatric dosage Handbook 1999-2000, p.119)

Survanta

Administration Procedure: Tracheal bronchial lavage was performed with 15 mL/kg of diluted surfactant saline suspension (Survanta [Ross Laboratories, Ohio, USA] 25 mg phospholipid/mL) at a phospholipid concentration of 5 mg/mL. This is equivalent to a dose of 75 mg/kg of phospholipids (Survanta, 3 mL/Kg). The lavage solution was instilled through the side hole of a Trach-care surfactant administration system (Ballard) so that ventilation could be maintained during the administration procedure. Because all were term-size infants, the lavage solutions were administrated in standard aliquots of 2 mL to the distal end of the endotracheal tube. The administration was stopped if there were signs of desaturation as shown by continuous O2 saturation monitoring. Manual bagging was performed until the oxygen saturation returned to normal. Suctioning was then done after each aliquot by a French size 8 catheter with a negative pressure of 80 mm Hg (10KPa) until clear. All aspirated fluid was collected for meconium content analysis. The lavage and suctioning was done in the usual four positions as for surfactant replacement therapy (SRT). Ventilation by manual bagging was performed in between suctioning until the oxygen saturation was >90.

Conclusion: Our experience suggested that surfactant lavage seems to be an effective and safe method for treatment of severe MAS. A multicenter randomized control trial is indicated to further study the efficacy of this treatment.

(Lam: Surfactant Lavage for Meconium Aspiration Syndrome: A Pilot Study. Pediatrics 1999;103:1014-1018)

<u>Surfactant, Pulmonary/Beractant</u>

Dose & Route: Prophylactic therapy: 4 ml/kg/dose intratracheally as soon as possible; up to 4 doses may be given at intervals no shorter than Q6 hr during the first 48 hr of life.
Rescue therapy: 4 ml/kg/dose intratracheally, immediately following the diagnosis of respiratory distress syndrome (RDS). May repeat dose as needed Q6 hr to maximum of 4 doses total.
Method of administration for above therapies: Each dose is divided into four 1 ml/kg aliquots; administer 1 ml/kg in each of four different positions (slight downward inclination with head turned to the right, head turned to the left; slight upward inclination with the head turned to the right, head turned to the left).

Remarks: All doses are administered intratracheally. If the suspension settles during storage, gently swirl the contents-do not shake.

Transient bradycardia, O_2 desaturation, pallor, vasoconstriction, hypotension, endotracheal tube blockage, hypercarbia, hypercapnea, apnea, and hypertension may occur during the administration process. Other side effects may include pulmonary interstitial emphysema, pulmonary air leak, and post-treatment nosocomial sepsis. Monitor heart rate and transcutaneous O_2 saturation during dose administration; and arterial blood gases for post-dose hyperoxia and hypocarbia after administration.

(Siberry: The Harriet Lane Handbook 2000, p.858)

COLFOSCERIL PALMITATE (Exosurf Neonatal, Synthetic Lung Surfactant)

Supplied: Lyophilized powder for injection 108mg in 10ml vials with 10ml SWFI and 2.5, 3, 3.5, 4 and 4.5mm endotracheal tube adapters

For prophylactic treatment, administer the first dose as soon as possible after birth

Administration: Colfosceril is best reconstituted immediately before use because it does not contain antibacterial preservatives. Reconstitute each vial with 8 ml of the accompanying diluent (preservative-free sterile water for injection). Reconstituted colfosceril is a milky white suspension with a total volume of 8 ml per vial. If the suspension separates, gently shake or swirl the vial to resuspend the preparation. Inspect the reconstituted product visually for homogeneity immediately before administration; if persistent large flakes or particulates are present, do not use the vial. (1) Suction the infant prior to administration, but do not suction for 2 hours after colfosceril is administered, except when clinically necessary. (1)

Surfactant (Exosurf Neonatal)

Indications and use:
Surfactant therapy is indicated for the prophylactic treatment of infants with a birth weight <1350 g who are at risk for the development of any type of RDS, or for infants with a birth weight >1350 g with coexisting, proven pulmonary immaturity or compromise. Exosurf Neonatal is also indicated for neonates with established surfactant deficiency syndrome.

Actions: Surfactant acts to decrease the work of breathing, increase lung compliance, and increase alveolar expansion and stability by decreasing surface tension, preventing atelectasis at end expiration. As a result, surfactant directly acts to reverse surfactant deficiency syndrome, prevent or reduce the development of pulmonary interstitial edema, which may progress to other forms of RDS, and reduce oxygen positive-pressure mechanical ventilation requirements. The pharmacologic activity of commercial surfactant results from the combined action of three synthetic components dipalmitoylphosphatidylcholine (DPPC), cetyl alcohol, and tyloxapol. DPPC, the major component of natural surfactant, rapidly and efficiently acts to dramatically decrease alveolar surface tension. Cetyl alcohol facilitates the dispersion and adsorption of DPPC onto the air: liquid interface of the alveoli. Cetyl alcohol modulates this physiologically essential function without the increased risk or immunogenicity of infectious potential associated with foreign protein substances. Tyloxapol provides the product with a hydrophilic agent that allows for reconstitution of the lyophilized powder. Tyloxapol also plays a minor role in distribution of the active components into the smaller airways.

Route: Surfactant can only be administered endotracheally using a special ET tube adaptor supplied with the drug kit, without the interruption of mechanical ventilation and after radiographic confirmation of the location of the ET tip in the trachea unless impractical due to time restraints.

Dosage and administration: Prior to administration of surfactant, the infant should be well suctioned, and suctioning should be withheld for 2 h following the dose unless clinically necessary. Prophylactic surfactant is administered as a single 5 mL/kg dose as soon as RDS is clinically confirmed after birth. Second and third doses may be subsequently administered if necessary while the infant remains mechanically ventilated and under respiratory distress. Rescue treatment for infants who acutely develop RDS is administered as two 5 mL/kg doses, with the first dose given at the time of diagnosis and the second administered 12-24 h later.

Administration of the dose requires intubation and should be done in 1/2 doses, with the first half given over 1-2 min using the appropriately sized endotracheal tube adaptor with the infant positioned at the midline position. The adaptor fits into the ventilator line and has a Leur lock syringe port, through which the drug is administered while maintaining the closed system of the respirator. The infant's head and torso are then rotated 45 degrees to the right and held in that position for 30 s. The infant is then returned to midline and the remaining drug is administered in the same manner, with the head and torso rotated to the left for 30 s. Wean ventilator pressures rapidly after administration.

Adverse effects: Significant adverse effects associated with Exosurf neonatal during clinical use to this point include increased incidence of pulmonary hemorrhage, apnea, and methylxanthine dosage requirements. Other adverse effects associated with the use of the drug involve increased risk of PDA, thrombocytopenia, and acute changes in respiratory status, the latter of which may be a direct result of the pharmacologic activity of the drug and require rapid adjustment of mechanical ventilatory parameters.

Comments: Administration of surfactant requires close and continuous monitoring during and 30 min after administration of the dose to ensure maximum safety, efficacy, and benefit. This should include blood gas monitoring, rapid weaning of mechanical ventilatory parameters, and monitoring of changes in clinical signs and symptoms consistent with changes in oxygenation and pulmonary function.

(Gomella: Neonatology 1999, pp. 592-593)

<u>Exosurf</u> (colfosceril)

Dose/kg: 5 mL

Route & frequency: Endoctracheal rescue treatment:
One dose as soon as RDS diagnosis is confirmed. May repeat 12 h after first dose if baby is still ventilator dependent

Comments: Adverse effects include pulmonary hemorrhage, apnea, and mucous plugging. Adjust ventilatory parameters to prevent hyperoxia and hypocarbia.

Route & frequency: Prophylaxis:
First dose given as soon as possible after birth; a second and third dose may be given 12 and 24 h after the first dose

Comments: May open ductus

(Avery: Neonatology Pathophysiology and Management of the Newborn 1999, p.1560)

Surfactant Pulmonary/Colfosceril Palmitate

Dose & Route: Prophylaxis therapy: 5 mg/kg intratracheally as soon as possible; 2 additional doses are given to infants remaining on ventilators at 12 and 24 hrs later.

Rescue therapy: 5 ml/kg intratracheally as soon as the diagnosis of RDS is made. A second 5 ml/kg dose should be administered 12 hr later as two 2.5 ml/kg aliquots.

Remarks: For intratracheal use only. Pulmonary hemorrhage, apnea, mucous plugging, and decrease in transcutaneous 0_2 of >20% may occur. Drug needs to be reconstituted with preservative-free sterile water for injection. Suction infant prior to administration. Suction only if necessary until 2 hours after administration. Monitor 0_2 saturation, EKG, and blood pressure during dose administration; and arterial blood gases for post-dose hyperoxia and hypocarbia after administration.

(Siberry: The Harriet Lane Handbook 2000, p.858)

CALFACTANT (Infasurf)

Supplied: 35mg phospholipids per ml suspended in 0.9% sodium chloride solution and 0.65mg proteins, in single-use vials containing 6ml suspension.

Administration: For intratracheal administration only. Calfactant does not require reconstitution. DO NOT dilute or sonicate. DO NOT shake. Gently swirl or agitate the vial for redispersion. Visible flecks in the suspension and foaming at the surface are normal. Unopened, unused vials that have warmed to room temperature can be returned to refrigerated storage within 24 hours for future use. Avoid repeated warming to room temperature (1).

Infasurf

This study compared the relative efficacy of administering second and subsequent doses of Infasurf surfactant at a low threshold (FI02> 30%, still requiring endotracheal intubation) versus a high threshold (FI02>40%, mean airway pressure > 7 cm H2O) of respiratory support. For all doses, 100 mg/kg of Infasurf was given as a 33-mg/mL solution (3.0 mL/kg). The surfactant was administered in 1/4 dose aliquots as a bolus down the endotracheal tube, with hand bagging or mechanical ventilation between each aliquot and 90 degree rotation of the patient between each aliquot.

Conclusions: We conclude that equal efficacy can be realized by delaying surfactant retreatment of infants with uncomplicated RDS until they have reached a higher level of respiratory support than is the current standard. We speculate that this would result in a substantial cost-saving from less utilization of drug. Conversely, we believe that infants with complicated RDS should continue to be treated by the low-threshold retreatment strategy, which is currently recommended by the manufacturers of the commerically available surfactants.

(Kattwinkel: High-Versus Low-Threshold Surfactant Retreatment for Neonatal Respiratory Distress Syndrome. Pediarics 2000;106:282-288)

Infrasurf

Inborn premature infants delivered to mothers at an estimated gestational age of 24[0/7] to 28[6/7] weeks.

Interventions. Those infants who were randomized to the immediate bolus strategy were intubated as rapidly as possible after birth, and a 3-mL intratracheal bolus of calf lung surfactant extract (Infasurf) was administered before the initiation of positive pressure ventilation. Those infants who were randomized to the postventilatory aliquot strategy received standard resuscitation measures with intubation by 5 minutes of age, if not required earlier. At 10 minutes after birth, 3 mL of surfactant was administered in 4 divided aliquots of 0.75 mL each. Patients in both groups were eligible to receive up to three additional doses of surfactant as rescue therapy in the neonatal intensive care unit, if needed.

Infants in both groups were eligible to receive a second dose of surfactant, as rescue therapy, (100 mg/kg in 4 aliquots with 2 minutes of hand bagging between each aliquot) after 4 hours of age if there was radiographic evidence of respiratory distress syndrome and the fraction of inspired oxygen (FIO2) was 0.4 or greater and the mean airway pressure was 0.686 kPa (7.0 cm of water) or greater. Patients were eligible to receive third and fourth doses (100 mg/kg in 4 aliquots) at 8-hour intervals if the FIO2 was 0.4 or greater and the mean airway pressure was 0.686 kPa (7.0 cm of water) or greater.

(Kendig: Comparison of Two Strategies for Surfactant Prophylaxis in Very Premature Infants: A Multicenter Randomized Trial. Pediatrics 1998;101:1006-1012)

Calfactant (Infasurf)

Synonyms: Bovine Lung Surfactant
Therapeutic Category: Lung Surfactant
Generic Available: No

Use: Prevention and treatment of respiratory distress syndrome (RDS) in premature infants

Prophylactic therapy: Infants <29 weeks at significant risk for RDS

Treatment: Infants ≤72 hours of age with RDS (confirmed by clinical and radiologic findings and requiring endotracheal intubation)

Warnings: Rapidly affects oxygenation and lung compliance and should be restricted to a highly supervised use in a clinical setting with immediate availability of clinicians experienced with intubation and ventilatory management of premature infants; if transient episodes of bradycardia and decreased oxygen saturation occur, discontinue the dosing procedure and initiate measures to alleviate the condition; produces rapid improvement in lung oxygenation and compliance that may require immediate reductions in ventilator settings and FiO_2; for intratracheal administration only

Precautions: Transient episodes of reflux of calfactant into the endotracheal tube, cyanosis, bradycardia, or airway obstruction have occurred during dosing procedures; such episodes may require stopping administration and taking appropriate measures to alleviate the condition before resuming therapy

Adverse Reactions:

Most adverse reactions occur during the dosing procedure
Cardiovascular: Bradycardia, cyanosis
Respiratory: Airway obstruction, pneumothorax, pulmonary hemorrhage, apnea

Stability: Refrigerate; protect from light; unopened, unused warmed vials of calfactant may be returned to refrigerator within 24 hours for future use; repeated warming to room temperature should be avoided

Mechanism of Action:

Replaces deficient or ineffective endogenous lung surfactant in neonates with RDS or in neonates at risk of developing RDS; surfactant prevents the alveoli from collapsing during expiration by lowering surface tension between air and alveolar surfaces

Usual Dosage: Intratracheal: Neonates: 3 mL/kg every 12 hours up to a total of 3 doses; repeat doses have been administered as early as 6 hours after the previous dose for a total of up to four doses (if the infant was still intubated and required at least 30% inspired oxygen to maintain a $PaO_2 \leq 80$ torr)

Administration: Intratracheal: Gently swirl to redisperse suspension; do not shake; administer dosage divided into two aliquots of 1.5 mL/kg each into the endotracheal tube; after each instillation, reposition the infant with either the right or left side dependent; administration is made while ventilation is continued over 20-30 breaths for each aliquot, with small bursts timed only during the inspiratory cycles; a pause followed by evaluation of the respiratory status and repositioning should separate the two aliquots; calfactant dosage has also been divided into four equal aliquots and administered with repositioning in four different positions (prone, supine, right and left lateral)

Monitoring Parameters:

Continuous heart rate and transcutaneous O_2 saturation should be monitored during administration; frequent ABG sampling is necessary to prevent postdosing hyperoxia and hypocarbia

(Taketomo: Pediatric dosage Handbook 1990-2000, pp.148-149

TERBUTALINE (Brethine, Bricanyl, Brethaire)

Supplied: Brethaire Aerosol 200mcg/spray
Injection 1mg/ml
Tablets 2.5mg, 5mg

Administration: Inhalation, Sub Q, PO

Terbutaline (Brethine)

Aerosol Therapy in Neonates, Indicating Dosing, Receptor Effects, and Common Side Effects

0.01-0.02 mg/kg. Dilute with NS to 3 mL.
Dose: every 2-8 h. Minimum dose: 0.1 mg

Side Effects: Hypertension
Hyperglycemia
Tachycardia

(Gomella: Neonatology: Management, Procedures, On-call Problems, Diseases and Drugs 1999, p.56)

Terbutaline

Dosage: 0.01 mg/kg SC for acute bronchospasm;
0.1 mg/kg in 2 ml normal saline by nebulization for inhalation. For continuous infusion
Loading dose: 2.0-5.0 μg/kg
Maintenance dose: 2 to 12 μg/kg/hr

Comments: Selective β_2 agonist

(Fanaroff: Neonatal-Perinatal Medicine 1997, p.1749)

Terbutaline (Brethine, Brethaire)

Dose: Nebulization:

- Intermittent: 0.01-0.03 mg/kg given every 2-6 hours. Dilute to a final total volume of 3 ml with normal saline or other concurrent medications.
  Minimum: 0.1 mg. Maximum: 1 mg/dose.
- Continuous: 0.4 mg/kg/hour by continuous nebulization. In a study by Portnoy and Aggarwal, continuous nebulization for 1-24 hours (mean=8 hours) was not associated with signs of toxicity such as tachycardia or arrhythmia. They considered it a safe and effective mode of treatment.

MDI: Two puffs every 4-12 hours. Use with a spacer.

Nursing Implications:
Monitor for tachycardia and cardiac arrhythmias.
Monitor blood pressure and respiratory status.

Comments: Monitoring and Dose Titration:

- Reduce the dose to the next smaller dose and/or increase the dosing interval to the next longer interval when the heart rate exceeds 180 bpm (if baseline HR was <150 bpm) or 200 bpm (if baseline HR was >150 bpm). A moderate increase in heart rate is expected and may indicate absorption and therapeutic response.

Lengthening the interval between doses should be tried when respiratory status has improved. Taper to the lowest effective dose.

- Increase the dose to the next large dose and/or decrease the dosing interval to the next shorter interval if the infant is still in respiratory distress after a trial of 1-3 doses. Do not increase dose if infant is experiencing adverse effects from existing dose. In severe airway obstruction, frequent small doses of bronchodilator by nebulizer may be more effective than larger, less frequent doses.

Discontinuation of Treatment: Monitor heart rate and blood pressure. Discontinue terbutaline if adverse effects occur or if the drug is no longer needed. If there has been no improvement in respiratory status as measured by pulmonary mechanics, blood gases, change in respiratory support, or clinical status after 3 doses, discontinue the drug.

(Zenk: Neonatal Medications & Nutrition. A Comprehensive Guide 2000; pp.457-458)

Terbutaline

Dose & Route: PO:
≤12 yr: Initial: 0.05 mg/kg/dose TID, increase as required.
Max dose: 0.15 mg/kg/dose TID or total of 5 mg/24 hr.
>12 yr and adults: 2.5-5 mg/dose PO Q6-8 hr.
Max dose: 12-15 yr, 7.5 mg/24 hr: >15 yr, 15 mg/24 hr
Nebulization:
<2 yr: 0.5 mg in 2.5 ml NS Q4-6 hr
SC:
≤12 yr: 0.005-0.01 mg/kg/dose Q15-20 min x 2;
Max dose: 0.4 mg/dose
Inhalations: 1-2 inhalations Q4-6 hr
Continuous Infusion, IV: 2-10 mcg/kg loading dose followed by infusion of 0.1-0.4 mcg/kg/minute. May titrate in increments of 0.1-0.2 mcg/kg/minutes Q30 min depending on clinical response. To prepare infusion: see inside front cover.

Remarks: Nervousness, tremor, headache, nausea, tachycardia, arrhythmias, palpitations may occur. Paradoxical bronchoconstriction may occur with excessive use; if it occurs, discontinue drug immediately. Injectable product may be used for nebulization. For acute asthma, nebulizations may be given more frequently than Q4-6 hr. **Adjust dose in renal failure**.

(Siberry: The Harriet Lane Handbook 2000, p.860)

TETANUS ANTITOXIN (TAT)

Supplied: No longer commercially available in United States (3).

Tetanus Antitoxin

In countries where TIG is not available, equine tetanus antitoxin may be available. This product is no longer available in the United States. Tetanus antitoxin is administered as a single dose of 50 000 to 100 000 U after appropriate testing for sensitivity and desensitization if necessary. Part of this dose (20 000 U) should be given intravenously. Doses as small as 10 000 U may be as effective as larger doses.

(AAP: Report of the Committee on Infectious Disease 2000, pp. 564-565)

Tetanus Antitoxin

Route and Dose: IM, IV: 10,000-20,000 units/day for 2 successive days

Adverse Effects, Cautions: Optimal dosage not established for newborns.

(Taeusch: Schaffer and Avery's Diseases of the Newborn 1991, p.1054)

TETANUS IMMUNE GLOBULIN, HUMAN (HYPER-TET, TIG)

Supplied: Injection 250 unit vial.

Administration: IM, DO NOT INJECT IV.

Tetanus Immune Globulin

Tetanus Immune Globulin (human) (TIG) is recommended for treatment. A single total dose of 3000 to 6000 U is recommended for children and adults. The optimum therapeutic dose, has not yet been established, and doses as small as 500 U have been effective in treatment of infants with tetanus neonatorum. Available preparations must be given intramuscularly. Some authorities recommend infiltration of part of the dose locally around the wound, although the efficacy of this approach has not been prove. Results of studies on the benefit from intrathecal TIG are conflicting. The TIG formulation in use in the United States is not licensed or appropriate for intrathecal or intravenous use.

In countries where TIG is not available, equine tetanus antitoxin may be available. This product is no longer available in the United States. Tetanus antitoxin is administered as a single dose of 50 000 to 100 000 U after appropriate testing for sensitivity and desensitization if necessary. Part of this dose (20 000 U) should be given intravenously. Doses as small as 10 000 U may be as effective as larger doses.

Immune Globulin Intravenous contains antibodies to tetanus and can be considered for treatment if TIG is not available. Approval by the US Food and Drug Administration has not been given for this use, and the dosage has not been determined.

Oral (or intravenous) metronidazole (30 mg/kg per day, given at 6-hour intervals) is effective in reducing the number of vegetative forms of *C tetani* and is the antibiotic of choice. Parenteral penicillin G (100 000 U /kg per day, given at 4- to 6-hour intervals) is an alternative treatment. therapy for 10 to 14 days is recommended.

(American Academy of Pediatrics: Report of the Committee on Infectious Diseases. Red Book 2000, pp.564-565)

Tetanus Immune Globulin

Route & Dose: IM: 250-500 units/dose

Adverse Effects, Cautions:

Optimal dosage not established for newborns

(Taeusch: Avery's Diseases of the Newborn 1998, p.1347)

Tetanus Immune Globulin, Human (Hyper-TET, TIG)

Indications: Prevention and/or treatment of tetanus neonatorum.

Dosage/Dosage Interval:

IM: 3000-6000 U x 1; optimal dosage not established for newborns.

Clinical Considerations:

Tetanus immune globulin is preferred over tetanus antitoxin for the prevention and/or treatment of tetanus neonatorum. The formulation in use in the United States is not licensed for intrathecal or intravenous use.

(Cloherty: Manual of Neonatal Care 1998, p.739)

TETRACYCLINE

Tetracycline

Comments: Contraindicated in newborns.

Toxicity: The use of tetracycline during the period of tooth development (from the last half of pregnancy through the eighth year of life) may cause permanent discoloration (yellow-gray-brown) of deciduous and permanent teeth. (1)

Decreased fibula growth rate occurred in premature infants given 25mg/kg oral TCN every 6 hrs. This was reversible when drug was discontinued. (1)

Tetracycline

Prevention of Neonatal Ophthalmia

Gonococcal Ophthalmia

For newborn infants, topical 1% silver nitrate solution, 0.5% erythromycin ointment, and **1% tetracycline ointment** are considered equally effective for prophylaxis of ocular gonorrheal infection. Each is available in single-dose tubes. Povidone-iodine in a 2.5% solution also might be useful for preventing gonococcal ophthalmia, but more studies are required, and a product for this purpose currently is not available in the United States. Silver nitrate causes more chemical conjunctivitis than other agents but is recommended in areas where the incidence of penicillinase-producing *Neisseria gonorrhoeae* (PPNG) is appreciable. The efficacy of erythromycin or povidone-iodine prophylaxis against PPNG is not known; 1 study has demonstrated tetracycline to be effective for prophylaxis of

PPNG infections. Infants born to women with untreated gonococcal infection should receive 1 dose of ceftriaxone (25-50 mg/kg) or cefotaxime (100 mg/kg), as well as topical prophylaxis. Infants who have gonococcal ophthalmia should be hospitalized and evaluated for signs of disseminated infection.

Chlamydial Ophthalmia
Neonatal ophthalmia due to *Chlamydia trachomatis*, although not as severe as gonococcal conjunctivitis, is common in the United States. Results of studies on the clinical efficacy of erythromycin and of **tetracycline ointment** for prophylaxis of chlamydial conjunctivitis have been conflicting. Topical antibiotics and silver nitrate do not have proven efficacy in preventing conjunctivitis or nasopharyngeal colonization. One study has shown that 2.5% povidone-iodine is likely to be more effective than either topical erythromycin or silver nitrate for preventing chlamydial conjunctivitis but does not prevent nasopharyngeal colonization and subsequent risk of pneumonia. Infants with ophthalmia neonatorum caused by *C trachomatis* should be evaluated and treated.

(American Academy of Pediatrics: Report of the Committee on Infectious Diseases. Red Book 2000, pp.735-736)

Tetracycline

Antibacterial Drugs for Pediatric Patients Beyond the Newborn Period
Dosage per kg/d
Route: IV
Mild to Moderate Infections: Inappropriate

Severe Infections: 10-25 mg in 2-4 doses

Comments: Responsible for staining of developing teeth; use only in children 8 years of age or older except in circumstances in which the benefits of therapy exceed the risks and alternative drugs are less effective or more toxic

Route: PO
Mild to Moderate Infections: 20-50 mg in 4 doses
Severe Infections: Inappropriate

(American Academy of Pediatrics: Report of the Committee on Infectious Diseases. Red Book 2000, pp.661-662)

TETRACYCLINE OPHTHALMIC OINTMENT (Achromycin)

Supplied: Ophthalmic Ointment 1% 3.5gms
Administration: Ophthalmic

Tetracycline

Recommendations: For prophylaxis of gonococcal ophthalmic neonatorum, a 1% silver nitrate solution in single-dose ampules or single-use tubes of an ophthalmic ointment containing 0.5% erythromycin or 1% tetracycline are each effective and acceptable. The effectiveness of erythromycin or tetracycline in the prevention of ophthalmia caused by penicillinase-producing Neisseria gonorrhoeae is not established.

Comment: Prophylaxis should be given shortly after birth...(including infants born by cesarean section).

Administration: Before administering local prophylaxis, each eyelid should be wiped gently with sterile cotton. Two drops of a 1% silver nitrate solution or a 1-cm ribbon of antibiotic ointment are placed in each lower conjunctival sac. The eyelids are then massaged gently to spread the ointment. After 1 minute, excess solution or ointment may be wiped away with sterile cotton. None of the prophylactic agents should be flushed from the eye after instillation.

(AAP: Report of the Committee on Infectious Diseases 1994, p. 533-534)

DOXYCYCLINE (Vibramycin)

Supplied: Oral suspension: powder for 25 mg/5 ml in 60 ml.
Syrup: 50 mg/5 ml in 60 ml.
Injection: 100 mg, 200 mg vial

Administration: PO, IV.
IV administration: dilute 100 mg vial with 10 ml SWFI, for a concentration of 10 mg/ml. Further dilute to a concentration of 0.1 to 1 mg/ml in D5W, NS and infuse over 1 to 4 hours (3).

Do not inject IM or SC.

Doxycycline (numerous types)

Antibacterial Drugs for Pediatric Patients Beyond the Newborn Period:
Dosage per kg/d
Route: PO, IV
Mild to Moderate Infections: 2-4 mg in 1-2 doses
Severe Infections: Inappropriate

Comments: Side effects similar to those of other tetracycline products except the risk of dental staining in children younger than 8 years of age is less

(American Academy of Pediatrics: Report of the Committee on Infectious Diseases. Red Book 2000, p.662)

THAM (TROMETHAMINE)

Supplied: Injection 18gm (150mEq) in 500ml (0.3M)

Administration: IV infusion
Severe hemorrhagic liver necrosis has occurred in neonates. Hypoglycemia may occur when administered to premature or even full term neonates (1).

Tromethamine (THAM)

Indications and use: Metabolic acidosis when sodium bicarbonate is contraindicated because of elevated serum sodium (eg, metabolic acidosis in persistent fetal circulation treated with multiple doses of sodium bicarbonate).

Actions: Alkalinizing agent that acts as a proton (hydrogen ion) acceptor; combines with hydrogen ions and their associated anions of acids (lactic, pyruvic, carbonic, and other metabolic acids). The resulting salts are then renally excreted.

Route: IV

Dosage: Loading dose: 3-5 mL/kg of undiluted solution infused over 1 h, or dose = weight (kg) x 1.1 x base deficit (meq/L).

Maintenance dose: 3 mL/kg/h (undiluted solution) as continuous infusion. Titrate dose to desired response via frequent blood gas monitoring.

Adverse effects: Respiratory depression, thrombophlebitis, venospasm, alkalosis, transient hypocalcemia or hypoglycemia, and hyperkalemia. Extravasation may cause sloughing of the skin.

Comments: Contraindicated in anuria, uremia, and chronic respiratory acidosis. Do not administer for periods >24 hours. Hyperkalemia is a problem especially with decreased renal function.

(Gomella: Neonatology 1999, p.595)

Tromethamine (THAM)

Dose/kg: 3 mL

Route and frequency:
IV slow infusion
Max rate: 1 ml/h

Comments: 1 mL = 0.3 mEq; 1 mM = 1 mEq
Infuse preferably in large blood vessel; may cause hypoglycemia, hyperkalemia, apnea, and fluid overload

(Avery: Neonatology Pathophysiology and Management of the Newborn 1999, p.1561)

THAM

Dose: 300 mg/kg

Comments: Possible use in respiratory acidosis

(Garson: The science and practice of pediatric cardiology 1998, p.2956)

THEOPHYLLINE (Elixophyllin, Theolair, Accurbron)

Supplied:

Elixophyllin Elixir	80mg/15ml	20% alcohol
Theolair Liquid	80mg/15ml	alcohol free
Accurbron Elixir	150mg/15ml	7.5% alcohol

IV Theophylline/Dextrose 5%: 0.8mg/ml in 500ml, 1.6mg/ml in 250ml, 2.0mg/ml in 100ml, 4.0mg/ml in 50ml

IV Theophylline/D5W physically and chemically compatible with dopamine, dobutamine, and tolazoline (8)

Administration: PO, IV

Theophylline (Various)

Indications and use: Apnea of prematurity. There is evidence that theophyline can improve lung compliance and aid in

	weaning infants from respiratory support in diseases such as BPD.
Actions:	A methylxanthine. Probably acts by virtue of adenosine antagonism. Neonates have the unique ability to convert theophylline to caffeine in a ration of 1:0.3, respectively, and caffeine may approach 50% of theophylline serum levels. Thus, it is impossible to distinguish the pharmacodynamic effects of theophylline from those of caffeine in the neonate. Theophylline produces excitation throughout all levels of the CNS; produces modest decreases in peripheral vascular resistance; increases cardiac output; relaxes pulmonary airway smooth muscle, with a resultant increase in vital capacity; decreases diaphragmatic fatigue; and may cause marked increases in cerebrovascular resistance, resulting in decreased cerebral blood flow. In premature infants at risk for ventricular hemorrhage, the latter effect may be deleterious.
Route:	IV, PO.
Dosage:	Apnea of prematurity: 5-6 mg/kg PO or IV (infused over 15-30 min) as a loading dose, followed by a maintenance dose of 2 mg/kg q12h starting 12 h after the loading dose. Ventilator weaning: 6.5 mg/kg PO or IV as a loading dose, followed by a maintenance dose of 3-4 mg/kg q 12h.
Adverse effects:	Side effects and toxicity include hyperglycemia, diuresis, dehydration, feeding intolerance, tachycardia and other arrhythmias, hyperreflexia, jitteriness, and seizures.
Comments:	Levels for apnea are 6-11 mcg/mL. Toxicity is associated with levels > 15-20 mcg/mL. Monitor serum levels on day 4 of therapy: peak level 1 h after an IV dose is completed or 2 h after an oral dose, and trough level 30 min before the next dose. Levels of caffeine and theophylline should ideally be monitored any time toxicity is suspected or when apnea spells appear to be increasing in frequency.

(Gomella: Neonatology 1999, p.593)

Theophylline

Theophylline Serum Levels (µg/mL)*	Adverse Reactions
15-25	GI upset, GE reflux, diarrhea, nausea, vomiting, abdominal pain, nervousness, headache, insomnia, agitation, dizziness, muscle cramp, tremor
25-35	Tachycardia, occasional PVC
>35	Ventricular tachycardia, frequent PVC, seizure

*Adverse effects do not necessarily occur according to serum levels. Arrhythmia and seizure can occur without seeing the other adverse effects.

Usual Dosage:	Oral Loading dose: Neonates: Apnea of prematurity: 4 mg/kg/dose

Guidelines for Drawing Theophylline Serum Levels

Dosage Form	Time to Draw Level*
I.V. bolus	30 min after end of 30-min infusion
I.V. continuous infusion	12-24 h after initiation of infusion
P.O. liquid, fast-release formulation	Peak: 1 h postdose after at least 1 day of therapy Trough: Just before a dose after at least 1 day of therapy
P.O. slow-release formulation	Peak: 4 h postdose after at least 1 day of therapy Trough: Just before a dose after at least 1 day of therapy

*The time to achieve steady-state serum levels is prolonged in patients with longer half-lives (eg. Premature neonates, infants and adults with cardiac or liver failure .... In these patients, serum theophylline levels should be drawn after 48-72 hours of therapy; serum levels may need to be done prior to steady-state to assess the patients current progress or evaluate potential toxicity.

Monitoring Parameters:
Respiratory rate, heart rate, serum theophylline level, arterial or capillary blood gases (if applicable); number and severity of apnea spells (apnea of prematurity)
(Taketomo: Pediatric Dosage Handbook 1999-2000, pp.864-869)

Theophylline

Route & Dose: PO, IV: loading dose: 5-6 mg/kg; maintenance dose; 1-2.5 mg/kg/dose q 6-12 h; aminophylline (IV) dose = theophylline (IV) dose x 1.25

Adverse Effects and Cautions:
Blood level monitoring indicated (therapeutic range: apnea, 7-12 µg/ml; bronchospasm, 10-20 µg/ml). Tachycardia at 15-20 µg/ml, seizures >40 µg/ml. Avoid rectal dosing owing to variable absorption. Clearance decreased by asphyxia and prematurity
(Taeusch: Avery's Diseases of the Newborn 1998, p.1347)

Theophylline

Dose & Route: Dosing intervals are for immediate release preparations. For sustained release preparations divide daily dose QD-TID based on product.
Neonatal apnea:
Load: 5 mg/kg/dose PO x 1
Maintenance: 3-6 mg/kg/24 hr PO ÷ Q6-8 hr

Bronchospasm: PO:
Loading dose: 1 mg/kg/dose for each 2 mg/L desired increase n serum theophylline level.
Maintenance, infants (<1 yr):
Preterm:
<24 days old (postnatal): 1 mg/kg/dose PO Q12 hr
≥24 days old (postnatal): 1.5 mg/kg/dose PO Q12 hr
Full-term up to 1 hr old: Total daily dose (mg) + [(0.2 x age in weeks) + 5] x (kg body weight)
≤26 weeks old: divide daily dose Q8 hr
>26 weeks old: divide daily dose Q6 hr

Remarks: Drug metabolism varies widely with age, drug formulation, and route of administration. Most common side effects and toxicities are nausea, vomiting, anorexia, abdominal pain, gastroesophageal reflux, nervousness, tachycardia, seizures, and arrhythmias.

Serum levels should be monitored. Therapeutic levels: bronchospasm: 10-20 mg/L; apnea: 7-13 mg/L. Half-life is age-dependent: 30 hr (newborns); 6.9 hr (infants); 3.4 hr (children). See aminophylline for guidelines for serum level determinations. Theophylline is a substrate for CYP 450 1A2. Levels increased with allopurinol, alcohol, ciprofloxacin, cimetidine, clarithromycin, disulfiram, erythromycin, estrogen, propranolol, thiabendazole, and verapamil. Levels decreased with carbamazepine, isoproterenol, phenobarbital, phenytoin, and rifampin.

(Siberry: The Harriet Lane Handbook 2000, pp.861-863)

THIOPENTAL (Pentothal)

Supplied: Powder for Injection 2% (20mg/mL)
400 mg vials; 1, 2.5 and 5 gm kits
Powder for Injection 2.5% (25 mg/mL)
250, 500 mg vials; 1, 2.5, 5 and 10 gm kits

Administration: IV

Thiopental

Indication: For Neonatal Seizures

Thiopental was reported to be highly effective in the treatment of seizures in nine asphyxiated term newborns who continued to convulse despite mean phenobarbital levels of 28 µg/ml. Dose was 10 mg/kg, administered intravenously over 2 minutes, and response occurred "promptly." However, a 27% decrease (mean) of arterial blood pressure occurred in six of the nine infants, and each was treated with pressor agents or volume expansion. The adjunctive value of this mode of therapy remains to be established conclusively.

(Volpe: Neurology of the Newborn 2001, p.206)

Thiopental

Usual Dosage: Induction anesthesia: I.V.:
Neonates: 3-4 mg/kg
Infants: 5-8 mg/kg

Administration: Parenteral: Avoid rapid I.V. injection (may cause hypotension or **decreased** cardiac output); may administer by intermittent infusion over 10-60 minutes at a maximum concentration of 50 mg/mL

Monitoring Parameters: Respiratory rate, heart rate, blood pressure
Nursing Implications: Avoid extravasation, necrosis may occur

(Taketomo: Pediatric Dosage Handbook 1999-2000, pp.874-875)

Thiopental Sodium

Dose & Route: Cerebral edema: 1.5-5 mg/kg/dose IV. Repeat PRN for increased ICP.
Anesthesia induction, children and adults:
IV: 2-6 mg/kg: Use lower doses in patients with hemodynamic instability.
Deep Sedation:
Children: 30 mg/kg PR x 1; **max** 1 g/dose

Remarks: **Contraindicated** in acute intermittent porphyria. May cause respiratory depression, hypotension, anaphylaxis, decreased cardiac output. Dee sedation is used for diagnostic imaging studies.

Onset of action: 30-60 sec for IV; 7-10 min for PR. Duration of action: 5-30 min for IV; 90 min for PR. **Adjust dose in renal failure**.

(Siberry: The Harriet Lane Handbook 2000, p.864)

THROMBIN, TOPICAL (Thrombinar, Thrombogen, Thrombostat)

Supplied: 1,000, 5,000, 10,000, 20,000 and 50,000 unit vials

Administration: Topical
Use solutions immediately upon reconstitution. If necessary, refrigerate at 2°–8° C for up to 3 hours (1).
The recipient surface should be sponged (not wiped) free of blood before thrombin is applied. A spray may be used or the surface may be flooded using a sterile syringe and small gauge needle. The most effective hemostasis results when the thrombin mixes freely with the blood as soon as it reaches the surface. Avoid sponging of treated surfaces to ensure that the clot remains securely in place (1).

Thrombin, Topical

Use: Hemostasis whenever minor bleeding from capillaries and small venules is accessible

Usual Dosage: Topical: Apply powder directly to the site of bleeding or on oozing surfaces or use 1000-2000 units/mL of solution where bleeding is profuse; use 100 units/mL for bleeding from skin or mucosal surfaces

Administration: Topical: May be applied directly as a powder or as reconstituted solution; use sterile water or NS to reconstituted powder to desired concentration; sponge surface free of blood prior to application, if possible

Additional Information: One unit is amount required to clot 1 mL of standardized fibrinogen solution in 15 seconds

(Taketomo: Pediatric Dosage Handbook 1999-2000, p.879)

Thrombin (Thrombinar, Thrombostat)

Administration & Dose:
Apply powder directly to the site of bleeding or oozing, or dissolve powder in sterile water or NS to a concentration of 100 units/ml (for bleeding from skin or mucosal surfaces)

to 1000 units/ml (for bleeding from exposed parenchyma of visceral organs). Blood should be sponged from the bleeding site immediately prior to application of thrombin; sponging should be avoided after treatment.

Toxicity: Allergic reactions.

(Benitz: The Pediatric Drug Handbook 1995, p.405)

Thrombin Fibrin Glue

The fibrin glue is formed by mixing components from separate syringes. Syringe A: 10 ml of single donor cryoprecipitate (cryoprecipitate serves as a concentrated source of fibrinogen-approximately 40 mg/ml), and Syringe B: contains 5 ml of 10% Calcium chloride solution mixed with 5 mg Bovine Thrombin (1000 U/ml)-Thrombinar. The fibrin glue is applied topically to the open wound using the two separate syringes. A gelatinous fibrin polymer begins to form after component mixing. The fibrin glue is applied a second time to the cannula exit site once the wound is closed completely. A total of 4-5 ml of fibrin glue was used for each patient.

The authors of this article applied fibrin glue to the cannulation sites in 11 neonatal ECMO patients during reexploration for excessive bleeding. No specific source of bleeding could be identified in any instance. After the application of fibrin glue, the diffuse bleeding was completely controlled with the use of sutures or electrocautery.

(Moront: The use of topical fibrin glue at cannulation sites in neonates. Surg Gynecol Obstet 1988;166:358-359)

THYROID DESICCATED

Supplied: Tablets 15mg, 30mg, 60mg
Administration: PO

Thyroid USP is composed of desiccated animal thyroid glands. (1)

SEE ALSO: LEVOTHYROXINE

Thyroid (Desiccated thyroid)

Dosage: Initial: 8-15 mg/day as a single dose PO.

Comments: Titrate dosage at weekly intervals to normalize serum T_4; usual maintenance 50-200 mg/day.

(Fanaroff: Neonatal-Perinatal Medicine 1997, p.1750)

TICARCILLIN-DISODIUM (Ticar)

Supplied: Injection, powder for 1gm, 3gm vial
Administration: IV, IM
Contains 5.2mEq Na/gm
IM Administration: Add 2ml SWFI or NS for each gm of Ticarcillin to obtain 1gm ticarcillin per 2.6ml. Use promptly.(3)

For direct IV injection add 4ml NS or D5W per gram for approximate concentration of 200mg/ml. To reduce vein irritation, injections should be made slowly and concentrations of 50mg/ml or less should be used.

For intermittent infusion dilute to a concentration of 10 to 100mg/ml. Infuse over 10-20 minutes in neonates. (Adults 30 minutes - 2 hours). Stable in D5W, NS (3).

<u>Ticarcillin</u>

Antibacterial Drugs for Newborn Infants
Dose (mg/kg or Units [U]/kg) and Frequency of Administration
Route: IV, IM
Dose: <u>Infants 0.4 wk</u>
BW <1200 g: 75 every 12 h

<u>Infants <1 wk old</u>
BW ≤1200-2000 g: 75 every 12 h
BW >2000 g: 75 every 8 h

<u>Infants ≥1 wk old</u>
BW ≤2000-2000 g: 75 every 8 h
BW >2000 g: 75 every 6 h

Antibacterial Drugs for Pediatric Patients Beyond the Newborn Period
Dosage per kg/d
Route: IV, IM
Mild to Moderate Infections: 100-200 mg in 4 doses
Severe Infections: 200-300 mg in 4-6 doses
Comments: Contains 5.2 mEq of Na per gram
Notes: In patients with history of allergy to penicillin or one of its many congeners, alternative drugs are recommended. In some circumstances, a cephalosporin or other β-lactam class drug may be acceptable. However, these drugs should not be used in patients with an immediate hypersensitivity (anaphylaxis) to penicillin because approximately 5% to 15% of penicillin-allergic patients will also be allergic to the cephalosporins.

(American Academy of Pediatrics: Report of the Committee on Infectious Diseases. Red Book 2000, pp.652,659,662)

<u>Ticarcillin</u>

Route: IV, IM
Dosage (mg/kg) and Interval of Administration:

<u>Weight <1200 g</u>
Age 0-4 Wk: 75 q12h

<u>Weight 1200-2000 g</u>
Age 0-7 Days: 75 q12h
Age >7 Days: 75 q8h

<u>Weight >2000 g</u>
Age 0-7 Days: 75 q8h
Age >7 Days: 75 q6h

(Remington: Infectious Diseases of the Fetus and Newborn Infant 2001, p.1454)

Ticarcillin

Route: IV, IM

Dosages (mg/kg/day) and Intervals of Administration:

Body weight <2000g
0-7 days old: 150 div q12h
8-28 days old: 225 div q8h

Body weight >2000g
0-7 days old: 225 div q8h
8-28 days old: 300 div q6h

>28 days old: 300 div q6h

(Nelson: Pocket Book of Pediatric Antimicrobial Therapy 2000-2001, p.16)

Ticarcillin

Condition: Urinary Tract Infection, Pseudomonas aeruginosa
Therapy: Mezlocillin or ticarcillin IV, IM AND aminoglycoside IV, IM x 10 days.
Comment: Ceftazidime is a suitable alternative

(Nelson: Pocket Book of Pediatric Antimicrobial Therapy 2000-2001, p.13)

Ticarcillin Disodium (Ticar)

Classification: Semisynthetic extended-spectrum penicillin.
Action and spectrum: See Mezlocillin Sodium.

Route: IM, IV (infuse over 30 min).
Dosage: < 2000 g and 0-7 days old: 150 mg/kg/day divided q 12h.
< 2000 g and >7 days old: 225 mg/kg/day divided q 8h.
> 2000 g and 0-7 days old 225 mg/kg/day divided q 8h.
> 2000 g and >7 days old: 300 mg/kg/day divided q 6h.

Elimination and metabolism: Renally excreted.
Adverse effects: See Mezlocillin Sodium. Hypokalemia is pronounced.
Comments: Drug of first choice when considering an extended-spectrum penicillin.
Avoid IM use if possible. Contains 5.2 meq of sodium per gram.

(Gomella: Neonatology 1999, p.593)

Ticarcillin (Ticar)

Dose & Route: Neonates, IM/IV:
≤7 days:
<2 kg: 150 mg/kg/24 hr ÷ Q12 hr
≥2 kg: 225 mg/kg/24 hr ÷ Q8 hr
>7 days:
<1.2 kg: 150 mg/kg/24 hr ÷ Q12 hr
1.2-2 kg: 225 mg/kg/24 hr ÷ Q8 hr
>2 kg: 300 mg/kg/24 hr ÷ Q6-8 hr

Infants and Children: (IM/IV): 200-300 mg/kg/24 hr ÷ Q4-6 hr. **Max dose**: 24 g/24 hr

Cystic Fibrosis. (IM/IV): 300-600 mg/kg/24 hr ÷ Q4-6 hr. **Max dose**: 24 g/24 hr

Remarks: May cause decreased platelet aggregation, bleeding diathesis, hypernatremia, hematuria, hypokalemia, hypocalcemia, allergy, rash, increased AST. Like other penicillins, CSF penetration occurs only with inflamed meninges. Do not mix with aminoglycoside in same solution. **Adjust dose in renal failure**.

(Siberry: The Harriet Lane Handbook 2000, p.866)

TICARCILLIN/CLAVULANATE (Timentin)

Supplied: 3.1gm vials (3gm Ticarcillin, 0.1gm clavulanate

Administration: IV infusion over 30 minutes

Contains 4.75 mEq Na^+/gm.

Add 13ml SWFI to vial (Each ml will contain ≈200mg ticarcillin and 6.7mg clavulanic acid). Further dilute to a concentration between 10-100 mg/ml (1).

Administer over 30 minutes.

Ticarcillin-clavulanate

Antibacterial Drugs for Pediatric Patients Beyond the Newborn Period

Dosage per kg/d

Route: IV, IM

Mild to Moderate Infections: 100-200 mg of ticarcillin in 4 doses (4-6 g)

Severe Infections: 200-300 mg of ticarcillin in 4 doses (12-24 g)

Note: In patients with history of allergy to penicillin or one of its many congeners, alternative drugs are recommended. In some circumstances, a cephalosporin or other β-lactam class drug may be acceptable. However, these drugs should not be used in patients with an immediate hypersensitivity (anaphylaxis) to penicillin because approximately 5% to 15% of penicillin-allergic patients will also be allergic to the cephalosporins.

(American Academy of Pediatrics: Report of the Committee on Infectious Diseases. Red Book 2000, pp.659,662)

Ticarcillin and Clavulanate Potassium

Route: IV

Dosage: 200-300 mg/kg/day

Interval: q4-q6h

NON-NEWBORN SECTION

(Nelson: Pocket Book of Pediatric Antimicrobial Therapy 2000-2001, p.85)

Ticarcillin Disodium and Clavulanate Potassium (Timentin)

Classification: Combination antibiotic of ticarcillin (a carboxypenicillin) and clavulanic acid (a β-lactamase inhibitor).

Spectrum: Good antipseudomonal activity similar to that of ticarcillin except for additional coverage of lactamase-producing species, particularly Gram-positive cocci (eg, *Staphylococcus aureus*, *Streptococcus pneumoniae*, and group B streptococcus). Good coverage against Gram-negative organisms, including *Escherichia coli*, *Klebsiella* spp, and *Proteus* spp. Also demonstrated activity against anaerobes such as *Clostridium* spp and *Peptostreptococcus* spp.

Route: IV.

Dosage: <2000 g and 0-7 days old: 150 mg/kg/day divided q 12h.
<2000 g and >7 days old: 225 mg/kg/day divided q 8h.
>2000 g and 0-7 days old: 225 mg/kg/day divided q 8h.
>2000 g and >7 days old: 300 mg/kg/day divided q 6h.

Elimination: Ticarcillin, renal (tubular secretion); clavulanic acid, hepatic and renal.

Adverse effects: See Ticarcillin Disodium.

(Gomella: Neonatology 1999, pp.593-594)

TISSUE PLASMINOGEN ACTIVATOR (TPA, Alteplase, Recombinant, Activase)

Supplied: Injection, powder for 50 mg, 100mg vial

Administration: IV
Reconstitute with accompanying SWFI. (Do not use bacteriostatic water for injection.) The resultant concentration will be 1 mg/ml may be administered as reconstituted at 1mg/mL. May be further diluted with D5W or NS for a concentration of 0.5 mg/ml. Stable for 8 hours at room temperature (1).
Avoid excessive agitation during dilution.

Tissue Plasminogen Activator

For treatment of aortic thrombosis.

Patient was a 4-day-old, 820 gm twin born at 28 weeks of gestation. A grade II intraventricular hemorrhage was documented on day 2 of life. The authors chose a dose used for reperfusion of coronary arteries, infusing 1 mg for 3 hours (1.4 or 0.47 mg/kg/hr). Clinical improvement was apparent within 20 minutes of the start of infusion. There was no progression of the IVH after t-PA treatment.

t-PA induces clot-sensitive fibrinolysis without producing a wide-spread systemic proteolytic state. The number of reported hemorrhagic complications with t-PA is similar to or fewer that with other agents.

Comments: The plasma half-life of streptokinase and urokinase are 23 and 16 minutes, respectively; that of t-PA is only 5 minutes.

(Kennedy: Successful treatment of neonatal aortic thrombosis with tissue plasminogen activator. J Pediatr 1990;116:798-801)

Tissue Plasminogen Activator

We describe the use of altplase in 17 infants and children with femoral artery thrombosis after cardiac catheterization...Femoral artery thrombosis was diagnosed, if after 24 hours of heparin...300 U/kg/day...therapy the leg was still pulseless, blood pressure was low or unrecordable, and if there was poor skin perfusion and pallor compared with the other leg...After 24 hours heparin was stopped and alteplase (Actilyse) was infused at a rate of 0.5 mg/kg/h for the first hour followed by 0.25 mg/kg/h until pulses were palpable and blood pressure in both legs was similar or bleeding complications occurred. Except for those cases with severe bleeding complications, the heparin infusion (300 U/kg/day) was continued to 24 hours after alteplase treatment was stopped.

(Zenz: Tissue plasminogen activator (alteplase) treatment for femoral artery thrombosis after cardiac catheterisation in infants and children. Br Heart J 1993;70:382-85)

Tissue Plasminogen Activator

...three neonates and one infant with arterial or venous thrombotic occlusion using rTPA (Genentech, San Francisco, CA) were managed at this institution...rTPA administratioon consisted of an initial bolus of 0.5 mg/kg over 20 minutes followed by a continuous infusion at rates ranging from 0.04 to 0.5 mg/kg/h. The infusion was continued until there was evidence of clot lysis by Doppler examination, angiogram, or venogram...Infusion rates of rTPA were adjusted in order to maintain fibrinogen levels above 100 mg/dL.

(Dillon: Recombinant tissue plasminogen activator for neonatal and pediatric vascular thrombolytic therapy. J Ped Surg 1993;28:1264-69)

Tissue Plasminogen Activator

TPA was given as bolus intraventricular injections of 1.0 mg to 21 of the infants, with 0.5 mg being used in two infants because of concern over low plasma fibrinogen concentrations. The dose of 1 mg was not chosen on the basis of body weight, but, rather, on the large amount of intraventricular blood clot present in some neonates.

The means by which tPA was delivered to the ventricle varied from centre to centre, according to the availability of a paediatric neurosurgeon.

Twenty two preterm infants, aged 7 to 26 days, with progressive posthaemorrhagic ventricular dilatation (ventricular width >4 mm over 97th centile) received one to five intraventricular bolus injections of 1.0 mg or 0.5 mg tPA at intervals of one to seven days.

Intraventricular tPA resulted in survival without a shunt for most of the infants, but with some risk. Failure may have been due to plasminogen deficiency, an inhibitor, or late intervention.

(Whitelaw: Phase I study of intraventricular recombinant tissue plasminogen activator for treatment of posthaemorrhagic hydrocephalus. Arch Dis Child 1996;75:F20-F26)

TOBRAMYCIN (Nebcin)

Supplied: Injection, Pediatric 20mg/2ml in 2ml
Injection, 80mg/2ml in 2ml
Ophthalmic, Ointment 0.3%, Solution 0.3%
Nebulizer solution: 300mg/5ml, 5ml ampules

Administration: IV, IM, Ophthalmic, Inhalation
For INTRAVENOUS INHALATION ADMINISTRATION, the usual volume of diluent (NS or D5W) is 50ml, or 100ml for adult doses. For children, the volume of diluent should be proportionately less than for adults. The diluted solution should be infused over 20 to 60 minutes (1).

The usual duration of infusion is 30 minutes (6).

Tobramycin

Antibacterial Drugs for Newborn Infants
Dose (mg/kg or Units [U]/kg) and frequency of Administration
Route: IV, IM
Dose: Infants 0-4 wk
BW <1200 g: 2.5 every 18-24 h

Infants <1 wk old
BW ≤1200-2000 g: 2.5 every 12 h
BW >2000 g: 2.5 every 12 h

Infants ≥1 wk old
BW ≤2000-2000 g: 2.5 every 8 or 12 h
BW >2000 g: 2.5 every 8 h

Note: Optimal dosage should be based on determination of serum concentrations, especially in low-birth-weight (<1500 g) infants. In very low-birth-weight Infants (<1200 g) every 18 to 24 hours dosing may be appropriate in the first week of life

Dosages for the aminoglycosides may differ from those recommended by the manufacturer in the package insert.

Antibacterial Drugs for Pediatric Patients Beyond the Newborn Period:
Dosage per kg/d
Route: IV, IM
Mild to Moderate Infections: Inappropriate
Severe Infections: 3-7.5 mg in 3 doses
Note: Once daily dosing (5-6 mg/kg every 24 h) is investigational in children
Dosages for the aminoglycosides may differ from those recommended by the manufacturers (see package insert).
(American Academy of Pediatrics: Report of the Committee on Infectious Diseases. Red Book 2000, pp.651,653,662)

Tobramycin

Route: IV, IM
Dosage (mg/kg) and Interval of Administration:
Weight <1200 g
Age 0-4 wk: 2.5 q18h

Weight 1200-2000 g
Age 0-7 days: 2 q12h
Age >7 days: 2 q8h

Weight >2000 g
Age 0-7 days: 2 q12h
Age >7 days: 2 q8h

(Remington: Infectious Diseases of the Fetus and Newborn Infant 2001, p.1454)

Tobramycin

Route: IV, IM

Dosage (mg/kg/dose) by Gestational age plus weeks of life:

≤26 Wks: 2.5 q24h
27-34 Wks: 2.5 q18h
35-42 Wks: 2.5 q12h
≥43 Wks: 2.5 q8h

Comment: Desired serum concentrations: 5-10 mg/ml (peak), < 2.5 mg/ml (trough)

(Nelson: Pocket Book of Pediatric Antimicrobial Therapy 2000-2001, p.17)

Tobramycin Sulfate (Nebcin)

Classification: Aminoglycoside.

Action and spectrum: Mechanism of action and spectrum identical to those of gentamicin sulfate.

Route: IM, IV (infuse over 30 min), topical (ophthalmic).

Dosage: IM or IV: Monitor and adjust by pharmacokinetics. Initial empiric dosing based on body weight.

< 1.2 kg: 2.5 mg/kg/dose q 18-24h.
<2 kg and 0-7 days old: 2.5 mg/kg/dose q12-18h.
< 2 kg and >7 days old: 2.5 mg/kg/dose q8-12h.
> 2 kg and 0-7 days : 2.5 mg/kg/dose q12h.
> 2 kg and >7 days old: 2.5 mg/kg/dose q8h.

Ophthalmic: Instill 1-2 drops into each eye 2-6 times a day or more often prn, or apply a small amount of ointment into each eye q 3-4h.

Elimination and metabolism: Renal.

Adverse effects: See Gentamicin Sulfate.

Comments: Reserve for cases resistant to gentamicin sulfate. Obtain serum peak and trough concentrations at about the fourth maintenance dose. Desired serum peak concentration is 4-10 mcg/mL (sample obtained 30 min after the infusion is complete); desired serum trough concentration is < 2 mcq/mL (sample obtained 30 min to just before the next dose).

(Gomella: Neonatology 1999, p.594)

Tobramycin (Nebcin, Tobrex)

Dose & Route: Neonates, IM/IV:

Post-conceptional (weeks)	Postnatal age (days)	Dose (mg/kg/dose)	Interval (hours)
≤29*	0 to 28	2.5	24
	>28	3	24
30 to 36	0 to 14	3	24
	>14	2.5	12
≥37	0 to 7	2.5	12
	>7	2.5	8

*Or significant asphyxia

Child: 6-7.5 mg/kg/24 hr ÷ Q8 hr IV/IM
Cystic Fibrosis: 7.5-10 mg/kg/24 hr ÷ Q8 hr IV
Ophthalmic: Apply thin ribbon of ointment to affected eye BID-TID; or 1-2 drops of solution to affected eye Q4 hr

Remarks: Use with **caution** in patients receiving anesthetics or neuromuscular blocking agents, and in patients with neuromuscular disorders. May cause ototoxicity, nephrotoxicity, myelotoxicity, allergy. **Ototoxic effects synergistic with furosemide**. Higher doses are recommended in patients with cystic fibrosis neutropenia, or burns. **Adjust dose in renal failure**. Monitor peak and trough levels.
Therapeutic peak levels:
6-10 mg/L in general
8-10 mg/L in pulmonary infections, neutropenia, and severe sepsis.
Therapeutic trough levels: <2 mg/L.
Recommended serum sampling time at steady-state: trough within 30 minutes prior to the 3rd consecutive dose and peak 30-60 minutes after the administration of the 3rd consecutive dose.

For inhalation use with other medications in cystic fibrosis, use the following order of administration: bronchodilator first, chest physiotherapy, other inhaled medications, then tobramycin last.

(Siberry: The Harriet Lane Handbook 2000, pp.867-868)

TOLAZOLINE HCL (Priscoline)

Supplied: Injection 25mg/ml in 4ml amp

Administration: IV
Administer loading dose over 10 minutes via a scalp vein. This is followed by a continuous IV infusion.(3) Physically compatible in D5W, NS, D10W (5).

Response to tolazoline therapy, if it occurs, can be expected within 30 minutes after the initial dose (1).

In treating hypotension induced by tolazoline, it is most important to place the patient's head low and administer intravenous fluids.

Large doses of tolazoline administered concurrently with epinephrine or norepinephrine may cause a paradoxical fall in blood pressure followed by an exaggerated rebound increase in blood pressure.

IV Tolazoline is physically and chemically compatible with Dopamine, Dobutamine, and Theophylline. (8)

Tolazoline (Priscoline)

Dose: Pulmonary Hypertension:

- Loading Dose: 1-2 mg/kg/dose infused over 10-15 minutes into a vein that drains into the superior vena cava, such as a scalp or upper-arm vein. Taper dose gradually when arterial blood gases stabilize.
- Maintenance Dose: 1-2 mg/kg/hour. For therapy longer than a few hours, use 0.16 mg/kg/hour for each 1 mg/kg loading dose to prevent accumulation and adverse effects.

Vasospasm Associated with Umbilical Arterial Catheters: A single dose of 1-2 mg/kg IV has been recommended. Fewer adverse effects would be expected, however, with the lower dose recommended by Health: Tolazoline 0.25 mg/kg/hour at a concentration of 0.1 mg/ml was infused via the umbilical artery catheter while leaving the catheters in place in two infants who required frequent arterial blood gas analyses. Catheters were positioned in the lower lumbar area to ensure perfusion to the arterial supply of the lower extremities. The regimen was also effective when given into a peripheral vein in a third infant using this dose. Venospasm improved within 10-30 minutes, but infusion should be continued to avoid recurrence. Infusion was continued for 34 hours, 72 hours, and 5 days in the three infants reported. None of the patients experienced adverse effects.

Management of Aortic Thrombosis Associated with Umbilical Catheterization: 0.1-0.2 mg/kg intra-arterially.

Reduce dose in patients with oliguria and/or renal dysfunction.

Administration: IV—Rate: The loading dose should be infused over 10-15 minutes. The continuous infusion should be given using a neonatal syringe pump.

IV—Concentration: May be given undiluted or diluted based on the infant's fluid requirements.

IV—Compatibility: See Appendix E: Y-Site Compatibility of Common NICU Drugs.

Adverse Effects: The overall incidence of adverse effects in neonates is 30 percent. Increasing the dose to higher than that indicated, especially in patients with renal dysfunction, may increase adverse effects to 80 percent. Use of the lower continuous infusion doses suggested previously should reduce accumulation and markedly minimize adverse effects.

Cardiovascular: Hypotension. Although tolazoline has been used for pulmonary hypertension, it is not a selective pulmonary vasodilator, and systemic hypotension may occur. The risk may be minimized by ensuring that the infant is in good fluid balance prior to initiation of tolazoline and using concomitant dopamine and a low-dose continuous infusion. Do not attempt to reverse hypotension with norepinephrine or epinephrine. (See Interactions under Comments.) Large doses may cause tachycardia, arrhythmias.

CNS: Seizures.

GI: increased abdominal girth, increased secretions and motility, gastric hemorrhage, perforation. Pretreatment with antacids may be beneficial.

Pulmonary: Hemorrhage.

Renal: Oliguria, hematuria, hyponatremia.

Nursing Implications:

Monitor EKG and blood pressure continuously.

Also monitor blood gases, urine output, fluid and electrolyte status.

Watch for signs of bleeding from GI tract or lung.

Comments: If tolazoline is administered by peripheral IV, the drug may preferentially cross into the systemic circulation by means of a right-to-left shunt. This would result in peripheral vasodilation rather than pulmonary vasodilation. Reduction of systemic vascular resistance may aggravate right-to-left shunting and worsen hypoxemia.

Interactions: Tolazoline may reverse the effects of epinephrine (further reduction in blood pressure, followed by exaggerated rebound). systemic acidosis may reduce the effectiveness of tolazoline because acidosis increases pulmonary vasoconstriction.

(Zenk: Neonatal Medications & Nutrition. A Comprehensive Guide 2000; pp.468-470)

Tolazoline Hydrochloride (Priscoline)

Indications and use:

Hypoxia caused by persistent pulmonary hypertension.

Actions: α-Adrenergic blocking agent with histaminergic properties. Results in pulmonary and systemic vasodilator effects. Histaminic effects stimulate gastric secretion and peripheral vasodilation and increase salivary, lacrimal, respiratory tract, and pancreatic secretions. Response is marked by cutaneous flushing followed by increased Pao_2.

Route: IV.

Dosage: 1-2 mg/kg IV as the initial dose (infused over 5-10 min), followed by a continuous infusion of 0.3-0.6 mg/kg/h. Some infants respond rapidly; others may require 30 min or more.

Adverse effects: Tachycardia, nausea, vomiting, diarrhea, GI bleeding, increased GI secretions, increased pilomotor activity, sweating, thrombocytopenia, agranulocytosis, and hypotension.

Comments: Contraindicated in renal failure, hypotension shock, and intraventricular hemorrhage. Dopamine and dobutamine are often used to support systemic pressure in neonates with persistent pulmonary hypertension; both drugs may have adverse effects on peripheral vascular resistance, especially at higher dosages. For severe hypotension, use ephedrine (0.2 mg/kg/dose) to increase peripheral vascular resistance or dopamine (< 10 mcg/kg/min) to improve cardiac output. Epinephrine administered with tolazoline may cause a paradoxic reduction in blood pressure followed by an exaggerated rebound blood pressure elevated.

(Gomella: Neonatology 1999, pp.594-595)

Tolazoline

Route & Dose: IV loading dose: 0.5-1 mg/kg over 10 min; maintenance dose 0.2-2 mg/kg/h

Adverse Effects and Cautions:
Hypotension; gastrointestinal and pulmonary bleeding; renal dysfunction. Accumulates with oliguria; no antidote

(Taeusch: Avery's Diseases of the Newborn 1998, p.1347)

Tolazoline (Priscoline)

Dose: 1-4 mg/kg/hr IV
Mode of Action: α-Blocking agent
Adverse Effects: Hypotension, flushing, impaired renal function

(Garson: The science and practice of pediatric cardiology 1998, p.2951)

Tolazoline

Dose & Route: Pulmonary hypertension, newborn:
Test dose: 1-2 mg/kg IV over 10 minutes
Maintenance infusion: 0.5-2 mg/kg/hr IV
Administer via upper extremity or scalp vein.
Dissolve 50 mg/kg x (wt in kg) in 50 ml of D_5W (ml/hr = mg/kg/hr)
Acute Vasospasm: 0.25 mg/kg/hr IV (no loading dose)

Remarks: Monitor BP, renal function, and CBC. May cause GI and pulmonary hemorrhage. If hypotension occurs, use dopamine (not epinephrine or norepinephrine). Reduce dose in renal impairment (decrease dose 50% if urinary output is <0.9 ml/kg/hr).

(Siberry: The Harriet Lane Handbook 2000, pp.868-869)

Tolazoline

Use: Persistent pulmonary hypertension of the newborn (PPHN) also known as persistent fetal circulation (PFC); peripheral vasospastic disorders

Adverse Reactions:

Cardiovascular: Hypotension, flushing, tachycardia, arrhythmias
Endocrine & metabolic: Hypochloremic alkalosis
Gastrointestinal: Increased secretions, nausea, vomiting, diarrhea, epigastric discomfort, GI bleeding
Hematology: Agranulocytosis, thrombocytopenia, pancytopenia
Ocular: Mydriasis
Renal: Oliguria
Respiratory: Pulmonary hemorrhage
Miscellaneous: Increased pilomotor activity

Usual Dosage: Neonates: I.V.:
Initial: 1-2 mg/kg over 10-15 minutes via scalp vein or upper extremity

Maintenance: I.V. continuous infusion: 1-2 mg/kg/hour; **Note**: some neonatal centers use lower maintenance doses (eg, 0.15-0.3 mg/kg/hour or 0.5-1 mg/kg/hour)

Acute vasospasm "cath toes": 0.25 mg/kg/hour (no load)

Administration: Parenteral: I.V.: Usual maximum concentrations: 0.1 mg/mL

Monitoring Parameters:

Heart rate, blood pressure, respiratory rate, blood gases, serum chloride and bicarbonate

Additional Information:

Little experience with infusions >48 hours; acidosis may decrease tolazoline's effects

(Taketomo: Pediatric dosage Handbook 1999-2000, pp.890-891)

TRACE MINERALS

Trace Minerals

Currently, the importance of iron, zinc, copper, and selenium in nutrition of ELBW infants is well established. The importance of iodine, manganese, molybdenum, chromium, fluoride, and cobalt also is recognized, but deficiency states are not a current concern in the United States. Vanadium, boron, arsenic, silicon, lead, and nickel may be important, but a need for these minerals has not been established. Several lines of evidence suggest that ELBW infants probably require more zinc than term infants. For example, increasing dietary zinc from moderate to high levels over the first year of postnatal life has been shown to improve growth and motor development as well as development and function of the immune system, especially in ELBW infants with IUGR. In addition, acute zinc deficiency occurs more readily in the ELBW preterm infant. Also, optimization of maternal zinc status during pregnancy appears to reduce the incidence of prematurity. Despite increased zinc needs, the ELBW infant has a remarkable ability to conserve endogenous zinc (bound to hepatic metallothionein) by 30 to 32 weeks postconceptional age. Hence, the need for zinc is very modest until rapid growth is established. Whether increased zinc supply can augment increased protein and energy intake to promote growth more rapidly and earlier remains unknown. Although the optimal range of zinc intake remains incompletely defined, it appears to be limited. Too much zinc, for example, impairs immune function and interferes with copper metabolism. Less is known about the ELBW infant's need for other trace minerals. The optimal iron intake, particularly that to be administered in conjunction with erythropoietin therapy, is still uncertain. The efficiency of utilization of fetal hepatic copper stores, including the extent of reabsorption of endogenous copper that has been secreted in the bile, also is not known. Both iron and copper are potent oxidants in biological systems, and the ELBW infant is especially vulnerable to oxidant stress. Selenium, on the other hand, is an essential component of one of the glutathione peroxidase enzymes and, hence, is an important antioxidant. Recent reports have linked selenium deficiency in ELBW infants with impaired pulmonary function and, possibly, retinopathy.

(Hay: Workshop Summary: Nutrition of the Extremely Low Birth Weight Infant. Pediatrics 1999;104:1360-1368)

<u>Zinc Supplements</u>

Usual Dosage: Clinical response may not occur for up to 6-8 weeks

RDA: Oral:

Neonates and Infants <12 months: 5 mg **elemental** zinc/day

Zinc deficiency: Oral:

Infants and Children: 0.5-1 mg **elemental** zinc/kg/day divided 1-3 times/day; larger doses may be needed if impaired intestinal absorption or an excessive loss of zinc (eg, excessive, prolonged diarrhea)

Supplement to parenteral nutrition solutions (clinical response may not occur for up to 6-8 weeks): I.V. (all doses are mcg of **elemental** zinc):

Premature Infants: 400 mcg/kg/day

Term Infants <3 months: 300 mcg/kg/day

Infants ≥3 months and Children ≤5 years: 100 mcg/kg/day (maximum: 5 mg/day)

Administration: Oral: Administer oral formulation with food if GI upset occurs

Parenteral: Dilute as component of daily parenteral nutrition or maintenance fluids; do not give undiluted by direct injection into a peripheral vein due to potential for phlebitis land tissue irritation, and potential to increase renal losses of minerals form a bolus injection

Monitoring Parameters:

Patients on parenteral nutrition or chronic therapy should have periodic serum copper and serum zinc levels; alkaline phosphatase, taste acuity, mental depression, wound healing (if indicated), growth (if indicated), skin integrity

(Taketomo: Pediatric Dosage Handbook 1999-2000, pp.948-949)

TRIAMCINOLONE

Supplied: Tablets: 4 mg, 8 mg

Syrup: 4 mg/5 ml

Injection (All injections are for IM use):

as Acetonide salt:

- 3 mg/ml suspension
- 10 mg/ml suspension
- 40 mg/ml suspension

as Diacetate salt:

- 25 mg/ml suspension
- 40 mg/ml suspension

as Hexacetonide salt:

- 5 mg/ml suspension
- 20 mg/ml suspension

Aerosol: 20 gm inhaler; each activation delivers ≈ 100 mcg from mouthpiece. Inhaler contains 60 mg Triamcinolone acetonide.

Topicals:
Cream: 0.025%, 0.1%, 0.5%
Ointment: 0.025%, 0.1%, 0.5%
Lotion: 0.025%, 0.1%

Administration: PO
Topical
IM (Not for IV use)
Intra-articular and intrasynovial

<u>Triamcinolone Acetonide</u>

Case Report: A female infant, born at 34 weeks gestation (birth weight 1765 g) developed a pink macule on her left axilla that enlarged rapidly and became ulcerated. The lesion continued to proliferate and the ulcers failed to heal despite treatment with antibiotics and dressings. At 3.5 months, under general anesthesia, the hemangioma was treated with intralesional triamcinolone acetonide (4 mg/kg), which was repeated 5 weeks later. An incisional biopsy was obtained just before each of the steroid injections, and hence samples from the same patient before and at 5 weeks after initial steroid injection were available for analyses.

(Hasan: Steroid therapy of a proliferating hemangioma: Histochemical and molecular changes. Pediatrics 2000;105:117-121)

TRICLOSAN (Septi-Soft, Septisol, Irgasan)

Administration: Topical
Septi-Soft: 0.25% solution - skin cleanser
Septisol: 0.25% solution - Health Care personnel handwash and skin degermer (1).

Triclosan

The single additional measure of changing handwashing and bathing soap to a preparation containing 0.3% triclosan (Bacti-Stat) was associated with the immediate termination of the acute phase of the MRSA outbreak.

(Zafar: Use of 0.3% triclosan (Bacti-Stat*) to eradicate an outbreak of methicillin-resistant Staphylococcus aureus in a neonatal nursery. Am J Infect Control 1995;23:200-208)

TRIFLURIDINE OPHTHALMIC DROPS (Viroptic)

Supplied: Ophthalmic solution 1% in 7.5ml

Administration: Ophthalmic
Solution must be refrigerated.
Continuous administration of Viroptic for periods greater than 21 days should be avoided because of potential ocular toxicity.

Trifluridine

Condition: Herpes simplex infection

Therapy: Acyclovir 60 mg/kg/day as 1-2 hr IV infusion div q8h x 21 days for CNS and disseminated disease, or x 14 days for other types; PLUS trifluridine ophthalmic solution topically q2h for conjunctivitis (max 9 times/day)

Comment: Larger dosages of acyclovir and more days of Rx than previously recommended may be beneficial

(Nelson: Pocket Book of Pediatric Antimicrobial Therapy 2000-2001, p.8)

TRIMETHOPRIM / SULFAMETHOXAZOLE
(Septra, Bactrim)

Supplied: Oral suspension: 40 mg trimethoprim and 200 mg sulfamethoxazole per 5 ml.
Injection: Trimethoprim 16 mg/ml and Sulfamethoxazole 80 mg/ml in 5, 10 ml

Administered: PO:
Not recommended for infants <2 months old (1).

IV: Administer over 60-90 minutes.
Manufacturers recommend only dextrose 5% in water for dilution.

Add 5ml of drug to 75-125ml of D5W. Mix solution just prior to use and administration.

STABILITY:
5ml diluted in D5W 125ml: 6 hrs.
5ml diluted in D5W 100ml: 4 hrs.
5ml diluted in D5W 75ml: 2 hrs.

Avoid rapid infusion or bolus injection.
Do not give IM.

Trimethoprim-sulfamethoxazole

Chemoprophylaxis for Pneumocystis Carinii Pneumonia

Prophylaxis against a first episode of PCP is indicated for many patients with significant immunocompromise, including persons with HIV infection and those with primary or acquired immunodeficiency, such as from chemotherapy or other immunosuppressive therapy.

Because half of all cases of PCP in children with perinatally acquired HIV occur in infants 3 to 6 months of age, identification as early as possible of infants who have been exposed perinatally to HIV is essential so that prophylaxis can be initiated before they are at risk. The most effective means to implement this recommendation is by diagnosing maternal HIV infection before or during pregnancy. Prophylaxis for PCP is recommended for all infants born to HIV-infected women beginning at 4 to 6 weeks of age. Prophylaxis for PCP should be discontinued for children in whom HIV infection has been excluded. Children whose HIV infection status is not determined should continue prophylaxis throughout the first year of life.

Table: Recommendations for *Pneumocystis carinii* Pneumonia (PCP) Prophylaxis for Human Immunodeficiency Virus (HIV)-Exposed Infants and Children, by Age and HIV-Infections Status*

Age and HIV Infection Status	PCP Prophylaxis †
Birth to 4-6 wk, HIV-exposed	No prophylaxis
4-6 wk to 4 mo, HIV-exposed	Prophylaxis
4-12 mo	
HIV-infected of indeterminate	Prophylaxis
HIV-infection excluded ‡	No prophylaxis

*Modified from Centers for Disease Control and Prevention. 1999 USPHS/IDSA guidelines for the prevention of opportunistic infections in persons infected with human immunodeficiency virus. *MMWR Morb Mortal Wkly Rep.* 1999;48(RR-10):1-59, 61-66

‡ HIV infection can be excluded reasonably among children who have had 2 or more negative results of HIV diagnostic tests (ie, HIV culture or polymerase chain reaction), both of which are performed at ≥1 month of age and 1 of which is performed at ≥4 months of age; or 2 or more negative results of HIV immunoglobulin G antibody tests performed at ≥6 months of age among children who have no clinical evidence of HIV disease.

Other drugs with potential for prophylaxis include pyrimethamine plus dapsone plus leucovorin, pyrimethamine-sulfadoxine, and oral atovaquone. Experience with these drugs in adults and children is limited. These agents should be considered only in unusual situations in which the recommended regimens are not tolerated or can not be used. The safety of discontinuing any prophylaxis in HIV-infected children receiving highly active antiretroviral therapy has not been studied.

Although prophylaxis substantially reduces the risk of PCP, pulmonary and extrapulmonary *P carinii* infections have occurred in HIV-infected adults and children receiving prophylaxis.

Drug Regimens for *Pneumocystis carinii* Pneumonia Prophylaxis for Children 4 Weeks of Age or Older:

Recommended regimen:

Trimethoprim-sulfamethoxazole, 150 mg/m^2 per day of trimethoprim with 750 mg/m^2 per day of sulfamethoxazole administered orally in divided doses twice a day 3 time per week on consecutive days (eg, Monday-Tuesday-Wednesday)

Acceptable alternative trimethoprim-sulfamethoxazole dosage schedules:

150 mg/m^2 per day of trimethoprim with 750 mg/m^2 per day of sulfamethoxazole administered orally **as a single daily dose** 3 times per week on consecutive days (eg, Monday-Tuesday-Wednesday)

150 mg/m^2 per day of trimethoprim with 750 mg/m^2 per day of sulfamethoxazole administered orally in divided doses twice a day and **administered 7 days per week**.

150 mg/m^2 per day of trimethoprim with 750 mg/m^2 per day of sulfamethoxazole administered orally in divided doses twice a day and administered 3 times per week on alternate days (eg, Monday-Wednesday-Friday).

Alternative regimens if trimethoprim-sulfamethoxazole is not tolerated

Dapsone (children ≥1 mo of age)

2 mg/kg (maximum 100 mg) administered orally once a day or 4 mg/kg (maximum 200 mg) orally every week

(American Academy of Pediatrics: Report of the Committee on Infectious Diseases. Red Book 2000, pp.463-465)

Trimethoprim-sulfamethoxazole

For treatment of Pneumocystis Infections

The drug of choice is trimethoprim-sulfamethoxazole (15 to 20 mg/kg per day of trimethoprim; 75 to 100 mg/kg of sulfamethoxazole daily in divided doses every 6 hours), usually given intravenously. Oral therapy should be reserved for patients with mild disease who do not have malabsorption or diarrhea. The rate of adverse reactions is higher in HIV-infected patients than in patients without HIV infection; the incidence in HIV-infected children treated with trimethoprim-sulfamethoxazole is approximately 15%

but may be as high as 60% in adults with HIV infection. If the adverse reaction is not severe, continuation of therapy is recommended, because 50% of patients with adverse reactions subsequently have been treated successfully with trimethoprim-sulfamethoxazole.

Parenterally administered pentamidine (4 mg/kg per day of salt given once a day) is an alternative drug for children and adults who cannot tolerate trimethoprim-sulfamethoxazole or who have severe disease and who have not responded to trimethoprim-sulfamethoxazole after 5 to 7 days of therapy. the therapeutic efficacy of parenteral pentamidine in adults with PCP has been similar to that of trimethoprim-sulfamethoxazole. However, pentamidine is associated with a high incidence of adverse reactions, including pancreatitis, renal dysfunction, hypoglycemia, hyperglycemia, hypotension, fever, and neutropenia. Pentamidine should not be used concomitantly with didanosine, since both drugs can cause pancreatitis. If a recipient of didanosine develops PCP and requires pentamidine, didanosine should be discontinued until 1 week after the pentamidine therapy has been discontinued.

Atovaquone is approved for the oral treatment of mild to moderate PCP in adults who are intolerant of trimethoprim-sulfamethoxazole. Experience with the use of atovaquone in children is limited.

Other potentially useful drugs identified by in vitro studies, animal models, and clinical trials in adults include dapsone with trimethoprim, trimetrexate with leucovorin, and clindamycin with primaquine. Experience with the use of these combinations in children is limited.

A minimum duration of 2 weeks of therapy is recommended; many experts advise 3 weeks of therapy for patients with AIDS. In patients with AIDS, continuous lifelong prophylaxis should be initiated at the end of therapy for acute infection.

Corticosteroids seem to be beneficial in the treatment of HIV-infected adults with moderate to severe PCP (as defined by an arterial oxygen pressure [PaO_2] of less than 70 mm Hg or an arterial-alveolar gradient of more than 35 mm Hg). For adolescents older than 13 years of age and adults, 80 mg/d of oral prednisone in 2 divided doses for the first 5 days of therapy, 40 mg once a day on days 6 through 10, and 20 mg once a day on days 11 through 21 is recommended. Although no controlled studies of the use of corticosteroids in young children have been performed, most experts would include corticosteroids as part of therapy for children with moderate to severe PCP. The optimal dose and duration of corticosteroid therapy for children have not been determined, but most experts suggest 2 mg/kg per day of prednisone or its equivalent for 7 to 10 days, followed by a tapering dose during the next 10 to 14 days.

(American Academy of Pediatrics: Report of the Committee on Infectious Diseases. Red Book 2000, pp.462-463)

Trimethoprim-sulfamethoxazole

For treatment of Pneumocystis Infections
Antibacterial Drugs for Pediatric Patients Beyond the Newborn Period
Dosage per kg/d

Route: PO

Mild to Moderate Infections: 8-12 mg trimethoprim—40-60 mg sulfamethoxazole in 2 doses

Severe Infections: 20 mg trimethoprim—100 mg sulfamethoxazole in 4 doses (for use only in pneumocystis carinii pneumonia)

Comments: For prophylaxis in immunocompromised patients, recommended daily dose is 5 mg trimethoprim—25 mg sulfamethoxazole per kg/d in 2 doses

Route: IV

Mild to Moderate Infections: Inappropriate

Severe Infections: 8-12 mg trimethoprim—40-60 mg sulfamethoxazole in 4 doses

OR

20 mg trimethoprim—100 mg sulfamethoxazole in 4 doses (for treatment of *Pneumocystis* infection)

Comment: Use intravenous formulation when oral formulation cannot be administered

(American Academy of Pediatrics: Report of the Committee on Infectious Diseases. Red Book 2000, p.661)

TRIPLE DYE See Skin and Cord Care

TUBOCURARINE (Curare)

Supplied: Injection 3mg/ml in 10ml (20 units/ml)
Administration: IV, IM

Administer as a sustained IV injection over 1 to 1.5 minutes.

Although rapid injection may be dangerous, curarization can be accomplished with a smaller dose if given more rapidly (1).

Tubocurarine (Curare)

Indications and use:

To improve oxygenation in the uncooperative neonate during mechanical ventilation. To provide muscle relaxation during general anesthesia.

Actions: Nondepolarizing (competitive) neuromuscular blocking agent. Rapid IV administration may cause hypotension, bradycardia, and possibly circulatory collapse. Atropine is an effective prophylactic agent. Onset of paralysis is generally 1-2 min after IV administration. Duration of paralysis depends on the number of doses and the total dosage delivered and may persist for 20-90 min.

Route: IV, IM (only if IV access is not available.)

Dosage: Infuse undiluted over 1 min or more to minimize cardiovascular effects.

Initial dosage: 0.25-0.5 mg/kg IV.
Maintenance dosage: 0.15 mg/kg/dose IV prn.

Adverse effects: Hypotension, bradycardia, possibly circulatory collapse and allergic reactions.

Comments: For reversal, give neostigmine with atropine IV.
(Gomella: Neonatology 1999, p.595)

UROKINASE (Abbokinase)

Supplied: Injection, powder for 250,000 I.U. per vial
Open cath, powder for 5000 I.U./ml in 1ml, 1.8ml vials.

Administration: IV, IV catheter clearance

For IV ADMINISTRATION, reconstitute vial with 5ml SWFI, without preservatives. To minimize formation of filaments, avoid shaking the vial during reconstitution. The solution may be terminally filtered, e.g. through a 0.45 micron or smaller cellulose filter. For further dilution procedures consult manufacturer's literature.

IV CATHETER CLEARANCE: follow package insert (1).

Urokinase

Dose: Lysis of Large-vessel Thrombus: 4,400 units/kg IV over 10 minutes, then 4,400 units/kg/hour for 4-72 hours. Response is usually seen within 48 hours.

- Success may be increased by pretreatment with fresh-frozen plasma.
- Gal and Ransom use urokinase 100 units/kg/hour for local infusion to a thrombus. For systemic therapy of neonatal thrombosis, they begin with 100 units/kg/hour (no loading dose) and increase in increments of 400-1,000 units/kg/hour every 2-4 hours, depending on the urgency of the clinical situation (range: 1,000-10,000 units/kg/hour). Hustead and Wicklund stated that the optimal dose in newborns is unknown and has varied in reports from 4,000 to 20,000 units/kg/hour for continuous infusion. Therapy is guided by clinical response and serial D-dimer values. Therapy with thrombolytics is reserved for neonates who do not respond to heparin therapy.

Regional Arterial Infusion: 100 units/kg/hour.

Occluded Central Venous Catheter: Use only sufficient volume to fill the lumen of the catheter, usually 0.3-0.6 ml of 5,000 units/ml, as described in Table 1-40.

Administration: IV: for lysis of large-vessel thrombus. Can be given intra-arterially for regional clot lysis. May also be given locally by infusing through the tip of the UAC around which a clot has developed. (Table below).

IV—Rate: Infuse loading dose over 10 minutes.

IV—Concentration:

- For systemic use: 1,250-1,500 units/ml; Maximum: 3,300 units/ml.
- For catheter patency: 5,000 units/ml.

IV—Preparation: Refrigerate powder for reconstitution. to minimize filament formation, avoid shaking the vial;

instead, roll and tilt vial to enhance reconstitution. May filter with 0.45 or 0.22 micron filter.
Storage: Refrigerate both the powder for reconstitution and the reconstituted solution. Reconstituted solution is stable for 24 hours at room temperature or under refrigeration.

Table: Procedure for Restoring Patency to Central Venous Catheters Using Urokinase:

Prepare Urokinase (Abbokinase Open-Cath): Reconstitute immediately before use to 5,000 units/ml following the manufacture's directions.

Gently roll and tilt rather than shake to minimize filament formation.

Withdraw 1 ml of the reconstituted solution into a tuberculin syringe. One vial may be used for several attempts to restore patency of the same catheter; however, the solution contains no preservative, so any unused portion should be discarded after 24 hours under refrigeration or at room temperature.

Instill Urokinase

- Aseptically disconnect the IV tubing connection at the catheter yb, and replace with a 1 ml tuberculin syringe filled with the urokinase solution.
- Carefully and slowly instill an amount of urokinase solution equal to the volume of the catheter – usually 0.3-0.6 ml.
- Fill catheter until slight resistance is felt. Avoid excessive pressure or volume to reduce risk of rupturing the catheter or forcing the clot and drug into the systemic circulation.
- Wait 5-10 minutes; then attempt to aspirate using a 5 ml syringe. Repeat every 5-10 minutes for 30 minutes (3-6 times).
- If patency is not restored in 30 minutes, cap the catheter and allow urokinase to remain in the catheter for an additional 30-60 minutes before again attempting to aspirate.
- If patency is not restored in 1-2 hours, try a second instillation of urokinase.

Follow-up

- After patency is restored and blood return is achieved, aspirate 1-2 ml of blood to remove residual clot and urokinase.
- Gently irrigate the catheter with sodium chloride 0.9 percent; then aseptically reconnect IV tubing to catheter hub.

Cautions/Contraindications:

A drug warning was issued by the Food and Drug Administration (FDA) on January 25, 1999, stating that

that Abbokinase be reserved for only those situations where a physician has considered the alternatives and has determined that the product's use is critical to the care of a specific patient in a specific situation. Abbott is working to correct the Good Manufacturing Practice deficiencies noted during the FDA inspections. Updated information may be obtained via the Internet at www.fda.gov/cber

Do not use for systemic therapy in infants who have undergone major surgery in the preceding 10 days, who have pre-existing severe bleeding, or who have had a recent cerebrovascular accident.

Adverse Effects: When Used for Occluded Central Line: Bleeding, if excessive amounts of urokinase are inadvertently injected into the systemic circulation. Excessive pressure of force on instillation may force the clot into the systemic circulation.

When Used for Systemic Therapy: Bleeding from puncture sites or internally, such as intracranial hemorrhage. If bleeding occurs secondary to hyperplasminemia, stop the infusion and consider replacement therapy with cryoprecipitate and fresh-frozen plasm.

Rare Effects: Rash, bronchospasm, fever.

Nursing Implications:

Recommendation is for infusion by a physician when used for occluded central venous catheters. Monitor vital signs continuously.

Reduce dose if signs of bleeding from nonpuncture sites are observed. Monitor for clinical improvement.

Monitoring: Gal and Ransom measured baseline and serial D-dimer (the final breakdown product from fibrin clots) levels to guide systemic fibrinolytic therapy. The end point was a D-dimer level of >1 mcg/ml or a raising D-dimer level if the baseline was >1 mcg/ml. Others have recommended serial measurements of fibrinogen, fibrin split products, and euglobulin lysis time for monitoring the status of newborns given fibrinolytic therapy.

Comments: Interactions: Increases risk of bleeding in infants concurrently on heparin, warfarin (Coumadin), or indomethacin.

(Zenk: Neonatal Medications & Nutrition. A Comprehensive Guide 2000; pp.475-478)

Urokinase

Eligibility included (1) age >1 month and <18 years and (2) venous thrombosis confirmed by ultrasonography, venography, or ventilation-perfusion scan.

The treatment guidelines for combination therapy are as follows. Urokinase is given as a bolus infusion of 4400

U/kg over a 20-minute period, followed by a maintenance infusion of 4400 U/kg/h for a 48-hour period. Heparin is given as an infusion of 10 U/kg/h during urokinase infusion without a bolus; at 48 hours a heparin bolus of 50 U/kg is given, and the rate of infusion is increased to achieve a plasma heparin level of 0.4 to 0.7 U/mL. Heparin is continued to maintain this therapeutic level for at least 5 days; heparin is discontinued when the international normalized ratio is >2. Warfarin is given to maintain the international normalized ration >2 for 3 months to indefinitely.

Plasma concentrations of plasminogen, fibrinogen, and platelets were monitored at least daily during thrombolytic therapy. Transfusion support was administered routinely on the following schedule: plasminogen <0.50 U/mL was replaced with fresh-frozen plasma, 10 mL/kg; fibrinogen <50 mg/dL was replaced with cryoprecipitate, 10 mL/kg; platelet count <50,000/µL was replaced with single donor platelet concentrates, 10 mL/kg.

Conclusions: Combination therapy in children (urokinase and unfractionated heparin) was safe and efficacious. A prospective, randomized, controlled study in children is needed.

(Manco-Johnson: Combined thrombolytic and anticoagulant therapy for venous thrombosis in children. J Pediatr 2000;136:446-53)

<u>Urokinose</u>

Dosage: Clotted catheter: 5,000-10,000 µ/mL instilled in catheter using a volume equal to the internal volume of the catheter; clamp for 1-4 h and then aspirate contents

(Allen: Moss and Adam's Heart Disease in Infants, children and Adolescents 2001, pp.1460-1468)

<u>Urokinase</u>

Dose & Route: Deep vein thrombosis and pulmonary emboli: **Should be used in consultation with a hematologist**. 4400 U/kg over 10 min, followed by 4400 U/kg/hr for 12-72 hr. Titrate to effect.

Occluded IV catheter:
Aspiration method: Use 5,000 U/ml conc. Instill into catheter a volume equal to the internal volume of catheter over 1-2 min, leave in place for 1-4 hr, then aspirate; may repeat with 10,000 U/ml in each lumen if no response. **DO NOT infuse into patient**.
IV infusion method: 150-200 U/kg/hr in each lumen for 8-48 hr at a rate of at least 20 ml/hr.
For dialysis patients: 5,000 U in each lumen administered over 1-2 min; leave drug in for 1-2 days, then aspirate.

Remarks: **Contraindicated** for patients with active internal bleeding, bacterial endocarditis, intracranial neoplasm, arteriovenous malformation, or aneurysm, history of cerebrovascular accident, or recent trauma/surgery. Monitor hematocrit, platelets, PT and aPTT before and during continuous infusion therapy.

Discontinue administration if signs of bleeding occur. Side effects include allergic reactions, fever, rash, and bronchospasm.

(Siberry: The Harriet Lane Handbook 2000, pp.874-875)

Urokinase

Catheter occlusion may be caused by the following:
(1) a clot or thrombus,
(2) fat deposition, or
(3) calcium phosphorus deposition.

The most common cause of occlusion is thrombus formation. Such an occlusion usually clears with urokinase infusion (e.g., Abbokinase Open Cath, Abbott Laboratories). The urokinase dose equals the catheter volume; for small catheters use the 1-ml vial-5000 IU of urokinase activity per milliliter (when mixed); for larger volume catheters use the 1.8 ml vial-5000 IU of urokinase activity per milliliter (when mixed). The manufacturer allows two such bolus infusions after appropriate waiting periods (see product information). Urokinase boluses have been shown to be successful in pediatric patients. Should bolus therapy fail, alternative causes of occlusion should be considered. Bagnall and others evaluated the efficiency of the continuous infusion of low-dose urokinase (200 units/kg/hr) in clearing catheters that had not cleared after two boluses of urokinase in a pediatric oncology population. Patency was reestablished in 11 of 12 catheters with a mean infusion time of 28.7 hours. No coagulation abnormalities or clinical bleeding associated with the urokinase infusion occurred.

An 11-month-old infant on TPN developed superior vena cava syndrome, with head and neck swelling, secondary to a thrombus at the catheter tip occluding the superior vena cava. A 48-hour transfusion of urokinase (4400 U/kg/h) resulted in clinical and radiographic evidence of clearance of the thrombus.

(Walker: Pediatric Gastrointestinal Disease 1996, p.1927)

Urokinase

Use: Thrombolytic agent used in treatment of recent severe or massive deep vein or arterial thrombosis, pulmonary emboli, and occluded arteriovenous cannulas

Precautions: Systemic use: Use with caution in patients with severe hypertension, recent lumbar puncture, patient receiving I.M. administration of medications. If indicated, febrile patients should receive antibiotics for at least 24 hours prior to urokinase therapy; obtain an echocardiogram in febrile patients prior to therapy to rule out intracardiac vegetations; pretreatment lab studies should include platelet count, PT/PTT, fibrinogen, fibrin degradation products, plasminogen, antithrombin III, protein S, protein C.

Stability: Store 250,000 unit vials in refrigerator, powder for 5000 unit/mL ("open-cath") should be stored below 77°F; avoid freezing; reconstitute by gently rolling and tilting, **do not shake**; does not contain preservative; the 5000 unit vial should be reconstituted just prior to use; discard unused portion; a reconstituted 250,000 unit vial is stable for 24 hours under refrigeration

Usual Dosage: Infants, Children:
Arterial or venous thrombosis or pulmonary emboli: I.V.: Loading dose: 4400 units/kg over 10 minutes, followed by 4400 units/kg/hour for 12-72 hours; continuous infusion doses of 4000-10,000 units/kg/hour have been used; titrate urokinase dose to bring level of plasma fibrinogen to 75% of fibrinogen measured after FFP infusion; reassess clot size every 12-24 hours

Occluded I.V. catheters:
5000 units/mL concentration; (use only Abbokinase Open Cath), the volume to instill into the catheter is equal to the internal volume of the catheter; administer in each lumen over 1-2 minutes, leave in lumen for 1-4 hours, then **aspirate out of catheter**, flush catheter with NS; may repeat with 10,000 units in each lumen if 5000 units fails to clear the catheter; **do not infuse into the patient**

Continuous I.V. infusion: 150-200 units/kg/hour in each lumen for 8-48 hours; infuse at a rate of at least 20 mL/hour in children and adults

Administration: Parenteral: I.V. infusion: Usual concentration: 1250-1500 units/mL; maximum concentration not yet defined
Abbokinase Open Cath 5000 unit product is **not** for systemic administration, it must be aspirated out of the catheter; do **not** dilute Abbokinase Open Cath for I.V. infusion

Monitoring Parameters:
CBC, reticulocyte, platelet count; fibrinogen level, plasminogen, fibrin/fibrinogen degradation products, D-dimer, PT, PTT, ATIII, protein C, U/A, ACT, urinalysis

Nursing Implications:
Use 0.22 or 0.45 micron filter during I.V. systemic therapy
(Taketomo: Pediatric Dosage Handbook 1999-2000, pp.918-919)

URSODEOXYCHOLIC ACID (Ursodiol, Actigall)

Supplied: 300mg capsule

Ursodiol (Actigall)

Dose: 10-18 mg/kg/day PO as a single daily dose or divided into 2 or 3 doses. Duration of therapy is usually weeks to months. Consider discontinuing the drug when the direct bilirubin is <2.5 mg/dl.

Administration: Preparation: An oral liquid is not commercially available; however, a suspension can be compounded by the pharmacist. Two are described below: 25 mg/ml and 60 mg/ml.

Pharmacist Compounding Directions
Ursodiol Oral Liquid 25 mg/ml Empty contents of ten 300 mg capsules into a glass mortar. Mix with 10 ml glycerin; then mix in 60 ml of Ora-Plus (Paddock Laboratories, Minneapolis, Minnesota), and levigate until a smooth mixture is obtained. Pour into a light-resistant prescription bottle; then add Orange syrup, NF, to bring to a final volume of 120 mg. shake vigorously. Stability: 60 days Storage: Refrigerate or store at room temperature
Ursodiol Oral Liquid 60 mg/ml Empty contents of twelve 300 mg capsules into a glass mortar. Triturate with a small amount of glycerin to wet the powder; then add simple syrup in portions to a final volume of 60 ml. Transfer to an amber glass bottle. Shake well. Stability: 35 days Storage: Refrigerate

Alternatively, these procedures have been used:

- *preparation of Capsules by Pharmacist*: Dosage standardization is sometimes feasible with this drug. some centers prepare 50 and 100 mg capsules and around off doses to these increments.
- *Preparation of solution by Nurse*: Empty contents of one 300 mg capsule into a 60 ml screw-cap vial. Dilute with 10 ml water and shake well (= 30 mg/ml concentration). Withdraw appropriate volume for mg dose ordered. Date, time and initial; then refrigerate. Discard unused portion after 24 hours.

Use: For cholestatic liver diseases, including parenteral nutrition cholestasis and biliary atresia, to induce hypercholeresis, stimulate bile flow, and thereby facilitate canalicular secretion of the accumulated atypical bile acids. UDCA therapy improves the biochemical markers of liver function. May improve and delay end-stage liver disease, making it possible for the child to grow to a sufficient size for liver transplantation to become feasible.

Adverse Effects: Usually well tolerated

Dose-related diarrhea, as well as nausea, vomiting, and abdominal pain, may occur.

(Zenk: Neonatal Medications & Nutrition 2000, pp.479-480)

<u>Ursodiol</u> (Actigall)

Adverse Reactions:

Central nervous system: Headache, fatigue, anxiety, depression, sleep disorder

Dermatologic: Rash, pruritus, hair thinning

Gastrointestinal: Diarrhea, biliary pain, constipation, stomatitis, flatulence, nausea, vomiting

Hepatic: Increased liver enzymes

Usual Dosage: Oral:

Biliary atresia: Infants: 10-15 mg/kg/day (once daily)

Improvement in the hepatic metabolism of essential fatty acids in cystic fibrosis: Children: 30 mg/kg/day

TPN-induced cholestasis: Infants and Children: 30 mg/kg/day in 3 divided doses

Monitoring Parameters:

ALT, AST, sonogram, oral cholecystogram before therapy and every 6 months during therapy; obtain ultrasound images of gallbladder at 6-month intervals for the first year of therapy.

Dosage Forms: Capsule: 300 mg

Extemporaneous Preparations:

A 25 mg/mL ursodiol suspension may be made by opening ten 300 mg capsules; mix with 10 mL Glycerin, USP until smooth mixture is obtained. Add 60 mL Ora-Plus and continue to levigate until a smooth mixture is achieved. Transfer mixture to a light-resistent bottle; add a small amount of Orange Syrup, NF to wash remaining drug from the mortar to bottle. Add additional syrup to make final volume of 120 mL. Label "shake well"; stable 60 days at room temperature or refrigerated.

A 60 mg/mL ursodiol suspension may be made in a similar method by opening twelve 300 mg capsules and wetting with sufficient glycerin and triturating to make a fine paste; gradually add simple syrup to make a final volume of 60 mL. Label "shake well"; stable 35 days in refrigerator.

(Taketomo: Pediatric Dosage Handbook 1988-99: pp.1111-1113)

Ursodiol (Actigall)

Gallstone solubilizing agent, cholelitholytic agent

Dose: Children: 10-15 mg/kg/24 hr QD PO

Contraindicated: in calcified cholesterol stones, radiopaque stones, bile pigment stones, or stones >20 mm in diameter. Limited data for use in TPN induced cholestasis at 30 mg/kg/24 hr ÷ TID PO (see Gastroenterology 1996; 111(3):716-719)

(Siberry: The Harriet Lane Handbook 2000, p.875)

SEE ALSO: CHOLECYSTOKININ

(Rintala: Total Parenteral Nutrition-Associated Cholestasis in Surgical Neonates May Be Reversed by Intravenous Cholecystokinin: A Preliminary Report. J Pediatr Surg 1995;30:827-830)

VALPROIC ACID (Depakene)

Supplied: Oral syrup 250mg/5ml in 480ml
Administration: PO

Valproic Acid

Indication: For Neonatal Seizures
Valproic acid administered orally as adjunctive therapy led to control of neonatal seizures recalcitrant to phenobarbital (mean blood level >40 μg/ml) in five of six cases. However, elevation of blood ammonia required cessation of therapy in three infants. Because of the risk of valproate hepatotoxicity in this age group, the value of this drug in the treatment of neonatal seizures is uncertain.

(Volpe: Neurology of the Newborn 2001, p.206)

Valproic Acid

Dosage: 10-60 mg/kg/day divided every 12 hr PO; initial dose 10-15 mg/kg/day; may be given rectally.

Comments: Little data available for newborns; optimum seizure control in children reported at serum concentrations between 50 and 100 μg/ml; may be administered rectally.

(Fanaroff: Neonatal-Perinatal Medicine 1997, p.1747)

Valproic Acid

Route: PO

Neonatal Dose: Preterm: 15 mg/kg/24 h q12H
Term: 40 mg/kg/24 h q12H

Pediatric Dose: Initial: 15 mg/kg/24 h once daily, titrate to effect up to 60 mg/kg/24 h

Discussion: Increase dose at weekly intervals to desired effect; therapeutic serum levels are generally between 50-100 μg/mL; interacts with other anticonvulsants so need to obtain levels when adding other drugs; also has hematologic and hepatic toxicity.

(Rudolph: Rudolph's Pediatrics 1996, p.2208)

Valproic Acid

Dose & Route: Oral:
Initial: 10-15 mg/kg/24 hr ÷ QD-TID
Increment: 5-10 mg/kg/24 hr at weekly intervals to **Max dose** of 60 mg/kg/24 hr

Maintenance: 30-60 mg/kg/24 hr ÷ BID-TID. Due to drug interactions, higher doses may be required in children or other anticonvulsants.

Intravenous (use only when PO is not possible:
Use same PO daily dose ÷ Q6 hr.
Convert back to PO as soon as possible.

Rectal (Use syrup, diluted 1:1 with water, given PR as a retention enema):
Load: 20 mg/kg/dose
Maintenance: 10-15 mg/kg/dose Q8 hr

Remarks: **Contraindicated** in hepatic disease. May cause GI, liver, blood, CNS toxicity, weight gain, transient alopecia, pancreatitis, nausea, sedation, vomiting, headache, thrombocytopenia, platelet dysfunction, and rash. Can cause hyperammonemia. Hepatic failure has occurred especially in Children <2 yrs. Valproic acid increases phenytoin, diazepam, and phenobarbital levels. Phenytoin, phenobarbital, and carbamazepine decrease valproic acid levels.

Do not give syrup with carbonated beverages. Use of IV route has not been evaluated for >14 days of continuous use. Infuse IV over 1 hr up to a maximum rate of 20 mg/min.

Therapeutic levels: 50-100 mg/L.
Recommendations for serum sampling at steady-state: obtain trough level within 30 minutes prior to the next scheduled dose after 2-3 days of continuous dosing.
Monitor CBC, LFTs prior to and during therapy.
(Siberry: The Harriet Lane Handbook 2000, pp.876-877)

VANCOMYCIN (Vancocin)

Supplied: Pulvules: 125mg, 250mg capsules
Powder for oral solution: 1gm, 10gm
Injection, powder for 500mg vial, 1gm

Administration: IV, PO

IV administration: reconstitute the 500mg vial with 10ml SWFI. This provides a concentration of 50mg/ml. After reconstitution, the vials may be stored in a refrigerator for 14 days without significant loss of potency. Further dilution is required. Dilute to a concentration of 2.5mg to 5.0mg/ml (decreased incidence of thrombophlebitis) in D5W or NS.

Administer each dose over at least 60 minutes. (1)

The recommended final concentration for administration is 5mg/ml (6).

Redneck syndrome is characterized by a sudden and profound fall in blood pressure with or without a maculopapular rash over the face, neck, upper chest, and extremities. The reaction appears to be at least partially mediated through a histaminergic response. The reaction is usually stimulated by a too rapid IV infusion (dose given over a few minutes), but it has been reported rarely when given a recommended (up to a 2 hour infusion) and following oral or intra peritoneal administration. This is not an allergic type reaction (1).

<u>Vancomycin</u>

Antibacterial Drugs for Newborn Infants
Dose (mg/kg or Units [U]/kg) and Frequency of Administration
Route: IV

Dose: <u>Infants 0-4 wk</u>
BW <1200 g: 15 every 24 h

<u>Infants <1 wk old</u>
BW ≤1200-2000 g: 10-15 every 12-18 h
BW >2000 g: 10-15 every 8-12 h

<u>Infants ≥1 wk old</u>
BW ≤2000-2000 g: 10-15 every 8-12 h
BW >2000 g: 10-15 every 6 or 8 h

Note: Optimal dosage should be based on determination of serum concentrations, especially in low-birth-weight (<1500 g) infants. In very low-birth-weight infants (<1200 g) every 18 to 24 hour dosing may be appropriate in the first week of life.

For meningitis, the larger dosage is recommended

Antibacterial Drugs for Pediatric Patients Beyond the Newborn Period
Dosage per kg/d
Route: IV

Mild to Moderate Infections: 40 mg in 3-4 doses

Severe Infections: 40-60 mg in 4 doses

Comment: In meningitis, 60 mg/kg dose should be given during at least 60 min; routine monitoring of serum concentrations is unnecessary

(American Academy of Pediatrics: Report of the Committee on Infectious Diseases. Red Book 2000, pp.652,662)

<u>Vancomycin</u>

Route: IV
Dosage (mg/kg) and Interval of Administration:

<u>Weight <1200 g</u>
Age 0-4 wk: 15 q24h

<u>Weight 1200-2000 g</u>
Age 0-7 days: 10 q12h
Age >7 days: 10 q12h

<u>Weight >2000 g</u>
Age 0-7 days: 10 q8h
Age >7 days: 10 q8h

(Remington: Infectious Diseases of the Fetus and Newborn Infant 2001, p.1454)

Vancomycin

Indication: Ventriculitis

Ventriculostomy (with intermittent intraventricular instillation of an antibiotic, usually through a reservoir) is indicated when the ventricular tap demonstrates purulent fluid with persistent infection. Antibiotics should be instilled in concentrations that generally exceed those usually sought in serum. Table shows the commonly used intraventricular antibiotics and the concentrations sought. Serial measurements of the CSF concentrations of the antibiotics are important. the best approach is to administer the agent at a dose calculated to produce a concentration approximately 20-fold greater than the measured minimal bactericidal concentration.

Ventriculostomy, with external drainage, may be required in neonatal bacterial meningitis when ventriculitis has caused obstruction to CSF flow and acute hydrocephalus, manifested by increased intracranial pressure and dilated lateral ventricles. This condition may develop despite eradication of the ventricular infection by the systemic antibiotics and therefore with a sterile ventricular CSF. In such a circumstance, intraventricular instillation of antibiotic is not needed, and the task is management of the intracranial hypertension by CSF drainage, as described in Chapter 11 in relation to rapidly progressive posthemorrhagic hydrocephalus.

TABLE
Intraventricular Antibiotics for Ventriculitis

Antibiotic	Dose (mg)	Desired Peak Cerebrospinal Fluid concentration (μg/ml)
Gentamicin	1-5	80-120*
Vancomycin	4-5	80-100
Polymyxin	1-2	Unknown

*Histological change in white matter observed with concentrations >150 μg/ml.

(Volpe: Neurology of the Newborn 2001, p.798)

Vancomycin

Route: IV, IM

Dosage (mg/kg/dose) by Gestational age plus weeks of life:

≤26 wks	27-34 wks	35-42 wks	≥43 wks
15 q24h	15 q18h*	15 q12h*	15 q8h*

*At 28 days of life (4 weeks) vancomycin is dosed at 20 mg/kg/dose. The interval remains the same.

Comment: Desired serum concentrations: 20-40 mg/ml (peak), < 10 mg/ml (trough)

(Nelson: Pocket Book of Pediatric Antimicrobial Therapy 2000-2001, p.17)

Vancomycin Hydrochloride (Vancocin, others)

Action and spectrum:

Bactericidal action by interference with bacterial cell wall synthesis. Active against most Gram-positive cocci and bacilli, including streptococci, staphylococci (including methicillin-resistant staphylococci), clostridia (including *Clostridium difficile*), *Corynebacterium* spp, and *Listeria monocytogenes*. Bacteriostatic against enterococci. No cross-resistance between vancomycin and other antibiotics has been reported. The drug of choice against methicillin-resistant staphylococci and *C difficile*.

Route: IV, PO.

Dosage: IV: Monitor and adjust by pharmacokinetics. Initial empirical dosing based on body weight:

<1.2 kg and 0-4 weeks' postnatal age:
15 mg/kg/dose q24h.
1.2-2 kg and 0-7 days: 15 mg/kg/dose q12-18h.
1.2-2 kg and >7 days: 15 mg/kg/dose q8-12h.
>2 kg and 0-7 days: 15 mg/kg/dose q12h.
>2 kg and >7 days: 15 mg/kg/dose q8h.

PO: To treat pseudomembranous colitis due to *C difficile* or staphylococcal enterocolitis, 20-40 mg/kg/day divided q6h for 5-7 days.

Elimination and metabolism: Renally excreted. Half-life 7-9 h.

Adverse effects: Allergy (rash, fever), ototoxicity (with serum peak levels >40 mcg/mL), thrombophlebitis at site of injection. Too rapid infusion may cause rash, chills, and fever ("red-man" syndrome) mimicking anaphylactic reaction. Rapid infusion may cause apnea and bradycardia without other signs of "red-man" syndrome. Infuse dose over at least 60 min.

Comments: Therapeutic range: 20-40 mcg/mL (sample drawn 60 min after infusion complete) and serum trough levels of 5-10 mcg/mL (sample drawn 30 min to just before next dose). In general, draw serum peak and trough levels at about the fourth maintenance dose. Monitor serum creatinine. If staphylococci exhibit tolerance to the drug, combine it with an aminoglycoside with or without rifampin. Oral doses are poorly absorbed. Powder for injection, diluted and flavored, is the most economical means of oral dosing.

(Gomella: Neonatology 1999, pp.595-596)

Vancomycin

Usual Dosage: Initial dosage recommendations:
Neonates: I.V.:

Postnatal age ≤ 7 days:
<1200 g: 15 mg/kg/day given every 24 hours
1200-2000 g: 10-15 mg/kg/dose given every 12-18 hours
> 2000 g: 10-15 mg/kg/dose given every 8-12 hours

Postnatal age >7 days:
<1200 g: 15 mg/kg/day given every 24 hours
1200-2000 g: 10-15 mg/kg/dose given every 8-12 hours
>2000 g: 15-20 mg/kg/dose given every 8 hours

Infants >1 month and Children: I.V.: 40 mg/kg/day in divided doses every 6-8 hours

Staphylococcal central nervous system infection: I.V.: 60 mg/kg/day in divided doses every 6 hours; maximum dose: 1 g/dose

Administration: Parenteral: Administer vancomycin by I.V. intermittent infusion over 60 minutes at a final concentration not to exceed 5 mg/mL; if a maculopapular rash appears on face, neck, trunk, and upper extremities, slow the infusion rate to administer dose over 1 ½ to 2 hours and increase the dilution volume; the reaction usually dissipates in 30-60 minutes; administration of antihistamines just before the infusion may also prevent or minimize this reaction.

Intrathecal/Intraventricular: Dilute in NS without preservatives to a final concentration between 2-5 mg/mL.

Monitoring Parameters:
Periodic renal function tests, urinalysis, serum vancomycin concentrations, WBC; audiogram (in patients who concurrently receive ototoxic chemotherapy)

Reference Range: Peak: 25-40 µg/mL
Trough: 5-10 µg/mL

Patient Information:
Report pain at infusion site; dizziness, fullness or ringing in ears with I.V. use.

Nursing Implications:
Do not administer I.M.; peak levels are drawn 30 minutes to 1 hour after the completion of a 1-hour infusion; troughs are obtained just before the next dose.

(Taketomo: Pediatric Dosage Handbook 2000-2001, pp.969-971)

VARICELLA-ZOSTER IMMUNE GLOBULIN (Human) (V-ZIG)

Supplied: 125 Units in 2.5ml OR less

Administration: IM, DEEP
One vial containing 125 Units is given for each 10kg of body weight (AND IS THE MINIMUM DOSE). Maximum dose is 625 units (5 vials). Inject 125 units per 10kg, up to a maximum dose of 625 units. The minimum dose is 125 units, do not give fractional doses (1).

Administer by deep IM injection in the gluteal muscle, or in another large muscle mass. Do not inject IV. (1)

Varicella-Zoster Immune Globulin (VZIG)

Types of Exposure to Varicella or Zoster for Which VZIG Is Indicated for Susceptible Persons

- Newborn Infant: Onset of varicella in the mother 5 d or less before delivery or within 48 h after delivery; VZIG is not indicated if the mother has zoster

Candidates for VZIG, Provided Significant Exposure Has Occurred.*

- Immunocompromised children† without history of chickenpox‡
- Susceptible pregnant women
- Newborn infant whose mother had onset of chickenpox within 5 d before delivery or within 48 h after delivery
- Hospitalized premature infant (≥wk of gestation) whose mother lacks a reliable history of chickenpox or serologic evidence of protection against varicella
- Hospitalized premature infants (<28 wk of gestation or ≤1000 g), regardless of maternal history of varicella or varicella-zoster virus serostatus

---

* VZIG indicates Varicella-Zoster Immune Globulin.

† Including those who are infected with the human immunodeficiency virus.

‡ Immunocompromised adolescents and adults known to be susceptible also should receive VZIG.

Administration and Dose:

Varicella-Zoster Immune Globulin is given by intramuscular (IM) injection. VZIG contains between 10% and 18% globulin; VZIG does not contain thimerosal. One vial (approximate volume, 1.25 mL) containing 125 U is given for each 10 kg of body weight and is the minimal dose. The suggested maximal dose of VZIG is 625 U (ie, 5 vials).

Local discomfort after IM injection, the most frequent adverse effect, is common and can be lessened if the VZIG is at room temperature when administered. Use of VZIG for patients with a bleeding diathesis should be avoided, as with other IM injections, if possible. Immune Globulin Intravenous would be an acceptable alternative in this situation. VZIG never should be given intravenously.

Indications for VZIG:

Tables (above) indicate susceptible persons who should receive VZIG, including immunocompromised persons, susceptible pregnant women, and certain newborn infants.

For healthy, full-term infants exposed postnatally to varicella, including infants whose mother's rash developed more than 48 hours after delivery, VZIG is not indicated. Some experts advise use of VZIG for any exposed susceptible newborn who has severe skin disease.

(American Academy of Pediatrics: Report of the Committee on Infectious Diseases. Red Book 2000, pp.629-632)

Varicella-Zoster Immune Globulin (VZIG)

Indications and use: For protection of infants of mothers with varicella-zoster infections (chickenpox) within 5 days before or 48 h after delivery; of postnatally exposed preterm infants <1000 g or < 28 weeks regardless of maternal history; and of postnatally exposed premature infants whose maternal history is negative for varicella.

Actions: Passive immunity through infusion of IgG antibody. Protection lasts 1 month or longer. VZIG does not reduce the incidence but acts to decrease the risk of complications.

Route: IM only.

Dosage: 0-10 kg: 125 units IM as a single dose injected at one site.

Adverse effects: Pain, erythema, swelling, and rash at the site of injection and, rarely, anaphylaxis.

Comments: Best results are achieved if VZIG is given within 96 h after exposure. It is obtained through the American Red Cross Blood Services.

Note: Do not give IV.

(Gomella: Neonatology 1999, p.596)

SEE ALSO: ACYCLOVIR

VASOPRESSIN (Pitressin)

Supplied: Injection, pitressin synthetic, 20 pressor units/ml in 1ml

Administration: Injection, pitressin synthetic 20 U/ml: IM or SC

Vasopressin

Route & Dose: IM, SC: 2.5-10 U 2-4 times daily

Adverse Effects and Cautions: 20 units/ml aqueous injection

(Taeusch: Avery's Diseases of the Newborn 1998, p.1348)

Vasopressin (aqueous)

Dose/kg: 2.5-10 U total dose

Route and frequency: IM, SC q12h-q16h

Comments: May cause bronchoconstriction, diarrhea and electrolyte imbalance

(Avery: Neonatology Pathophysiology and Management of the Newborn 1999, p.1561)

Vasopressin

Antidiuretic hormone analog

Inj: 20 U/ml (aqueous) 0.5, 1 ml)

Dose: Children: 2.5-10 U BID-QID

Continuous infusion, children: Start at 0.5 mU/kg/hr (0.0005 U/kg/hr). Double dosage every 30 minutes PRN up to max dose of 10 mU/kg/hr (0.01 U/kg/hr)

GI hemorrhage (IV):

Children: Start at 0.002-0.005 U/kg/min. Increase dose as needed to 0.01 U/kg/min.

Comments: Side effects include tremor, sweating, vertigo, abdominal discomfort, nausea, vomiting, urticaria, anaphylaxis, hypertension, and bradycardia. May cause vasoconstriction, water intoxication, and bronchoconstriction. Drug interactions: lithium, demeclocycline, heparin, and alcohol reduce activity; carbamazepine, tricyclic antidepressants, fludrocortisone, and chlorpropamide increase activity.

Do not abruptly discontinue IV infusion (taper dose). Patients with variceal hemorrhage and hepatic insufficiency may respond to lower dosages. Monitor fluid intake and output, urine specific gravity, urine and serum osmolality and sodium.

(Siberry: The Harriet Lane Handbook 2000, p.879)

<u>Vasopressin</u>

We report three cases of hemorrhagic gastritis in term infants that led to massive bleeding of life-threatening proportions in the first 24 hours of life. In all three cases, bleeding was controlled by conservative therapeutic management...

Case Report 1: A 3820 gm female ...at 18 hours of age she had two episodes of bloody emesis ...she was treated with intravenous cimetidine (10mg/kg per dose every 6 hours) and a continuous vasopressin drip was started at 0.3 units/hr by the umbilical arterial line.

(Madan: Acute hemorrhagic gastritis in the newborn infant. J Perinatol 1992;12:377-380)

VECURONIUM (Norcuron)

Supplied: Injection, powder for 10mg/vial, 20mg/vial

Administration: IV

Diluent supplied by manufacturer contains benzyl alcohol which is not intended for use in newborns.

Use SWFI (without preservatives) 10ml to reconstitute the 10mg vial to yield final concentration of 1mg/ml. This product is stable for 24 hours-single use only-discard unused portion. Vecuronium is physically and chemically stable for 24 hours in D5W, NS (5).

<u>Vecuronium Bromide</u> (Norcuron)

Indications and use: Skeletal muscle relaxation and paralysis in infants requiring mechanical ventilation.

Actions: Nondepolarizing muscle relaxant that competitively antagonizes autonomic cholinergic receptors. Onset of action is 1-2 min with a duration that varies with dose and age.

Route: IV

Dosage: 0.03-0.15 mg/kg IV push q1-2h to maintain paralysis.

Adverse effects: May cause hypoxemia.

Comments: Causes less tachycardia than pancuronium bromide. When used with narcotics, decreases in heart rate and blood pressure have been observed.

(Gomella: Neonatology 1999, p.596)

Vecuronium

Route & Dose: IV: 0.08-0.1 mg/kg/dose, repeat prn at 0.03-0.15 mg/kg/dose q 1-2 h

Adverse Effects and Cautions:
Neuromuscular blockade potentiated by calcium channel blockers such as verapamil

(Taeusch: Avery's Diseases of the Newborn 1998, p.1348)

Vecuronium Bromide

Dose & Route: Neonates:
Initial: 0.1 mg/kg/dose IV
Maintenance: 0.03-0.15 mg/kg/dose IV Q1-2 hr PRN

>7 wk-1 yr:
Initial: 0.08-0.1 mg/kg/dose IV
Maintenance: 0.05-0.1 mg/kg/dose IV Q1 hr PRN;

>1 yr-adults:
Initial: 0.08-0.1 mg/kg/dose IV
Maintenance: 0.05-0.1 mg/kg/dose IV Q1 hr PRN; may administer via continuous infusion at 0.1 mg/kg/hr IV

Remarks: Use with **caution** in patients with renal or hepatic impairment, and neuromuscular disease. Infants from 7 wk to 1 yr are more sensitive to the drug and may have a longer recovery time. Children (1-10 yr) may require higher doses and more frequent supplementation than adults. Enflurane, isoflurane, aminoglycosides, magnesium salts, tetracyclines, bacitracin, and clindamycin may increase the potency and duration of neuromuscular blockade. May cause arrhythmias, rash, and bronchospasm.

Neostigmine, pyridostigmine, or edrophonium are antidotes. Onset of action within 1-3 minutes. Duration is 30-90 minutes.

(Siberry: The Harriet Lane Handbook 2000, p.880)

Vecuronium

Use: Adjunct to anesthesia, to facilitate endotracheal intubation, and provide skeletal muscle relaxation during surgery or mechanical ventilation

Usual Dosage: I.V.:
Neonates: 0.1 mg/kg/dose; maintenance: 0.03-0.15 mg/kg/dose every 1-2 hours as needed

Infants >7 weeks to 1 year: Initial: 0.08-0.1 mg/kg/dose; maintenance: 0.05-0.1 mg/kg every hour as needed.

Administration: Parenteral: I.V.: dilute vial to a maximum concentration of 2 mg/mL and administer by rapid direct injection; for continuous infusion, dilute to a maximum concentration 1 mg/mL

Monitoring Parameters:
Assisted ventilation status, heart rate, blood pressure, peripheral nerve stimulator measuring twitch response

Nursing Implications:
Does not alter the patient's state of consciousness; addition of sedation and analgesia is recommended
(Takemoto: Pediatric Dosage Handbook 2000-2001, pp.972-974)

Vecuronium (Norcuron)

Dose: 0.1 mg/kg/dose. May repeat every hour, as needed. Continuous Infusion: Begin with a loading dose of 0.1 mg/kg; then infuse at 0.05-0.1 mg/kg/hour. Individualize dose.

Dosing in Renal Impairment: Duration of action of this drug is prolonged in patients with renal impairment. Dose may need to be reduced with long-term use to prevent accumulation.

Dosing in Hepatic Dysfunction: Significant decreases in clearance and a longer elimination half-life (approximately double) may occur in severe hepatic dysfunction.

Administration: IV—Rate: Infuse IV push over 1-2 minutes or by continuous infusion.

IV—Concentration: Maximum: 1 mg/ml. May dilute further with saline or dextrose as desired. Note; Use nonbacteriostatic saline to reconstitute. Do not use the diluent provided with the product because it contains benzyl alcohol.

IV—Compatibility: See Appendix E: Y-Site Compatibility of Common NICU Drugs.
Storage: Refrigerate.

Cautions/Contraindications:
Infants with congenital myasthenia gravis may have exaggerated pharmacologic effects (e.g., neuromuscular blockade), even with small doses. Use with extreme caution, if at all.

Use only when equipment for intubation, artificial respiration, and oxygen are available and reversal agents are present.

May mask seizures in asphyxiated infants.

Vecuronium has no analgesic or sedative effects, and the paralysis it produces may mask signs and symptoms of pain. Assess for and treat pain and agitation, if needed.

Precautions should be used to prevent corneal abrasion (tape eyelids shut, use ocular lubricant ointment).

Adverse Effects: May cause pain during injection.

Cardiovascular: Tachycardia and hypertension are less likely to occur with vecuronium than with use of other neuromuscular blockers, such as pancuronium.
From Prolonged Use: May cause fluid retention and negative effects on pulmonary mechanics (decreased pulmonary dynamic compliance and increased pulmonary resistance, resulting in the need for increased ventilatory support.) Muscle atrophy and weakness caused by disuse, joint contractures, decubitus ulcers, and accumulation of pulmonary secretions also may occur.
Histamine Release from Mast Cells (displayed as bronchospasm, vasodilation, hypotension, cutaneous flushing): Vecuronium does not release clinically significant amounts of histamine, so cardiovascular effects are minimal. Tubocurarine releases the most histamine, followed by atracurium, then vecuronium, metocurine, and pancuronium. The latter 3 drugs cause the least histamine-releasing effects and are approximately equal in this respect.

Nursing Implications:

Have reversal agents available at bedside.

All paralyzed infants need analgesia and/or sedation in conjunction with paralyzation-consider concomitant infusion of fentanyl, morphine, or midazolam.

Provide range of motion, position changes, and eye lubrication to avoid side effects of paralyzation.

Consider need for bladder catheterization or Credé if urine output decreases.

Monitor for movement.

When drug is taken on transport, refrigerate immediately upon return.

Comments: Mechanical ventilation must be provided during use. Drug does not provide analgesia or sedation, only paralysis.

Reversal of Neuromuscular Blockade:

- Mechanism of Reversal: Neostigmine inhibits acetylcholinesterase at the neuromuscular junction, allowing the accumulation of acetylcholine, which can successfully compete with the neuromuscular blocker at the neuromuscular junction, thus restoring muscle activity. Atropine is also given to avert the nonneuromuscular effects of neostigmine, such as increased secretions, bronchoconstriction, and bradycardia.

- Dose: Neostigmine 0.06 mg/kg IV plus atropine 0.02 mg/kg/IV. Onset of reversal is approximately 10 minutes.

(Zenk: Neonatal Medications & Nutrition. A Comprehensive Guide 2000; pp.487-489)

VERAPAMIL (Isoptin, Calan)

Supplied: Injection 5mg/2ml in 2ml, 4ml
Tablets 40mg, 80mg, others

Administration: IV, PO
IV administration: Administer IV as a slow intravenous injection, for at least a two-minute period of time, under continuous ECG and blood pressure monitoring (1).

Extemporaneous Compounding (Recipe)

Dosage form: Oral suspension
Made from: Tablets
Concentration: 50mg/mL
Stability: 60 days
Store: Refrigerate
Label: Shake well

Ingredient	Strength	Quantity
Verapamil tablets	80 mg	75
Ora-Sweet or Ora-Sweet SF		
Ora-plus		aa qs 120 mL

Instructions: Crush the tablets in a mortar and reduce to a fine powder. Add a small amount of vehicle and mix to a uniform paste. Add geometric amounts of vehicle to almost desired volume while mixing. Transfer to a graduate and qs to volume while mixing. (11)

Verapamil

It is useful for SVT, for verapamil-sensitive ventricular tachycardias, and for hypertrophic cardiomyopathy.

Dosing: PO: 4-17 mg/kg/day
Warnings: Bradycardia, constipation, hypotension

Oral Administration, Kinetics, Metabolites:

Verapamil levels are not generally useful guidelines but range from 0.1 to 0.4 µg/ml.

Dosing and Interactions:

The oral preparation has been used with a wide range of reported effective daily doses, from 4 to 17 mg/kg/day. The drug is usually given on a schedule of three to four times daily. When the sustained-release preparation is given, the total daily dose is generally reduced slightly to account for the higher bioavailability.

The intravenous form of the drug should not be provided for patients younger than 1 year.

The use of concomitant calcium blockers with beta blockers is unwise because of the synergistic negative effects on ventricular function and sinus rate. A mild increase in digoxin levels has been reported.

Side Effects: With the oral preparation of verapamil, one of the more commonly reported adverse effects is constipation. Headaches, dizziness, rashes, and pruritus are other adverse reactions. Cardiovascular side effects include bradycardia, AV block, postural hypotension, and worsening of congestive heart failure.

The most significant side effect occurs with the intravenous preparation. Serious hypotension may occur, especially in young patients, resulting in asystole and cardiovascular collapse. Intravenous administration should be considered as contraindicated in patients younger than 1 year. In either the oral or intravenous preparation, verapamil may increase the ventricular response rate of atrial fibrillation in patients with Wolff-Parkinson-White syndrome.

(Gillette: Clinical Pediatric Arrhythmias 1999, pp.231-248)

Verapamil

Class: IV
Ca^{++} blockers

Uses: SVT (acute, in patient >1 year old and not on –blockers)
AVN reentry SVT
Hypertrophic cardiomyopathy
Some patients with PVCs, VT

Dose (Level): IV: 0.15 mg/kg over 3 min, may repeat once (have IV $CaCl_2$ ready)
PO: 2-7 mg/kg/day divided TID, QID

Mode of Action: Slow channel blockade; negative inotropism

ECG/EP Changes: Broad P wave, ↑ PR, Increased AH. No change SACT, CSNRT; increased AVNERP

Side Effects: Hypotension (IV); contraindicated with β-blockers; constipation, flushing; contraindicated in pulmonary hypertension, SSS, poor LV function; Dig.-↑ dig. level; warfarin ↑ PT

(Garson: The science and practice of pediatric cardiology 1998, p.2954)

Verapamil

Route & Dose: IV: 0.1-0.2 mg/kg infused over 2 min; if response is inadequate, repeat in 30 min
PO: 2-5 mg/kg/day in 3 divided doses

Adverse Effects and Cautions:
Monitor electrocardiogram during infusion. Bradycardia, atrioventricular block, asystole. Contraindicated in patients with 2nd and 3rd degree atrioventricular block during treatment with beta blockers

(Taeusch: Avery's Diseases of the Newborn 1998, p. 1348)

Verapamil

Use: Angina, hypertension; I.V. for supraventricular tachyarrhythmias (PSVT, atrial fibrillation, atrial flutter)

Contraindications:
Sinus bradycardia; advanced heart block; ventricular tachycardia; cardiogenic shock; hypersensitivity to verapamil or any component; atrial fibrillation or flutter associated with accessory conduction pathways

Warnings: Avoid I.V. use in neonates and young infants due to severe apnea, bradycardia, hypotensive reactions, and cardiac arrest; monitor EKG and blood pressure closely in patients receiving I.V. therapy; have I.V. calcium chloride 10 mg/kg available at bedside to treat hypotension

I.V. administration, hypertrophic cardiomyopathy, sick sinus syndrome, moderate to severe CHF, concomitant therapy with beta-blockers or digoxin can all increase the incidence of adverse effect

Adverse Reactions:
Cardiovascular: Hypotension, bradycardia; first, second, or third degree A-V block, worsening heart failure
Central nervous system: Dizziness, fatigue, seizures (occasionally with I.V. use), headache
Gastrointestinal: constipation, nausea, abdominal discomfort
Hepatic: Increase in hepatic enzymes
Respiratory: **May** precipitate insufficiency of respiratory muscle function in Duchenne muscular dystrophy

Usual Dosage: Infants <1 year: I.V.: Usually not used, (see Warnings); administer with continuous EKG monitoring, have I.V. calcium available at bedside: 0.1-0.2 mg/kg (usual: 0.75-2 mg/dose) may repeat dose in 30 minutes if adequate response not achieved

(Taketomo: Pediatric Dosage Handbook 1999-2000, pp.;928-930)

Verapamil

Dose & Route: IV: Give over 2-3 minutes. May repeat once after 30 mins.
0-1 yr: 0.1-0.2 mg/kg, using continuous ECG monitoring.
1-15 yr: 0.1-0.3 mg/kg; **max dose**: 5 mg 1st dose, 10 mg 2nd dose.
PO: Children: 4-8 mg/kg/24 hr ÷ TID

Remarks: **Contraindications** include hypersensitivity, cardiogenic shock, severe CHF, sick-sinus syndrome, or AV block. Due to negative inotropic effects, verapamil should **not** be used to treat SVT in an emergency setting in infants. **Avoid** IV use in neonates and young infants due to apnea, bradycardia, hypotension. Monitor ECG. Have calcium and isoproterenol available to reverse myocardial depression.

Like other calcium channel antagonists, drug is a substrate of CYP 450 3A4. Barbiturates, sulfinpyrazone, phenytoin, vitamin D, and rifampin may decrease serum levels/effects of verapamil; quinidine may increase serum levels/effects. Verapamil may increase effects of beta-blockers (severe myocardial depression), carbamazepine, cyclosporine, digoxin, fentanyl, nondepolarizing muscle relaxants, and prazosin. Reduce dose in renal insufficiency.

(Siberry: The Harriet Lane Handbook 2000, pp.880-881)

VIDARABINE (Vira-A, Adenine arabinoside)

Supplied: Injection: no longer available in United States.
Ophthalmic Ointment 3%

Administration: Opthalmic

Vidarabine

For Herpes Simplex Virus Infection:

A comparison of vidarabine with acyclovir suggests that these compounds have a similar level of activity for this disease, but vidarabine is no longer available for clinical use. Acyclovir is safe for use in newborns and is familiar to pediatricians from its other clinical uses.

(Remington : Infectious Diseases of the Fetus and Newborn Infant 2001, p.437)

Vidarabine

For Treatment of Herpes Simplex and Ocular Lesions

For recommended antiviral dosages and duration of therapy with acyclovir, valacyclovir, famciclovir, and penciclovir for different HSV infections. Neither valacyclovir nor famciclovir is approved by the US Food and Drug Administration (FDA) for use in children.

Neonatal Parenteral acyclovir is the treatment of choice for neonatal HSV infections. Acyclovir should be administered to all neonates with HSV infection, irrespective of presenting clinical findings. The best outcome in terms of morbidity and mortality is observed among infants with disease limited to the skin, eyes, and mouth. Although most neonates treated for HSV encephalitis survive, the majority suffer substantial neurologic sequelae. Approximately 50% of neonates with disseminated disease die despite antiviral therapy. The dosage of acyclovir is 60 mg/kg per day in 3 divided doses, given intravenously for 14 days if disease is limited to the skin, eye, and mouth and for 21 days if disease is disseminated or involves the CNS. Relapse of skin, eyes, and mouth and CNS disease can occur after cessation of treatment. The optimal management of these recurrences is not established. The value of long-term suppressive or intermittent acyclovir therapy for neonates with disease of the skin, eyes, and mouth is being evaluated.

Infants with ocular involvement due to HSV infection should receive a topical ophthalmic drug (1% to 2%

trifluridine, 1% iododeoxyuridine, or 3% vidarabine), as well as parenteral antiviral therapy.

Ocular Treatment of eye lesions should be undertaken in consultation with an ophthalmologist. several DNA inhibitor drugs, such as 1% to 2% trifluridine, 1% iododeoxyuridine, and 3% vidarabine, have proven efficacy for topical therapy of superficial keratitis. Topical corticosteroids are contraindicated in suspected HSV conjunctivitis; however, ophthalmologists may choose to use corticosteroids in conjunction with antiviral drugs to treat locally invasive infections. For children with recurrent ocular lesions, oral suppressive therapy with acyclovir (20 mg/kg every 6 hours) may be of benefit.

(American Academy of Pediatrics: Report of the Committee on Infectious Diseases. Red Book 2000, pp.313-315)

Vidarabine

Indication: For neonatal herpes simplex infection

Vidarabine, a purine nucleotide, proved to be beneficial in reducing mortality and morbidity of neonatal herpes simplex infections in controlled studies. The drug crosses the blood-brain barrier efficiently and exerts its antiviral activity with less systemic toxicity than Ara-C. Moreover, vidarabine has little of the deleterious effect on rat brain growth exhibited by Ara-C. The drug is administered in a dose of 15 mg/kg/day or 30 mg/kg/day (similar clinical effect in one study). Even with severe disease, i.e., disseminated or localized CNS, a sharp decrease in both mortality (from approximately 75% to 40%) and morbidity (approximately threefold increase in normal survivors) has been observed. The benefits of therapy in patients with localized skin disease were particularly striking. A major disadvantage of vidarabine is the relatively low solubility of the drug and the need for administration of relatively large volumes of fluid with each dose.

(Volpe: Neurology of the Newborn 2001, p.746)

Vidarabine (Vira-A)

Action and spectrum:

Antiviral agent for treatment of herpes encephalitis. Inhibits viral DNA formation. Good activity against herpes simplex type 1, poor activity against adenoviruses or RNA viruses. Activity against varicella-zoster virus unconfirmed.

Route: Ophthalmic, IV
(dilute to 1 mg/2.2 mL and infuse over 12-24 h).

Dosage: Ophthalmic: Instill a small amount into each eye q3h
IV:
< 1 month: 15-30 mg/kg/day as an 18-to 24-hr infusion.
> 1 month: 10-15 mg/kg/day as a 12 h or longer infusion.

Adverse effects: Rash, pain at injection site. Decreased reticulocyte count, white cell count, and platelet count. Elevated total bilirubin and AST (SGOT).

Comments: Rarely used. Volume necessary for IV infusion may cause fluid overload. Acyclovir is usual agent of choice. Must filter final solution (use 0.45-micron filter).

(Gomella: Neonatology 1999, pp.596-597)

Vidarabine (Adenine Arabinoside, Ara-A, Vira-A)

Dose & Route: Keratoconjunctivitis (HSV, VZV): Apply 1/2 in. ribbon of ointment to lower conjunctival sac Q3 hr, 5 x/24 hr until complete re-epithelialization has occurred, then decrease dose to BID for additional 7 days.

If there are no signs of improvement after 7 days, or if complete re-epithelialization has not occurred in 21 days, consider other forms of therapy.

Remarks: Ophthalmic product may cause burning, lacrimation, keratitis, photophobia, blurred vision.

(Siberry: The Harriet Lane Handbook 2000, p.881)

VITAMIN A (Aquasol A, see also Vitamins)

Supplied: Oral Drops 5,000 IU/0.1ml in 30ml
Injection 50,000 IU/ml in 2ml

Administration: PO, IM

Vitamin A

We studied 807 infants with birth weights ranging from 401 to 1000 g who received mechanical ventilation or supplemental oxygen at hours of age in one of the participating centers (see the Appendix) between January 1996 and July 1997. To reduce the likelihood of early death that was unrelated to vitamin A status and to facilitate enrollment, we enrolled infants 24 to 96 hours after birth. We excluded infants with major congenital anomalies, those with congenital nonbacterial infection, those thought to have a terminal illness (indicated by a pH below 6.80 or by the presence of hypoxia with bradycardia for more than two hours), and those who were to receive vitamin A in a parenteral fat emulsion or in doses exceeding recommendations for multivitamin preparations.

The infants were stratified according to center and birth weight (401 to 750 g or 751 to 1000 g) and assigned to the vitamin A or control group by a hospital pharmacist using a randomization list (or at four centers, by a research nurse using sealed envelopes containing the treatment assignments). Vitamin A was given intramuscularly because of its poor enteral absorption and unreliable delivery in crystalloid solutions: a dose of 5000 IU (0.1 ml) was given on Mondays, Wednesdays, and Fridays for four weeks (study days 0 to 25 or 26) in a 0.3-ml insulin syringe (Becton Dickinson, Cockeysville, Md.) with a 29-gauge needle. The same dose was used regardless of birth weight, because the smallest infants have the highest incidence of chronic lung disease, the lowest vitamin A stores at birth, and the lowest enteral intakes. The vitamin A preparation (Aquasol A, Astra USA, Westborough, Mass.) was refrigerated and shielded at all times from direct light.

Conclusions: Intramuscular administration of 5000 IU of vitamin A three times per week for four weeks reduced biochemical evidence of vitamin A deficiency and slightly decreased the risk of chronic lung disease in extremely-low-birth-weight infants.

(Tyson: Vitamin A supplementation for extremely low birth weight infants. N Engl J Med. 1999;340:1962-68)

Vitamin A

Indication: Treatment of BPD

Dexamethasone Treatment:

A dexamethasone preparation (Decadron, Merck, West Point, PA) containing .4 mg/mL dexamethasone-sodium-phosphate was used. The dosage of dexamethasone included .5 mg/kg/d on days 1 and 2 of treatment, .25 mg/kg/d on days 3 and 4, and .1 mg/kg/d on days 5,6, and 7. Each daily dose of dexamethasone was administered by bolus intravenous infusion in 2 equally divided doses at 12-hour intervals. This dosage regimen was patterned after the study by Durand et al, in which both short-term and long-term pulmonary benefits and minimal side effect were shown in response to dexamethasone treatment.

Vitamin A Intake:

The vitamin A concentration of human milk was estimated to be 300 IU/dL, and that of preterm infant formula ws estimated to be 970 IU/dL. In addition, before the initiation of dexamethasone treatment, each infant received supplemental vitamin A in the form of retinyl palmitate (Aquasol A, Astra, Wastboro, MA) by either intramuscular injection or orogastric administration beginning shortly after birth. The dosage of supplemental vitamin A by intramuscular route was 2000 IU/kg/dose administered every other day, and that by orogastric route was 4000 IU/kg/dose administered daily. This supplemental vitamin A was withheld during the week of dexamethasone treatment and also during the following week.

Conclusion: In summary, we examined the changes in plasma vitamin A and RBP concentrations in response to postnatal dexamethasone treatment, and correlated these changes with the pulmonary outcome in a cohort of VLBW neonates with BPD. Postnatal dexamethasone treatment induced a significant, yet short-term, increase in plasma concentrations of both vitamin A and RBP. This increase was independent of the total intake of vitamin A and probably resulted from endogenous mobilization of vitamin A from the liver. Our data suggest that the beneficial

pulmonary response to dexamethasone in infants with BPD is influenced, at least in part, by the vitamin A status, and that gender plays a role in this response. Additional studies are needed to determine the optimal usage of dexamethasone and vitamin A nutrition in these infants.
(Shenai: Vitamin A Status and Postnatal Dexamethasone Treatment in Bronchopulmonary Dysplasia. Pediatrics 2000;106:547-553)

Vitamin A

Evidence of Vitamin A Deficiency: Measurement of plasma concentration of vitamin A is the most commonly used biochemical marker of vitamin A status. In healthy adult humans, the plasma vitamin A concentration ranges from 20 to 80 *u*g/dL. In children, including infants, a plasma vitamin A concentration < 20 *u*g/dL is considered to be indicative of vitamin A deficiency. Most VLBW neonates are born with plasma vitamin A concentrations that are in the deficient range. Most VLBW neonates are born with plasma RBP concentrations that are in the deficient range.

Vitamin A Supplements: For intramuscular supplementation, a water-miscible preparation (Aquasol A Parenteral, Astra, Westboro, MA) containing 50,000 IU/mL of vitamin A as retinyl palmitate is used. This preparation is unstable when diluted and therefore is used in its undiluted form. A unit dose of this preparation is dispensed from pharmacy in a plastic insulin syringe (U100 Becton Dickinson, Franklin Lakes, NJ). For orogastric supplementation, a vitamin A preparation (Pharmaceutical Compounding Centers of America, Houston, TX) containing 10,000 IU/mL of vitamin A as retinyl palmitate is used. A unit dose of this preparation is dispensed from pharmacy in a plastic oral dispenser (Exacta-Med, Baxa Corporation, Englewood, CA). All unit doses are administered to the infants within 30 minutes of dispensing. To prevent photodegradative loss of vitamin A, each unit dose is shielded from light until administration.

Dosage: The supplemental doses of vitamin A are provided in 2 phases. During the first phase, supplemental vitamin A (2000 IU/kg/dose) is provided by intramuscular injection on postnatal day 1 and on alternate days thereafter until establishment of full enteral feeding. Full enteral feeding is considered established when energy intake by enteral route exceeds 75% of total energy intake. This intramuscular dosage of supplemental vitamin A is based on previous clinical trials, in which normalization of plasma vitamin A indexes was demonstrated using this dosage. The intramuscular route is selected for administration of supplemental vitamin A during the first phase, because of the greater efficacy in normalizing plasma vitamin A indexes with intramuscular supplements, relative to orogastric supplements, in young immature infants. During the second phase, supplemental vitamin A (4000

IU/kg/dose) is provided by orogastric administration daily from the day of establishment of full enteral feeding until discharge from the neonatal intensive care unit.

This orogastric dosage of supplemental vitamin A is based on the trial by Landman et al, in which orogastric supplements (5000 IU daily) were demonstrated to be comparable to intramuscular supplements (2000 IU on alternate days) in normalizing plasma vitamin A indexes. In the event enteral feeding is withheld because of evidence of intolerance, orogastric administration of supplemental vitamin A is discontinued and substituted by intramuscular supplementation until resumption of enteral feeding.

Biochemical Monitoring: Plasma concentrations of vitamin A and RBP are monitored weekly throughout the period of vitamin A supplementation. Plasma vitamin A concentration is determined by spectrofluorometry, and plasma RBP concentration by quantitative radial immunodiffusion (Binding Site, Inc, San Diego, CA). The desired range of plasma vitamin A concentrations is 30 to 60 *u*g/dL, and the desired plasma RBP concentration is >2.5 mg/dL. Vitamin A toxicity has not been reported in humans when the plasma vitamin A concentration is <100 *u*g/dL. The dosage of supplemental vitamin A is adjusted weekly based on plasma vitamin A concentrations.

In summary, BPD is a disease of multiple causes, and its incidence among VLBW neonates is unacceptably high. In addition to the prevention of prematurity as the primary perinatal health care goal, the strategies for reducing the occurrence of BPD among VLBW survivors are clearly warranted. These strategies involve the modulation of a delicate balance between injury and healing of the immature lung. Optimal vitamin A nutrition is one such strategy to complement a host of other approaches. Although with clinical trials to date, significant strides have been made toward understanding the role of vitamin A in BPD among VLBW neonates, much remains to be studied. The precise requirement of vitamin A in these infants, and the optimal mode and duration of its administration warrant further investigation. Diagnostic measures that can evaluate molecular mechanisms of vitamin A action in the developing lung need to be explored for their clinical applications. Likewise, the therapeutic role of vitamin A metabolites, including retinoic acid, in promoting lung healing awaits further investigation.

(Shenai: Vitamin A Supplementation in Very Low Birth Weight Neonates: Rationale and Evidence. Pediatrics 1999;104:1369 - 1374)

VITAMIN B_1 (Thiamine)

Supplied: PO: 50mg
Injection; 100mg/ml, 1ml, 2ml, 10ml vials

Route: PO, IM, IV (slowly)
Incompatibility: B_1 is unstable in neutral or alkaline solutions, do not use in combination with alkaline solutions (eg, carbonates, citrates, barbiturates, erythromycin lactobionate IV). Solutions containing sulfites are incompatible with thiamine.

Vitamin B_1

Route & Dose: PO: preventive, 0.5-1.0 mg q day;
PO: therapeutic, 5-10 mg q 6-8 h
(Taeusch: Avery's Diseases of the Newborn 1998, p.1348)

VITAMIN B_2 (Riboflavin)

Supplied: 25mg, 50mg tables

A deficiency of riboflavin affects glucose, fatty acid, and amino acid metabolism.

PolyViSol or ViDaylin 1 ml supplies 600 mcg.

Vitamin B2 (Riboflavin)

Indications: Riboflavin daily requirements (RDA)
Dosage/route/frequency:
Premature: 400 μg PO
Full-term: 60 μg PO

Indications: Riboflavin deficiency: therapy
Dosage/route/frequency:
IV therapy (VLWB): 0.15 mg/mg/day

Indications: Riboflavin sources
Dosage/route/frequency:
Human milk supplies 88 μg/day
1 ml PolyViSol or ViDaylin supplies 600μg

Clinical Considerations:
Riboflavin deficiency affects glucose, fatty acid, and amino acid metabolism.

Drug Interactions:
GI absorption of riboflavin is increased with food intake and decreased with liver dysfunction and concurrent probenecid usage.

Test Interactions:
Large doses may interfere with urinalysis based on spectrometry and may cause false elevations in fluorimetric determinations of catecholamines and urobilinogen.
(Cloherty: Manual of Neonatal Care 1998 pp.745-746)

Riboflavin

For Treatment of Glutaric Aciduria Type II

After confirming the diagnosis of GA II and implementing therapy with IV carnitine (200 to 300 mg/kg per day) and oral riboflavin (100 mg/kg per day), the patient was weaned off the ventilator within 3 days. His atelectasis disappeared. His blood glucose, lactate, bilirubin, prothrombin time and partial thromboplastin time, platelet count, and liver and muscle enzymes normalized after 6 days of therapy. He regained his strength gradually and his seizures and apneic episodes resolved. After 4 weeks, the hepatosplenomegaly and ascites had completely resolved. Repeated chest x-ray and echocardiography indicated normal heart size and function and complete disappearance of the inferior vena cava thrombus. He was discharge from the hospital at 2 months of age in good condition on high-caloric formula low in fat and protein, oral riboflavin, and high-dose oral carnitine.

The patient's adhered to the treatment. However, between 2 and 4 months of age, the patient's clinical condition deteriorated due to repeated acidotic hypoglycemia attacks, vomiting associated with poor weight gain, and worsening hypotonia. At 4 months of age, a repeated MS/MS study showed a low free carnitine level and slightly increased acylcarnitines species typical of GA II. Because of his clinical deterioration and low plasma carnitine level, a central venous line (Infuse-A-Port, distributed by Horizon Medical Products, Manchester, GA) was inserted and IV carnitine (200 mg/kg three times per week) was started and maintained for 6 months. After IV carnitine therapy, the patient's condition stabilized; he started babbling, socially interacting, rolling over, had relatively good head control, and could maintain sitting balance for 3 seconds. His follow-up developmental assessment at the age of 6 months showed a playful child with good social interaction who could sit with support; apart from mild hypotonia, his neurologic examination was essentially normal. Brain magnetic resonance imaging (MRI) showed mild brain atrophy and delayed myelination. Repeated electroencephalography, visual-evoked potentials, brainstem evoked potentials, electromyography, and nerve conduction studies were normal. At 10 months of age, a repeated MS/MS showed a normal acylcarnitine profile; however, free carnitine was significantly elevated, so he was switched from an IV to an oral carnitine preparation. Later on, however, his clinical condition deteriorated with increased hypotonia and loss of previously acquired milestones. The Port-A-Cath was reinserted, and IV carnitine therapy was resumed at 12 months of age. Meanwhile, his blood free carnitine level was maintained in the high range, which was closely monitored through repeated MS/MS testing.

(Al-Essa: Glutaric Aciduria Type II: Observations in Seven Patients With Neonatal- and Late-Onset Disease. J Perinatol 2000;2:120-128)

VITAMIN B_6

SEE PYRIDOXINE

VITAMIN C (Ascorbic acid) (Ce-Vi-Sol, Cecon)

Supplied: Ce-Vi-Sol 35mg/0.6mL; Cecon 100mg/mL

Vitamin C (ascorbic acid)

Route & Dose: IM, IV, PO: preventive, 25-50 mg/day (term infants): 100 mg/day (premature infants)

(Taeusch: Avery's Diseases of the Newborn 1998, p.1348)

Vitamin C

A double-blind, randomized, controlled trial of vitamin C supplementation (50 mg/day) was undertaken in premature neonates (birth weight, 1000 to 1500 gm)

....supplementation of premature infants with vitamin C is not associated with evidence of increased erythrocyte destruction, hyperbilirubinemia, or other morbidity.

(Doyle: Does vitamin C cause hemolysis in premature newborn infants? Results of a multicenter double-blind, randomized, controlled trial. J Pediatr 1997;130:103-109)

VITAMIN D_2 (Calciferol, Drisdol, Ergocalciferol)

Supplied: ERGOCALCIFEROL (D_2) Liquid 8000 IU/ml in 60ml
Injection 500,000 U/ml in 1ml

Administration: PO, IM

Ergocalciferol (D_2) 1.25mg provides 50,000 IU of vitamin D activity (1).

Vitamin D_2 (Ergocalciferol, Calciferol)(Drisdol)

Indications and use:

To prevent or treat rickets and to manage hypocalcemia due to vitamin D deficiency.

Actions: Regulation of plasma calcium and phosphate, supporting normal mineralization of bone.

Route: PO, IM

Dosage: 400-800 units/day

Comments: Excessive doses may lead to hypervitaminosis D, manifested by hypercalcemia and its associated complications.

(Gomella: Neonatology 1999, p.597)

Vitamin D_2

Route & Dose: PO: preventive, 400-1000 IU/day (premature infants), 40-100 IU/day (term infants)

(Taeusch: Avery's Diseases of the Newborn 1998, p.1348)

Vitamin D_2 (Ergocalciferol)

Dose & Route: Dietary supplementation:
Preterm: 400-800 IU/24 hr PO
Infants/Children: 400 IU/24 hr PO

Renal Failure:
Children: 4000-40,000 IU/24 hr PO

Rickets: Vitamin D dependent:
Children: 3000-5000 IU/24 hr PO;
max dose: 60,000 IU/24 hr

Nutritional Rickets:
Children with Normal GI absorption: 2000-5000 IU/24 hr PO x 6-12 wk

Malabsorption:
Children: 10,000-25,000 IU/24 hr PO

Vitamin D resistant rickets (with phosphate supplementation):
Children: Initial dose 400,000-800,000 IU/24 hr PO; increase daily dose by 10,000-20,000 IU PO Q3-4 mo if needed.

Hypoparathyroidism (with calcium supplementation):
Children: 50,000-200,000 IU/24 hr PO

Remarks: Monitor serum Ca, PO_4, and alkaline phosphate. Serum Ca = PO_4 product should be <70 mg/dl to avoid ectopic calcification. Titrate dosage to patient response. Watch for symptoms of hypercalcemia: weakness, diarrhea, polyuria, metastatic calcification, nephrocalcinosis. Vitamin D_2 is activated by 25-hydroxylation in liver and 1-hydroxylation in kidney.

Oral route is preferred. May use IM route in cases of fat malabsorption. Injectable for IM administration only.

(Siberry: The Harriet Lane Handbook 2000, p.707)

VITAMIN E (Aquasol E)

Supplied: Oral Drops 50mg/ml in 12 and 30ml

Administration: PO

Aquasol E is supplied as dl-alpha tocopherol acetate. 1mg of dl-alpha tocopherol acetate = 1 IU of Vitamin E (1). Vitamin E should not be administered IV, since the role of IV Vitamin E in the deaths of 38 infants receiving the drug remains unclear. (1)

Vitamin E (DL-α -Tocopherol Acetate)
(Aquasol E)

Indications and use:

Investigational for treatment or prevention of anemia of prematurity, retinopathy of prematurity, BPD, and intraventricular hemorrhage.

Actions: A potent free radical scavenger. An antioxidant to prevent destruction of unsaturated fatty acids and cell membranes by uncontrolled free radicals. At birth, tissue stores of α-tocopherol (active form) are low.

Route: PO

Dosage: Requirements: The following recommendations are currently followed in infant formulas.

Full-term infants: 0.3 unit/100 kcal or 0.7 units/g of linoleic acid.

Premature infants: 1 units/g of linoleic acid.

Anemia of prematurity: Prevention or treatment requires only adequate nutritional intake of vitamin E.

Alternative: Prophylaxis: 25-50 units/day PO until 2-3 months of age. Treatment: 50-200 units/day PO for 2 weeks.

Comments: Physiologic serum levels for premature infants are 1-3 mg/dL. Serum levels should be monitored when pharmacologic doses of vitamin E are administered. Liquid preparation is very hyperosmolar (3000 mosm/L) and should be diluted (1 mg of DL-α -tocopherol acetate = 1 unit).

(Gomella: Neonatology 1999, p.598)

Vitamin E

Usual Dosage: 1 unit vitamin E = mg *dl*-alpha-tocopherol acetate. Oral:

Recommended daily allowance (RDA) and
Estimated Average Requirement (EAR)

Age	RDA (mg/day)	EAR (mg/day)
0-6 mo	--	4* (6 units)
7-12 mo	--	6* (9 units)

Vitamin E deficiency:

Neonates, premature, low birth weight: 25-30 units/day results in normal levels within 1 week

Prevention of vitamin E deficiency:
Neonates:
Low birth weight: 5 units/day
Full-term: 5 units/L of formula ingested

Prevention of retinopathy of prematurity or BPD secondary to O_2 therapy: Neonates and Infants: (American Academy of Pediatrics considers this use investigational and routine use is not recommended): 15-30 units/kg/day to maintain plasma levels between 1.5-2 mcg/mL (may need as high as 100 units/kg/day)

Administration: Oral: May administer with or without food

Monitoring Parameters: Plasma tocopherol concentrations

Reference Range Plasma tocopherol : 6-14 µg/mL

(Takemoto: Pediatric Dosage Handbook 2000-2001, pp.982-983)

Vitamin E (*d*-alpha tocopherol)

Route & Dose: PO: prevention of hemolysis- 25-50 IU/day (1 IU = 1 mg)

Adverse Effects and Cautions: Some preparations are hyperosmolar (Taeusch: Avery's Diseases of the Newborn 1998, p.1348)

VITAMIN K_1 (Aquamephyton, Phytonadione, Mephyton)

Supplied: Tablets: 5mg
Injection 1mg/0.5ml
Injection 10mg/ml

Administration: IM, IV
CAUTION: Use appropriate strength injection 1mg/0.5mL.

IV Use: WARNING: severe reactions, including fatalities, have occurred during and immediately after IV injection, even with precautions to dilute the injection and to avoid rapid infusion. Therefore restrict the IV route to those situations where other routes are not feasible and the serious risk involved is justified. (1)

Vitamin K

To prevent vitamin K-dependent hemorrhagic disease of the newborn, every neonate should receive a single parenteral dose of 0.5-1.0-mg of natural vitamin K_1 oxide (phytonadione) within 1 hour of birth. Oral administration of vitamin K has not been shown to be as efficacious as parenteral administration. Furthermore, no commercial oral vitamin K preparations are approved for use in the United States.

(AAP/ACOG: Guidelines for Perinatal Care 1997, p.157)

Vitamin K_1 (Phytonadione)(AquaMEPHYTON, Mephyton)

Indications and use:
Prevention and treatment of hemorrhagic disease of the newborn, and vitamin K deficiency.

Actions: Required for the synthesis of blood coagulation factors II, VII, IX, and X. Because vitamin K_1 may require 3 h or more to stop active bleeding, fresh-frozen plasma, 10 mL/kg, may be necessary when bleeding is severe. The drug has no antagonistic effects against heparin.

Route: PO, IM, IV, SC. (For IV use, dilute in D_5W and infuse over 30 minutes or longer.)

Dosage: Neonatal hemorrhagic disease:
Prevention: 1 mg/ IM at birth; if infant <1500 g, give 0.5 mg IM at birth.

Treatment: 1 mg as single dose.

Deficiency state: 1 mg/dose PO, IM, or slowly IV.

Oral anticoagulant overdose: 1-2 mg/dose IV q4-8h prn (Follow serial prothrombin time and partial thromboplastin time for response).

Adverse effects: Relatively nontoxic. Hemolytic anemia and kernicterus have been reported in neonates given menadiol sodium diphosphate (vitamin K_3 [Synkayvite]); however, vitamin K_1 has not been associated with toxic symptoms or hypersensitivity. No association between exposure to vitamin K at birth and an increased risk for any childhood cancer or of all childhood cancers combined were found using data from the Collaborative Perinatal Project, although a slightly increased risk could not be ruled out.

(Gomella: Neonatology 1999, pp.597-598)

Phytonadione

Dose/kg: Neonatal hemorrhagic disease:
Prophylaxis: 0.5-1 mg total dose

Route & frequency:
IM, SC once within 1 hour of birth; may repeat 6-8 h later

Dose/kg: Treatment: 1-2 mg total dose
Route & frequency: IV, SC once

Comments: IV route should be used only when other routes are not available: infuse rate at a max rate of 1 mg/min; severe reactions resembling anaphylaxis may occur with IV administration

(Avery: Neonatology Pathophysiology and Management of the Newborn

Vitamin K_1 (phytonadione)

Route & Dose: SC, IM: preventive, 0.5-1.0 mg, single dose; therapeutic, 1-2 mg/kg/dose q 6-12 h according to prothrombin time

Adverse Effects and Cautions:
With thrombocytopenia, slow IV infusion at same dose. Anaphylaxis observed with rapid injection IV

(Taeusch: Avery's Diseases of the Newborn 1998, p.1348)
1999, p.1559)

VOLUME EXPANDERS

Volume Expanders

Volume expanders may be necessary to resuscitate a newly born infant who is hypovolemic. Suspect hypovolemia in any infant who fails to respond to resuscitation. Consider volume expansion when there has been suspected blood loss or the infant appears to be in shock (pale, poor perfusion, weak pulse) and has not responded adequately to other resuscitative measures (Class I). The fluid of choice for volume expansion is an isotonic crystalloid solution such as normal saline or Ringer's lactate (Class IIb, LOE 7). Administration of O-negative red blood cells may be indicated for replacement of large-volume blood loss (Class IIb, LOE 7). Albumin-containing solutions are less frequently used for initial volume expansion because of limited availability, risk of infectious disease, and an observed association with increased mortality.

The initial dose of volume expander is 10 mL/kg given by slow intravenous push over 5 to 10 minutes. The dose may be repeated after further clinical assessment and observation of response. Higher bolus volumes have been recommended for resuscitation of older infants. However, volume overload or complications such as intracranial hemorrhage may result from inappropriate intravascular volume expansion in asphyxiated newly born infants as well as in preterm infants.

(International Guidelines for Neonatal Resuscitation: An Excerpt From the Guidelines 2000 for Cardiopulmonary Resuscitation and Emergency Cardiovascular Care: International Consensus on Science. Pediatrics 2000;106:11of16)

WARFARIN (Coumadin)

Supplied: Tablets 1mg, 2mg, others
Powder for injection 5mg vial

Administration: PO, IV
IM route not recommended

Warfarin

Eligibility included (1) age >1 month and <18 years and (2) venous thrombosis confirmed by ultrasonography, venography, or ventilation-perfusion scan.

The treatment guidelines for combination therapy are as follows. Urokinase is given as a bolus infusion of 4400 U/kg over a 20-minute period, followed by a maintenance infusion of 4400 U/kg/h for a 48-hour period. Heparin is given as an infusion of 10 U/kg/h during urokinase infusion without a bolus; at 48 hours a heparin bolus of 50 U/kg is given, and the rate of infusion is increased to achieve a plasma heparin level of 0.4 to 0.7 U/mL. Heparin is continued to maintain this therapeutic level for at least 5 days; heparin is discontinued when the international normalized ratio is >2. Warfarin is given to maintain the international normalized ratio >2 for 3 months to indefinitely.

Plasma concentrations of plasminogen, fibrinogen, and platelets were monitored at least daily during thrombolytic therapy. Transfusion support was administered routinely on the following schedule: plasminogen <0.50 U/mL was replaced with fresh-frozen plasma, 10 mL/kg; fibrinogen <50 mg/dL was replaced with cryoprecipitate, 10 mL/kg; platelet count <50,000/µL was replaced with single donor platelet concentrates, 10 mL/kg.

Conclusions: Combination therapy in children (urokinase and unfractionated heparin) was safe and efficacious. A prospective, randomized, controlled study in children is needed.

(Manco-Johnson: Combined thrombolytic and anticoagulant therapy for venous thrombosis in children. J Pediatr 2000;136:446-53)

Warfarin

Dosage: Pediatrics: 0.05-0.3 mg/kg/day p.o. (do not exceed adult dose)

Comments: Monitor INR for PT; INR should be approximately 2.5-3.5 for mechanical valves (controversy exists and some authorities recommend higher-intensity anticoagulation). Limited data in infants and children; contraindicated in pregnancy

INR, International Normalized Ratio; PT, prothrombin time; TPN, total parenteral nutrition

(Allen: Moss and Adam's Heart Disease in Infants, children and Adolescents 2001, pp.1460-1468)

Warfarin (Coumadin)

Dose: 10-30 mg/day IV, then 1-5 mg/day PO

Mode of Action: Inhibits prothrombin synthesis, vitamin K-dependent factors

Comments: Vitamin K antidote; effect potentiated by quinidine, phenytoin, amiodarone

(Garson: The science and practice of pediatric cardiology 1998, p.2955

Warfarin

Route: IV, IM, PO

Neonatal Dose: 0.05-0.34 mg/kg/24 h as a single dose; adjust dose to maintain desired prolongation of prothrombin time (PT)

Pediatric Dose: 0.05-0.34 mg/kg/24 h as a single dose; adjust dose to maintain desired prolongation of PT

Discussion: Should be administered orally and used IV or IM only in situations where it cannot be used orally; patients with liver dysfunction may require lower doses; consistent anticoagulation may be difficult to achieve in children <5y

(Rudolph: Rudolph's Pediatrics 1996, p.2209)

ZALCITABINE (Hivid, DDC)

Supplied: Tablets 0.375 mg and 0.75 mg
Administration: PO
Indications: Combination therapy with Zidovudine. (3)

Zalcitabine (ddc) / Hivid

Dosage: Pediatric range: 0.005 to 0.01 mg/kg q 8 h
Neonatal: Unknown

Major Toxic Effects:
Most frequent: Headache, malaise. Unusual (more severe): Peripheral neuropathy, pancreatitis, hepatic toxic effects, skin rashes, oral ulcers, esophageal ulcers, hematologic toxic effects

Drug Interactions:
Cimetidine, amphotericin, foscarnet and aminoglycosides may decrease renal clearance of zalcitabine.

Antacids decrease absorption.

Concomitant use with ddl is not recommended because of the increased risk of peripheral neuropathy.

Special Instructions:
Administer on an empty stomach (1 h before or 2 h after a meal)
Decrease dosage in patients with impaired renal function

(American Academy of Pediatrics: Report of the Committee on Infectious Diseases. Red Book 2000, p.680)

Zalcitabine (ddC)

Route: PO
Dosage: 2.25 mg/day (adult dosage)
Interval: q8h
NON-NEWBORN SECTION

(Nelson: Pocket Book of Pediatric Antimicrobial Therapy 2000-2001, p.86)

Zalcitabine

Dose & Route: Children <13 yr (NIH Pediatric HIV Working Group Guidelines):
Usual dose: 0.01 mg/kg/dose PO TID
Dosage range: 0.005-0.01 mg/kg/dose PO TID

Remarks: Use with **caution** in patients with liver disease, pancreatitis, or severe myelosuppression. Peripheral neuropathy, headaches, GI disturbances, and malaise are common side effects. Other side effects include bone marrow suppression, hepatitis, pancreatitis, hypertension, rash, oral and esophageal ulcers, myalgias, and fatigue.

Amphotericin, cimetidine, foscarnet, and aminoglycosides may reduce clearance and increase chances of peripheral neuropathy. In addition, drugs which cause peripheral neuropathy (ddl) should not be used in combination with ddC. Concurrent use of IV pentamidine can increase risk of pancreatitis. Antacids can decrease absorption. **Adjust dose in renal dysfunction**. Administer doses on an empty stomach; 1 hour before or 2 hours after meals.

(Siberry: The Harriet Lane Handbook 2000, p.888)

ZIDOVUDINE (Retrovir, AZT)

Supplied: PO: 300mg tablets, 100mg capsules
Syrup: 50 mg/5 ml in 240 ml
Injection: 10mg/ml in 20 ml

Administration: PO, IV
IV administration: Dilute prior to administration. Remove the calculated dose from the vial; add to D5W to achieve a concentration less than 4mg/mL. Infuse this dose over 1 hour. Stable for 24 hours at room Temperature or 48 hours refrigerated (1). Avoid rapid infusion or bolus injection. Do not give IM. (1)

Zidovudine (ZDV, AZT) Retrovir

Preparations: Syrup: 10 mg/mL syrup

Dosage: Usual pediatric:
Oral: 160 mg/m^2 q 8 h

IV (intermittent infusion): 1-2 mg/kg q 4 h
IV (continuous infusion): 20 mg/m^2 per hour

Pediatric range: 90 mg/m^2 to 180 mg/m^2 q 6-8 h

Neonatal:
Oral: 2 mg/kg q 6 h
IV: 1.5 mg/kg q 6 h

Premature infants:
(Standard neonatal dose may be excessive for premature infants)

Under study in PACTG 331:1.5 mg/kg q 12 h from birth to 2 wk of age; then increase to 2 mg/kg q 8 h after 2 wk of age

Major Toxic Effects:

Most frequent: Hematologic toxic effects, including granulocytopenia and anemia, headache

Unusual: Myopathy, myositis, hepatic toxic effects

Drug Interactions:

Increased toxic effects may be observed with concomitant administration of the following drugs (therefore, more intensive monitoring for toxic effects may be warranted): ganciclovir, interferon $\propto$, TMP-SMX. acyclovir.

The following drugs may increase ZDV concentration (and therefore potential toxic effects): probenecid, atovaquone, methadone, valproic acid

Decreased renal clearance may be observed with coadministration of cimetidine (may be significant inpatients with renal impairment)

ZDV metabolism any be increased with coadministration of rifampin and rifabutin; clarithromycin decreases concentrations of ZDV probably by interfering with absorption (administer 4 h apart)

Ribavirin decreases the intracellular phosphorylation of ZDV (conversion to active metabolite).

Phenytoin concentrations may increase or decrease.

Should not be administered in combination with stavudine (poor antiretroviral effect).

Special Instructions:

Can be administered with food (although the manufacturer recommends administration 30 min before or 1 h after a meal).

Decrease dosage for patients with severe renal impairment

Significant granulocytopenia or anemia may necessitate interruption of therapy until marrow recovery is observed; use of erythropoietin or reduced ZDV dosage may be necessary for some patients.

Reduced dosage may be indicated for patients with significant hepatic dysfunction.

For IV solution: Refrigerated diluted solution stable for 24 h Some experts use a dosage of 180 mg/m^2 q 12 h when used in combination with other antiretroviral compounds, but data on this dosing in children are limited.

(American Academy of Pediatrics: Report of the Committee on Infectious Diseases. Red Book 2000, pp681-682)

<u>Zidovudine</u> (AZT) (Retrovir)

Indications and use:

Management of patients with HIV infection. Prevention of maternal-fetal HIV transmission.

Actons: Virostatic. Inhibits HIV viral polymerases and DNA replication.

Route: IV, PO.

Dosage: 0-2 weeks old: 2mg/kg/dose PO q6h.
2-4 weeks old: 3 mg/kg/dose PO q6h.
>4 weeks old: 90 -180 mg/m^2/dose PO q 6h;
0.5-1.8 mg/kg/h IV continuous infusion; 100-120 mg/m^2/dose q6h over 1 h with a maximum concentration of 4 mg/mL in D_5W.

Reduce the dose by 30% in children with zidovudine toxicity with hemoglobin <8 g/dL.

Give the PO dose 30 min before or 1 h after feedings with water.

Adverse effects: The most frequent are granulocytopenia and severe anemia. Others include thrombocytopenia, leukopenia, diarrhea, fever, seizures insomnia, and cholestatic hepatitis.

Comments: Use with caution in patients with impaired hepatic function, bone marrow compromise, or folic acid or vitamin B_{12} deficiency. Interactions: Concurrent acetaminophen, probenecid, cimetidine, indomethacin, morphine, and benzodiazepines may increase toxicity due to decreased glucuronidation or reduced renal excretion of zidovudine. Concomitant acyclovir may cause neurotoxicity; gancyclovir may cause severe hematologic toxicity due to synergistic myelosuppression. Ribavirin and zidovudine are antagonistic and should not be used concurrently.

(Gomella: Neonatology 1999, p.598)

<u>Zidovudine</u> (AZT)

Route: IV, PO
Dose: 480 mg/m² /day (max 600 mg/day)
Interval: q6h

(Nelson: Pocket Book of Pediatric Antimicrobial Therapy 2000-2001, p.86)

<u>Zidovudine</u>

Condition: Human immunodeficiency virus infection
Therapy: Term baby: zidovudine 8 mg/kg/day PO div q6h <u>OR</u> 6 mg/kg/day IV div q6h; Preterm baby (≤ 34 wks): 3 mg/kg/day IV, PO div q12h x 2 wks, then 6 mg/kg/day IV, PO div q8h x 6 wks.

Comment: For infants born to HIV-positive mothers; Single dose nivirapine 2 mg/kg PO being tested

(Nelson: Pocket Book of Pediatric Antimicrobial Therapy 2000-2001, p.8)

<u>Zidovudine</u>

Children between the ages of 3 months and 18 years were eligible for enrollment. Children were included when the plasma HIV-1 RNA test result was positive on 2 subsequent occasions (children <18 months old)...

Medication was given in following doses: indinavir, 400 mg/m² every 8 hours; zidovudine, 120 mg/m² every 8 hours; and lamivudine, 4 mg/kg every 12 hours. Indinavir was administered as standard capsules of 200 mg and 400mg or as capsules of 150 mg and 300 mg, which were prepared at the pharmacy. When patients were too young to swallow capsules, indinavir capsules had to be opened by the caregivers and dissolved in 5 to 10 mL of water. In children in whom problems were encountered with the ingestion of indinavir, the drug was changed to nelfinavir (30 mg/kg every 8 hours). Zidovudine was administered either as syrup (10 mg/mL) or as capsules of 100 mg and

250 mg, depending on the child's age. Lamivudine was administered as syrup (10 mg/mL) or as tablets of 150 mg. The importance of taking the indinavir 1 hour before or 2 hours after meals was repeatedly emphasized.

Conclusions: Highly active antiretroviral therapy consisting of indinavir, zidovudine, and lamivudine in children reduced HIV-1 RNA to less than 500 copies/mL in 70% of the children within 6 months. Improved CD4 cell counts were observed in most patients, as was a better clinical condition (no invasive or opportunistic infections, increased weight gain). Side effects of the triple therapy were mild. Highly active antiretroviral therapy can be used as successfully in children as in adults.

(van Rossum: Clinical and virologic response to combination treatment with indinavir, zidovudine, and lamivudine in children with human immunodeficiency virus-1 infections: A multicenter study in The Netherlands. J Pediatr 2000;136:780-8)

<u>Zidovudine</u>

Usual Dosage: Premature Infants: (Standard neonatal dose may be excessive in premature infants) Under investigation in PACTG 331: Oral: 1.5 mg/kg/dose every 12 hours from birth to 2 weeks of age; then increase to 2 mg/kg/dose every 8 hours after 2 weeks of age

Neonates:
Oral: 2 mg/kg/dose every 6 hours
I.V.: 1.5 mg/kg/dose every 6 hours

Administration: Oral: May administer with food (although the manufacturer recommends administration 30 minutes before or 1 hour after a meal with a glass of water); the patient should be in an upright position while taking zidovudine capsules to minimize the risk of esophageal ulceration

Monitoring Parameters:
CBC with differential, hemoglobin, MCV, reticulocyte count, serum creatine kinase, CD4 cell count, HIV RNA plasma levels, renal and hepatic function tests

Patient Information: Take zidovudine exactly as prescribed

Additional Information:
Conversion from oral to I.V. dose: I.V. dose = 2/3 of the oral dose

(Takemoto: Pediatric Dosage Handbook 1999-2000, pp.944-946)

<u>Zidovudine</u> (Retrovir, AZT)

Dose & Route: Prevention of vertical transmission:
14-34 weeks of pregnancy:
Until labor: 100 mg PO 5 x/24 hr or 600 mg/24 hr PO ÷ BID-TID
During labor: 2 mg/kg/dose IV over 1 hour followed by 1 mg/kg/hr IV infusion until umbilical cord clamped.

Neonate: 2 mg/kg/dose Q6 hr PO or 1.5 mg/kg/dose Q6 hr IV over 60 min. Begin within 12 hr of birth and continue until 6 wk of age.

Premature Infant (investigational dose from ACTG 331): 1.5 mg/kg/dose IV/PO Q12 hr from birth to 2 weeks of age; then increase to 2 mg/kg/dose IV/PO Q8 hr thereafter.

Needle stick prophylaxis: 200 mg/dose PO TID or 300 mg/dose PO BID x 28 days. Use in combination with lamivudine 150 mg/dose PO BID, and indinavir 800 mg/dose PO TID x 28 days.

(Siberry: The Harriet Lane Handbook 2000, p.889)

ZINC SULFATE (also as Chloride)

Supplied: 1mg/mL, 5mg/mL as sulfate
1mg/mL as chloride

Administration: Supplement to IV solutions given for TPN

Zinc sulfate

Route: IV

Neonatal Dose: Maintenance dose for parenteral nutrition:
Preterm: (<1500-3000 g): 300 μg/kg/24 h as a continuous infusion in parenteral nutrition solution

Full-term: 100 μg/kg/24 h as a continuous infusion in parenteral nutrition solution

Pediatric Dose: Maintenance dose for parenteral nutrition: <5 y: 100 μg/kg/24 h as a continuous infusion in parenteral nutrition solution

Route: PO

Neonatal Dose: Not recommended

Pediatric Dose: Deficiency: 0.3 mg/kg/24 h (usually 3 mg given)

Discussion: Administer additional parenteral nutrition for increased amounts of small bowel fluid loss

(Rudolph: Rudolph's Pediatrics 1996, p.2209)

Zinc Sulfate

Indication: Suspected zinc deficiency

Dose: Mild def: 1 to 2 mg/kg/day of zinc. One milligram of the zinc ion (ZN^{++}) is equivalent to 4.5 mg zinc sulfate ($ZnSO_4$)

Severe def: 2 to 4 mg/kg/day

Comment: Zinc supplements can be discontinued when other zinc-containing foods are introduced into the diet. In treatment of classic acrodermatitis enteropathica, permanent zinc therapy is necessary to achieve and maintain a complete clinical remission. Doses of 20 to 30 mg zinc are likely to be needed in infants.

(Hay: Neonatal Nutrition and Metabolism 1991, pp.213-214)

SEE ALSO: TRACE MINERALS

TABLES and GUIDELINES

Congenital Toxoplasma Infection

Therapy for Neonatal Seizures

Medications for Neonatal Resuscitation

Drug Dilution Guidelines

Blood Level Sampling Time Guidelines

CONGENITAL *TOXOPLASMA* INFECTION

Congenital *Toxoplasma* infection in the infant [d]

Medication	Dosage	Duration of Therapy
Pyrimethamine [d] plus	Loading dose: 2 mg/kg per day for 2 days, then 1 mg/kg per day for 2 or 6 mo, [e] then this dose every Monday, Wednesday, Friday [d]	1yr [f]
Sulfadiazine [d] plus	100 mg/kg per day in two divided doses	1 yr [f]
Leucovorin [d] plus	10 mg three times weekly [c]	During and for 1 wk after pyrimethamine therapy
Corticosteroids [g] (prednisone) have been used when cerebrospinal fluid protein is ≥ 1 g/dl and when active chorioretinitis threatens vision	B = 1 mg/kg per day in two divided doses	C = Until resolution of elevated (≥ 1 g/dl) cerebrospinal fluid protein level or active chorioretinitis that threatens vision.

c Adjusted for megaloblastic anemia, granulocytopenia, or thrombocytopenia; blood cell counts, including platelets, should be monitored as describe in text.

d Optimal dosage, feasibility, and toxicity currently being evaluated or planned in ongoing Chicago-based National Collaborative Treatment Trial, telephone number 773-834-4152

e These two regimens are currently being compared in a randomized manner in the National Collaborative Treatment Trial. Data are not yet to determine which, if either, is superior. Both regimens appear to be feasible and relatively safe.

f The duration of therapy is unknown for infants and children, especially those with AIDS. See discussion in the Congential Taxoplasma Infection and AIDS section.

g Corticosteroids should be used only in conjunction with pyrimethamine, sulfadiazine, and leucovorin treatment and should be continued until signs of inflammation (high cerebrospinal fluid protein > 1 g/dl) or active chorioretinitis that threatens vision have subsided-dosage can then be tapered and discontinued; use only with pyrimethamine, sulfadiazine, and leucovorin.

(Remington: Infectious Diseases of the Fetus and Newborn Infant 2001 pp.292-293)

Infection: Toxoplasmosis (Toxoplasma gondii)[87] Drug of choice[88]

Drug	Pediatric Dosage
Pyrimethamine [89]	2 mg/kg/d x 3d, then 1 mg/kg/d (max. 25 mg/d) x 4 wks
plus	
Sulfadiazine	100-200 mg/kg/d x 3-4 wks
Spiramycin	50-100 mg/kg/d x 3-4 wks

87. In ocular toxoplasmosis with macular involvement, corticosteroids are recommended for an anti-inflammatory effect on the eyes.

88. To treat CNS toxoplasmosis in HIV-infected patients, some clinicians have used pyrimethamine 50 to 100 mg daily (after a loading dose of 200 mg) with a sulfonamide and, when sulfonamide sensitivity developed, have given clindamycin 1.8 to 2.4 g/d in divided doses instead of the sulfonamide (JS Remington et al, Lancet, 338:1142, 1991; BJ Luft et al, N Engl J Med, 329:995, 1993). Atovaquone plus pyrimethamine appears to be an effective alternative in sulfa-intolerant patients (JA Kovacs et al, Lancet, 340:637, 1992). Treatment is followed by chronic suppression with lower dosage regimens of the same drugs. For primary prophylaxis in HIV patients with <100 CD4 cells, either trimethoprim-sulfamethoxazole, pyrimethamine with dapsone or atovaquone with or without pyrimethamine can be used (USPHS/IDSA, MMWR, Morbid Mortal Weekly Report, 48, RR-10:41, 1999).

89. Plus leucovorin 10 to 25 mg with each dose of pyrimethamine.

(American Academy of Pediatrics: Report of the committee on Infectious Diseases. Red Book 2000, p.715)

THERAPY OF NEONATAL SEIZURES

Acute Therapy of Neonatal Seizures
HYPOGLYCEMIA Glucose, 10% solution: 2 ml/kg, IV
NO HYPOGLYCEMIA Phenobarbital: 20 mg/kg, IV If necessary: additional phenobarbital: 5 mg/kg IV to a maximum of 20 mg/kg (consider omission of this additional phenobarbital if infant is severely "asphyxiated") phenytoin*: 20 mg/kg, IV (1mg/kg/min) lorazepam: 0.05-0.10 mg/kg, IV
OTHER (AS INDICATED) Calcium gluconate, 5% solution: 4 ml/kg, IV Magnesium sulfate, 50% solution: 0.2 ml/kg, IM Pyridoxine: 50-100 mg, IV

IM, Intramuscularly; IV, intravenously
*Fosphenytoin may be a preferred form of phenytoin (see text).

Maintenance therapy:

For *maintenance* of anticonvulsant action, I utilize phenobarbital in a dose of 3 to 4 mg/kg/day (Table). If phenytoin is also needed for the acute episode, this drug is also used for maintenance, initially in a similar dose (Table). The maintenance doses are begun 12 hours following administration of the loading dose and given in divided doses every 12 hours. Intravenous, intramuscular, or oral administration is adequate for phenobarbital, although the parenteral routes should be used in the seriously ill infant. Only intravenous therapy should be utilized for phenytoin; intramuscular administration is associated with erratic absorption (because of precipitation of the drug) and possible muscle necrosis.

Fosphenytoin can be administered intramuscularly effectively. Oral administration of phenytoin is less desirable than intravenous, although pharmacokinetic data have corrected the prior notion that phenytoin absorption is poor in the newborn.

Drug accumulation results within 5 to 10 days when maintenance doses of *phenobarbital* of 5 mg/kg/day are utilized. This effect may depress the infant significantly and relates to relatively slow elimination rates in the first 1 to 2 weeks of therapy. These rates are particularly slow in some asphyxiated infants, presumably secondary to hepatic involvement, renal involvement, or both, and lead more readily to drug accumulation than in nonasphyxiated infants. It is for this reason that administration of less than a maximal loading dose (40 mg/kg) of phenobarbital to the asphyxiated newborn with seizures before adding phenytoin is an appropriate alternative (see earlier discussion). However, elimination rates do increase with increasing duration of therapy, and dose requirements may increase.

Maintenance administration of *phenytoin* in the newborn is particularly difficult because of its nonlinear kinetics and rapid decrease in elimination rates in the first weeks of life. Thus the apparent half-life of the drug decreases from 57 hours in the first week of life to 20 hours in the fourth weeks. Careful attention to blood levels is particularly necessary when this drug is utilized for maintenance. Similar concern is appropriate if fosphenytoin is utilized for maintenance.

Two reports suggest that carbamazepine may be a useful alternative to phenobarbital or phenytoin in maintenance therapy. Oral doses of 10 to 15 mg/kg/day have been associated with good seizure control. More data are needed.

Overly vigorous maintenance therapy can cause as many problems as under treatment and must be avoided . Correlation of clinical, EEG, and blood level determinations are necessary for rational therapy of the newborn with seizures.

Maintenance Therapy of Neonatal Seizures
Glucose: as high as 8 mg/kg/min, IV
Phenobarbital: 3-4 mh/kg/24 hr [sic], IV, IM, or PO
Phenytoin: 3-4 mg/kg/24 hr, IV
Calcium gluconate: 500 mg/kg/24 hr, PO
Magnesium sulfate (50%): 0.2 ml/kg/24 hr, IM

IM, Intramuscularly; IV, intravenously, PO, by mouth

(Volpe: Neurology of the Newborn 2001, pp.203,206,207)

MEDICATIONS FOR NEONATAL RESUSCITATION

Medication	Concentration to Administer	Preparation	Dosage/ Route**	Rate/ Precautions
Epinephrine	1:10,000	1:10,000 solution in 1 mL syringe	0.01– 0.03 mg/kg (0.1– 0.3 mL/kg) ET or IV	Give rapidly Flush catheter / ET tube with 0.5 – 1 mL normal saline
Volume expanders	Normal saline (recommended) Ringer's Lactate O negative blood	Estimated volume drawn into large syringe(s)	10 mL/kg IV (Umbilical vein)	Give over 5 – 10 minutes
Sodium Bicarbonate	0.5 mEq/mL (4.2% solution)	Estimated volume drawn into prefilled or prepared syringe(s)	2 mEq/kg (4 mL/kg) IV only (Umbilical vein)	Give slowly, over at least 2 minutes (1 mEq/kg/mim) Give only if newborn is being effectively ventilated

Postresuscitation medications (including post delivery room):

- Naloxone hydrochloride . . . . 0.1 mg/kg; give rapidly; IV or ET (preferred); IM, SQ (acceptable)
  (for narcotic-induced respiratory depression)
- Glucose / D10W . . . . 2 mL/kg (200 mg/kg) IV over 1-2 minutes; followed by continuous IV glucose infusion
  (for hypoglycemia)
- Phenobarbital (for seizures) . . . . 20 mg/kg slow IV push (1 mg/kg/min); may depress respiratory effort
- Dopamine (for hypotension) . . . . 2 – 20 mcg/kg/min by continuous IV infusion

Drip Calculation: $\frac{6 \text{ X Wt (kg) X desired mcg/kg/min}}{\text{desired mL/hr}}$ = mg in 100 mL D5W

**IM – Intramuscular; ET – Endotracheal; IV – Intravenous; SQ – Subcutaneous
(American Academy of Pediatrics and American Heart Association, NRP 2000)

DRUG DILUTION GUIDELINES

Drug	Available Concentration	Infusion solution	Dilution Instructions	Final Concentration	IV Push max conc @ max rate	Intermittent infusion Max conc @ max rate	Comments	Reference
Acetazolamide	500 mg powder	sterile water	Add at least 5 ml sterile water	100 mg/ml	100 mg/ml at 100 mg/min	Not recommended	Direct IV injection is preferred, IM is painful and not recommended	1
Acyclovir	25 mg/ml solution	D5W, NS	Dilute to final conc of 7mg/ml or less	7mg/ml or less	Not recommended	Infuse over at least 1 hour	Avoid rapid administration	1, 10
Adenosine	3 mg/ml	NS	Dilute 1 ml with 5 ml diluent	0.5 mg/ml	Rapid IV Push (over 1-2 seconds)	Not recommended	Administered in injection site as close as possible to patient. Flush with NS immediately after administration	1, Manufacturer
Albumin	5%	none			Undiluted at 2-4 ml/min			1
Albumin	25%	none			Undiluted at 1ml/min		A 5% soln may be prepared from the 25% product by adding 1 volume of 25% albumin to 4 volumes of an infusion solution such as D5W or NS.	1

Drug	Available Concentration	Infusion solution	Dilution Instructions	Final Concentration	IV Push max conc @ max rate	Intermittent infusion Max conc @ max rate	Comments	Reference
Allopurinol	500 mg powder	D5W, NS	Reconstitute vial with 25 ml sterile water. Dilute further to 6mg/ml or less.	6 mg/ml or less	Not recommended			Manufacturer
Amikacin	50 mg/ml, 250 mg/ml	D5W, NS	Dilute to final conc of 2.5 - 5 mg/ml	2.5 mg to 5 mg/ml	Not recommended	Infuse over 30-60 minutes		1
Aminophylline	25 mg/ml	D5W, NS	Dilute to 1-25 mg/ml	1-25 mg/ml	0.36 mg/kg/min and no greater than 20 mg/minute	Infuse over 20-30 minutes		1, 10
Amiodarone	50 mg/ml	D5W,NS	Dilute to 1-6 mg/ml	1-6 mg/ml	Not recommended	Continuous infusion	May precipitate, inline filter recommended. Conc <0.6 mg/ml unstable. Increase phlebitis may occur with peripheral solutions of >3 mg/ml in D5W.	1, 10
Amphotericin B Lidid Complex (Abelcet)	5 mg/ml	D5W only	Dilute with D5W to 1-2 mg/ml	1-2 mg/ml	Not recommended	1-2 mg/ml at 2.5 mg/kg/hr	If infusion exceeds 2 hours, shake IV bag to mix contents.	Manufacturer
Amphotericin B Deoxycholate (Fungizone)	powder	D5W only	Dilute 50 mg vial with 10 ml Sterile water without preservatives.	5 mg/ml	Not recommended	0.1 mg/ml over 4 - 6 hours	Dilute reconstituted drug further with D5W only.	1

DRUG DILUTION GUIDELINES

Drug	Available Concentration	Infusion solution	Dilution Instructions	Final Concentration	IV Push max conc @ max rate	Intermittent infusion Max conc @ max rate	Comments	Reference
Amphotericin B Lyposomal (AmBisone)	50 mg powder	D5W cnly	Reconstitute with sterile water, further dilute with D5W only.	1-2 mg/ml	Not recommended	Infuse over 2 hours; may be reduced to 60 minutes if well tolerated.	Final concentration of 0.2-0.5 mg/ml may be appropriate for infants and small children to provide sufficient volume for infusion. Use within 6 hours after dilution	Manufacturer
Ampicillin	125 mg, 250 mg, 500 mg, 1 gram, 2 grams powder	D5W, NS	See Manufacturer's recommendation	100 mg/ml or less	100 mg/ml over 3-5 minutes	30 mg/ml over 10-15 minutes	More stable in NS, rapidly degrades in D5W.	1
Ampicillin/ Sulbactam (Unasyn)	Powder, 1.5 gm vial (1gm ampicillin +0.5gm sulbactam)	D5W,NS	Add 3.2 ml sterile water to make 250 mg/ml of ampicillin. Dilute further to 2-30 mg/ml	2-30 mg/ml	30 mg/ml over 10-15 minutes	30 mg/ml over 15-30 minutes		1
Amrinone	5 mg/ml of base	0.45NS, NS	Dilute to 1 to 3 mg/ml	1-3 mg/ml	3 mg/ml over 2 -3minutes	1-3 mg/ml as continuous infusion	Unstable in D5W. Use controlled infusion device.	1
Atropine	0.5 mg/ml, 1 mg/ml			0.5-1 mg/ml	Undiluted over 1 min	Not recommended		1

Drug	Available Concentration	Infusion solution	Dilution Instructions	Final Concentration	IV Push max conc @ max rate	Intermittent infusion Max conc @ max rate	Comments	Reference
Aztreonam	500 mg, 1 gram	D5W, NS	Reconstitute with 6-10 ml sterile water	50-83 mg/ml	66 mg/ml over 2-3 minutes	20 mg/ml over 30-60 minutes	Reconstitute with 6-10 ml of sterile water.	1
Bretylium	50 mg/ml	D5W, NS	Dilute to 2-4 mg/ml		Undiluted IV push over <30 seconds	Dilute to 10 mg/ml; administer slow IV push over at least 8-10 minutes (for non-life threatening situations).		1, 10
Calcium Chloride 10%	100 mg/ml (1.4 mEq Ca++/ml)	D5W, NS	Can be given undiluted, or diluted to a convenient volume	20-100 mg/ml	50-100 mg/min	Dilute to convenient volume over 30-60 minutes at no greater than 45-90 mg/kg/hour.	Severe necrosis and sloughing may result if injected into perivascular tissue. Do not use scalp veins or small veins in hand or foot.	1, 10
Calcium Gluconate 10%	93-96 mg/ml (0.465 mEq Ca/ml)	D5W,NS	Can be given undiluted, or diluted to a convenient volume.	20-96 mg/ml	1.5 - 2 ml/min	Dilute to 50 mg/ml; infuse over 1 hour or no greater than 120-240 mg/kg/hour.	Tissue irritation and necrosis may occur from extravasation, especially in infants and children.	1, 10
Cefazolin	500 mg, 1gram powder	D5W, NS	Add 5 ml sterile water to 500 mg vial, or 10 ml sterile water to 1 gram vial.	100 mg/ml	100 mg/ml over 3 – 5 minutes	20 mg/ml over 20-30 minutes		1, 73

DRUG DILUTION GUIDELINES

Drug	Available Concentration	Infusion solution	Dilution Instructions	Final Concentration	IV Push max conc @ max rate	Intermittent infusion Max conc @ max rate	Comments	Reference
Cefotaxime	500 mg, 1 gram powder	D5W, NS	Dissolve with 10 ml sterile water	50 mg/ml, 95 mg/ml respectively	95 mg/ml over 3-5 minutes	10-40 mg/ml over 20-30 minutes		1
Cefotetan	1gram, 2 gram powder	D5W, NS	Dissolve with 10 ml sterile water	95 mg/ml, 182 mg/ml respectively	95 mg/ml over 3-5 minutes	10-40 mg/ml over 20-30 minutes		1
Cefoxitin	1gram, 2 gram powder	D5W, NS	Dissolve with 10 ml sterile water	95 mg/ml, 180 mg/ml respectively	95 mg/ml over 3-5 minutes	10-40 mg/ml over 20-30 minutes		1
Ceftazidime	500 mg, 1 gram powder	D5W, NS	Dissolve 500 mg vial with 1.5 ml sterile water; 1 gram vial with 3 ml sterile water. Dilute further to 100 mg/ml	280 mg/ml	70-100 mg/ml over 3-5 minutes	10-40 mg/ml over 15-30 minutes	Dilute further to 100 mg/ml. Carbon dioxide is formed during dissolution. Use of a vented needle reduces spraying or leaking of the solution.	1
Ceftriaxone	250 mg, 500 mg powder	D5W, NS	Dissolve 250 mg vial with 2.4 ml sterile water, 500 mg vial with 4.8ml sterile water.	100 mg/ml	Not recommended	10 - 40 mg/ml over 10-30 minutes		1
Cefuroxime	750 mg, 1.5 gram powder	D5W NS	Dissolve 750mg vial with 8 ml sterile water; 1.5 gram vial with 16 ml sterile water	90 mg/ml	76 mg/ml over 3-5 minutes	15-30 mg/ml over 15-60 minutes		1

Drug	Available Concentration	Infusion solution	Dilution Instructions	Final Concentration	IV Push max conc @ max rate	Intermittent infusion Max conc @ max rate	Comments	Reference
Chloramphenicol	1 gram powder	D5W, NS	Dissolve with 10 ml sterile water	100 mg/ml	100 mg/ml at > 1 minute	20 mg/ml over 30-60 minutes		1
Cimetidine	150 mg/ml	D5W, NS	Dilute to 6-15 mg/ml	6-15 mg/ml	15 mg/ml over 5 minutes	6 mg/ml over 15-20 minutes		1
Clindamycin	150 mg/ml	D5W, NS	Dilute to18 mg/ml or less	18 mg/ml or less	Not recommended	18 mg/ml over 10-60 minutes	Do not exceed rate of 30 mg/min.	1
Dexamethasone	4 mg/ml	D5W, NS		4 mg/ml	4 mg/ml over 1-5 minutes	Dilute to convenient volume, over 10-20 minutes		1
Dextrose 50%	50% (500 mg/ml)		Dilute 1:1 with sterile water	25%	over 5-10 minutes	Not recommended		
Diazepam	5 mg/ml		undiluted	5 mg/ml	2 -5 mg/min	Not recommended		1
Diazoxide	15 mg/ml		undiluted	15 mg/ml	over 30 seconds or less			10
Digoxin	100 mcg/ml	D5W, NS	Dilute 4 fold or greater volume, can be given undiluted	25 mcg/ml - 100 mcg/ml	100 mcg/ml (undiluted) over 1-5 minutes	25 mcg/ml over 5-10 minutes	Dilution to a more concentrated solution than this fourfold volume of dilution may lead to precipitation of digoxin.	1

DRUG DILUTION GUIDELINES

Drug	Available Concentration	Infusion solution	Dilution Instructions	Final Concentration	IV Push max conc @ max rate	Intermittent infusion Max conc @ max rate	Comments	Reference
Diltiazem	5 mg/ml	D5W, NS	Dilute to final conc of 0.45-1 mg/ml	1 mg/ml	1 mg/ml over 2 minutes	1 mg/ml as continuous infusion		1
Diphenhydramine	50 mg/ml	D5W,NS	Dilute to convenient volume	10-50 mg/ml	50 mg/ml over 5 minutes	10-50 mg/ml over 15-20 minutes		1
Dobutamine	12.5 mg/ml, 5 mg/ml concentrate	D5W,NS	Dilute to 250 -6000 mcg/ml		Not recommended	Continuous infusion, concentration dependent on pt's fluid restrictions	Administer with pump or infusion device. Administer into large vein.	1
Dopamine	40 mg/ml, 80 mg/ml	D5W, NS	Dilute to convenient volume up to max conc 3200 mcg/ml	1600-3200 mcg/ml	Not recommended	Continuous infusion concentration dependent on pt's fluid restrictions	Administer with pump or infusion device. Infiltrates may cause tissue necrosis.	1
Doxapram	20 mg/ml	D5W,NS	Dilute to 1-2 mg/ml	1-2 mg/ml	Not recommended	Infuse over 15-30 minutes.		1,
Enalapril	1.25 mg/ml	D5W,NS	Undiluted, or diluted to convenient volume	1.25 mg/ml or less	1.25 mg/ml over 5 minutes			1
Epinephrine	1:10,000 (0.1 mg/ml)	D5W,NS	Undiluted	1mg/10 ml	Bolus over 3-5 seconds		For resuscitation use.	

Drug	Available Concentration	Infusion solution	Dilution Instructions	Final Concentration	IV Push max conc @ max rate	Intermittent infusion Max conc @ max rate	Comments	Reference
Epinephrine	1:1000 (1mg/ml)	D5W,NS	Dilute to convenient volume			Constant infusion, final conc based on fluid needs of pt.		
Erythromcyin Lactobionate	500 mg, 1 gram powder	NS	Reconstitute with sterile water, further dilute to 1mg/ml-5 mg/ml	1mg/ml – 5 mg/ml	Not recommended	Infuse over 20-60 minutes	To minimize venous irritation, use the most dilute solution as possible, 1-2.5 mg/ml or less.	
Ethacrynate Na	50 mg powder	D5W,NS	Reconstitute with D5W or NS to make 1 mg/ml	1 mg/ml	1 mg/ml over 5-10 minutes	<1 mg/ml over 20-30 minutes	Discard unused vial after 24hrs	1
Fentanyl	50 mcg/ml	D5W, NS	Dilute to 5-40 mcg/ml	5-40 mcg/ml	Undiluted over 1-2 minutes	Not recommended	Can be given as continuous infusion.	1
Fluconazole	2 mg/ml	D5W, LR	Undilute, or dilute to convenient volume	2 mg/ml or less	Not recommended	Do not exceed 3.3 mg/min (200mg/hr)		1
Flumazenil	0.1 mg/ml	D5W, NS,LR	Undiluted	0.1 mg/ml	Over 15-30 seconds	Not recommended	Avoid Extravasation	1
Furosemide	10 mg/ml	D5W, NS, RL	Undiluted, or diluted to convenient volume	10 mg/ml or less	Over 1-2 minutes, not exceeding 4 mg/min	Dilute to convenient volume, over 20 minutes, not exceeding 4 mg/min	Avoid mixing with acidic drugs or solutions. Precipitation may result.	1

DRUG DILUTION GUIDELINES

Drug	Available Concentration	Infusion solution	Dilution Instructions	Final Concentration	IV Push max conc @ max rate	Intermittent infusion Max conc @ max rate	Comments	Reference
Gentamicin	10 mg/ml, 40 mg/ml	D5W, NS	Dilute to 1-2 mg/ml	1-2 mg/ml or less	Not recommended	Infuse over 30 minutes	Administer penicillin-like or cephalosporin-like drugs at least 1 hour before or 1 hour after aminoglycosides.	1
Glucagon (rDNS origin)	1 mg powder		Reconstitute with 1ml sterile water	1 mg/ml (do not use solution with conc >1mg/ml)	Undiluted over 1 minute	Not recommended	1 unit = 1 mg, use immediately after reconstituting. (Usual route is IM).	Manufacturer
Hydralazine	20 mg/ml	NS, LR, D5W	Undiluted	20 mg/ml	Undiluted over 1-2 minutes Do not exceed rate of 0.2 mg/kg/minute	Not recommended	The manufacturer (Solopak) does not recommend admixture in IV infusion solutions.	Manufacturer
Hydrocortisone Na Succinate	100 mg powder	D5W,NS, LR	Reconstitute with 2 ml sterile water	50 mg/ml	Undiluted over 30 seconds to several minutes	0.1-1 mg/ml over 20-30 minutes		1
Imipenem-Cilastin (1:1 ratio) (Primaxin)	250 mg, 500 mg powder	NS	Reconstitute with 10 ml NS, further dilute with NS to final concentration of 2.5-5 mg/ml (Agitate final dilution until all suspension is dissolved).	2.5 mg/ml; 5 mg/ml respectively	Not recommended	≤5 mg/ml over 20-60 minutes (depending on dose).	Solution is colorless to yellow, but may become deeper yellow over time. Potency is not affected by color variations in this range. However, brown solutions should be discarded.	1

Drug	Available Concentration	Infusion solution	Dilution Instructions	Final Concentration	IV Push max conc @ max rate	Intermittent infusion Max conc @ max rate	Comments	Reference
Indomethacin I.V.	1 mg powder		Reconstitute with 1-2 ml sterile water or NS	0.5-1 mg/ml	1mg/ml over 5-10 seconds	Not recommended	Reconstitution with solutions with pH <6 may result in precipitation of free indomethacin	1
Isoproterenol 1:5000	0.2 mg/ml	D5W, NS	For direct IV injection: 1 ml of 1:5000 diluted to 10 ml with NS or D5W to provide a 20 mcg/ml soln. IV solutions are prepared by adding 1-10 ml of 1:5000 injection to 500 ml of compatible diluent.	20 mcg/ml	20 mcg/ml over 2-3 minutes	Not recommended	Also given as continuous infusion at a concentration of 4 mcg/ml in D5W or NS. Maximum concentration for continuous infusion is 20 mcg/ml.	1, 10
Kanamycin	37.5 mg/ml, 250 mg/ml, 333 mg/ml	D5W, NS, LR	Dilute to 5 mg/ml for peripheral use, 6 mg/ml for central use.	5-6 mg/ml	Not recommended	Infuse over 30-60 minutes		1, 6
Ketamine	10 mg/ml, 50 mg/ml, 100 mg/ml	D5W, NS	10 mg/ml or 50 mg/ml may be given undiluted. Dilute 100 mg/ml with equal volume of sterile water, D5W, or NS.	10-50 mg/ml	Infuse over 60 seconds.	Not recommended	For IV infusion, a 1-2 mg/ml solution may be prepared in D5W or NS.	1

DRUG DILUTION GUIDELINES

Drug	Available Concentration	Infusion solution	Dilution Instructions	Final Concentration	IV Push max conc @ max rate	Intermittent infusion Max conc @ max rate	Comments	Reference
Lebetalol	5 mg/ml	D5W, NS, LR	Dilute with D5W or NS to 1 mg/ml	1 mg/ml	5 mg/ml over 2-3 minutes at max rate of 2 mg/min		Undiluted Lebetalol has been administered to a very small number of adult patients who were extremely fluid restricted.	1, 10
Levothyroxine	200 mcg, 500 mcg powder	NS	Reconstitute with 5 ml NS only	40 mcg/ml, 100 mcg/ml respectively	over 2-3 minutes	Not recommended	Use immediately after reconstitution. Do not add to other IV fluid.	Manufacturer
Lidocaine	10 mg/ml, 20 mg/ml ampules	Premixed bags of 2, 4, and 8 mg/ml in D5W	10-20 mg/ml undiluted, higher concentrations must be diluted prior to administration.		10-20 mg/ml at a rate not exceeding 0.7 mg/kg/min or 50 mg/min, whichever is less.	Not recommended	Products containing epinephrine should not be used to treat arrhythmias.	1, 10
Lorazepam	2 mg/ml		Dilute 1:1 with NS immediately prior to use.	1 mg/ml	1 mg/ml over 2 minutes not exceeding 2 mg/minute	Not recommended		1
Magnesium Sulfate 50%	500 mg/ml	D5W, NS	Dilute to convenient volume to 200 mg/ml or less	200 mg/ml or less	Over 3-5 minutes. Do not exceed 150 mg/min	20 mg/ml over 30-60 minutes, max infusion rate = 125 mg/kg/hr	Beware of hypotension, respiratory depression, or complete heart block. Calcium gluconate IV should be available as antidote.	1, 10, 155

Drug	Available Concentration	Infusion solution	Dilution Instructions	Final Concentration	IV Push max conc @ max rate	Intermittent infusion Max conc @ max rate	Comments	Reference
Mannitol	20%, 25%			200 mg/ml, 250 mg/ml respectively		Undiluted over 30-60 minutes	Use a 5 micron filter for solutions ≥20%. Do not use a mannitol solution containing crystals.	1
Meropenem	500mg, 1gram powder	NS, D5W	Reconstitute 500 mg vial with 10ml and 1 gram vial with 20ml sterile water.	50 mg/ml	May dilute to 5-20 ml. Over 3-5 minutes.	1- 20 mg/ml. Infuse over 15-30 minutes	Use immediately after reconstitution.	1
Methyldopate	50 mg/ml	D5W, NS, LR	Dilute to 10 mg/ml or less	10 mg/ml or less	Not recommended	Infuse slowly over 30-60 minutes		1
Methyl-prednisolone	40 mg/ml	D5W, NS		40 mg/ml	Undiluted over 1-5 minutes	5 mg/ml over 20-30 minutes		1
Metoclopramide	5 mg/ml	D5W, NS		5 mg/ml or less	Undiluted over 1-2 minutes	Dilute to convenient volume, infuse over 15 minutes		1
Metronidazole (RTU)	5 mg/ml	RTU = Ready to Use	None	5 mg/ml	Not recommended	Infuse over 60 minutes	It is recommend to stop the primary IV infusion solution during administration.	1
Mezlocillin	1, 2, 3, 4 gram powder	D5W, NS	Reconstitute with 10 ml sterile water for each gram of mezlocillin.	100 mg/ml	Undiluted over 3-5 minutes	10-20 mg/ml over 15-30 minutes		1, 10

DRUG DILUTION GUIDELINES

Drug	Available Concentration	Infusion solution	Dilution Instructions	Final Concentration	IV Push max conc @ max rate	Intermittent infusion Max conc @ max rate	Comments	Reference
Midazolam	5 mg/ml	D5W, NS	Dilute to 1 mg/ml for more accurate dose titration		1 mg/ml over 2-5 minutes		Also given as continuous infusion.	1, 10
Milrinone	1 mg/ml	D5W, NS	Dilute to 100, 150, or 200 mcg/ml	100, 150, or 200 mcg/ml	Undiluted or dilute to 10-20 ml, infuse over 10 minutes.		Dilute to 100,150, or 200 mcg/ml and give as continuous infusion	1
Morphine	1 mg/ml, 10 mg/ml, 15 mg/ml, others	D5W, NS	Dilute to convenient volume	0.1 - 1 mg/ml	Slowly over 3 - 5 minutes	0.1-1 mg/ml for continuous infusion.	Neonates and infants <3 mos of age are more susceptible to respiratory depression, use with caution and at reduced doses in this age group. Use infusion control device for continuous infusion.	1, 10
Naloxone	0.4 mg/ml, 1 mg/ml	D5W, NS	Dilute to convenient volume	4 mcg/ml	Undiluted over 30 seconds		As continuous infusion diluted to 4 mcg/ml.	1, 10
Nafcillin	500 mg, 1gram, 2 gram powder	D5W, NS	Dilute to 250 mg/ml with sterile water or NS, dilute further to 66 mg/ml	66 mg/ml	66 mg/ml over 5-10 minutes into tubing of running IV solution	2-40 mg/ml over 30-60 minutes	Elimination will be decreased in the neonate; avoid using in during the first 2 weeks of life. Avoid extravasation.	1, 10

Drug	Available Concentration	Infusion solution	Dilution Instructions	Final Concentration	IV Push max conc @ max rate	Intermittent infusion Max conc @ max rate	Comments	Reference
Nitroglycerin	0.5 - 5 mg/ml	Must be diluted before use. Dilute with D5W or NS in glass bottles to convenient volume.	Dilute to 50-100 mcg/ml. The concentration should not exceed 400 mcg/ml	50 - 400 mcg/ml	Not recommended	Not recommended	Administer as continuous infusion using NTG approved tubing.	1
Nitroprusside	10 mg/ml, 25 mg/ml	D5W only		200 mcg/ml (1000 mcg/ml has been use in fluid restricted patients)	Not recommended	Not recommended	As continuous infusion only with controlled infusion device. Do not mix with other medications or solutions.	10
Norepinephrine	1 mg/ml	D5W, NS	Standard dilution: 4 mg/D5W 500ml, but 8 mg/500 ml has been used.	8 mcg/ml - 16 mcg/ml	Not recommended	Not recommended	As continuous infusion with a controlled infusion device. Administer into large vein to avoid potential extravasation.	1, 10
Octreotide	0.05, 0.1, 0.2, 0.5, 1 mg/ml	D5W , NS		Dilute to convenient volume, over 3 minutes	Over 3 minutes	Dilute to convenient volume with NS or D5W, infuse over 15-30 minutes		1

DRUG DILUTION GUIDELINES

Drug	Available Concentration	Infusion solution	Dilution Instructions	Final Concentration	IV Push max conc @ max rate	Intermittent infusion Max conc @ max rate	Comments	Reference
Ondansetron	2 mg/ml	D5W, NS		2 mg/ml or less	Undiluted over 2-5 minutes	Infuse over 15 minutes		1
Oxacillin	250 mg, 500 mg, 1gram, 2 gram powder	D5W, NS	See Manufacturer's recommendation for reconstitution instructions.	0.5-40 mg/ml	100 mg/ml over 10 minutes	Dilute further to final concentration of 0.5-40 mg/ml infuse over 15-30 minutes.		1
Penicillin G (Na, K)	1, 5, 20 million units, powder (various)	D5W, NS	See Manufacturer's recommendation for reconstitution instructions.		Not recommended	50,000 units/ml over 15-30 minutes		1
Phenobarbital	D5W, NS		Dilute to convenient volume		Undiluted no faster than 1 mg/kg/min with max of 30 mg/min	Dilute in equal volume, infuse over 20 minutes.	Do not administer intra-arterially, avoid extravasation	1, 10
Phenytoin	50 mg/ml	NS only	Dilute to <6 mg/ml with NS	<6 mg/ml	Undiluted at 1-3 mg/kg/min, max of 50 mg/min	Dilute to <6 mg/ml, over 30 minutes	Use in-line filter; afterwards flush tubing with NS to avoid local irritation.	1, 10

Drug	Available Concentration	Infusion solution	Dilution Instructions	Final Concentration	IV Push max conc @ max rate	Intermittent infusion Max conc @ max rate	Comments	Reference
Phytonadione	1 mg/0.5 m , 10 mg/ml	D5W, NS	Dilute in 5-10 ml of D5W or NS	0.1-1 mg/ml		Infuse over 15-30 minutes; maximum rate of infusion = 1 mg/minute	IM or SC routes are preferred.	1, 10
Piperacillin	2 gram, 3 gram, 4 gram powder	D5W, NS, LR	Reconstitute each gram with 5 ml sterile water to make 200 mg/ml.	200 mg/ml	200 mg/ml over 3-5 minutes	Dilute to 80 mg/ml or less, infuse over 20-30 minutes.		1
Piperacillin / Tazobactam (Zosyn)	2.25 gram, 3.375 gram powder	D5W, NS	Reconstitute each gram of piperacillin with 5 ml sterile water	200 mg/ml of piperacillin	Not recommended	Dilute to 80 mg/ml or less, infuse over 30 minutes.	Concentration of 20 mcg/ml or less is preferred for intermittent infusion.	1, 10
Potassium Chloride	2 mEq/ml	D5W, NS	Must be diluted prior to infusion.	0.04 - 0.1 mEq/ml	Not recommended	0.5 mEq/kg over 1-2 hours.	Maximum infusion rate of 1 mEq/kg/hr in critical situations. Extreme care must be taken to avoid extravasation.	1, Harriet Lane Handbook.
Potassium Phosphate	3 mm/ml	D5W, NS	Dilute to 0.05 mm/ml or less	For peripheral line: 0.05 mm/ml or less. For central line: 0.12 mm/ml.	Not recommended	0.06 mm/kg/hr	Do not infuse with calcium containing IV solutions. 1 mm P = 31 mg P	1, 10

DRUG DILUTION GUIDELINES

Drug	Available Concentration	Infusion solution	Dilution Instructions	Final Concentration	IV Push max conc @ max rate	Intermittent infusion Max conc @ max rate	Comments	Reference
Procainamide	100 mg/ml, 500 mg/ml	NS	Dilute to 20-30 mg/ml for loading dose; dilute to 2-4 mg/ml for maintenance infusions	4-30 mg/ml	20-30 mg/min over at least 5 minutes	2-4 mg/ml over 25-30 minutes	Do not administer faster than 20-30 mg/minute; severe hypotension can occur with rapid IV administration.	1, 10
Propranolol	1 mg/ml	D5W, NS			Undiluted at 1 mg/min or less for life-threatening arrhythmias	Dilute to convenient volume and infuse over 10-15 minutes.		1, 10
Ranitidine	25 mg/ml	D5W, NS	Dilute to 2.5 mg/ml or less	2.5 mg/ml	2.5 mg/ml over 5 minutes	0.5 mg/ml over 15 - 20 minutes.		1
Rifampin	600 mg powder	D5W	Reconstitute with 10 ml sterile water to make 60 mg/ml: dilute further to 6 mg/ml or less.	6 mg/ml or less	Not recommended	Dilute to 6 mg/ml or less; infuse over 30 minutes to 3 hours.	The IV solution should be administered within 4 hours of preparation to avoid precipitation.	1, 10
Sodium Bicarbonate	0.5-1 mEq/ml	D5W, NS	Dilute to convenient volume	0.5-1 mEq/ml	Undiluted; maximum rate in neonates and infant of 10 mEq/minute.	Dilute to convenient volume and infuse over 2 hours: maximum infusion rate of 1 mEq/kg/hr	In neonates, use 0.5 mEq/ml for direct IV infusion or dilute the 1 mEq/ml solution 1:1 with sterile water.	1, 10

Drug	Available Concentration	Infusion solution	Dilution Instructions	Final Concentration	IV Push max conc @ max rate	Intermittent infusion Max conc @ max rate	Comments	Reference
Ticarcillin	1gram, 3 grams, 6 grams powder	D5W, NS	Reconstitute each gram of ticarcillin with 4 ml sterile water to make 200 mg/ml.		Dilute to 50 mg/ml or less, over 10-20 minutes	Dilute to 10-100 mg/ml; infuse over 30 -120 minutes.	Concentration of 50 mg/ml or less is preferred to avoid venous irritation.	1, 10
Ticarcillin 3grams/ Clavulanate 0.1 grams (Timentin)	3.1 grams	D5W, NS		Reconstitute powder with 13 ml sterile water to make 200 mg/ml (ticarcillin)+ 6.7mg/ml (clavulanate)	Not recommended	Dilute further to 10-100 mg/ml, infuse over 30 minutes	Solutions of 50 mg or less are recommended.	1, 10
Tobramycin	10 mg/ml, 40 mg/ml	D5W, NS	Dilute to convenient volume to achieve concentration of 10 mg/ml or less	10 mg/ml or less	Not recommended	Infuse over 20-60 minutes	Concentrations of 1-2 mg/ml are preferred. Administer penicillin-like or cephalosporin-like drugs at least 1 hour before or 1 hour after aminoglycosides.	1, 10
Trimethoprim/ Sulfamethoxazole (Bactrim IV, Septra IV)	Trimethoprim 16 mg/ml-Sulfamethoxazole 80mg/ml	D5W , NS	Dilute each 5ml with 75-125 ml D5W.		Not recommended	Infuse over 60-90 minutes		1

DRUG DILUTION GUIDELINES

Drug	Available Concentration	Infusion solution	Dilution Instructions	Final Concentration	IV Push max conc @ max rate	Intermittent infusion Max conc @ max rate	Comments	Reference
Vancomycin	500 mg, 1 gram powder	D5W, NS	Reconstitute 500mg vial with 10ml, or 1 gram vial with 20 ml of sterile water to make 50 mg/ml.	Dilute to final concentration of 2.5-10 mg/ml.	Not recommended	5-10 mg/ml, infuse over at least 1 hour.	Thrombophlebitis can be minimized by using dilute solutions of 2.5 - 5 mg ml.	1
Vecuronium	10 mg powder	D5W, NS	Reconstitute with 10 ml sterile water to make 1 mg/ml.	1 mg/ml	Rapid IV administration over 1-2 minutes	Not recommended	For continuous infusion, dilute to 0.1 - 1 mg/ml; administer with controlled delivery device.	1, 10
Verapamil	2.5 mg/ml	D5W, NS		2.5 mg/ml or less	Undiluted over 2-3 minutes.		Intravenous infusions of concentrations of 0.5 - 2.5 mg/ml have been performed.	1, 10
Zidovudine	10 mg/ml	D5W, NS	Dilute to 4 mg/ml or less.	4 mg/ml or less	Not recommended	Dilute to 4 mg/ml or less; infuse over 1 hour.	Do not give IM or by rapid IV push.	1, 10

BLOOD LEVEL SAMPLING TIME GUIDLINES

Drug	Infusion Time	Therapeutic Range	When to Draw Levels
Amikacin Sulfate I.V. I.M.	30 min	Peak: 20-30 μg/mL Trough: <10 μg/mL	Peak: 30 min after end of 30 min infusion Trough: Within 30 min before next dose Peak: 1 h after I.M. injection Trough: Within 30 min before next dose
Digoxin I.V./P.O.		Age and disease related: 0.8-2 ng/mL	6 h postdose to just before next dose
Flucytosine P.O.		25-100 μg/mL	Peak: 2 h postdose after at least 4 d of therapy
Fosphenytoin (measure phenytoin levels) I.V. I.M.		Phenytoin: 10-20 μg/mL	Peak: 2 h after end of an infusion Peak: 4 h after I.M. injection
Gentamicin I.V. I.M.	30 min	Peak: 4-10 μg/mL Trough: 0.5-2 μg/mL	Peak: 30 min after end of 30 min infusion Trough: Within 30 min before next dose Peak: 1 h after I.M. injection Trough: Within 30 min before next dose
Phenobarbital		15-40 μg/mL	Trough: just before next dose
Phenytoin P.O., I.V. I.V.		10-20 μg/mL	Trough: Just before next dose Post-load/Peak: 1 h after end of infusion
Theophylline I.V. bolus Continuous infusion	30 min	10-20 μg/mL	Peak: 30 min after end of 30 min infusion 16-24 h after the start or change in a constant I.V. infusion
Tobramycin I.V. I.M.	30 min	Peak: 4-10 μg/mL Trough: 0.5-2 μg/mL	Peak: 30 min after end of 30 min infusion Trough: Within 30 min before next dose Peak: 1 h post-I.M. injection Trough: Within 30 min before next dose
Valproic acid P.O.		50-100 μg/mL	Trough: Just before next dose
Vancomycin	60 min	Peak: 25-40 μg/mL Trough: 5-15 μg/mL	Peak: 20-30 min after end of 60 min infusion* Trough: Within 30 min before next dose

*Some institutions may draw vancomycin peak 1 hour after 1-hour infusion and accept the lower range of therapeutic.

ABBREVIATIONS

Conc	Concentration
Div	Divided
ET	Endotracheal
g, gm	Gram
H, hr	Hour
IA	Intraarterial
IC	Intracardiac
IM	Intramuscular
INJ	Injection
IT	Intratracheal
IV	Intravenous
Kg	Kilogram
Maint	Maintenance
Max	Maximum
μg, mcg	Microgram
Min	Minute
Ng	Nasogastric
OU	Each eye
p	Page
pp	Pages
PN	Parenteral Nutrition
PO	Orally
PR	Per Rectum
PRN	If needed
Q	Every
QD	Everyday
SC, SQ	Subcutaneous
[sic]	When a writer quotes information containing an error and wishes to make clear that the original was copied accurately, [sic] is inserted beside the error.
Sol, soln	Solution
Top	Topical
U	Unit
Yr	Year
>	Greater Than
<	Less Than
≥	Equal to or greater than
≤	Equal to or less than

REFERENCES

1. DRUG Facts and Comparisons 2000, Fifty-fourth Edition. Facts and Comparison, A Wolters Kluwer Comapny 1999.
2. Pagliaro LA, Pagliaro AM. Problems in Pediatric Drug Therapy. Second Edition. Drug Intelligence Publications, 1987.
3. American Hospital Formulary Service. AHFS Drug Information 2000. American Society of Hospital Pharmacists Inc, 2000.
4. Ford DC, Leist ER. Guidelines for Administration of Intravenous Medications to Pediatric Patients. Second Edition. American Society of Hospital Pharmacists, 1984.
5. Trissel LA. Handbook on Injectable Drugs. Eleventh Edition. American Society of Health-System Pharmacists, 2001.
6. Nelson JD, Bradley JS. Nelson's Pocket Book of Pediatric Antimicrobial Therapy. Fourteenth Edition. Lippincott Williams & Wilkins, 2000-2001.
7. Prober CG, Stevenson DK, Benitz WE. The use of antibiotics in neonates weighing less than 1200 grams. Pediatr Infect Dis J 1990;9:119.
8. Bhatt-Mehta V, Nahata MC. Stability of dopamine hydrochloride injection in the presence of dobutamine hydrochloride, tolazoline hydrochloride, and theophylline injections. J Perinatol 1990;10:129-133.
9. Zenk KE. Y-site compatibility of drugs used in the NICU. Neonatal Pharmacol Q 1992;1:13-22.
10. Taketomo CK, Hodding JH, Kraus DM. American Pharmaceutical Association, Pediatric Dosage Handbook 1997-1998. Fourth Edition Lexi-Comp Inc 1997
11. Nahata MC, Hipple TF. Pediatric Drug Formulations. Third Edition. Harvey Whitney Books Company 1997
12. Al-Essa MA, Rashed MS, Bakheet SM, Patay ZJ, Ozand PT. Glutaric Aciduria Type II: Observations in Seven Patients With Neonatal- and Late-Onset Disease. J Perinatol 2000;2:120-128)
13. Allen HD, Clark EB, Gutgesell HP, Driscoll DJ.: Moss and Adams' Heart Disease in Infants, Children, and Adolescents: Including the Fetus and Young Adult. Sixth Edition, Volume Two. Lippincott Williams & Wilkins, 2001.
14. American Academy of Pediatrics Committee on Fetus and Newborn: Use of Inhaled Nitric Oxide. Pediatrics 2000; 106:344-345.
15. American Academy of Pediatrics. American Heart Association. Pediatric Advanced Life Support. 1997.
16. American Academy of Pediatrics. American Heart Association: International Guidelines for Neonatal Resuscitation: An excerpt from the guidelines 2000 for cardiopulmonary resuscitation and emergency cardiovascular care: International consensus on science. Pediatrics 2000;106:1-16.

17. American Academy of Pediatrics. Policy Statement: Recommendations for the Prevention of Pneumococcal Infections, Including the Use of Pneumococcal Conjugate Vaccine (Prevnar), Pneumococcal Polysaccharide Vaccine, and Antibiotic Prophylaxis. Committee on Infectious Disease: 2000;106:362-366

18. American Academy of Pediatrics. The American College of Obstetricians and Gynecologist. Guidelines for Perinatal Care. Fourth Edition. 1997.

19. American Academy Of Pediatrics: Committee on Fetus and Newborn. Surfactant Replacement Therapy for Respiratory Distress Syndrome. Pediatrics 1999;103:684-865

20. American Academy of Pediatrics: Report of the Committee on Infectious Diseases. Red Book . Twenty-Fifth Edition. 2000.

21. American Academy Of Pediatrics: Section on Endocrinology and Committee on Genetics. Technical Report: Congenital Adrenal Hyperplasia. Pediatrics 2000;106:1511-1518.

22. American Heart Association: Part 11: Neonatal Resuscitation 2000;102:(suppl I):I-343 - I-357.

23. Avery GB, Fletcher MA, MacDonald MG. Neonatology: Pathophysiology and Management of the Newborn. Fifth Edition. Lippincott Williams & Walkins, 1999.

24. Banks B, Seri I, Ischiropoulos H, Merrill J, Rychik J, Ballard RA. Changes in Oxygenation With Inhaled Nitric Oxide in Severe Bronchopulmonary Dysplasia. Pediatrics 1999;103:610-618.

25. Baram TZ, Mitchell WG, Tournay A, Snead III OC, Hanson RA, Horton EJ. High-dose Corticotropin (ACTH) Versus Prednisone for Infantile Spasms: A Prospective, Randomized, Blinded Study. Pediatrics 1996;97:375-379.

26. Barst RJ, Maislin G, Fishman AP. Vasodilator Therapy for Primary Pulmonary Hypertension in Children. Circulation 1999;99:1197-1208.

27. Belik J, Musey J, Trussell RA. Continuous Infusion of Glucagon Induces Severe Hyponatremia and Thrombocytopenia in a Premature Neonate. Pediatrics 2001;107:595-597.

28. Benini D, Johnston CC, Faucher D, Aranda JV. Topical Anesthesia During Circumcision in Newborn Infants. JAMA 1993;270:850-853.

29. Benitz WE, Tatro DS. The Pediatric Drug Handbook. Third Edition. Year Book Medical Publishers, 1995.

30. Berkovitch M, Akilesh MR, Gerace R, Verjee Z, McGuigan M, Whyte H, Koren G. Acute Digoxin Overdose in a Newborn with Renal Failure: Use of Digoxin Immune Fab and Peritoneal Dialysis. Ther Drug Monit 1994;16:531-533.

31. Berkovitch M, Akilesh MR, Gerace R, Verjee Z, McGuigan M, Whyte H, Koren G. Acute Digoxin Overdose in a Newborn with Renal Failure: Use of Digoxin Immune Fab and Peritoneal Dialysis. Ther Drug Monit 1994;16:531-533.

32. Bibi H, Seifert B, Oullette M, Belika J. Intratracheal N-acetylcysteine use in infants with chronic lung disease. Acta Paediatr 1992;81:335-339.

33. Blickman H. Pediatric Radiology 1998; pp.78-80

34. Bongers-Schokking JJ, Koot H, Wiersma D, Verkerk PH, deMuinck Keizer-Schrama S. Influcence of timing and dose of thyroid hormone replacement on development in infants with congenital hypothyroidism. J Pediatr 2000;136:292-7.

35. Brand JM, Greer FR. Hypermagnesemia and intestinal perforation following antacid administration in a premature infant. Pediatrics 1990;85:121-123.

36. Brown MS, Keith II, JF. Comparison Between Two and Five Doses a Week of Recombinant Human Erythropoietin for Anemia of Prematurity: A Randomized Trial. Pediatrics 1999;104:210-215.

37. Caglayan S, Candemir H, Aksit S, Kansoy S, Asik S, Yaprak I. Superiority of Oral Agar and Phototherapy Combination in the Treatment of Neonatal Hyperbilirubinemia. Pediatrics 1993;92:86-89.

38. Cairo MS, Agosti J, Ellis R, Laver JJ, Puppala B, deLemos R, Givner L, Nesin Mirjana, Wheeler JG, Seth T, van de Ven C, Fanaroff A, the Very Low Birthweight Neonate GM-CSF Consortium. A randomized, double-blind, placebo-controlled trail of prophylactic recombinant human granulocyte-macrophage colony-stimulating factor to reduce nosocomial infections in very low birth weight neonates. J Pediatr 1999;134:64-70.

39. Calhoun DA, Christensen RD, Edstrom CS, Juul SE, Ohls RK, Schibler KR, Sola MC, Sullivan SE. Consistent approaches to procedures and practices in neonatal hematology. Clinics in Perinatology 2000, 27:733-753.

40. Calhoun DA, Lunøe M, Du Y, Hutson AD, Veerman M. Christensen RD. Granulocyte Colony-Stimulating Factor Serum and Urine Concetrations in Neutropenic Neonates Before and After Intravenous Administration of Recombinant Granulocyte Colony-Stimulating Factor. Pediatrics 2000;105:392-397.

41. Campbell J, Zaccaria E, Baker C. Systemic Candidiasis in Extremely Low Birth Weight Infants Receiving Topical Petrolatum Ointment for Skin Care: A Case-Control Study. Pediatrics 2000;105:1041-1045

42. Carey Cf, Lee HH, Woeltje KF. The Washington Manual of Medical Therapeutics. Twenty Ninth Edition. Lippincott Raven, 1998.

43. Carr R, Modi N, Doré CJ, El-Rifai R, Lindo D. A Randomized, controlled Trial of Prophylactic Granulocyte-Macrophage Colony-Stimulating Factor in Human Newborns Less Than 32 Weeks Gestation. Pediatrics 1999;103:796-802.

44. Cheung P, Tyebkhan JM, Peliowski A, Ainsworth W, Robertson CMT. Prolonged use of pancuronium bromide and sensorineural hearing loss in childhood survivors of congential diaphragmatic hernia. J Pediatr 1999;135:233-9)

45. Christensen RD. Hematologic Problems of the Neonate. W.B. Sanuders Company, 2000.

46. Christian SL, Rich BH, Loebl C, Israel J, Vasa R, Kittikamron K, Spiro R, Rosenfield R, Ledbetter DH. Significance of genetic testing for paternal uniparental disomy of chromosome 6 in neonatal diabetes mellitus. J Pediatr 1999;134:42-6.

47. Christou J, Van Marter LJ, Wessel D, Allred EN, Kane JW, Thompson JE, Stark AR, Kourembanas S. Inhaled nitric oxide reduces the need for extracorporeal membrane oxygenation in infants with persistent pulmonary hypertension of the newborn. Crit Care Med 2000; 28:3722-3727.

48. Clark RH, Kueser TJ, Walker MW, Southgate WM, Huckaby JL, Perez JA. Low-dose nitric oxide therapy for persistent pulmonary hypertension of the newborn. N Engl J Med. 2000;342:469-74.

49. Cloherty JP, Stark AR. Manual of Neonatal Care. Fourth Edition. Lippincott Raven, 1998.

50. Cole Ch, Shab B, Abbasi S, Demissie S, MacKinnon B, Colton T, Frantz III ID. Adrenal function in premature infants during inhaled beclomethasone therapy. J Pediatr 1999;135:65-70.

51. Cornfield DN, Maynard RC, deRegnier RO, Guiang III, SF, Barbato JE, Milla CE. Randomized Controlled Trial of Low-dose Inhaled Nitric Oxide in the Treatment of Term and Near-term Infants With Respiratory Failure and Pulmonary Hypertension. Pediatrics 1999;104:1089-1094.

52. Koumbourlis AC, Mutich RL, Motoyama EK. Contribution of airway hyperresponsiveness to lower airway obstruction after extracorporeal membrane oxygenation for meconium aspiration syndrome. Crit Care Med 1995;23:749-54)

53. da Silva O, Alexandrou D, Knoppert D, Young GB. Seizure and Electroencephalographic changes in the Newborn Period Induced by Opiates and Corrected By Naloxone Infusion. J Perinatol 1999;19(2):120-123.

54. Darlow B, Winterbourn CC, Inder TE, Graham PT, Harding JE. The effect of selenium supplementation on outcome in very low birth weight infants: A randomized controlled trial. J Pediatr 2000;136:473-80

55. Davidson D, Barefield ES, Kattwinkel J, Dudell G, Damask M. Safety of Withdrawing Inhaled Nitric Oxide Therapy in Persistent Pulmonary Hypertension of the Newborn. Pediatrics 1999;104:231-236.

56. Dillon PW, Fos PS, Berg CJ, Cardella JF, Krummel TM. Recombinant tissue plasminogen activator for neonatal and pediatric vascular thrombolytic therapy. J Ped Surg 1993;28:1264-69.

57. Dix D, Andrew M, Marzinotto V, Charpentier K, Bridge S, Monagle P, deVeber G, Leaker M, Chan AK, Massicotte MP. The use of low molecular weight heparin in pediatric patients: A prospective cohort study. J Pediatr 2000;136:439-45.

58. Dobyns EL, Cornfield DN, Anas NG, Fortenberry HJD, Tasker RC. Multicenter randomized controlled trial of the effects of inhaled nitric

oxide therapy on gas exchange in children with acute hypoxemic respiratory failure. J Pediatr 1999;134:406-12.

59. Doyle J, Vreman HJ, Stevenson K, et al. Does vitamin C cause hemolysis in premature newborn infants? Results of a multicenter double-blind, randomized, controlled trial. J Pediatr 1997;130:103-109.

60. Elpeleg ON, Ruitenbeek W, Jakobs C, Barash V, De Vivo Dc, Amir N. Congenital lacticacidemia caused by lipoamide dehydrogenase deficiency with favorable outcome. J Pediatr 1995;126:72-74.

61. Ezekowitz RAB, Mulliken JB, Folkman J. Interferon alfa-2a therapy for life-threatening hemangiomas of infancy. N Engl J Med 1992;326:1456-1463.

62. Fahnenstich H, Steffan J, Kau N, Bartmann P. Fentanyl-induced chest wall rigidity and laryngospasm in preterm and term infants. Crit Care Med 2000;28:836-839.

63. Fanaroff AA, Martin RJ. Neonatal-Perinatal Medicine: Diseases of the Fetus and Infant Edition. Mosby Year Book, 1997.

64. Feigin RD, Cherry JD. Textbook of Pediatric Infectious Diseases. Fourth Edition. W. B. Saunders Company, 1998.

65. Finer NN, Tierney A, Etches PC, Peliowski A, Ainsworth W. Congenital Diaphragmatic Hernia: Developing a Protocolized Approach. J Pediatr Surg 1998;33:1331-1337.

66. Fortuna RS, Chinnock RE, Bailey LL, Loma Linda Pediatric Heart Transplant Group. Heart transplantation among 233 infants during the first six months of life: the Loma Linda Experience. Loma Linda Pediatric Heart Transplant Group. Clin Transpl 1999;263-272.

67. Friel JK, Andrews WL, Hall MS. Intravenous Iron Administration to Very-Low-Birth-Weight Newborns Receiving Total and Partial Parenteral Nutrition. Journal of Parenteral and Enteral Nutrition 1995;19:114-118.

68. Gaissmaier RE, Poblandt F. Single-dose dexamethasone treatment of hypotension in preterm infants. J Pediatr 1999;134:701-5.

69. Garland JS, Alex CP, Pauly TH, Whitehead VL, Brand J, Winston JF, Samuels DP, McAuliffe TL. Three-day Course of Dexamethasone Therapy to Prevent Chronic Lung disease in Ventilated Neonates: A Randomized Trial. Pediatrics 1999;104:91-99.

70. Garland JS, Buck RK, Maloney P, et al. Comparison of 10% povidone-iodine and 0.5% chlorhexidine gluconate for the prevention of peripheral intravenous catheter colonization in neonates: a prospective trial. Pediatr Infect Dis J 1995;14:510-516

71. Garson, Jr. A, Bricker TJ, Fisher DJ, Neish SR. The science and practice of pediatric cardiology. Second Edition. Williams & Wilkins, 1998.

72. Gillette PC, Garson Jr. A. Clinical Pediatric Arrhythmias. Second Edition. W.B. Saunders Company, 1999.

73. Gomella TL, Cunningham MD, Eyal FG, Zenk KE. Neonatology: Management, Procedures, On-call Problems, Diseases and Drugs. Fourth Edition. Appleton & Lange, 1999.

74. Gordon P, Rutledge J, Sawin R, Thomas S, Woodrum D. Early Postnatal Dexamethasone Increases the Risk of Focal Small Bowel Perforation in Extremely Low Birth Weight Infants. J Perinatol 1999;19(8)1:573-577.

75. Gouyon JB, Benoit A, Bétremieux P, et al. Cardiac Toxicity of Intravenous Erythromycin Lactobionate in Preterm Infants. Pediatr Infect Dis J 1994;13:840-841.

76. Gregory GA. Pediatric Anesthesia. Third Edition. Churchill Livingstone, 1994.

77. Gunasekaran t, Hassall EG. Efficacy and safety of omeprazole for severe gastroesophageal reflux in children. J Pediatr 1993;123:148-154.

78. Hall: High Dose Phenobarbital Therapy In Term Newborn Infants With Severe Perinatal Asphyxia: A Randomized, Prospective Study With Three Year Follow-Up. Pediatrics 1996;98(3):582)

79. Hallman M, Bry K, Hoppu K, Lappi M, Pohjavuori M. Inositol supplementation in infants with respiratory distress syndrome. N Engl J Med 1992;326:1233-1239.

80. Hammerman C, Glaser J, Schimmel MS, Ferber B, Kaplan M, Eidelman A. Continuous Versus Multiple Rapid Infusions of Indomethacin: Effects on Cerebral Blood Flow Velocity. Pediatrics 1995;95:244-248.

81. Hamosh A, McDonald JW, Valle D, Francomano CA, Niedermeyer E, Johnston MV. Dextromethorphan and high-dose benzoate therapy for nonketotic hyperglycinemia in an infant. J Pediatr 1992;121:131-135.

82. Hasan Q, Tan ST, Gush J, Peters SG, Davis PF. Steroid therapy of a proliferating hemangioma: Histochemical and molecular changes. Pediatrics 2000;105:117-121

83. Hay, Jr WW. Neonatal Nutrition and Metabolism. Mosby Year Book, 1991.

84. Hay, Jr WW, Lucas A, Heird WC, Ziegler E, Levin E. Workshop Summary: Nutrition of the Extremely Low Birth Weight Infant. Pediatrics 1999;104:1360 –1368.

85. Heldrich FJ, Salcedo UT, Salcedo JR, Herrera AJ. Aminocaproic acid (EACA) therapy for neonatal post-renal biopsy bleeding with renal failure. MD State Med J 1982;31:32-33.

86. Helton E, Darragh R, Francis P, Fricker FJ, Jue Kenneth, Koch G, Mair Douglas, Pierpont ME, Prochazka JV, Linn LS, Winter Sc. Metabolic Aspects of Myocardial Disease and a Role for L-Carnitine in the Treatment of Childhood Cardiomyopathy: Pediatrics 2000;105:1260-1270.

87. Herting E, Gefeller O, Land M, van Sonderen L, Harms K. Surfactant Treatment of Neonates With Respiratory Failure and Group B Streptococcal Infections. Pediatrics 2000;106:957-964

88. Hill A. Neonatal Seizures. Pediatrics in Review 2000;21:117-121.

89. Hocker JR, Saving KL. Fatal Aortic Thrombosis in a Neonate During Infusion of Epsilon-Aminocaproic Acid. J Pediatr Surg 1995;30:1490-1492.

90. Hrachovy RA, Frost Jr. JD, Glaze DG. High-dose, long-duration versus low-dose, short-duration corticotropin therapy for infantile spasms. J Pediatr 194;124:803-806.

91. Hurvitz CH, Alkaly AL, Sloninsky L, Kallus M, Pomerance JJ. Cyclophosphamide therapy in life-threatening vascular tumors. J Pediatr 1986;109:360-363.

92. Iafolla AK, Gale DS, Roe CP. Citrate therapy in argininosuccinate lyase deficiency. J Pediatr 1990;117:102-105.

93. International Guidelines for Neonatal Resuscitation: An Excerpt From the Guidelines 2000 for Cardiopulmonary Resuscitation and Emergency Cardiovascular Care: International Consensus on Science. Pediatrics 2000;106:11of16)

94. Isenberg SJ, APT L, Wood M. A controlled Trial Of Povidone-Iodine As Prophylaxis Against Ophthalmia Neonatorum. N Engl J Med 1995;332:562-566.

95. Jobe A. Commentary on Surfactant Treatment of Neonates With Respiratory Failure and Group B Streptococcal Infection. Pediatrics 2000; 106:1135-1136)

96. Julia MV, Parri FJ, Albert A, Figuras J, Rovira J, Morales L. Treatment of an enteric fistula with somatostatin in a premature. Clin Pediatr 1989;28:149-150.

97. Kasabian NG, Bauer SB, Dyro FM, Colodny AH, Mandell J, Retik AB. The prophylactic value of clean intermittent catheterization and anticholinergic medication in newborns and infants with myelodysplasia at risk of developing urinary tract deterioration. AJDC 1992;146:840-843.

98. Kattwinkel J, Bloom BT, Delmore P, Glick C, Brown D. High-Versus Low-Threshold Surfactant Retreatment for Neonatal Respiratory Distress Syndrome. Pediarics 2000;106:282-288

99. Kaufman SS, Loseke CA, Anderson JB, Murray ND, Vanderhoof JA, Young RJ. Magnesium acetate vs. magnesium gluconate supplementation in short bowel syndrome. J Pedatr Gastroenterol Nutr 1993;16:104-105.

100. Kearns GL, Bradley JS, Jacobs RF, Capparelli EV, James LP. Single dose pharmacokinetics of pleconaril in neonates. Pediatr Infect Dis J, 2000;19:833-9)

101. Kendig JW, Ryan RM, Sinkin RA, Maniscalco WM, Notter RH. Comparison of Two Strategies for Surfactant Prophylaxis in Very

Premature Infants: A Multicenter Randomized Trial. Pediatrics 1998;101:1006-1012

102. Kennedy LA, Drummond WH, Knight ME, Millsaps MM, Williams JL. Successful treatment of neonatal aortic thrombosis with tissue plasminogen activator. J Pediatr 1990;116:798-801.

103. Khaneja M, Naprawa J, Kumar A, Piecuch S. Successful Treatment of Late-Onset Infection due to Resistant Klebsiella pneumoniae in an Extremely Low Birth Weight Infant Using Ciprofloxacin. J Perinatol 1999;19:311-314.

104. Khaneja M, Naprawa J, Kumar A, Piecuch S. Successful Treatment of Late-Onset Infection due to Resistant Klebsiella pneumoniae in an Extremely Low Birth Weight Infant Using Ciprofloxacin. J Perinatol 1999;19:311-314

105. Kicklighter SD, Springer SH, Cox T, Hulsey TC, Turner RB. Fluconazole for Prophylaxis Against Candidal Rectal Colonization in the Very Low Birth Weight Infant. Pediatrics 2001;107:293-298.

106. Kinsella JP, Abman SH. Clinical approach to inhaled nitric oxide therapy in the newborn with hypoxemia. J Pediatr 2000;136:717-26.

107. Kinsella JP, Walsh WF, Bose CL, Gerstmann DR, Labella JJ, Sardesai S. Inhaled nitric oxide for preterm infants-still an experimental therapy. J Pediatr 2000;136:416-417.

108. Klitzner. Pharmacology and Therapeutics in Pediatric Cardiology 1994, pp.1099-1125.

109. Konduri GG, Garcia DC, Kazzi NJ, Shankaran S. Adenosine Infusion Improves Oxygenation in Term Infants With Respiratory Failure. Pediatrics 1996;97:295-300.

110. Kopelman AE, Moise AA, Holbert D, Hegemier SE. A single very early dexamethasone dose improves respiratory and cardiovascular adaptation in preterm infants. J Pediatr 1999;135:345-50.

111. Korte C, Styne D, Merritt TA, Mayes D, Wertz A, Helbock HJ. Adrenocortical function in the very low birth weight infant: Improved testing sensitivity and association with neonatal outcome. J Pediatr 1996;128:257-263.

112. Kothadia JM, O'Shea TM, Roberts D, Auringer ST, Weaver III RG, Dillard RG. Randomized Placebo-controlled Trial of a 42-Day Tapering Course of Dexamethasone to Reduce the Duration of Ventilator Dependency in Very Low Birth Weight Infants. Pediatrics 1999;104:22-27.

113. Kurikka. Neonatal Immunization: Response to Haemophilus influenzae Type b-Tetanus Toxoid Conjugate Vaccine. Pediatrics 1995;95:815-821.

114. LaForce WR, Brudno DS. Controlled trial of beclomethasone dipropionate by nebulization in oxygen- and ventilator-dependent infants. J Pediatr 1993;122:285-288.

115. Lam BCC, Yeung CY. Surfactant Lavage for Meconium Aspiration Syndrome: A Pilot Study. Pediatrics 1999;103:1014-1018)

116. Lilleyman: JS, Hann IM, Blanchette VS.Pediatric Hematology. Second Edition. Churchill Livingstone, 1999.

117. Liu EA, Heldt GP. A trial of the safety of inhaled beclomethasone in ventilator-treated neonates. J Pediatr 1996;129:154-156.

118. Lundergan FS, Glasscock GF, Kim EH, Cohen RS. Once-daily Gentamicin Dosing in Newborn Infants. Pediatrics 1999;103:1228-1234.

119. Madan A, Lavine JE, Heyman MB, Townsend SF. Acute hemorrhagic gastritis in the newborn infant. J Perinatol 1992;12:377-380.

120. Manco-Johnson MJ, Nuss R, Hays T, Krupski W, Drose J, Manco-Johnson ML. Combined thrombolytic and anticoagulant therapy for venous thrombosis in children. J Pediatr 2000;136:446-53.

121. Marlow N, Weindling AM, Van Peer A, Heykants J. Alfentanil pharmacokinetics in preterm infants. Arch Dis Child 1990;80:304-307.

122. McGaurn SP, Davis LE, Krawxzeniuk MM, Murphy JD, Jacobs MI, Norwood WI, Clancy RR. The Pharmacokinetics of Injectable Allopurinol in Newborns With the Hypoplastic Left Heart Syndrome. Pediatrics 1994;94:820-823.

123. Meyer MP, Haworth C, Meyer JH, Commerford A. A comparison of oral and intravenous iron supplementation in preterm infants receiving recombinant erythropoietin. J Pediatr 1996;129:258-263.

124. Murphy BP, Inder TE, Huppi PS, Warfield S, Zientara GP, Kikinis R, Jolesz FA, Volpe JJ. Impaired Cerebral Cortical Gray Matter Growth After Treatment With Dexamethasone for Neonatal Chronic Lung Disease. Pediatrics 2001;107:217-221.

125. Narayanan M, Cooper B, Weiss H, Clyman RI. Prophylactic indomethacin: Factors determining permanent ductus arteriosus closure. J Pediatr 2000; 136:330-7.

126. Narayanan M, Schlueter M, Clyman RI. Incidence and outcome of a 10-fold indomethacin overdose in premature infants. J Pediatr 1999;135:105-7.

127. Neely MN, Schreiber JR. Fluconazole Prophylaxis in the Very Low Birth Weight Infant: Not Ready for Prime Time Pediatrics 2001;107:404-406.

128. Nelson JD. Therapy for Neonatal Sepsis. Seminars in Pediatric Infectious Diseases 1994;5:15-19.

129. Nopper AJ, Horil KA, Sookdeo-Drost S, Wang TH, Mancini AJ, Lane AT. Topical ointment therapy benefits premature infants. J Peditr 1996;128:660-669.

130. Odim J, Laks H, Burch C, Komanapalli C, Alejos JC. Transplantation for Congenital Heart Disease. Adv Card Surg 2000;12:59-76.

131. Ohls RK, Veerman MW, Christensen RD. Pharmacokinetics and effectiveness of recombinant erythropoietin administered to preterm infants by continuous infusion in total parenteral nutrition solution. J Pediatr 1996;128:518-523.

132. O'Shea TM, Kothadia JM, Klinepeter KL, Goldstein DJ, Jackson BG, Weaver III RG, Dillard RG. Randomized Placebo-controlled Trial of a 42-Day Tapering Course of Dexamethasone to Reduce the Duration of Ventilator Dependency in Very Low Birth Weight Infants: Outcome of Study Participants at 1-Year Adjusted Age. Pediatrics 1999;104:15-21.

133. Pabst RC, Starr KP, Qaiyumi S, Schwalbe RS, Gewolb IH. The Effects of Application of Aquaphor on Skin Condition, Fluid Requirements, and Bacterial Colonization in Very Low Birth Weight Infants. J Perinatol 1999;19(4):278-283.

134. Pezzati M, Vanji V, Biagiotti R, Bertini G, Cianciulli D, Rubaltelli FF. Effects of indomethacin and ibuprofen on mesenteric and renal blood flow in preterm infants with patent ductus arteriosus. J Pediatr 1999;135:733-8.

135. Pomeranz A, Wolach B, Bernheim J, Korzets Z, Bernheim J. Successful treatment of Finnish congenital nephrotic syndrome with captopril and indomethacin. J Pediatr 1995;126:140-142.

136. Powell C, Painter MJ, Pippenger CE. Primidone therapy in refractory neonatal seizures. J Pediatr 1984;105:651-654.

137. Prober CG, Long SS, Pickering LK. Principles and Practice of Pediatric Infectious Diseases. Churchill Livingstone Inc., 1997.

138. Raju NV, Bharadwaj RA, Thomas R, Konduri GG. Ibuprofen Use to Reduce the Incidence and Severity of Bronchopulmonary dysplasia: A Pilot Study. Journal of Perinatology 2000; 1:13-16.

139. Ramenghi LA, Wood CM, Griffith GC, Levene MI. Effect of non-sucrose sweet tasting solution on neonatal heel prick responses. Arch Dis Child 1996;74:F129-F131.

140. Ramenghi LA, Wood CM, Griffith GC, Levene MI. Reduction of pain response in premature infants using intraoral sucrose. Arch Dis Child 1996;74:F126-F128.

141. Rapaport R. Neonatal thyrotoxicosis. Pediatr Rev 1989;10:216.

142. Rasoulpour M, Marinelli KA. Systemic hypertension. Clin Perinatol 1992;19:121-137.

143. Reed MD, Buck ML, Stuphen JL. Drug therapy and the gastrointestinal tract. Semin Perinatol 1992;16:21-31.

144. Remington JS, Klein JO. Infectious Diseases of the Fetus and Newborn Infant. Fifth Edition. W. B. Saunders Company, 2001.

145. Rice AM, Rivkees SA. Etidronate therapy for hypercalcemia in subcutaneous fat necrosis of the newborn. J Pediatr 1999;134:349-51.

146. Rosenfeld: Safety and Pharmacokinetics of Recombinant Human Superoxide Dismutase Administered Itratracheally to Premature Neonates With Respiratory Distress Syndrome. Pediatrics 1996;97:811-817)

147. Rudolph AM, Hoffman JIE, Rudolph CD. Rudolph's Pediatrics. Twentieth Edition. Appleton & Lange, 1996.

148. Russell GAB, Cooke RWI. Randomized controlled trial of allopurinol prophylaxis in very preterm infants. Arch Dis Child 1995;73:F27-F31.

149. Saarenmaa E, Huttunen P, Leppäluoto J, Fellman V. Alfentanil as procedural pain relief in newborn infants. Arch Dis child 1996;75:F103-F107.

150. Saarenmaa E, Huttunen P, Leppäluoto J, Meretoja O, Fellman V. Advantages of fentanyl over morphine in analgesia for ventilated newborn infants after birth: a randomized trial. J Pediatr 1999;134:144-50.

151. Seri I, Tan R, Evans J. Cardiovascular Effects of Hydrocortisone in Preterm Infants With Pressor-Resistant Hypotension. Pediatrics 2001;107:1070-1074.

152. Shannon KM, Keith JF, Mentzer WC, et al. Recombinant human erythropoietin stimulates erythropoiesis and reduces erythrocyte transfusions in very low birth weight preterm infants. Pediatrics 1995;95:1-8.

153. Shenai JP, Mellen BG, Chytil F. Vitamin A Status and Postnatal Dexamethasone Treatment in Bronchopulmonary Dysplasia. Pediatrics 2000;106:547-553.

154. Shenai JP. Vitamin A Supplementation in Very Low Birth Weight Neonates: Rationale and Evidence. Pediatrics 1999;104:1369 - 1374)

155. Siberry GK, Iannone R. The Harriet Lane Handbook. Fifteenth Edition. Mosby Inc., 2000.

156. Simeon PS, Geffner ME, Levin SR, Lindsey AM. Continuous insulin infusion in neonates: Pharmacologic availability of insulin in intravenous solutions. J Pediatr 1994;124:818-820.

157. Sinkin RA, Dweck HS, Horgan MJ, Gallaher K, Cox C, Maniscalco WM, Chess PR, D'Angio CT, Guillet R, Kendig JW, Ryan RM, Phelps DL. Early Dexamethasone-Attempting to Prevent Chronic Lung Disease. Pediatrics 2000;105:542-548.

158. Stajich WV, Lopez GP, Harry SW, Sexson WR. Iatrogenic exposure to mercury after hepatitis B vaccination in preterm infants. J Pediatr 2000;136:679-81.

159. Stapleton G, DiGeronimo RJ. Persistent Central Diabetes Insipidus Presenting in a Very Low Birth Weight Infant Successfully Managed With Intranasal dDAVP. J Perinatol 2000; 2:132-134.

160. Steward DJ. Manual of Pediatric Anesthesia. Fourth Edition. Churchill Livingstone, 1995.

161. Swaipman KF, Ashwal S. Pediatric Neurology. Third Edition. Mosby Inc.1999.

162. Taddio A, Shennan AT, Stevens B, Leeder JS, Koren G. Safety of Lidocaine-prilocaine cream in the treatment of preterm neonates. J Pediatr 1995:1002-1005.

163. Taeusch HW, Ballard RA. Avery's Diseases of the Newborn. Seventh Edition. W. B. Saunders Company, 1998.

164. Tagher RJ, Baumann R, Desai N. Failure of intravenously administered immunoglobulin in the treatment of neonatal myasthenia gravis. J Pediatr 1999;134:233-5.

165. Taketomo CK, Hodding JH, Kraus DM. Pediatric Dosage Handbook, Fourth Edition. Lexi-Comp Inc., 1997-1998.

166. Taketomo CK, Hodding JH, Kraus DM. Pediatric Dosage Handbook, Seventh Edition. Lexi-Comp Inc., 2000-2001.

167. Taketomo CK, Hooding JH, Kraus DM. Pediatric Dosage Handbook , Sixth Edition. Lexi-Comp Inc.1999-2000.

168. Tantivit P, Subramanian N, Garg M, Ramanathan R, deLemos RA. Low Serum Cortisol in Term Newborns With Refractory Hypotension. J Perinatol 1999;19:352-357.

169. Teitelbaum DH, Han-Markey T, Schumacher Re. Treatment of Parenteral Nutrition-Associated Cholestasis With Cholecystokinin-Octapeptide. J Pediatr Surg 1995;30:1082-1085.

170. The IMpact-RSV Study Group. Palivizumab, a Humanized Respiratory Syncytial Virus Monoclonal Antibody, Reduces Hospitalization From Respiratory Syncytial Virus Infection in High-risk Infants. Pediatrics 1998;102:531-537)

171. The Neonatal Inhaled Nitric Oxide Study Group: Inhaled nitric oxide in term and near-term infants: Neurodevelopmental follow-up of The Neonatal Inhaled Nitric Oxide Study Group (NINOS). J Pediatr 2000;136:611-7.

172. Thébaud B, Lacaze-Masmonteil T, Watterberg K. Postnatal Glucocorticoid in Very Preterm Infants: "The Good, the Bad, and the Ugly'? Pediatrics 2001;107:413-415.

173. Thureen PJ, Reiter PD, Gresores A, Stolpman NM. Kawato K, Hall DM. Once- Verses Twice-daily Gentamicin Dosing in Neonates > or = 34 Weeks' Gestation: Cost-effectiveness Analyses. Pediatrics 1999;03:594-598.

174. Tolsa JF, Cotting J, Sekarski N, Payot M, Micheli JL, Calame A. Magnesium sulphate as an alternative and safe treatment for severe persistent pulmonary hypertension of the newborn. Arch Dis Child 1995;72:F184-F187.

175. Transue D, Chan J, Kaplan M. Management of neonatal graves disease with iopanoic acid. J Pediatr 1992;121:472-474.

176. Treem WR, Davis PM, Hyams JS. Suppression of gastric acid secretion by intravenous administration of famotidine in children. J Pediatr 1991;118:812-816.

177. Truog R, Anand KJS. Management of pain in the postoperative neonate. Clin Perinatol 1989;16:61-78.

178. Tyson JE, Wright L, Oh W, Kennedy KA, Mele L, Ehrenkranz RA, Stoll BJ, Lemons JA, Stevenson DK, Bauer CR, Korones SB, Fanaroff AA.

Vitamin A supplementation for extremely low birth weight infants. N Engl J Med. 1999;340:1962-68)

179. Urea Cycle Disorders Conference Group: Consensus statement from a conference for the Management of Patients with Urea cycle Disorders. J Pediatr 2001;138:S1-S5)

180. Van Bel F, Shadid M, Moison RMW, Dorrepaal CA, Fontijn J, Monteiro L, Van De Bor M, Berger HM. Effects of Allopurinol on Postasphyxial Free Radical Formation, Cerebral Hemodynamics, and Electrical Brain Activity. Pediatrics 1998;101:185-193.

181. Van Overmeire B. Smets K, Lecoutere D, Van De Broek H, Weyler J, De Groote K, Langhendries J. A Comparison of Ibuprofen and Indomethacin for Closure of Patent Ductus Arteriosus. N Engl J Med 2000;343:674-81.

182. van Rossum AMC, Niesters HGM, Geelen SPM, Scherpbier HJ, Hartwig NG. clinical and virologic response to combination treatment with indinavir, zidovudine, and lamivudine in children with human immunodeficiency virus-1 infections: A multicenter study in The Netherlands. J. Pediatr 2000;136:780-8.

183. Varvarigou A, Bardin CL, Beharry K, Chemtob S, Papageorgiou A, Aranda JV. Early Ibuprofen Administration to Prevent Patent Ductus Arteriosus in Premature Newborn Infants. JAMA 1996;275:539-544.

184. Volpe JJ, Neurology of the Newborn. Fourth Edition. W.B. Saunders Company 2001.

185. Walker WA, Durie PR, Hamilton JR, Walker-Smith JA, Watkins JB. Pediatric Gastrointestinal Disease. Volume Two, Second Edition. Mosby-Year Book Inc., 1996.

186. Walker WA, Durie PR, Hamilton JR, Walker-Smith JA, Watkins JB. Pediatric Gastrointestinal Disease. Third Edition. B. C. Decker Inc., 2000.

187. Ward RM, Lemons JA, Molteni RA. Cisapride: A survey of the Frequency of Use and Adverse Events in Premature Newborns. Pediatrics 1999;103:469-472.

188. Watterberg KL, Gerdes JS, Gifford KL, Lin H. Prophylaxis Against Early Adrenal Insufficiency to Prevent Chronic Lung Disease in Premature Infants. Pediatrics 1999;104:1258 –1263.

189. Watterberg KL, Scott SM. Evidence of Early Adrenal Insufficiency in Babies Who Develop Bronchopulmonary Dysplasia. Pediatrics 1995;95:120-125.

190. Wheatcroft S, Sharma A, McAllister J. Reduction in mydriatic drop size in premature infants. Br J Ophthalmol 1993;77:364-365.

191. Whitelaw A, Saliba E, Fellman V, Mowinkel M-C, Acolet D, Marlow N. Phase I study of intraventricular recombinant tissue plasminogen activator for treatment of posthemorrhagic hydrocephalus. Arch Dis Child 1996;75:F20-F26.

192. Wilson JM, Bower LK, Fackler JC, Beais DA, Bergus BO, Kevy SV. Aminocaproic acid decreases in the incidence of intracranial hemorrhage and other hemorrhagic complications of ECMO. J Pediatr Surg 1993;28:536-541.

193. Wolff JA, Kulovich S, Yu AL, Qiao C, Nyhan WL. The effectiveness of benzoate in the management of seizures in nonketotic hyperglycinemia. Am J Dis Child 1986;140:596-602.

194. Wong AF, McCulloch LM, Sola A. Treatment of peripheral tissue ischemia with topical nitroglycerin ointment in neonates. J Pediatr 1992;121:980-983.

195. Wyllie R, Hyams JS. Pediatric Gastrointestinal Disease, Pathophysiology, Diagnosis, Management. Second Edition. W.B. Saunders Company, 1999.

196. Yeh TF. Neonatal Therapeutics. Second Edition. Mosby Year Book, 1991.

197. Zafar AB, Butler RC, Reese DJ, Gaydos La, Mennonna Pa. Use of 0.3% triclosan (Bacti-Stat*) to eradicate an outbreak of methicillin-resistant Staphylococcus aureus in a neonatal nursery. Am J Infect Control 1995;23:200-208.

198. Zenk KE, Sills JH, Koeppel RM. Neonatal Medications & Nutrition, A Comprehensive Guide. Second Edition. NICU Ink Book Publishers, 2000.

199. Zenz W, Muntean W, Beitzke A, Zobel G, Riccabona M, Gamilscheg A. Tissue plasminogen activator (alteplase) treatment for femoral artery thrombosis after cardiac catheterisation in infants and children. Br Heart J 1993;70:382-85.

B

C

D

E

F

G

H

I

J

- - - -

K

L

M

N

O

P

S

T

U

V

W

X

Y

Z